W9-AGT-799

# Clinical Electrotherapy

third edition

# *Clinical* ———————
# *Electrotherapy*

third edition

**Edited by**

**Roger M. Nelson, PhD, PT, FAPTA**
Professor and Chairman
Department of Physical Therapy
College of Allied Health Sciences
Thomas Jefferson University
Philadelphia, Pennsylvania

**Karen W. Hayes, PhD, PT**
Assistant Professor
Programs in Physical Therapy
Northwestern University Medical School
Chicago, Illinois

**Dean P. Currier, PhD, PT**
Professor Emeritus
Division of Physical Therapy
College of Allied Health Professions
University of Kentucky
Lexington, Kentucky

APPLETON & LANGE
Stamford, Connecticut

Notice: The authors and the publisher of this volume have taken care to make certain that the doses of drugs and schedules of treatment are correct and compatible with the standards generally accepted at the time of publication. Nevertheless, as new information becomes available, changes in treatment and in the use of drugs become necessary. The reader is advised to carefully consult the instruction and information material included in the package insert of each drug or therapeutic agent before administration. This advice is especially important when using, administering, or recommending new or infrequently used drugs. The authors and the publisher disclaim all responsibility for any liability, loss, injury, or damage incurred as a consequence, directly or indirectly, of the use and application of any of the contents of this volume.

Copyright © 1999 by Appleton & Lange
A Simon & Schuster Company
Copyright © 1991, 1987 by Appleton & Lange

All rights reserved. This book, or any parts thereof, may not be used or reproduced in any manner without written permission. For information, address Appleton & Lange, Four Stamford Plaza, PO Box 120041, Stamford, Connecticut 06912-0041.

www.appletonlange.com

99 00 01 02 03 / 10 9 8 7 6 5 4 3 2 1

Prentice Hall International (UK) Limited, *London*
Prentice Hall of Australia Pty. Limited, *Sydney*
Prentice Hall Canada, Inc., *Toronto*
Prentice Hall Hispanoamericana, S.A., *Mexico*
Prentice Hall of India Private Limited, *New Delhi*
Prentice Hall of Japan, Inc., *Tokyo*
Simon & Schuster Asia Pte. Ltd., *Singapore*
Editora Prentice Hall do Brasil Ltda., *Rio de Janeiro*
Prentice Hall, *Upper Saddle River, New Jersey*

**Library of Congress Cataloging-in-Publication Data**
Clinical electrotherapy / edited by Roger M. Nelson, Karen W. Hayes,
    Dean P. Currier. — 3rd ed.
        p.      cm.
    Includes bibliographical references and index.
    ISBN 0-8385-1491-X (case : alk. paper)
    1. Neuromuscular diseases—Treatment.    2. Electric stimulation.
3. Electrotherapeutics.      I. Nelson, Roger M.      II. Hayes, Karen W.
III. Currier, Dean P.
RC925.5.C58      1999
616.7´40645—dc21                                                98-50864
                                                                    CIP

Acquisitions Editor: Linda Marshall
Production Editor: Mary Ellen McCourt
Art Coordinator: Eve Siegel
Designer: Mary Skudlarek

ISBN 0-8385-1491-X
90000
9 780838 514917

PRINTED IN THE UNITED STATES OF AMERICA

To my wife Martha, our children, and their spouses:
Jennifer and Gary, David and Kristen.
*Roger M. Nelson*


To all the faculty and students with whom I have worked and
from whom I have learned so much.
*Karen W. Hayes*


To Joan.
*Dean P. Currier*

# Contributors

**Gad Alon, PhD, PT**
Department of Physical Therapy,
   University of Maryland
School of Medicine, Baltimore, Maryland

**Lucinda L. Baker, PhD, PT**
Department of Biokinesiology and
   Physical Therapy, University of Southern
   California
Los Angeles, California

**John O. Barr, PhD, PT**
Physical Therapy Program,
   St. Ambrose University
Davenport, Iowa

**Nancy N. Byl, PhD, PT**
Physical Therapy Graduate Program,
   University of California
San Francisco, California

**Dean P. Currier, PhD, PT**
Professor Emeritus, University of Kentucky
Lexington, Kentucky

**Stan Dacko, PhD, PT**
Department of Physical Therapy,
   Thomas Jefferson University
Philadelphia, Pennsylvania

**David G. Gerleman**
Physical Therapy Graduate Program,
   University of Iowa
Iowa City, Iowa

**Timothy Hanke, MS, PT**
Marianjoy Rehabilitation Hospital and
   Clinics
RehabLink
Wheaton, Illinois

**Karen W. Hayes, PhD, PT**
Programs in Physical Therapy,
   Northwestern University
Chicago, Illinois

**Roger M. Nelson, PhD, PT, FAPTA**
Department of Physical Therapy,
   Thomas Jefferson University
Philadelphia, Pennsylvania

**David E. Nestor, PT, MS, ECS**
Department of Physical Therapy, FMC
Lexington, Kentucky

**Neil I. Spielholz, PhD, PT**
Department of Orthopedics and
   Rehabilitation, University of Miami
Coral Gables, Florida

**Jane E. Sullivan, MS, PT**
Programs in Physical Therapy,
   Northwestern University Medical School
Chicago, Illinois

**Carrie Sussman, PT**
Sussman Physical Therapy, Inc.
Torrance, California

**Jessie Van Swearingen, PhD, PT**
Department of Physical Therapy,
   School of Health and Rehabilitation
Pittsburgh, Pennsylvania

# Contents

# Preface

The third edition of *Clinical Electrotherapy* has been developed in response to both the changing scope of health care and the publication of the *Guide to Physical Therapist Practice*, Parts I and II, by the American Physical Therapy Association (APTA). The arrival of managed care, with its associated cost-containment philosophy, has caused restrictions on the length and type of all physical therapy intervention. Electrotherapy treatments have also been closely scrutinized and in some cases challenged by local and federal reimbursement organizations. The *Guide to Physical Therapist Practice* is a major publication that for the first time in the history of our profession formalized both the development of a patient management conceptual framework and classification/standardization of terminology.

The third edition of *Clinical Electrotherapy* has been completely rewritten using the following published material as a guide:

- *Guide to Physical Therapist Practice*, Vol. 1; Description of Patient Management, published by APTA
- *Electrotherapeutic Terminology in Physical Therapy*, published by APTA
- Concepts of Health, Impairment, Disability, and Handicap, as described by the World Health Organization

There are three major sections to the third edition. The first section serves as a foundation for the remainder of the book. The chapters on physiology of excitable membranes, instrumentation and safety, and the principles of electrical stimulation all have had significant revision and use standardized terminology.

The second section contains chapters that relate to the application of electrical stimulation to improve tissue healing, increase muscle performance, improve neuromuscular function, and modulate pain. In this era of managed health care, these chapters will guide the student and clinician through a series of steps to enable them to become more effective and efficient as they use electrotherapeutic techniques. The use of APTA's Patient Management Framework in each of these chapters is intentional. These chapters were also developed using a problem-solving approach. Additionally, these chapters will help the clinician to answer questions about the usefulness of specific electrotherapeutic procedures on certain clinical manifestations when managed care organizations ask for documentation.

The third section contains chapters on the specialized uses of electrical stimulation, electrophysiologic evaluation, and electromyographic biofeedback for patients with specific problems. Additionally, there is a unique chapter that will enable the reader to evaluate critically existing and new electrical techniques in a scientific fashion.

We hope that clinicians and students will view the third edition as one that will lead electrotherapy into the new millennium.

# Section One

# Basic Principles of Electrotherapy

# Review of Physiology

Stan Dacko

## Introduction

 lectrical stimulation is utilized as a physical therapy intervention for various disorders. The therapist must understand not only the disorder to be treated, but also the mechanism by which electrical stimulation affects tissue. If such knowledge is either absent or ignored, the physical therapist will be unable to select safe and effective procedures of electrical stimulation.

This chapter discusses the basic properties of muscle and nerve cell membranes and their responses to electrical stimulation. The purpose of the chapter is to provide the therapist with the knowledge necessary to understand the phenomena of both natural and invoked discharge of excitable membranes.

## PROPERTIES OF EXCITABLE CELL MEMBRANES

### Resting Membrane Potentials

Excitable cells are enveloped by a membrane that separates a charge across the structure. This charge, or resting membrane potential, can be measured experimentally and is typically between 60 and 90 millivolts (mV), the inside of the cell being negative with respect to the outside. The charge on the membrane is a result of an unequal concentration of ions on either side of the structure. In a normal muscle or nerve cell, the sodium ($Na^+$) concentration is higher outside the cell, whereas the potassium ($K^+$) concentration is higher inside the cell. Each ion, however, will attempt to diffuse across the membrane passively in an attempt to equalize its concentration (Figure 1–1). The ability for an ion to diffuse across the membrane is primarily determined by the permeability of membrane to that ion. Because the membrane has a greater permeability to $K^+$ than to $Na^+$, a greater number of positively charged $K^+$ ions will leave, and a net negativity develops inside the cell. The diffusion of $K^+$ ions out of the cell is eventually retarded as the negative charge inside of the cell increases. The diffusion force acting on $K^+$ ions to move out of the cell to equalize the concentration is eventually matched by an opposing electrostatic force to return the ions to the cell, because of the negative charge inside. When these forces are equal, $K^+$ ions will be in a steady-state condition, with one $K^+$ ion leaving the cell for every one that enters. This exchange of ions occurs when the charge on the membrane potential is −100 mV and is called the **equilibrium potential** for $K^+$.

As mentioned earlier, the resting membrane potential is −60 to −90 mV. Therefore, in the typical resting excitable cell, $K^+$ ions are not in equilibrium, and more $K^+$ will be passively leaving the cell that entering it. Why does the resting membrane fail to remain at −100 mV, the equilibrium potential for potassium? The reason is that other ions will also be passively moving across the membrane. In the case of the $Na^+$ ions, passive diffusion will favor movement into the cell (Figure 1–1). The passive movement of $Na^+$ into the cell will not be as large as the passive movement of $K^+$ out of the cell because of the lower membrane permeability to $Na^+$. The inward movement of

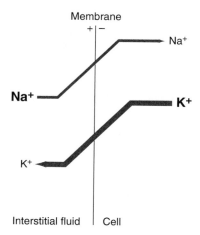

**FIGURE 1–1.** Passive movement of $Na^+$ and $K^+$ ions. Each arrow represents the direction of movement of each ion in a resting cell. The width of the arrow indicates the relative permeability for $Na^+$ and $K^+$.

the $Na^+$ ions will reduce the negative charge developed by the outward leak of the $K^+$ ions. The movement of the $Na^+$ and $K^+$ ions eventually reaches a steady state at approximately −60 to −90 mV, the resting membrane potential. At this potential, however, $Na^+$ has not equalized its concentration, and forces still exist to passively move it into the cell. In order for $Na^+$ to be at equilibrium, the membrane would have to be charged at +50 mV inside with respect to the outside, the equilibrium potential for $Na^+$. The resting membrane potential normally lies much closer to the equilibrium potential of $K^+$ because the excitable membranes are much more permeable to $K^+$.

In summary, the resting membrane potential of an excitable membrane is the consequence of both the concentration differences across the membrane and the different permeabilities of the resting excitable membrane to $Na^+$ and $K^+$.

## Discharge of an Action Potential

Most excitable cells in the body spend little time at their membrane potential because these cells are continuously subjected to events that change the membrane's permeability to $Na^+$ and $K^+$ ions. If a cell membrane is excited by chemical, electrical, or physical stimuli, the cell membrane may undergo a slight increase in its permeability to $Na^+$. As the number of $Na^+$ ions moving into the cell increases, the cell membrane will undergo a reduction of its negative charge (depolarization). If this depolarization reaches a certain critical membrane voltage (threshold), membrane permeability to $Na^+$ dramatically increases and $Na^+$ ions will rush into the cell. The membrane potential will rapidly change to +25 to +35 mV because of the influx of these positive ions (Figure 1–2). This increase in membrane permeability to $Na^+$ ions is brief, lasting 0.5 millisecond (msec).

The initial depolarization of the membrane also increases the membrane's permeability to $K^+$. This increase in permeability to $K^+$ peaks a little later in time than the increase to $Na^+$ ions (Figure 1–2). This latter change in the membrane's permeability to $K^+$ causes the membrane potential to become negative (hyperpolarization), approaching the equilibrium potential for potassium. This sudden, rapid alteration in the membrane's potential is known as an **action potential**. The ability of a membrane to generate an action potential is the property that defines an excitable membrane. An active $Na^+$–$K^+$ pump, which is present in the membrane, returns the ions to their original concentrations. This pump expels $Na^+$ from the cell and takes in $K^+$ on a 3 to 2 exchange (Figure 1–3). This exchange of ions by pump action not only maintains a concentration gradient but also helps to create a net negative charge inside the cell.

Although normal excitable cells exhibit action potentials very

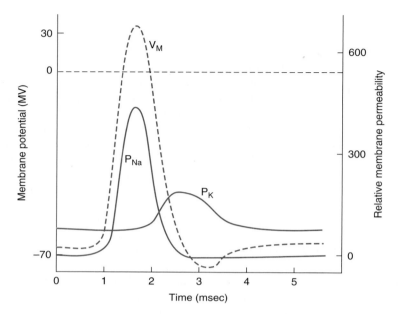

FIGURE 1–2. Changes in the permeability of K+ (P$_K$), Na+ (P$_{Na}$) and membrane voltage (V$_m$) during an action potential.

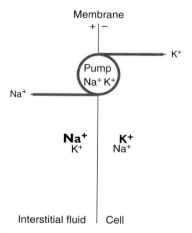

FIGURE 1–3. Active movement of Na+–K+ ions across an excitable membrane via an active Na+–K+ pump. Three Na+ ions are transported out for every two K+ transported in the cell.

frequently, there are conditions that will cause an excitable membrane to fail. If a membrane becomes sufficiently hyperpolarized, it may be unable to discharge an action potential, because the firing threshold cannot be easily reached. Also, if a membrane has been depolarized for a period of time, an action potential will not be evoked, even if the normal threshold depolarization is reached. The excitable membrane in these circumstances is said to have **accommodated** to the stimulus. An action potential can occur, however, if depolarization of the cell reaches a level that is much higher than the normal firing threshold. The prolonged depolarization apparently raises the threshold level for the sudden increase in permeability to $Na^+$ that normally occurs during an action potential. A slowly rising depolarization apparently inactivates many of the $Na^+$ gated channels, which limits the large influx of $Na^+$. Not all membranes accommodate to the same degree. For instance, the sarcolemma of muscle accommodates less to a stimulus than that of nerve.

## Propagation of an Action Potential

An action potential occurring in one region of an excitable membrane can trigger an action potential in a neighboring region of the membrane. The depolarization occurring in the beginning of an action potential causes a localized flow of current around the site of the action potential. This current may cause a threshold depolarization of the neighboring membrane, which may evoke an action potential. If the excitable membrane is very large, such as in a nerve axon or a muscle fiber, the action potential can be propagated over the entire membrane. If propagation is occurring in the normal direction (eg, progressing in a proximal direction for a sensory fiber), it is called **orthodromic conduction**. **Antidromic conduction** occurs when the action potential is progressing in the opposite direction, compared to normal. If a stimulus is applied to the middle of a nerve at a sufficient amplitude, the action potential travels both orthodromically and antidromically.

The speed at which an action potential is propagated varies from one excitable membrane to another. In nerve cell fibers that are unmyelinated, action potentials create localized eddy currents that cross the membrane (Figure 1–4A). The span encompassed by the eddy currents is small because of the high resistance of the membrane. In nerve membranes that are myelinated, the local current generated by an action potential travels inside the fiber, because the myelin prevents the eddy currents from crossing the membrane. The action potential occurs only at interruptions in the myelin (Figure 1–4B). Conduction in a myelinated fiber is much faster than in an unmyelinated fiber. For unmyelinated fibers, each portion of the

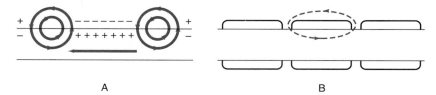

FIGURE 1–4. Local current flow generated by an action potential in axons. **(A)** Eddy currents produced by an action potential in an unmyelinated axon. **(B)** Local current flow evoked by an action potential in a myelinated axon. The current crosses only at the node.

membrane must sequentially undergo an action potential in order to propagate the full length of an excitable membrane. In myelinated fibers, the potential skips from node to node; thus, fewer action potentials will be propagated along the length of the membrane. Each action potential lasts approximately 1.0 msec; thus, the fewer action potentials produced during propagation of activity along the length of a nerve fiber, the less time it takes to conduct from one end to the other end of the fiber.

Conduction velocity within a group of either unmyelinated or myelinated fibers will vary as well. The larger the diameter of the fiber, the less resistance offered to conduction currents generated by action potentials and, thus, the faster the speed of conduction of an action potential. Other factors influence conduction velocity. For example, nerve fibers conduct faster if the temperature in the surrounding environment is raised.

An action potential along a nerve fiber can be prevented in a number of ways. If a nerve fiber is exposed to local pressure or to anoxia, that region of fiber will begin to slowly depolarize. If this adverse condition occurs, the sudden increase in permeability to $Na^+$ ions will not occur; therefore, propagation of an action potential will cease in this area. An injection of a local anesthetic (eg, novocaine) will block conduction of an action potential in the region by decreasing $Na^+$ permeability. Extreme cooling can also stop conduction.

## RESPONSE OF AN EXCITABLE MEMBRANE TO ELECTRICAL STIMULATION

The behavior of an excitable membrane can be modified by the application of electrical current through two external electrodes. The current passing between the electrodes can cause a depolarization of the membrane. If the amplitude of the electrical stimulus is too weak to produce a threshold depolarization, an action potential will not take place.

## Threshold for Excitation

If the applied current depolarizes the membrane to threshold, an action potential will result. Whether the membrane reaches the threshold partially depends on the stimulus amplitude. The stimulus amplitude required, however, varies from membrane to membrane and even from minute to minute in the same membrane. For example, narrow-diameter nerve fibers require a higher stimulus amplitude to reach threshold because of the high internal resistance of such fibers to current flow. In addition, a fiber that has been exposed to a continuous level of depolarization may eventually accommodate to the stimulus and become inexcitable unless the stimulus amplitude is increased.

The duration of the stimulus pulse also affects whether the membrane reaches firing threshold. A membrane exposed to an electrical stimulus does not immediately change its charge. When exposed to a maintained electrical stimulus, the excitable membrane will eventually reach a steady state in which the charge on the membrane reaches its peak in response to the externally applied current. The amount of time that it takes an applied current to change the cell membrane's voltage is directly related to the capacitance and resistance of the membrane. Membranes with a larger capacitance (eg, denervated skeletal muscle) take longer to charge than those with a smaller capacitance (nerve fibers). If the stimulus duration is too short, the membrane voltage will not reach threshold no matter how high the stimulus amplitude. Likewise, critical stimulus amplitude is required to achieve threshold level for an action potential. The relationship between the threshold stimulus amplitude (strength, an old term) and the stimulus duration needed to evoke a consistent response is plotted as a strength–duration curve. A change in the shape of the curve is used to determine the extent of reinnervation following injury.

## Refractory Periods

When an electrical current is applied to a nerve cell membrane, the stimulation may be applied in pulses separated by time. Even if the stimuli are of sufficient duration and amplitude, the membrane may not discharge to the second stimulus if it occurs too close in time to the first stimulus. A membrane needs approximately 0.5 msec to recover its excitability after an action potential. This recovery time is called the **absolute refractory period**. A higher-amplitude stimulus may be needed before the membrane will again fire for a period of time between 0.5 and 1 msec after having discharged an action potential. This time of recovery is called the **relative refractory period**, which to some extent limits the maximum frequency of discharge of an excitable membrane.

## Stimulating Nerve Trunks

When physical therapists apply electrodes for electrical stimulation, the path of current will most likely include nerve fibers of different diameters. Fibers having large diameters require the lowest stimulus amplitude and shortest stimulus duration to reach threshold because of their lower resistance. Fibers having small diameters require a higher stimulus amplitude and longer duration to reach threshold than the large fibers. Fibers that provide the sensation of cutaneous pain are typically of small diameter. Thus, use of short stimulus duration, lower stimulus amplitude, or both, may reduce the painful sensation accompanying stimulation.

When stimulating a nerve to evoke a muscle contraction, not all of the alpha motor axons in the nerve will discharge at the same threshold or stimulus amplitude. Because of difference in both axonal diameter and anatomical orientation to the current, the stimulus amplitude may have to be quite high (sometimes beyond tolerance) to recruit all of the motor axons.

# SPECIFIC RESPONSES OF MUSCLE TO ELECTRICAL STIMULATION

In a normally innervated muscle, electrical stimulation evokes a contraction by excitation of the nerve rather than by excitation of the muscle fibers directly. This is because nerve fibers have a lower threshold to stimulation compared to muscle fibers. Only when a muscle is denervated will electrical stimulation specifically excite muscle fibers.

## Temporal Summation

If a motor nerve is exposed to a single stimulus of adequate duration and amplitude, a single twitch muscle contraction results. The evoked twitch is a synchronous contraction of all of the motor units whose alpha motor axons are excited by the stimulus. The tension produced by a group of motor units may be increased if a volley of stimuli, rather than a single stimulus, is used. When muscle twitches are evoked in rapid succession, there may not be enough time for complete relaxation between twitches. If the tension during one twitch fuses with that of the successive twitch, the tension will be additive. When the frequency of stimuli is high enough, the contraction will not show alterations in contraction and relaxation. At this point, the contraction produced is described as **tetanic** or **fused** (Figure 1–5).

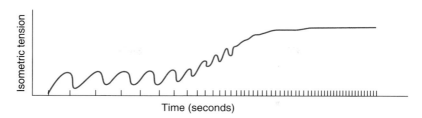

FIGURE 1–5. Accumulated tension in skeletal muscle from isometric twitches produced by gradually increasing the frequency of electrical stimulation.

The frequency at which tetanic contraction occurs depends on the physiological properties of the muscle. Postural muscles generally have motor units with slow contraction times (> 40 msec), and individual motor unit responses will fuse at low stimulus rates (~ 20 pulses per second [pps]). By contrast, muscles that are typically used for movement requiring additional speed or force have motor units with faster contraction times (< 35 msec), thereby undergoing a tetanic contraction at higher (~ 40 pps) stimulus rates.

Although stimulation at a frequency to excite all motor units to produce a tetanic contraction is possible, this is not how voluntary movement occurs. With a voluntary contraction, motor units fire asynchronously. During asynchronous activation, each unit's force is summated to cause a smooth contraction, even though an individual unit may be firing at a rate that does not cause a tetanic contraction.

## Regulation of Muscle Force

The active regulation of muscle force is thought to be the result of the number of active motor units (recruitment) and the rate at which each activated unit is firing (rate coding). Voluntary activation of motor units is thought to occur in an orderly, fixed recruitment pattern: low-force-producing, slow-contracting, fatigue-resistant (type S) motor units are activated before more forceful, faster-contracting, fatigable (type F) units. Electrical stimulation of a motor nerve, however, appears to activate motor units in the opposite sequence, preferentially activating the low-threshold, large-diameter axons generally belonging to the more forceful, fatigable type F units. Simplistically, it may seem that an external electrical stimulus applied to a nerve will excite all the large motor axons before the small ones. However, spatial orientation of the axon within the nerve affects the amount of current delivered and, together with fiber size, ultimately determines whether the applied current is sufficient to excite a particular motor unit. In this way, multiple and unpredictable combinations of motor units are activated with external current. Thus, contractions evoked by electrical stimulation are nonphysiological, in that they do not duplicate normal recruitment and firing patterns of motor units and may cause *premature* muscle fatigue.

# Summary

Nerve and muscle cells are excitable cells because they are able to discharge action potentials. Prior to discharge, an excitable membrane has a resting potential of −60 to −90 mV because of differences in concentration and permeability of $Na^+$ and $K^+$ ions across the membrane. During an action potential, the permeability mostly to $Na^+$ but also $K^+$ ions increases momentarily and there is a sudden reversal in the membrane's charge. An action potential is conducted along an excitable membrane by triggering discharge in adjacent resting zones of the membrane. Conduction speed in a nerve fiber is enhanced by myelinization or by increased diameter of the fiber.

Electrical stimulation of nerve or muscle membranes can evoke action potentials. For an action potential to be evoked, stimulus amplitude and pulse duration must be sufficient to overcome the threshold. Threshold amplitude is lowest for large-diameter axons. Stimulus amplitude for threshold may need to be increased if the membrane has been depolarized for a period of time. Following an action potential, all excitable membranes pass through a recovery period, which limits maximal frequency of discharge.

Motor units will undergo a twitch contraction in response to a brief application of electrical stimulation to their motor axons. Fusion of the twitch occurs as frequency of electrical stimulation increases. Contraction evoked by electrical stimulation is not normal, in that motor units are recruited in the opposite pattern compared to voluntary activation and that the rate of firing is synchronous and the same for all units.

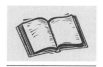

## REVIEW QUESTIONS

1. Describe the movement of $K^+$ and $Na^+$ ions in an excitable membrane at rest and during an action potential.
2. Discuss the differences in the way impulses are conducted in myelinated vs. unmyelinated nerve fibers.

3. What is the relationship between the strength and duration of a stimulus and the ability of an excitable membrane to reach threshold for an action potential?
4. Describe the effect of stimulus frequency on the generation of muscle force.
5. How is electrical stimulation of a muscle–nerve complex different from normal voluntary activation of muscle?

## Bibliography

Hille B. Ionic Channels of Excitable Membranes (2nd ed). Sunderland, MA, Sinauer and Associates, 1992.

Kandel ER, Schwartz JH, Jessell TM (eds). Principles of Neural Science (3rd ed). New York, NY, Elsevier Science, 1991.

Lieber R. Skeletal Muscle Structure and Function. Baltimore, MD, Williams & Wilkins, 1992.

Sunderland S. Nerve Injuries and Their Repair: A Critical Appraisal. New York, NY, Churchill Livingstone, 1991.

# 2

# Instrumentation and Product Safety

David G. Gerleman and John O. Barr

## Introduction

An excitable membrane can generate an action potential as a consequence of normal physiological stimulation or in response to a variety of chemical and physical agents. Electrical stimulation of muscle and nerve membranes is among the most common methods of stimulation because it is very controllable. This chapter reviews the fundamental descriptors of electrical phenomena and terminology relevant to the electrical stimulation of excitable membranes. The discussion of instrumentation will focus on functional stimulator components and controls. This framework will serve as a basis for the understanding of application-specific instrumentation. Emphasis is given to electrode–electrolyte electrochemistry because of its importance to the clinician's safe and effective use of electrotherapy. Finally, attention will be given to the safety considerations common to all therapeutic applications of electricity.

## ELECTRICAL PHENOMENA

### Charge

A fundamental concept of electrical phenomena is **charge.** What is known about charge has been learned by observing how it behaves. Early experiments with charged objects allowed investigators to discern that there exist two kinds of charge. When two objects that have been charged similarly are brought into close proximity to each other, they repel each other; two objects with opposite charges will attract each other when brought near each other. The two kinds of charge have been named negative and positive.

## Electrons and Ions

All matter is made up of atoms containing positively charged nuclei, and negatively charged electrons held in orbits around them. An atom is electrically neutral in that there is an equality of charge between the nucleus and the orbiting electrons. When acted upon by an outside force (such as chemical reactions, electrostatic fields, heat, light, and magnetic fields), an atom can lose or gain electrons, thus altering its neutral charge and causing it to take on electrical properties. An atom that is no longer in its original neutral state is called an **ion,** and the process of changing the electrical state of an atom is called **ionization.** A **negative ion** is an atom that has gained one or more electrons, giving it a net negative charge; a **positive ion** is an atom that has lost one or more electrons, giving it a net positive charge. Ions are present in electrolytic solutions of acids, bases, and salts such as those of which biological tissues are composed. Acid radicals tend to form negative ions, whereas alkaloids, bases, and metals tend to form positive ions. An ion has the same nucleus that the atom had prior to adding or losing electrons, and thus it possesses the basic characteristics of the original atom. The charge of a single electron has been defined as:

$$-e = 1.6 \times 10^{-19} \text{ coulombs}$$

Therefore, the charge on an object is a measure of the number of free electrons that it has lost or gained and is expressed as coulombs of charge. One coulomb (C) of charge (q) is equal to the combined charge of $6.25 \times 10^{18}$ electrons. (See Table 2–1.)

## Current

The directed flow of charge from one place to another within matter is termed **current.** The charge may consist of free electrons or ions. There is a naturally occurring random drift of free electrons, negative ions, and positive ions within all matter. Because of the composition of their orbital shells, some atoms tend to both give up and take on free electrons more readily than do others. Those materials that have their valence shells almost filled tend to be very stable, with very few free electrons **(insulators).** Materials (principally metals) with only one or two valence electrons tend to give up their electrons very easily **(conductors)** and readily allow electron movement, or flow, within them. Electrolytic solutions allow the free movement of positive and negative ions, as well as the free movement of electrons.

## TABLE 2–1. ELECTROPHYSICS TERMINOLOGY

| Term | Term Abbreviation | Unit | Unit Abbreviation |
|------|-------------------|------|-------------------|
| Capacitance | C | Farad | F |
| Charge | q | Coulomb | C |
| Conductance | G | Siemens | S |
| Current | I | Ampere | A |
| Impedance | Z | Ohm | Ω |
| Inductance | L | Henry | H |
| Power | P | Watt | W |
| Reactance | X | Ohm | Ω |
| Resistance | R | Ohm | Ω |
| Voltage | V | Volt | V |

In order to produce directed **current flow,** there must be a source of free electrons and positive ions, a conductive material that will allow the flow of charge, and an **electromotive force** (EMF) tending to move or concentrate the charge. The unit of current (I) is the **ampere** (A), which is defined as the rate at which charge flows past a fixed reference point in a conductor. An ampere is equal to 1 coulomb per second. Coulombs indicate the number of electrons; amperes indicate the rate of electron flow. An ampere is a large unit of current in the context of electrical stimulation, and smaller units are more commonly used. A **milliampere** (mA) is one thousandth of an ampere; a **microampere** (μA) is one millionth of an ampere.

In Chapter 1, the physiology of excitable cell membranes was discussed in terms of both the normal movement of ions into and out of the cell and of the resultant net charge difference that results from the unequal concentration of ions on either side of the membrane. A necessary condition for cell membrane depolarization from external electrical stimulation is the accumulation of negative charge on the exterior of the cell such that a critical excitation threshold is reached. While the minimum quantity of charge necessary to produce an action potential is largely dependent on the electrical properties of the particular cell type and is quite predictable, the actual quantity of charge needed in a particular application is dependent on the fraction of the charge delivered by the stimulator that actually reaches the target membranes. The path taken by the stimulating current is dependent on a number of factors including the type and size of electrode, the coupling of the electrode to the skin surface, the location of the electrodes, and the multitude of varied tissue impedances lying in the general vicinity of the target membrane. The stimulus charge delivered by the stimulator, measured in units of coulombs, is the integral of the stimulus current in amperes, integrated with respect to the time duration in seconds,

$$q = \int i(t)\,dt$$

For a monophasic, rectangular-shaped stimulus, stimulus charge is equal to the peak current amplitude multiplied by the phase duration,

$$q = I \times t$$

## Voltage

Associated with charge is an electrical field that fills the space around the charge such that when another charge is in the field, electrical forces act on it. If two similar charged particles are moved together, electrical forces act to keep them apart. The force becomes stronger the closer the charged particles are moved together. Work must be done to move the two similar charged particles together, thus converting kinetic energy to potential energy. The potential energy difference per unit charge between the particles is termed the **potential difference.** The unit of potential difference, or **voltage,** is the volt (V), defined as one joule/coulomb. Because the work in moving charge is relative to another charge, potential difference is always relative to a reference point. In cases in which the reference point is not explicitly given, an assumption is made that the reference point is **ground,** or the electrical potential of the earth. **Earth ground** is assigned a zero potential in that it can supply any practical quantity of charge without changing its electrical characteristics.

There are two contexts in which voltage or potential difference is used to describe the electrical stimulation of excitable membranes. The inequality of charge between the interior and exterior of a muscle or nerve cell results in a potential difference which is measured in units of millivolts. Potential difference can also be used to describe the electromotive force produced by the stimulator circuit in order to move charge from the stimulator output terminals, through the connecting leads and stimulating electrodes, and to force the flow of charge through the intervening body tissues en route to the target cells.

## Resistance

**Resistance** is the property of a material to resist or oppose the steady flow of current through it. Materials have different intrinsic resistivity based on their chemistry. The best conductors, such as gold, silver, and copper, have low resistivity. Insulators, such as plastic, paper, and cloth, have high resistivity. Some materials, such as silicon and germanium, are neither good conductors nor good insulators. These **semiconductor** materials can be made to act as both a conductor and insulator. The dual resistance personality of semiconductors is the basis for modern solid-state electronic components. The resistance of a material acting as a conductor of direct current may be calculated from **Ohm's law,** which relates the properties of current, resistance, and voltage. If one volt of potential difference causes a current of one ampere to flow in an electrical circuit, by Ohm's law, the limiting resistance is equal to one ohm ($\Omega$).

$$\text{Resistance } (\Omega) = \frac{\text{Voltage (V)}}{\text{Current (A)}}$$

Common values for resistance include kilohms (k$\Omega$) and megohms (M$\Omega$): thousands and millions of ohms, respectively. The term **resistor** refers to an electronic component used to introduce a desired amount of resistance in a circuit.

Sometimes it is more convenient to think in terms of how well a material conducts current rather than how well it opposes. **Conductance** is the term used to define the ease with which a material allows current flow; *it is the inverse of resistance.* The *unit* of conductance is the mho.

$$\text{Conductance } (S) = \frac{1}{\text{Resistance } (\Omega)}$$

## Capacitance

**Capacitance** is the property of an insulator that permits the storage of energy when opposite surfaces of the insulator are maintained at an electrical potential difference. The measure of capacitance, expressed in farads (F), is the ratio of the charge on either surface of the insulator to the potential difference between the surfaces. Mathematically, this may be expressed as

$$\text{Capacitance } (F) = \frac{\text{Charge (C)}}{\text{Voltage (V)}}$$

One farad of capacitance requires one coulomb of charge to raise the potential by one volt. An electrical component, a **capacitor** is composed of two metal plates separated by a very thin insulating material. The capacitance of a capacitor is dependent on the size and separation of the conductors and the type of material used as the insulator. The closer the conductors are moved together, the less work is required to move a unit charge through a shorter distance and the higher the capacitance between them.

Cells exhibit the electrical property of capacitance. A capacitor is formed with the interstitial and the extracellular fluids acting as conductors and the cell membrane acting as an insulator. The cell is not an ideal capacitor because the cell membrane is semipermeable and ions can penetrate the cell membrane. The charge across the membrane will eventually leak off if it is not restored by another means. Cell membrane capacitance is high because the membrane separating the charged ions is very thin. The capacitance of cell membranes of different types is expressed as capacitance per unit area because the capacitance of a parallel plate capacitor is proportional to its surface area. Thus, the capacitance of a muscle or nerve fiber is proportional to the diameter and length of the fiber as both affect membrane surface area. A farad is a large unit of capacitance. Cell membrane capacitance is expressed in units of microfarads (1 $\mu F = 1 \times 10^{-6}$ F) or picofarads (1 pF = $1 \times 10^{-12}$ F) per $cm^2$.

## Inductance

**Inductance** is a measure of the degree to which a varying current can induce an EMF in a circuit.[1,2] **Inductors** are electrical components that possess the property of inductance. Inductors are formed by coiling wire on a spool or iron core, thereby concentrating the magnetic field that exists around a current-carrying conductor. A varying magnetic field will induce an electromotive force in any conductors within the magnetic field, including itself. The induced electromotive force must act counter to the original EMF such that the net energy in the system is constant and energy is conserved. Thus, energy stored in the magnetic field acts to oppose a change in the current flow that produced it. The relationship between the magnitude of the induced counter EMF, the rate of change of current, and the inductance of the coil may be expressed as

$$-EMF = L \frac{dI}{dt}$$

where L is the inductance in henrys (H). An inductance of one henry will induce an electromotive force of one volt when the current is changing at the rate of one ampere per second. Note that the counter-EMF is given a negative sign to denote its reverse polarity.

While inductance is negligible in biological systems, it may be used to advantage in inducing currents into biological tissues without the need for electrodes on the surface of the skin (see Chapter 14). A special application of induction is the transformer, which is really two inductors wound together on the same core. Current flow in the primary coil forms a magnetic field which induces an EMF (V) in the secondary coil. The induced EMF is proportional to the ratio of the number of turns of wire in the secondary coil to the number of turns or wire in the primary coil. The transformer is an essential component of the power supply used in the design of electrical stimulators. The step-up voltage transformer is used to generate the high voltages necessary for electrical stimulation of excitable membranes via electrodes. The inherent electrical isolation of the primary from the secondary winding(s) of an isolation transformer is used to provide necessary electrical isolation of the patient from earth ground in isolated stimulator designs. Isolation of the patient from ground-referenced currents is desirable. Isolation limits the shock hazard of main-powered instrumentation by reducing ground-referenced electrical currents to extremely low levels. Isolation affords better control of the path of the desired stimulus current by eliminating the possibility of stimulus current returning to ground via multiple unknown paths. Stimulus isolation also greatly reduces the pickup of the stimulus, known as stimulus artifact, during the recording of an evoked bioelectrical response.[3]

## Frequency and Phase

All voltage waveforms that vary over time can be described as being composed of a series of periodic sinusoids of different amplitude, phase, and frequency, which together uniquely define the waveform. The frequency of a single sinusoid is defined by its period, or the amount of time that it takes to complete one cycle of the sinusoid, where

$$\text{Frequency (Hz)} = \frac{1}{\text{Period (sec)}}$$

In this context, phase refers to the fraction of the fundamental cycle that the zero reference point of each component sinusoid is displaced from the zero reference point of the fundamental frequency. There are 360 electrical degrees in one cycle of a sine wave, beginning with the zero reference point and returning to that same point after a positive and negative voltage excursion. If two sinusoids do not begin from the zero reference voltage together at the same point in time, the sinusoids are described as being out of phase. The phase difference is measured in electrical degrees. Taken together, the component sinusoids of any voltage waveform form the frequency spectrum of the waveform, ranging from the lowest frequency sinusoid, the fundamental, to the highest component frequency. Current flow that does not vary or alternate polarity is referred to as direct current (DC) and is assigned zero frequency (0 Hz).

## Impedance

An electrical circuit, the pathway in which charged ions or electrons flow, may consist of a complex combination of resistive, capacitive, and inductive elements. Capacitors and inductors offer opposition or **reactance** (X) to current flow that is frequency dependent. Capacitive reactance is infinite at DC (0 Hz) and decreases with increasing frequency. Conversely, inductive reactance is proportional to frequency. **Impedance** (Z) is defined as the total frequency-dependent opposition to electric current flow, where

$$Z = \sqrt{R^2 + X^2}$$

Like resistance and reactance, impedance is expressed in ohms. Because of the complex nature of the properties involved, impedance is a vector quantity. This vector quantity results in a phase difference between the applied voltage and resulting current in a circuit containing reactive components.

The circuit composed of an electrical stimulator and the human body is complex and contains resistive and reactive components. The impedance of the body tissue being stimulated has resistive and capacitive elements, while the stimulator output circuit impedance may include all three elements (ie, resistive, capacitive, and inductive).

## THERAPEUTIC CURRENTS

### Description of Currents

The description or classification of therapeutic currents begins with the simple division of all currents into two types: direct current (DC) and alternating current (AC). **Direct current** is the continuous flow of charged particles in one direction, the direction being dependent on the polarity of the applied EMF. **Alternating current** is the continuous bidirectional flow of charged particles. The term "AC" has been broadened to include both the classical symmetrical alternating current, in which the current flow in each direction is equal, and asymmetrical alternating current, in which the current flow in each direction is unequal. A third classification, **pulsed current,** also known as pulsatile or interrupted current, is defined as the noncontinuous flow of direct or alternating current. A pulse is a discrete electrical event, separated from other pulses by a period of time during which no electrical activity exists. Figure 2–1 shows examples of direct current, alternating current, and pulsed current.

### Waveform Terminology

This text has adopted the electrotherapeutic terminology recommended in a report by the Section on Clinical Electrophysiology of the American Physical Therapy Association. By clarifying and stan-

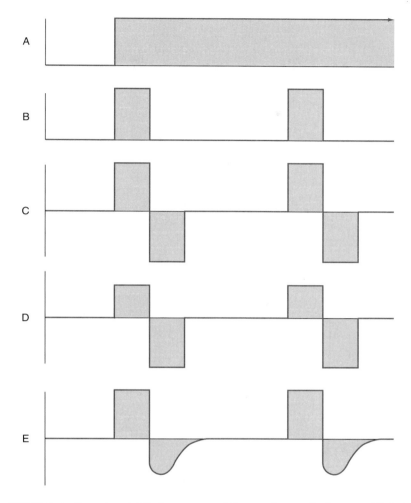

FIGURE 2–1. Examples of **(A)** direct current; **(B)** monophasic pulsed current; **(C)** balanced, biphasic, symmetric pusled current; **(D)** unbalanced, biphasic, symmetric pusled current; and **(E)** unbalanced, biphasic, asymmetric pulsed current.

dardizing terminology used to describe electrotherapeutic stimulator output characteristics and clinical application procedures, the report seeks to "foster uniformity of communication in product development and performance, clinical and research applications, and publications."[2] The names and definitions given in this chapter to electrotherapeutic waveforms are taken from the published report.

Because DC is constant and has no shape, the term **waveform** is properly used to describe the shape of an alternating or pulsed current. A current versus time plot or a voltage versus time plot is the typical method of conveying visual information about wave shape or waveform. The oscilloscope is the most common instrument for providing waveform information. The oscilloscope displays voltage versus time, although it can be adapted to display current versus time. Where the voltage displayed is the output of an electrical stimulator connected to a complex bioelectrical impedance, the current waveform will differ from the voltage waveform. This difference of waveforms can be a source of confusion because it is the current waveform, not the voltage waveform, that best describes the response of excitable tissue to stimulation. The electrotherapy terminology and units that are used in the remainder of this chapter are meant to refer to current waveforms, even though the same terms could be used to describe voltage waveforms.

The term *phase* has a special meaning when used to describe therapeutic currents, different from engineering usage. **Phase** is current flow in one direction for a definite period of time. A monophasic current, a current that flows in one direction from a zero current reference and returns to that reference after a period of time, is applicable only to the description of pulsed currents. Likewise, biphasic currents are applicable to alternating and pulsed currents. Figure 2–1B may be described as a monophasic pulsed current. Figures 2–1C and 2–1D are examples of a balanced biphasic symmetrical waveform and unbalanced biphasic symmetrical waveform, respectively. Figure 2–1E is termed an unbalanced biphasic asymmetrical waveform.

## Waveform Amplitude

The amplitude of a stimulus waveform is one of several measures of the magnitude of the stimulus current (or voltage) with reference to a zero baseline. The peak amplitude is the maximum current (or voltage) during a phase. For an unbalanced biphasic waveform, the peak amplitude is different for each phase and should be specified separately. Peak amplitude has been recommended as the preferred method of expressing amplitude.[2]

The peak-to-peak amplitude is the sum of the absolute value of the maximum current (or voltage) during the two phases of an alternating current. This term is not recommended for describing therapeutic currents because it does not give any information about the magnitude of the negative and positive amplitudes for an asymmetrical waveform.

The root-mean-square (RMS) amplitude represents the effective current applied to tissues. The effective current is an important value because it allows the calculation of power, measured in units of watts. Power is a measure of the rate at which work is done or energy is transferred.

$$\text{Power (W)} = \text{Voltage (V)} \times \text{Current (I)}$$

Because the energy transferred to the tissue impedance is converted to heat, the RMS amplitude of the stimulus current must be limited to safe levels to prevent tissue damage. The RMS amplitude may be calculated for a stimulus waveform of any shape. The instantaneous current (or voltage) is first squared, removing any sign, and then summed with the other squared values over a fixed time period in order to calculate a mean of the squared values. The final step is to take the square root of the mean of the squared values. The RMS value of a stimulus waveform may be computed with a computer program or with a special analog electrical circuit. Figure 2–2 gives some common conversions for sinusoidal and rectangular wave-forms.

The average current amplitude is another current magnitude descriptor that is widely used in engineering terminology. In comparing the average amplitude to the RMS amplitude, as in Figure 2–2, one can see that the values differ for certain waveforms and are identical for others. The equality of these different measures is unique to rectangular-shaped waveforms such as the square wave and pulse of Figure 2–2. This equality of magnitude is emphasized because of the wide use of rectangular current waveforms in electrotherapy and the inequality of the measures for other stimulus waveforms. The use of the RMS amplitude as a measure of stimulus magnitude is recommended over the average value.

## Duration

The duration of a stimulus has been divided into a number of interrelated time periods, which together make up the total time between the beginning and end of one stimulus pulse. Refer to Figure 2–3 for a graphic representation of the time-dependent terminology. **Phase duration** is the elapsed time from the beginning to the end of one phase of a pulse or a cycle of alternating current. Typical phase durations are short to prevent significant heating of biological tissue and are therefore expressed in fractions of a second such as microseconds (μsec) or milliseconds (msec).

Pulse duration, interphase interval and interpulse interval all refer to time characteristics of pulsed currents. **Pulse duration** is the total time elapsed from the beginning to the end of one pulse and includes the phase duration of all phases plus the interphase interval. The **interphase interval** is the period of no electrical activity between

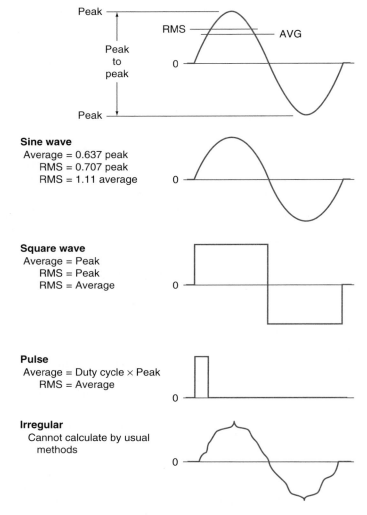

**Sine wave**
Average = 0.637 peak
RMS = 0.707 peak
RMS = 1.11 average

**Square wave**
Average = Peak
RMS = Peak
RMS = Average

**Pulse**
Average = Duty cycle × Peak
RMS = Average

**Irregular**
Cannot calculate by usual
methods

| From \ To | Peak | RMS | Average | Peak to peak |
|---|---|---|---|---|
| Peak | × 1.000 | × 0.707 | × 0.637 | × 2.000 |
| RMS | × 1.414 | × 1.000 | × 0.901 | × 2.829 |
| Average | × 1.570 | × 1.110 | × 1.000 | × 3.140 |
| Peak to peak | × 0.500 | × 0.354 | × 0.319 | × 1.000 |

FIGURE 2–2. Common descriptors of waveform amplitudes.

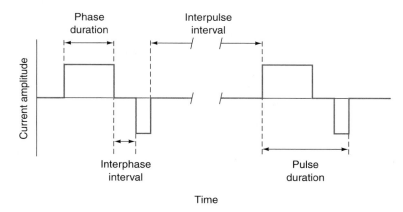

FIGURE 2–3. Time-dependent characteristics of pulsed current. *(Reprinted from Electrotherapeutic Terminology in Physical Therapy, Section on Clinical Electrophysiology, 1990, p 16, with the permission of the APTA.)*

two successive phases of a pulse. The **interpulse interval** is the period of no electrical activity between two successive pulses. The interphase interval cannot exceed the interpulse interval.

## Rise and Decay Times

**Rise time** is the time required for the leading edge of a phase to increase from the zero baseline to the peak amplitude of the phase. Rise time is an important descriptor of stimulus currents because of the physiological "accommodation" effect that can occur with repeated stimulation. Typical rise times range from billionths of a second, or nanoseconds, to hundreds of milliseconds, or longer. Similarly, the **decay time** is the time for the trailing edge of a phase to fall from the peak amplitude to the zero baseline. If the decay in current follows an exponential pattern, the time decay may be described in terms of a time constant. One time constant is the time required for the signal to decrease from the peak amplitude to approximately one third of its amplitude.

## Repetition Frequency

Pulses or alternating current in which the waveform repeats at regular intervals are described as having a repetition frequency, pulse repetition rate, or pulse frequency. The **repetition frequency** is the number of times per second the waveform repeats itself. The unit of measure for pulsed current is pulses per second (pps) and is hertz

(Hz) or cycles per second (cps) for alternating current. The reciprocal of repetition frequency is the period. The **period** is defined as the time from an arbitrary reference point on a pulse (or cycle) to the identical point on the following pulse (or cycle). Referring again to Figure 2–3, the period of a pulsed current is equal to the pulse duration plus the interpulse interval. For alternating currents, the duration of one cycle is equal to the period.

## Phase and Pulse Charge

Phase charge and pulse charge refer to the total charge within each phase or pulse, respectively. Charge is calculated by integrating the current amplitude with respect to time. Both phase and pulse charge are measured in microcoulombs ($\mu$C).

## Modulation

Modulation, or ordered variation, may occur in any of the previously noted waveform descriptors, such as amplitude, duration, or frequency. **Amplitude modulations** are variations in the peak amplitude in a series of pulses or cycles as in Figure 2–4A. **Phase** or **pulse duration modulations** are variations in phase or pulse duration in a series of pulses, as in Figure 2–4B. **Frequency modulations** are variations in frequency in a series of pulses, as in Figure 2–4C. **Ramp** or **surge modulations** are cyclical, sequential increases or decreases in phase charge over time. Figure 2–4D represents ramp modulation of phase duration, while Figure 2–4E represents ramp modulation of amplitude.

**Timing modulations** are variations in the delivery pattern of a series of pulses or alternating current. In many clinical applications, the periods of electrical stimulation (on time) are alternated with periods of rest (off time), measured in seconds. **Duty cycle** is defined as the ratio of the on time to the total time of the stimulation, expressed as a percentage. While different from duty cycle, the ON:OFF ratio conveys similar information. A 10-second on time with a 20-second off time equals a 1:2 ON:OFF ratio and a 33% duty cycle.

The term **burst** is used to describe the series of pulses or cycles of alternating current delivered during a stimulator ON period. (Refer to Figure 3–19.) Characteristics that further define the burst stimulation should be specified, including the **burst duration** (usually in msec), and the **burst frequency,** in bursts per second (bps). The **interburst interval** corresponds to the stimulator OFF time and is usually reported in milliseconds.

There are a seemingly unlimited variety of ways of modulating the amplitude, phase duration, frequency, and timing of a waveform. One method of timed modulation that has gained some popularity is

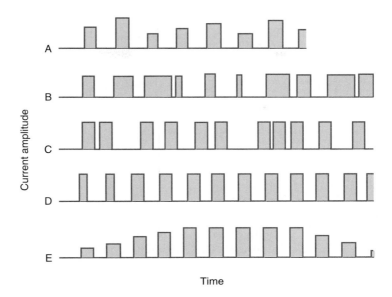

FIGURE 2–4. Waveform modulations of pulsed current: **(A)** random amplitute modulation; **(B)** random phase duration modulation; **(C)** random frequency modulation; **(D)** pulse duration ramp; **(E)** pulse amplitude ramp. *(Reprinted from the Electrotherapeutic Terminology in Physical Therapy, Section on Clinical Electrophysiology. 1990, p. 22, with the permission of the APTA.)*

the interferential current formed by mixing two sinusoidal waveforms of two different frequencies together. The mixing or temporal summation may occur in an electrical circuit of the stimulator or in the patient's tissues. The mixing of the frequencies causes a third frequency or beat frequency to be formed. The frequency of the beat is determined by the frequency difference between the two original sinusoids. The result of the mixing is a waveform that varies in frequency between the two original frequencies and varies in amplitude at the beat frequency. (See Figure 3–18.) Beat frequency is expressed in beats per second (bps).

# STIMULATORS

Stimulator design has undergone an evolution similar to most other electronic products. The ubiquitous application of the electronic computer in nearly every new design has made the stimulator safer to use, more adaptable to different uses, and more reliable. Irrespective of the name given the stimulator or type of waveform produced, all stimulators have the common functional components shown in Figure 2–5.

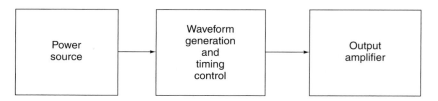

FIGURE 2–5. Stimulator functional components.

## Power Source

The EMF used to create stimulus currents must come from a power source. There are two basic sources used in electrotherapeutics: chemical energy stored in batteries and generated power distributed by connecting instrumentation to a building's electrical outlets. Neither of these sources is directly usable for electrotherapeutic stimulation, so transformation and regulation of voltages is necessary.

Batteries are a source of low-voltage direct current in the range of 1.5 to 12.0 volts. In order to provide the much higher voltages required for electrical stimulation, the voltage must somehow be multiplied. Such multiplication may be accomplished by placing many batteries in series or, more commonly, with an electronic circuit called a switching regulator. The switching regulator uses electromagnetic induction to increase the voltage of the battery to very high levels and capacitance to store charge at the high voltage for later use. A mechanical analogy to the switching regulator is the bicycle pump and tire. The pump (switcher) is used to increase the pressure (voltage) of the tire (capacitor) where air (charge) is stored. The switching regulator does not increase the battery power. In fact, a small percentage of the battery's power is lost in the switching regulator circuitry. The rest of the power is available at the output of the regulator as a higher voltage but smaller current. Charge must be removed from the battery at a high rate to provide the power needed by the stimulator. This charge removal limits the operating time of battery-powered stimulators before battery recharge is necessary. Battery power is usually limited to applications in which the advantages of portability, safety, and size outweigh the disadvantages.

The chief advantage of a line-powered stimulator is the quantity and reliability of the power available from the power company. In North America, the nominal line voltage is 120 volts of alternating sinusoidal current at a frequency of 60 Hz. In order to be used to power the various circuits needed to produce the stimulation waveform and the high-voltage switching regulator, the AC line power must be "converted" to direct current. This conversion occurs in a unit called a DC power supply, which usually consists of four major components: a transformer, a bridge rectifier, a filter, and a regulator. While the line-powered power supply requires more components, stimulator designs requiring a high-voltage output with significant current are not practical with battery power. The primary disadvantage of line-powered stimulators is their potential for producing hazardous shock currents. This topic will be covered in detail later under "Safety Considerations."

## Waveform Generation and Timing Control

The functional component of stimulators has undergone the most change in recent years. Before the wide-scale use of computers in instruments, the generation and timing control of stimulus waveforms was performed exclusively by specialized analog electrical circuits called oscillators. These circuits are still in use today, but they are gradually being replaced by computers. The key element in oscillators is the charge–discharge activity of a capacitor. The frequency of the generated waveform is determined by the rate at which the capacitor is charged and discharged. Other circuit components are used to shape the waveform to produce square waves and ramps. By combining several oscillators together, the production of a complex waveform is possible. For example, to generate the waveform of Figure 2–4E, a square wave oscillator can be used to control the pulse repetition frequency, while a second ramp oscillator with a lower frequency can modulate the amplitude of the pulse train by controlling the rate of surge buildup and decline. Separate controls for each of the oscillators may or may not be provided. Other timing and control operations are performed by logic circuits. Logic circuits can be used to count the number of pulses in a train of pulses or the number of bursts that are delivered before a unit turns itself off.

The uniqueness of the computer as a machine is its ability to change its character, or the work that it performs, based on how it is programmed. The combination of a computer with an analog-to-digital converter is capable of producing an arbitrary waveform of any shape or timing with great precision. In addition, the computer can monitor the pulse charge being delivered to a subject to control the stimulator output within safe levels. Some manufacturers are programming the stimulator computer to give instructions to the physical therapist as to the proper protocol for a type of treatment. Printed operation manuals are being replaced with computer-generated displays of text and graphics. The use of computers in stimulators is evolutionary in the sense that one stimulator can now be programmed and reprogrammed to replace a number of specialized stimulators.

## Output Amplifier

The final component in a stimulator circuit is the **output amplifier.** The function of this component is to amplify the power of the waveform generation and timing component to the amplitude needed for the treatment effect desired. Amplification is accomplished by using the limited power of the input waveform to proportionally control the amplitude of the stimulator output, which takes its power from the high-voltage power supply.

The control of the output waveform can take one of two different forms: **constant voltage** control or **constant current** control. These descriptors mean that the output voltage or current is directly proportional to the input signal and is unaffected by changes in impedance in the electrode–subject circuit to which it is connected. Stimulators of both types are in common use and many new designs allow the physical therapist to switch between control modes. A basic understanding of both types is necessary to evaluate the operation of a stimulator.

A simplified equivalent circuit representation of a stimulator output connected in series with the bulk electrode–subject impedance (Zs) is shown in Figure 2–6A. The waveform of the stimulus depicted in the circle represents the desired output waveform. The magnitude of the output impedance (Zo), located internal to the stimulator, determines the character of the output circuit as constant voltage or constant current. If the electrode–subject impedance was purely resistive, there would be no difference between the voltage and current waveforms. However, both the electrode–electrolyte interface and living tissue have capacitive and resistive components. The result of this complex impedance is that for any stimulus waveform other than a sine wave, the waveform for current and voltage will not be the same.

For the constant voltage output circuit of Figure 2–6B, the stimulator has a very low-output impedance, much smaller than the bulk electrode–subject impedance. This low-output impedance results in an inverse relationship between the impedance Zs and the current in the circuit. Note that the output voltage waveform is identical to the source waveform (constant voltage), whereas there is a peaking in the current pulse because of the charging of the capacitive component in the electrode–subject impedance.

The constant current circuit of Figure 2–6C provides the same current, irrespective of the impedance Zs. That is, the internal impedance of the stimulator, which is primarily resistive, is very high with respect to the electrode–subject impedance Zs. Note that the output current waveform is identical to the source waveform (constant current), whereas the leading edge of the voltage waveform is

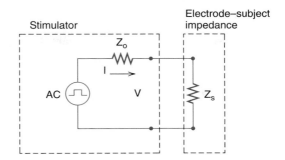

A. Simplified stimulator–subject circuit

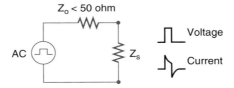

B. Constant voltage output circuit

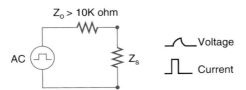

C. Constant current output circuit

FIGURE 2–6. **(A)** Circuit representation of a stimulator connected to the bulk electrode–subject impedance Zs. **(B)** Voltage and current waveforms for constant voltage ouput circuit. **(C)** Constant current output circuit.

rounded by the capacitive component in the electrode–subject impedance.

The extent to which any stimulator acts as an ideal constant voltage or constant current source depends on the magnitude of the difference in impedance between Zo and Zs. A pair of stimulating electrodes has a typical impedance of about 500 ohms at the frequencies contained in a rectangular pulse.[4] For a stimulator to act as either a constant voltage or constant current source, there must be at least a 10:1 difference in the impedance ratio. Designing a battery-powered constant current stimulator is difficult because a large portion of the output voltage is dropped across the large output impedance Zo, leaving less voltage to be dropped across the electrode–subject impedance. In a study of 10 battery-powered, constant current, trancutaneous nerve stimulators evaluated by Campbell,[5] most units displayed changes in current output ranging from 22 to 31 percent when different loads were applied to their outputs. Larger (and usually more expensive) AC-powered units would be expected to function better than battery-powered units in this regard.[5]

## Stimulator Controls

The largest physical components of small, portable, battery-powered stimulators tend to be the control knobs that determine amplitude, duty cycle, frequency, pulse duration, surge decline, and surge rate. Unfortunately, the markings for these controls are most often linear, usually from 0 to 10, but the actual control of these various functions may be quite nonlinear.[5] In practical applications, this means that a slight knob movement in the upper portions of the control range may produce disproportionate increases or decreases in comparison to the same control movement in the lower part of the range. Caution should be taken regarding abrupt, extreme changes in the upper part of the control range so as to avoid patient discomfort.

The introduction of the computer in stimulator design has also affected the type of controls needed. Instead of having one control for each function to be controlled, as was required in analog oscillator types, a computer-controlled stimulator can use one or two controls to input all the required control functions. Often, there will be a selection menu from which choices are picked. The computer can limit the settings for each type of stimulus to those that are relevant, which saves set-up time and decreases the likelihood of an improper setup.

# ELECTRODES

Electrodes are the means by which the electron flow of the stimulator output circuit is converted to an ionic current flow in living tissue. The most common electrical method employed as the means of making contact is to establish a direct ohmic contact with the tissue via an electrolyte. A minimum of two electrodes are required to direct the stimulator current to the target tissues and complete the electrical circuit. A variety of electrode materials are used for making ohmic contact. The size and shape of an electrode affects the distribution of charge in the stimulated tissues.

## Electrode–Electrolyte Interface

The electrode–electrolyte interface is the site of the electron-to-ion and ion-to-electron exchange. At any electrode–electrolyte interface, there is a tendency for the electrode to discharge ions into solution and for ions in the electrolyte to combine with the electrode. Living tissue is a rich source of ions and serves as the electrolyte in the interface. To establish an ionic current in living tissue, it is necessary for the electrodes to have opposite charges. The electrode with the greater concentration of electrons, referred to as the **cathode** or **negative electrode,** is negatively charged and therefore attracts positive ions from the underlying tissues. The electrode with the relative scarcity of electrons, the **anode** or **positive electrode,** attracts negative ions and free electrons from the underlying tissue.

Positive ions (mostly sodium and some potassium) flow oppositely to negative ions (principally chloride) and free electrons. The density of the ionic current is greatest proximal to the electrode sites because of the current spreading that occurs in the intervening tissues. The resting membrane potential of muscle fibers and nerve axons in the vicinity of the electrodes is affected by the concentration of charge at each electrode site. At the cathode, the membrane potential is reduced or depolarized. At the anode, the membrane potential is increased or hyperpolarized. If the transmembrane current at the cathode is sufficient to reduce the membrane potential to the threshold value, an action potential begins. Once the critical threshold has been reached and the depolarization wave begins propagating up and down the membrane, further infusion of negative ions and electrons will have no effect until the refractory period has been completed.

Because the cathode is the site of the lowest threshold for depolarization, it is also known as the **active electrode,** and is the site where stimulation is first perceived. The anode is sometimes referred to as the indifferent electrode. In the vicinity of the anode, the concentration of positive ions hyperpolarizes the cell membrane making it less sensitive to depolarization. With an AC waveform, each electrode is alternately the anode and cathode. If the waveform is symmetrically biphasic, the perception of stimulation is equal at both electrode sites. In the case of unbalanced waveforms, the quantity of charge delivered is unequal for the negative and positive phases of the signal. As a result, with identical electrodes, stimulation will be felt more strongly at one of the electrodes.

## Tissue Impedance

Different body tissues provide different impedances to current flow. Adipose tissue, bone, and skin tend to be poorer conductors than muscle and nerve tissues. Because the adipose and skin tissues are not pure insulators, DC does flow through these resistive elements. When good conductors, such as a metallic electrode and a bundle of muscle fibers, are separated by more insulating, less conductive, layers of skin and subcutaneous fat, a biological capacitor exists. As was discussed earlier, capacitors tend to impede DC flow and provide different impedances to different AC wave forms, depending on their frequency. The resulting biological circuit, therefore, is not a simple resistive one, but displays more complex impedance characteristics which are likely to vary from individual to individual.

The skin provides the greatest opposition element to current flow because it is composed primarily of keratin and contains very little fluid.[6,7] Skin lesions, such as open wounds and lacerations, and even minor irritation, such as from shaving, can significantly lower skin impedance. Conversely, skin impedance may be abnormally high in certain dermatologic conditions, such as icthyosis. Techniques to reduce skin impedance include hydration, mild abrasion, and tissue warming. In addition to mild physical abrasion to remove the superficial cell layers of the skin, another method has been suggested to avoid skin-heat buildup.[8] The use of high-voltage currents of approximately 100 V can cause sudden, spontaneous breakdown in skin impedance.[7,9] This initial resistance drop is followed by a continued, slower decrease in skin impedance.

The impedance effects of the skin and adipose layers can be minimized by the use of higher-frequency signals because, in general, the higher the frequency, the lower the impedance to current flow. Carrier frequencies of several kH are sometimes used for the express purpose of increasing current flow across the electrode–skin interface.

## Electrode Materials

Electrodes are the means of making an electrical connection to the body. Normally, they are mechanically attached to the skin's surface (transcutaneous stimulation), but can also be implanted below the skin (percutaneous stimulation). Electrodes have different roles. They may be used to detect biologically generated potentials as in electrocardiography and electromyography and to deliver current to biological tissue in therapeutic applications. The electrode material appropriate for a given use depends on its safety and effectiveness in the application. Other factors such as durability, ease of preparation, and initial versus long-term cost should be considered.

As discussed earlier, the electrode is the site of the electrode–electrolyte interface. For an electrode material to be perfectly effective, it must be capable of reacting chemically with a dilute chloride solution, such as found in the body, and to transfer charge in either direction with equal ease. Practical electrodes have electrical properties that fall short of ideal behavior. All electrode systems offer opposition to the transfer of charge between the electrode and electrolyte termed *electrode impedance*. Additionally, the movement of charge does not occur with equal ease in either direction, causing the electrode–electrolyte interface to become polarized like a battery after a period of time. The final magnitude of the electrode–electrolyte polarization potential is chiefly dependent on the electrode material, the electrolyte and the concentration of the electrolyte. For detection applications in which the electrodes are direct-coupled to a preamplifier, it is advantageous that both the absolute magnitude of the electrode–electrolyte polarization potential and the difference potential formed between a pair of monitoring electrodes be small. These conditions will produce the lowest level of long-term voltage change between the electrode pairs, termed *electrode offset potential drift*. If current is deliberately passed through electrodes, as in electrical tissue stimulation, the stimulation current will tend to charge the "battery" at the electrode–electrolyte junction. In cases in which the stimulation waveform is unbalanced, the magnitude of the electrode potential will increase as the electrodes become increasingly polarized. One of the advantages of a balanced stimulation waveform is that the net charge that flows in either direction is equal and this keeps the electrode–electrolyte junction from becoming overly polarized.

In addition to the necessary chemical behavior, electrodes must be good electrical conductors so that they offer little resistance to electron flow interior to the electrode where it is joined to a flexible wire lead. Metals such as copper, gold, platinum, silver, steel, and tin are excellent conductors and have traditionally been used as electrodes in both applications of detection and stimulation. Silver/silver chloride is favored as an electrode material for the detection of biogenerated potentials because it behaves as a near-perfect nonpolarizable reversible electrode. This property results in a low electrode offset potential interface, and low impedance between the electrode and body electrolyte.

The safety of the electrode material must be considered. Most metal electrodes form soluble metallic salts that are toxic, especially to exposed tissue. Silver and silver/silver chloride electrodes are minimally toxic as surface electrodes because silver chloride is nearly insoluble in a chloride-containing solution. As a result, there are very few free silver ions present, and the tissue damage from them is negligible. A number of studies have been performed in which non–current-carrying metals of different types were inserted in cat brains to assess long-term tissue response to implanted electrodes.[3,10] Gold and stainless steel and were found to evoke the least tissue response, whereas copper and silver produced a toxic reaction. Tissue responses to current-carrying electrodes have not been studied extensively to date, but the more vigorous electrolytic reactions typical of stimulating electrodes can radically alter the electrode environment by changing the local pH and ion concentrations and produce corrosion products of certain metals.[6]

A significant safety concern when electrodes are used to deliver stimulating currents is their potential to cause tissue burns at the site of the electrode–tissue interface. The temperature rise at an electrode is proportional to the square of the current density. **Current density** is the amount of current flow per unit area. Current density is a measure of the quantity of charged ions moving through a specific cross-sectional area of body tissue and is expressed in units of milliamperes per square centimeter or per square inch. One should not assume that the current density is uniform over the whole electrode surface. When an electrolytically coated metal electrode is placed on the skin and used to deliver current, the current density is much higher at the perimeter of the electrode than at its center. The current tends to spread out from the perimeter of the electrode. The perimeter of the electrode is where tissue burns would likely first occur. Adding to the potential burn risk at high levels of stimulating current is the effect of current density on the electrode–electrolyte impedance. The impedance of the electrode–electrolyte interface has been shown to decrease with increasing current density. This situation can cause a runaway condition in which a surge of current passes through a localized area of the skin, where the resistance of the skin is progressively decreased, resulting in a tissue burn.

Electrodes used in electrotherapeutic applications such as transcutaneous electrical nerve stimulation (TENS) and neuromuscular electrical stimulation (NMES) have undergone a significant evolution in recent years. These electrodes must be durable enough to be used repeatedly over a period of a week or more and adhere well enough to stay attached. Additionally, they should be flexible enough to conform to any body surface and still maintain their electrical conductance. A number of these electrodes use carbon as a conductive electrode material. Figure 2–7 illustrates three common flexible electrodes. Carbon has some advantages as an electrode material: It is inert and biocompatible and can be added to other materials such as silicone and synthetic rubber to produce a flexible, durable structure. Carbon has a much higher resisitivity than metal. This resisitive property would suggest that the current density from this type of electrode

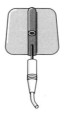

A. Flexible electrode with pin connector

B. Flexible electrode with pigtail connector

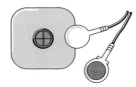

C. Flexible electrode with snap connector

FIGURE 2–7. Common flexible electrodes demonstrating three connection methods. *(From UNI-PATCH Medical Supplies, Wabasha, MN, 1997, with permission.)*

would be greatest where the resistance is the least. That condition would likely occur at the center of the electrode were the carbon-filled material is connected to a highly conductive metal lead wire, snap conductor, or other provisional connecting means. Even in this location, however, the current would be limited to some degree by the resistance of the carbon material. Some stimulation electrodes combine the favorable properties of carbon and silver by coating carbon film with a thin coat of silver to improve current dispersion while maintaining a high degree of flexibility.

Other types of electrodes include those made of sponge rubber over a metallic base that is encased in a nonconductive backing. Although these electrodes lack the glamour of other electrodes, they are durable, easy to prepare and maintain, and inexpensive. The sponge is used to absorb and contain the electrolytic medium, plain tap water. These electrodes can be quickly repositioned when handheld by the clinician, or are secured with fishnet surgical stockinet (one should note that solid stockinet or elastic bandages can become wet, thereby creating a conductive bridge between electrodes). Some clinicians have been impressed with the utility of this type of electrode in determining optimal electrode placement for treating pain and have described how these electrodes can be easily fabricated at low cost.[11,12] The electrode sponges should be kept clean and free of bacteria. Sponges should be separated from the electrode backing if possible, washed with mild soap, and rinsed thoroughly. The sponges can be air dried on a clean, flat surface after being gently compressed to remove the excess water.

## Electrode Coupling

For an electrode to function properly, it must be coupled to the tissue site both mechanically and electrically. Obviously, it is impossible to have good electrical coupling without good mechanical coupling. The total electrode surface area must be kept in contact with the target tissue to prevent an unintentional increase in current density at the stimulation site. The electrode surface area is of particular concern when constant current stimulation is used, because a one-half reduction in effective stimulation area will double the average current density. Painful sensations are likely to result. Electrode fixation is more difficult when rigid metal electrodes are employed. These electrodes are likely to lose some of their contact with the skin when a muscle contracts and changes its shape. Flexibility is an important electrode attribute that greatly reduces the demands on the method of electrode fixation and reduces the likelihood of an electrode's losing contact with the skin surface. The reusable carbonized rubber electrodes that are supplied with many commercial stimulators are commonly secured to the skin with surgical tape or a variety of commercial paper or foam adhesive patches. Although patches are often more convenient than tape, they are considerably more expensive. Electrode placement belts, which hold a pair of electrodes so that they can be secured in difficult-to-reach locations (the low back), are also commercially available.

Good mechanical coupling of the electrode does not ensure good electrical coupling. Recall that for an electrode to transfer charge, the electrode material must be in contact with the body electrolyte. Keratin is a protein formed at the outer layer of the skin epithelial tissue, which shields the fluid environment of the deeper epithelial layers. The large impedance of the keratin surface membrane is a barrier to the conduction of electrical charge and is a major component of the electrode–subject impedance. The application of an electrolytic liquid or gel medium between the electrode and skin surface is an effective way to reduce the electrode–subject impedance and facilitate the electron–ion exchange. Historically, water-soaked gauze or cotton pads have been used for this purpose. Improved water-soluble pastes and gels were introduced with better conductivity and less susceptibility to rapid drying. While manufacturers have their own formulation, each seeks to increase the conductivity by adding to the number of charge-carrying ions in the solution. Often, these are chlorides such as potassium chloride and sodium chloride that will not cause a toxic skin reaction.

Carbonized electrodes require a conductive medium. These may be either water based (moistened conductive pads, electrolytic gel, or karaya gum pads) or dry (a conductive "tac gel" adhesive). The conductive media should completely cover the electrode surface to avoid focal areas of high current density. The water-based media must be prevented from drying as this can potentially decrease the effective conductive area of the electrode and increase the current density. If too much medium is used, it can ooze from under the electrode and render the securing tape or other adhesives useless. The conductive medium should never be applied in such a way to span the area between the electrodes, creating an unintended low-impedance path on the surface of the skin for the stimulator current.

Gel conductive media should be applied in a thin, even layer on the electrode surface prior to attachment to the skin. The lead wire should be attached to the electrode prior to the application of the conductive media. A dab of gel, the quantity depending on the size of the electrode, can be quickly spread on the electrode by grasping the electrode with lead wire in one hand, while the other hand is used to spread the gel in a thin, even layer. Excess gel should be removed. The adequacy of the medium coverage can be confirmed by viewing the reflected room light from the gelled electrode surface.

Most recently, natural or synthetic hydrocolloids such as karaya gum and polyacrylamide have been introduced for application to carbon-based electrodes. These materials have the unique property of forming a semiliquid, adhesive conductive layer when wet and do not require the use of an additional conductive medium. Although very convenient to apply, they are not without their detractions. These materials are more expensive and often require a few drops of water to restore or maintain their conductivity and self-adhesion. Too much water, however, will turn their surfaces to nonadhering mush. Some of the newest electrodes of this type do not require additional wetting. Instead of adding water, reusable electrodes must be positioned on a nonporous backing and placed in an airtight container to prevent the conductive surface from drying out. Self-adhering electrodes are also available for single-use applications. Unfortunately, skin irritation and burns at high stimulation amplitudes have been noted with some karaya[13] and synthetic polymer gel electrodes.[14] Despite having self-adhesive properties, some electrodes require additional fixation in order to withstand the motion of patient activities. Self-adhesive electrodes should be reused with caution because their adhesive surfaces have the potential to harbor infective organisms.

## Size and Placement of Electrodes

Electrodes come in a wide variety of arrangements, sizes, and shapes. Each of these factors can affect a very important stimulation variable—current density. Current density is an important factor in determining the reaction of biological tissues to stimulation. In general, the greater the current density, the greater is the "effect" on the tissues in the current path. The determinants of current density are the total current flow in the stimulator output circuit and the size of the area of its application.

The area of an electrode affects the current density in two relevant ways. Increasing the surface area of an electrode decreases the electrode–subject impedance. That is, that for any given level of current, the polarization voltage at the electrode will be less for an electrode of greater surface area. Furthermore, larger electrodes will exhibit lower average current densities than smaller electrodes, because for a given current, the current will be dispersed over a larger area. The use of a porous electrode material with an electrolyte can dramatically increase the effective surface area of an electrode.

The practical importance of the current density to electrode size relationship is realized when an electrode size for a desired effect is selected. A small electrode will focus the current over a small area. A large electrode will disperse the current. The use of different-sized electrodes with a balanced AC waveform will produce selective effects in the area of the smaller electrode, even though the polarity is alternating equally between the electrodes. Therefore, the clinician can localize the effects of the stimulating current by using a smaller electrode at the "target area" and a much larger electrode at a location where the effects are to be minimized. In this case, the smaller electrode(s) would be termed the "active" or "stimulating" electrode, and the larger electrode would be termed the "dispersive" or "reference" electrode. Caution should be exercised in using too small an electrode for the intended application, because large current densities may elicit pain or cause tissue damage.

Electrode placement is another factor that influences current density and thus tissue response. Do not think of the current flowing between the electrodes as moving in a straight line; rather, consider the different impedances of the many anatomic structures lying in the path between the electrodes. The impeding properties of adipose tissue, bone, and skin have been previously mentioned. The greatest current flow will be through the tissues providing the least impedance (usually, muscle and nerve). Also, muscle tissues are nearly four times more conductive in the longitudinal direction of their fibers than in the transverse direction.[3,15]

Additionally, it is generally true that the greater the distance between stimulating electrodes, the lesser the current density in the intervening tissues. In other words, with more possible conductive routes, the current will disperse in its travel between electrodes. With large spacing between electrodes, it is difficult to estimate exactly what the current density might be for any particular structure. The tendency for current to disperse when wide electrode spacing is selected can be used to great advantage when the goal is to stimulate deeper tissues.

Electrode placement may be further complicated by the proximity of nerve axons and pain receptors to the target membrane but are not intended to be stimulated. Optimum placement is, therefore, part art and part science. Specific electrode orientations for a range of clinical applications are discussed in detail throughout the remainder of this book. Electrodes constructed in a wide variety of shapes and sizes so as to facilitate placements for specific applications are also described in the following chapters.

## Electrode Connections

Electrical connection is made between the stimulator output jacks and various stimulation electrodes via lead wires. Stimulators typically employ banana jacks, miniature phono jacks, or tip jacks as output connectors. Single and paired lead wires come in various lengths and are outfitted with connectors at each end to match their mating receptacle. The fit of jacks and plugs should be firm enough to prevent accidental disconnection during patient activities, yet connectors should allow for separation with minimum effort when desired by clinicians and patients. Paired wires may be attached by common separable insulation or movable plastic sleeves, or both, which limits tangling of the leads. The electrode end of the lead wires must be terminated with a connector to match the connection method of the electrode utilized. These lead wire terminations include the pin, pigtail pin, and snap connections. (Refer to Figure 2–7.) Consideration should be given to the convenience, intended use, patient comfort, and placement site in the selection process. Pin connectors are inserted directly into a receptacle molded into the back of the electrode, producing a secure, low-profile connection. Care must be taken not to drive the tip through the electrode surface, thus placing the tip in direct contact with the skin. This problem can be avoided by using electrodes with pigtail pin or snap connections. Pin-to-snap converters are available for various brands of lead wires. Some stimulation units permit electrodes to be "piggy-backed" so that more than two electrodes may be connected to an output channel. When using any connection scheme, be careful to prevent the metal connections from coming in contact with the patient's skin during treatment. This contact with the patient's skin can cause unintended local skin irritation or burns.

Stimulator output jacks are often marked with symbols such as − (negative) and + (positive) to indicate electrical polarity. Additionally, output jacks and associated lead wire connectors are often color coded, with black designating negative and red designating positive. Lack of conformance to industry standards by manufacturers can cause confusion. For example, one manufacturer refers to its red-coded connectors as being negative! Given that most electrical stimulators used for NMES have symmetric or balanced asymmetric biphasic waveforms that produce zero net current, and thus no polar effects, coding referenced to polarity makes no sense. Each lead is equally negative and positive in effect. Other waveform characteristics, however, such as rapid rise or fall times for one phase, may cause a lead to be more active than its paired partner. Units having DC, monophasic, or unbalanced asymmetric biphasic waveforms can produce polar effects associated with both *active* and *indifferent* electrodes, and thus benefit from color coding.

The effects of polarity or relative electrode activity are clinically significant. In order to standardize lead and electrode orientation for each stimulator output channel, the following technique has been suggested for determining whether one lead is more "active" than its partner.[16] Two equal-sized electrodes are prepared and secured to the clinician's skin, one over a known motor point and the other over a bony prominence. Lead wires from one output channel are then carefully attached to the electrodes. Using a low-frequency (2 pps) and narrow-pulse-duration (50 μsec) biphasic waveform, the amplitude control is slowly advanced to the point of initial sensation and then to initial muscle contraction. Amplitude dial settings at these two points are noted, as are differences in the qualities of sensation and contraction at the electrodes. The stimulator is then turned off and the lead wires are reversed at the electrodes, while the electrodes themselves remain in place. Stimulation amplitude is increased to the previous settings, and observations are again documented. This process can be repeated a number of times in order to discern whether a difference in lead wire activity exists, as opposed to effects resulting from the different electrode sites. If one lead is found to be more active, its output jack and connectors can be distinctively marked with paint or durable marker.

## SAFETY CONSIDERATIONS

Health care professionals work with patients in hazardous environments such as hospitals and private clinics. A number of sources of electrical hazards in health care settings have been described since the 1960s, and recommendations for promoting electrical safety in these settings have been outlined in a range of publications.[17-30] Twenty years ago, it was suggested that approximately 12,000 patients per year were being electrocuted in hospitals.[25] Since then, much stricter electrical safety standards have been instituted,[31,32] significantly reducing this hazard. At least one death from electrocution by common physical therapy equipment has been documented.[26] Shock and electrocution are not the only electrical hazards. Other hazards include electrical burns, interference with cardiac function, and disruption of implanted electrical devices such as cardiac pacers.

In 1969, Ben-Zvi reported that, over a two-year period, approximately 40 percent of all electronic and mechanical equipment inspected at his medical center was found to be either unsafe or did not meet manufacturer's safety specifications.[27] Over the intervening years, equipment preventive maintenance programs have become common in health care settings. A preventive maintenance program typically consists of a documented formal plan of regularly scheduled equipment inspection, performance tests, and required maintenance by a certified technician. Monitoring and compliance of hospital preventive maintenance programs is done through hospital accreditation commissions.

Economic pressures and concerns about efficient allocation of resources are currently stimulating the development of risk-based methodologies for preventive maintenance. Capuano and Koritko have noted that properly executed and cost-effective preventive maintenance focuses inspections on devices needing them most. Such a program can prevent device failures and poor performance, while minimizing treatment delays and the likelihood of patient discomfort, injury, and death.[33]

Not all electrical hazards are the result of defective equipment. Errors of judgment based on lack of knowledge concerning safety principles and regulations, and aggravated by clinician fatigue or patient medications, contribute significantly to the existence of electrical hazards.[34]

## Electrical Shock

Electrical shock is the primary concern of clinicians. Electrical shock involves the flow of current through human tissue, usually with adverse effects. Such effects are related to a number of factors including current amplitude, individual susceptibility, size of area contacted, and tissue impedance (presence of a cardiac pacemaker). For humans, tissue impedance may range from 500,000 ohms for dry skin to 1000 ohms for wet skin, whereas an intravenous line or a cardiac catheter running directly to the heart may present only a few ohms of impedance.[4,28] **Microshock** (generally imperceptible) is produced by low levels of current (< 1000 μA) applied to the surface of the heart that result in an unwanted physiologic response. Physiologic responses to electrical current include unwanted stimulation, muscle contractions, and tissue injury. Microshock on the order of 20 μA through a ventricular pacing catheter can induce fibrillation. **Macroshock** is the physiologic response to an electrical current applied to the surface of the body. The physiologic effects of macroshock are detailed in Table 2–2.

Electrical shock commonly results when current passes from a source of high electrical potential, through the body, and to a point of lower potential. Sources of high electrical potential (110 or 220 V) include electrical outlets, equipment power cords and plugs, and internal equipment circuitry. If damaged, these components may allow **fault current** to escape. Electrical shock may also result from **leakage current,** which is a normal characteristic of electrical circuits. Leakage current is produced by stray circuit capacitance. Leakage currents also may be induced in circuit wiring by electromagnetic fields from inductors and transformers. Standards have been established that limit the AC leakage current root-mean-square (RMS) amplitude to 300 μA on grounded equipment cases, to 50 μA

### TABLE 2–2. PHYSIOLOGICAL EFFECTS OF ELECTRICAL CURRENT*

| Current Amplitude | Physiological Effects |
| --- | --- |
| 1 mA | Threshold for tingling sensation |
| 16 mA | Cannot release grip on electrical conductor due to muscle contraction |
| 50 mA | Pain and possible fainting |
| 100 mA to 3 A | Ventricular fibrillation |
| 6 A | Sustained myocardial contraction, temporary respiratory paralysis, and burns |

*Modified from Bruner JMR, 1967, pp 396–425, for 1 second of 60-Hz AC stimulation of intact skin of the hands.[28]

on ordinary direct patient connections like an ultrasonic transducer head, and to 10 µA on isolated patient connections like electrocardiographic (ECG) electrodes or intra-aortic pressure monitors.[32]

## Grounding and Ground Fault Circuit Interrupters

Most electrical power systems are grounded; that is, one of the two conductors supplying current to an electrical appliance is physically connected to the earth. This grounding does not affect the operation of the appliance as long as the voltage difference between the two power conductors is the proper operating voltage of the appliance. Standard 120-V, 60-Hz electrical power is distributed in buildings via wall-mounted electrical outlets. (See Figure 2–8.) Each outlet contains two rectangular slots above one circular slot in a triangular arrangement. The two rectangular slots are used to distribute electrical power to the appliance and are of different sizes. The nongrounded "hot" wire (coated with black insulation) is attached to the narrow prong slot. The grounded "neutral" wire (coated with white insulation) is attached to the wide prong slot. Contemporary electrical codes and equipment specifications require that wall outlets and equipment plugs and power cables be equipped with a **safety ground** wire (coated with green insulation). The safety ground wire is attached to the metal parts of an appliance that are not intended to carry electrical current. Trace the path of the safety

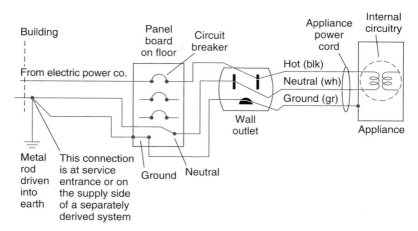

FIGURE 2–8. Grounding. *(Reprinted with permission from Healthcare Facilities Handbook (5th ed). Copyright 1996, National Fire Protection Association, Quincy, MA 02269. This reprinted material is not the complete and official position of the National Fire Protection Association on the referenced subject, which is represented only by the publication in its entirety.)*

ground wire from the chassis of the appliance in Figure 2–8 to the wall outlet. At the wall outlet, the ground wire runs from the circular prong hole socket to a common grounding buss, where it is connected to true **earth ground.** The safety ground wire provides a very low resistance pathway for fault and leakage currents to pass harmlessly to ground. If an equipment fault occurs that induces an electrical potential between the metal chassis and ground, without the existence of a low-resistance path to ground, a patient or clinician in contact with both the equipment chassis and earth ground would be shocked as current passed through him or her en route to ground. This unexpected shock is a significant hazard resulting from the large number of grounded structures, building services, and equipment found throughout any building such as cement floors, metal conduits, water pipes, or other grounded equipment.

Maintenance of the safety ground must be ensured. Wall outlets, including metal face plate and attaching screws, should be tested for ground continuity. One-piece, molded, three-prong plugs do not allow inspection of the wire to the ground prong. Underwriters Laboratories-approved hospital grade plugs (coded with a green dot) allow visual and physical inspection. "Cheater adapters," which allow a three-prong plug to be inserted into a two-prong outlet, should never be used. Extension cords are to be avoided.

A **ground fault circuit interrupter (GFCI)** is a device that can provide an extra margin of shock protection. The device monitors the power line current by comparing the amplitude of the current flowing in the "hot" wire versus the "neutral" wire. A difference in amplitudes indicates the loss of current to ground through an electrical fault. At a preset difference limit, usually 5 mA, the GFCI interrupts the circuit and shuts off power to the equipment in a fraction of a second. Such a device is beneficial for preventing most levels of macroshock, but it is not activated by currents which produce microshock. Also, the GFCI does not protect against shock arising from contact directly between hot and neutral wires. Available in models which can protect single or multiple outlets, this device should be installed wherever electrical equipment is used.[35] Some authorities have cautioned that GFCIs should not be used with life-sustaining equipment, or with other equipment vital to health and safety that rely upon continuous electrical power.[25]

## SUGGESTIONS FOR ENSURING ELECTRICAL SAFETY

The following suggestions are intended to facilitate consideration of electrical safety in the clinical environment. This listing is not all-inclusive; rather, it is meant to prompt development of safety policies and procedures that are in compliance with extant codes and standards for various clinical settings.[32,35,36]

We recommend that:

1. An adequate number of three-prong outlets attached to true earth ground should be installed in all clinical areas. Ground continuity and plug-pull tension should be regularly tested.

2. GFCIs should be incorporated in all outlets powering therapeutic and diagnostic equipment, and tested monthly.

3. Bibliographic sources that critically evaluate equipment safety and performance should be consulted prior to placing equipment in a clinical setting. ECRI (5200 Butler Pike, Plymouth Meeting, PA 19462) publishes *Health Devices, The Healthcare Product Comparison System,* and *The Health Devices Sourcebook.*

4. Equipment should be purchased on a trial basis, during which time it can be evaluated by trained biomedical personnel for compliance with safety standards and manufacturer's specifications. Professional staff should also assess the equipment for clinical utility and effectiveness.

5. Equipment should be tested at the correct interval as part of a preventive maintenance and safety program. Practitioners should comply with manufacturer-specified mandatory testing intervals should be complied with. Key specifications for line-powered equipment to which patients are connected include: chassis leakage current to ground ($\leq 300$ µA) and the lead leakage between patient lead(s) and ground ($\leq 50$ µA). The resistance between the equipment chassis or exposed conductive surface and the ground pin of the power plug ($< 0.50$ $\Omega$). For equipment with ground isolated inputs, the lead leakage between any patient lead and ground shall not exceed 10 µA with the ground intact and 50 µA with the ground open.[32]

6. Three-prong to two-prong "cheater" adapters and extension cords should never be used.

7. Metal equipment that might easily become grounded should be removed from the vicinity of the patient.

8. External cardiac pacing leads should not contact other electrical devices. Exposed metal lead heads should not be touched without rubber gloves, and the unattached heads should be kept insulated.

9. Power cord plugs should never be removed from an outlet by pulling on the power cord itself.

10. Shoes that provide good insulation should be worn by all personnel, especially in areas likely to have water on the floor.

11. Any equipment that is suspected of being defective should be immediately removed from service and clearly labeled as to

the problem, date, and personnel involved. An incident report filed with the clinical facility may be necessary. Entry of water into equipment cases, smoke, and unusual equipment odors or sounds should also prompt action. Equipment should be thoroughly inspected before it is returned to service.

12. Voluntarily share your experiences concerning equipment problems and hazards with trained biomedical personnel. Reports can be filed, either in writing or by fax, with the ECRI User Experience Network (ECRI, 5200 Bulter Pike, Plymouth Meeting, PA, 19462; fax 610-834-1275; phone 610-825-6000) and with the Adverse Event Product Problem Reporting Program (MEDWATCH, The FDA Medical Products Reporting Program, Food and Drug Administration, 5600 Fishers Lane, Rockville, MD 20852-9787; fax 1-800-FDA-0178; phone 1-800-FDA-1088).

13. Comply with the mandatory reporting requirements of the Safe Medical Devices Act of 1990 if practicing in settings other than a private office or patient home.[36] Device user facilities (eg, hospitals, nursing homes, nonprivate outpatient facilities) must report to the U.S. Food and Drug Administration (FDA) within 10 working days if there is reasonable suggestion that a medical device caused or contributed to the serious injury, illness, or death of a patient. Additionally, facilities must maintain device incident files and submit a semiannual report to the Secretary of Health and Human Services, summarizing related injuries, illnesses, or deaths. Noncompliance may result in both criminal and civil liabilities.

## Summary

The informed user of eletrotherapeutic equipment must have a fundamental understanding of electrical phenomena, of the wave forms produced and controlled by modern-day instrumentation, and of the factors affecting the choice and placement of electrodes. The competent practitioner must also be knowledgeable of safety hazards and pertinent safety standards and practices

## REVIEW QUESTIONS

1. It is typical of the physiology of excitable cell membranes that there be a continual movement of ions into and out of the cell. Which electrical phenomenon can be used to describe the un-

equal concentration of ions on either side of the cell membrane that results in the generation of an action potential?

2. A primary differentiating electrical characteristic of excitable membranes is their cell membrane capacitance. What are the chief factors that influence cell membrane capacitance?

3. A constant current amplitude stimulator is employed in a clinical application of electrotherapy. For a peak amplitude of 50 mA and a phase duration of 50 μsec, calculate the phase charge for a single phase of the stimulus waveform.

4. Explain why a patient can potentially receive a painful stimulus or burn if an electrode becomes partially unattached from the target membrane during stimulation with a constant current stimulator.

5. Often, electrodes of two different sizes will be employed in clinical electrotherapy. Explain the rationale for using different-sized electrodes.

6. Describe the primary safety hazard when utilizing line-powered patient care equipment such as electrical stimulators. List three policies or procedures that would reduce the electrical shock hazard.

## References

1. Jay F ed. IEEE Standard Dictionary of Electrical and Electronic Terms (2nd ed). New York, NY, IEEE Inc and Wiley-Interscience, 1977.

2. Electrotherapeutic Terminology in Physical Therapy. American Physical Therapy Association, 1990. Report by the Electrotherapy Standards Committee of the Section on Clinical Electrophysiology of the American Physical Therapy Association.

3. Geddes LA, Baker LE. Principles of Applied Biomedical Instrumentation (3rd ed). New York, NY, Wiley, 1989.

4. Strong P. Biophysical Measurements. Beaverton, OR, Tektronix, 1970.

5. Campbell JA. A critical appraisal of the electrical output characteristics of ten transcutaneous nerve stimulators. Clin Phys Physiol Meas, 3: 141–150, 1982.

6. Beard RB, Hung BN, Schmukler R. Biocompatibility Considerations at Stimulating Electrode Interfaces. Ann of Biomed Eng, 20:395–410, 1992.

7. Procacci P, Corte D, Zoppi M, et al. Pain threshold measurements in man. In Bonica JJ (ed), Recent Advances in Pain Therapy. Springfield, IL, Charles C Thomas, 1974, pp 105–147.

8. Newton RA, Karselis TC: Skin pH following high voltage pulsed galvanic stimulation. Phys Ther, 63:1593–1596, 1983.

9. Mueller EE, Loeffel R, Mead S. Skin impedance in relation to pain threshold testing by electrical means. J Appl Physiol, 5:746–752, 1952.

10. Collias JC, Manuelidis EE. Histopathological changes produced by implanted electrodes in cat brains. J Neurosurg, 14:302–328, 1957.

11. Mannheimer C, Lampe GN. Clinical Trancutaneous Electrical Nerve Stimulation. Philadelphia, PA, FA Davis, 1984.

12. Lamm KE. Optimal placement techniques for TENS: A soft tissue approach. Tucson, AZ, Workshop on TENS, 1986.

13. Ronnen M, Suster S, Kahana M et al. Contact dermatitis due to karaya gum and induced by the application of electrodes. Int J Dermatol, 25:189–190, 1986.

14. Henley EJ. Pain suppression device is explained: Henley responds (letter). PT Bulletin, Dec 7, 1988, p 8.

15. Shriber WJ. A Manual of Electrotherapy (4th ed). Philadelphia, PA, Lea & Febiger, 1975.

16. Barr JO. The Effect of Transcutaneous Electrical Nerve Stimulation Parameters on Experimentally Induced Acute Pain. Master's thesis. University of Iowa, Iowa City, IA, 1980.

17. The fatal current (clinic note). J Am Phys Ther Assoc, 46:968–969, 1966.

18. Tiny flaws in medical design can kill (clinic note). Phys Ther, 48:158–160, 1968.

19. Berger WH. Electrical hazards (letter to the editor). Phys Ther, 55:794, 1975.

20. Arledge RL. Prevention of electrical shock hazards in physical therapy. Phys Ther, 58:1215–1217, 1978.

21. Reeter AK, Jensen R. Nursing electrical safety (video tape). Medfilms Inc, 1983.

22. Berger WH. Electrical shock hazards in the physical therapy department. Clinical Management in Physical Therapy, 5:26–31, 1985.

23. American National Standard for Transcutaneous Electrical Nerve Stimulators. Arlington, Va. Association for the Advancement of Medical Instrumentation, 1986.

24. Robinson AJ. Instrumentation for electrotherapy. In Robinson AJ, Snyder-Mackler L (eds), Clinical Electrophysiology: Electrotherapy and Electrophysiologic Testing. Baltimore, MD, Williams & Wilkins, 1995.

25. Electrical Safety (special issue). Health Devices, January 1974.

26. Therapist dies in whirlpool. Progress Report, September 1984, p 30.

27. Ben-Zvi S. The lack of safety standards in medical instrumentation. Trans NY Acad of Sciences, 31:737–750, 1969.

28. Bruner JMR. Hazards of electrical apparatus. Anesthesiology, 28:396–425, 1967.

29. Day FJ. Electrical safety revisited: A new wrinkle. Anesthesiology, 80:220–221, 1994.

30. Moak E. AANA Journal Course: Update for nurse anesthetists—An overview of electrical safety. AANA J, 62:69–76, 1994.

31. Standard for medical and dental equipment. UL544 (3rd ed). Northbrook, IL, Underwriters Laboratories Inc, 1993.

32. Standard for Health Care Facilities. NFPA 99. Quincy, MA. National Fire Protection Association, 1993.

33. Capuano M, Koritko S. Risk-oriented maintenance. Biomedical Instrumentation & Technology, Jan/Feb:25–37, 1996.

34. Griffin JE, Karselis TC, Dean P. Physical Agents for Physical Therapists (3rd ed). Springfield, IL, Charles C Thomas, 1988.

35. Ritter HTM. Instrumentation considerations: Operating principles, purchase, managment, and safety. In Michlovitz SL (ed), Thermal Agents in Rehabilitation (3rd ed). Philadelphia, PA, FA Davis Co, 1996.
36. Center for Device and Radiological Health (U.S.). Division of Small Manufacturers Assistance. The Safe Medical Devices Act of 1990 and the Medical Device Amendments of 1992. Rockville, MD, U.S. Department of Health and Human Services, Public Health Service, Food and Drug Administration, Center for Devices and Radiological Health.

# 3

# Principles of
# Electrical Stimulation

Gad Alon

# Introduction

*T*he recognition that conduction of electricity through biologic systems alters physiologic and pathologic events is as old as the discovery that biologic systems are conductive media. The historical development and evolution of clinical electrical stimulators has been characterized by a cyclic pattern, alternating between popularity and disregard. The latest surge of interest has evolved around the use of electrical stimulation to modulate pain. Yet, since the mid-1980s, this surge of popularity has not only continued but expanded far beyond the application of electrical stimulation used to manage pain.

Many additional physical deficiencies have been reported to respond favorably to electrical energy. Among those are limb swelling and inflammatory reactions,[1–10] slow-to-heal wounds and ulcers,[11–30] muscle atrophy and impaired motor control associated with orthopedic[31–49] and neurologic damage,[50–62] circulatory impairments,[63–70] joint motion dysfunction,[71–76] postural disorders,[77–80] and incontinence associated with pelvic floor incapacity.[81–85]

These, as well as many other uses of electrical stimulation, can be found in historical and other reviews.[86–90] This latest surge of interest in electrical stimulation has attracted the attention of many professionals. Furthermore, numerous commercial stimulators have become available, creating a diversity of characteristics, properties, terminology, and many unsubstantiated claims for unique physiologic effects and superior clinical results.

Which type of stimulator should be used to manage each of various impairments is a daily decision the practicing clinicians must face. Questions such as which physical impairments indicate the need for electrical stimulation intervention and what treatment protocol(s) can provide predictive results can be problematic and rather confusing to most care providers. The dilemma is particularly true if the decisions are made based on information beliefs and anecdotal testimonies.[90] The present disarray, and the natural tendency to accept nonscientific, subjective, and commercially motivated claims, may threaten the substantive potential that electrical stimulation can offer as an objective clinical modality.

The goals of this chapter are to minimize confusion and to redirect clinicians and students toward a sound, systematic, objective, and predictive approach to the principles of electrical stimulation. To achieve these goals, a clinical model must be developed. By definition, such a model is dependent on the hypothesis that electrical, physiologic, physical, and procedural concepts are directly applied to clinical practice. The section on therapeutic currents offers functional definitions and is organized so as to provide a framework by which any present or future clinical electrical stimulator can be recognized for its clinical capabilities and limitations. The Electrophysiological Section of the American Physical Therapy Association (APTA) published a document that attempts to unify and standardize the terms and definitions used by biomedical engineers, researchers, educators, and clinicians. This chapter incorporates these terms and definitions as proposed in the document.[91] The section on physiologic responses delineates physiologic events and processes induced by the stimulation and associates them with the expected clinical results. Surface electrodes are an integral part of the electrical stimulation system, and their size, material, and placement technique dramatically affect physiologic responses and clinical results. The section on surface electrodes offers a functional approach to their application and will hopefully resolve many of the current misconceptions. The last section presents a clinical model for making decisions as to when, why, and how to incorporate electrical stimulation in the management of various impairments and physical dysfunctions.

This chapter is restricted to the transcutaneous (surface) application of electrical stimulation. Invasive electrodes may prove very beneficial in the future, particularly when inserted in denervated muscles, but because present clinical practice does not include them, they are not discussed in this chapter.

# THERAPEUTIC CURRENTS

## General Consideration

The custom has been to recognize electrical stimulators by the names of their inventors or by the (mostly) inappropriate names promoted by commercial companies. Galvanic, faradic, diadynamic, high voltage, low voltage, low frequency, medium frequency, TENS, and NMES are several examples. These names have created tremendous confusion relative to the physiologic effects and clinical benefits. The simple fact is that all are **transcutaneous electrical stimulators (TES)**, and the majority are also **transcutaneous electrical nerve stimulators (TENS)** because they are applied transcutaneously with the physiologic objective of exciting peripheral nerves.[89] Thus, as long as surface electrodes are utilized, and as long as the peripheral nerves are excited, the stimulator is a TENS unit.

Discrimination between TENS and transcutaneous muscle stimulators (TMS) or neuromuscular electrical stimulators (NMES) is also misleading, because the applied stimulation always excites the peripheral motor nerves, which in turn leads to muscle contraction. Direct activation of muscle fibers is possible only if the muscle is denervated,[92] and such condition require that the phase duration be set in milliseconds.[92,93] Indeed, only under such conditions may the term TMS be substituted for TENS. (With the exception of Chapter 8, where electrical stimulators of denervated muscles are discussed, all remaining chapters simply recognize TENS devices of different pulse characteristics, properties, and different current modulations.) In the field of physical medicine and rehabilitation, electrical stimulators should be classified as either direct current (DC), alternating current (AC), or pulsed current (PC). With the exception of subliminal (nonperceived) stimulation, all PC and most AC currents are TENS stimulators, regardless of their waveforms or commercial names.

All stimulators must provide sufficient voltage in order to conduct appropriate current against the impedance of the conductive medium. Most clinical stimulators are designed electronically as either **constant current** or **constant voltage** stimulators. Constant voltage means that the voltage output level set by the physical therapist will remain the same. If the impedance of the tissue or of the tissue–electrode interface (or both) is changed, the current will also change, but the voltage will remain constant. Conversely, any change of impedance during the application of a constant current stimulator will change the voltage output but will leave the current unaffected, provided that the stimulator is appropriately designed to function in the full range of tissue impedance.

Basic physiologic responses and clinical results are most likely to be identical whether constant voltage or constant current stimulators are used.[87,94,95] The clinical advantage of a constant voltage stimulator is the automatic diminution of current when electrode size is reduced or if electrode contact with the skin becomes loose. The disadvantage is apparent if the pressure between the tissue and the electrode is suddenly increased. Such increase causes reduction of impedance, and the current amplitude is automatically increased, thus intensifying the stimulation level. The advantage of constant current is the more consistent level of stimulation. The disadvantage is apparent when electrode size or their pressure against the skin, or both, are reduced and lead to a sudden increase of current concentrations. The result is a sudden discomfort of the stimulation and, in extreme cases, electrical burns. This hazard can be minimized by limiting the maximum voltage output.

The advanced clinician should also recognize that in a constant voltage design, the shape of the current waveform is altered because the impedance of the conductive medium and similarly the voltage waveform is altered in a constant current design (Figure 3–1). Only in a sine wave AC the shape of the waveform remains unchanged irrespective of a constant current or constant voltage design.

Another concept of general concern is the classical term **average current,** which each clinical stimulator provides. This generic term may not be the most appropriate relative to physiologic processes. Mathematically, current is calculated as coulombs/sec, where coulombs are the unit measure of electric charge, and 1 sec represents the time interval over which the rate of charge flow is calculated. Current flow per unit time may be better described by its absolute value, measured as root mean square (RMS) and averaged over 1 sec. Clinically, averaged $RMS_A$ current can be thought of as the amount of current flow averaged over one sec. Excessive $RMS_A$ current may cause harm, whereas insufficient $RMS_A$ current will not elicit the expected physiologic response. The upper limit of safe $RMS_A$ current depends largely on current density or current per area of electrode. Application of 10 mA/cm$^2$ of surface electrode has been suggested, but more conservative values of 1.5 to 4 mA/cm$^2$ are also recommended.[96] Because more specific guidelines are yet to be established, the prevailing clinical approach should be to use the lowest $RMS_A$ current density that is capable of producing the desired physiologic response. Excess, unnecessary current increases patient discomfort and decreases the efficiency of the stimulator.

Constant current design

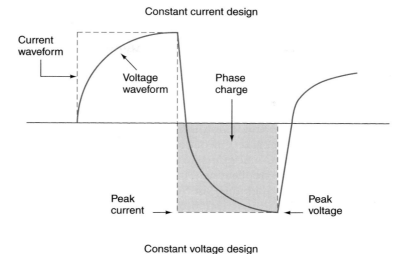

Constant voltage design

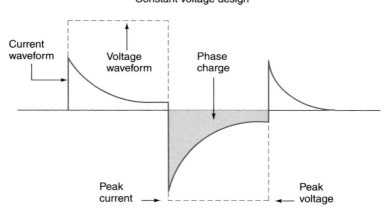

FIGURE 3–1. Voltage and current waveforms now both vary considerably with stimulator design. The differences are attributed to capacitative resistive characteristics of the conductive medium (body).

## Direct Current

Electrical current that flows in one direction for about 1 sec or longer can be defined as **direct current (DC)**. (Historically, DC is also termed **galvanic current**.) Current that flows unidirectionally for less than 1 sec, especially a few msec or less, is no longer a DC but rather a pulsed current.

The flow of a DC can be modulated for clinical purposes. The three most common modulations are:

1. Reversed DC
2. Interrupted DC
3. Ramped DC

In reversed DC, the direction of current flow is reversed. Since, by definition, DC should flow for about 1 sec or longer, reversal also occurs after about 1 sec or longer. Reversal of the current can be accomplished by using a hand switch or by an automatic switch inside the unit. Continuous DC and reversed DC are illustrated in Figure 3–2. A recent discovery that reversing DC (erroneously termed AC) can minimize skin irritation[97] may lead to fundamental changes in the application of DC, particularly in the attempt to deliver drugs through the skin (iontophoresis).

Interruption of current flow occurs when the current ceases to flow for about 1 sec or longer, and then flows again for about 1 sec or longer. Interruption is usually accomplished by a switch on the hand probe or by an automatic switch inside the stimulator. The most common classical purpose of interrupted DC is to cause twitch contraction of denervated muscles during electrodiagnosis or treatment (TMS). When the switch is closed, an ON current flow prevails; switching OFF arrests current flow. Switching ON and OFF occur abruptly. If one wishes to grade the ON and OFF so that current amplitude will increase and decrease gradually, a modulation termed **ramp** can be added. Classically, *ramp-up* and *ramp-down* were termed *surge-up* and *surge-down*, respectively. Ramping usually occurs over a period of time lasting from 0.5 sec to several seconds. Interruption without ramp, with ramp, and the combination of interruption coupled with reversed DC and ramp are illustrated in Figure 3–3.

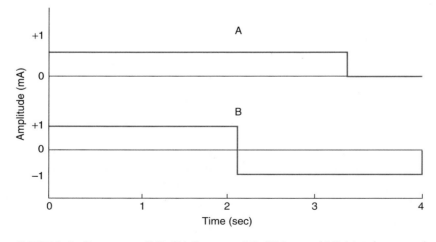

FIGURE 3–2. Direct current (DC). **(A)** Continuous DC. **(B)** Reversed DC. Note the time scale.

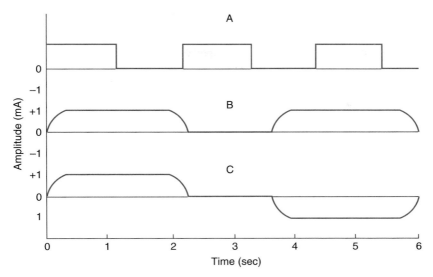

FIGURE 3–3. Direct-current modulation. **(A)** Interrupted DC. **(B)** Ramped, interrupted DC. **(C)** Ramped, reversed, interrupted DC.

With modern clinical methods, there is very little use for interrupted DC. In fact, most applications of electrical stimulation since the 1970s have been used to treat conditions where the peripheral nerves are intact and have employed to a limited degree alternating currents and to a large extent pulsed currents.

## Alternating Current

As defined, **alternating current (AC)** is a current that changes the direction of flow, with reference to the zero baseline, at least once every second. Continuous AC indicates no modulation and no intervals between cycles. The common AC is symmetric and can be delivered in various shapes, including sinusoidal, rectangular, trapezoidal, and triangular. Uncommon AC can be asymmetric and of various shapes (Figure 3–4).

Typical to AC are the inverse relations between frequency and pulse and phase durations. Inherent in this relationship is the phenomenon that as the frequency of AC is increased, phase and pulse durations are automatically decreased. The opposite occurs if the pulse frequency decreases (Figure 3–5). Phase and pulse duration then can be calculated as the reciprocal of frequency.

A growing body of knowledge on the physiologic and clinical effects of continuous, unmodulated AC is evident in the medical literature. The most common use to date is of a 60,000-Hz sine wave with

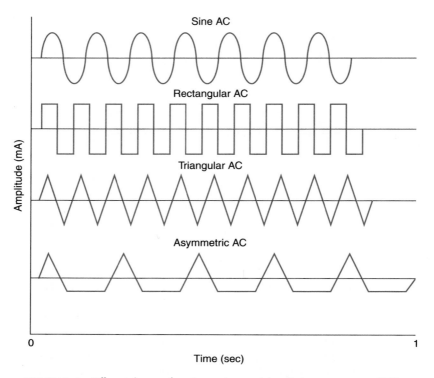

FIGURE 3–4.  Different shapes of continuous (nonmodulated) alternating current (AC).

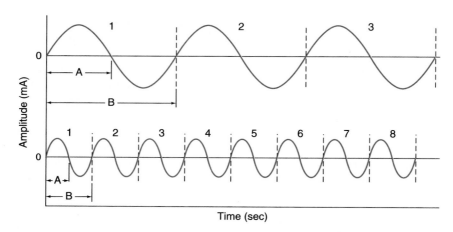

FIGURE 3–5. Frequency–pulse and –phase duration relationships of continuous sine waves. **(A)** Phase duration. **(B)** Pulse (1 cycle) duration. Note how both phase and pulse duration are shortened as frequency increases.

a 5- to 10-volt peak-to-peak (P-P) amplitude. Such AC is not designed to excite peripheral nerves and is aimed at promoting soft and osseous tissue regeneration.[98–100] Another common application of AC is for transcranial electrical stimulation (TCES). The frequency ranges between 5 and 2000 Hz,[101–103] and the clinical objectives include assistance in detoxification from alcohol and drug dependency[104–106] and as a method of treating traumatic brain injury and cerebral palsy.[107–111] Recently, AC has been also introduced as a method of inducing local skin anesthesia.[112–113] Typically, the frequency varies between 2000 and 30,000 Hz, and with adequate stimulus amplitude, the skin is anesthetized for a few minutes. The clinical benefit is purported to yield much greater and longer-lasting pain reduction, but objective clinical results as of this writing are not available.

## AC Modulation

AC modulation is recognized by time and amplitude variants. Time-modulated AC can be subgrouped into burst and interrupted modes. Bursting AC is created when the current is permitted to flow *for a few msec* and then ceases to flow for a few msec, in a repeated cycle (Figure 3–6). The interval between successive bursts is known as **interburst interval** and is synonymous with the interpulse interval of pulsed currents. The AC bursts have also been termed **polyphasic pulses**[89] because physiologically they seem to elicit the same excitation as monophasic or biphasic pulses.[114–115] The most common clinical stimulator that is designed to deliver bursts of time-modulated AC is the so-called "Russian current."

Alternating current can also be modulated as interrupted AC. This modulation prevails when the current ceases to flow *for 1 sec or*

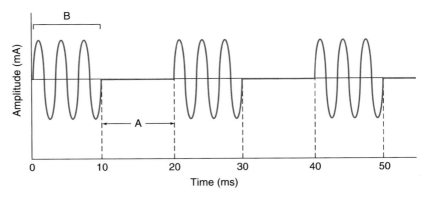

FIGURE 3–6.  Time-modulated AC to form bursts of pulses. **(A)** Interburst interval. **(B)** Single burst.

*longer* and then flows again for a few sec in a repeated cycle. Such modulation is different from burst in that the current ceases to flow for a long enough time to permit relaxation from a muscle contraction. The interruption modulation of AC is identical to the interruption of pulsed current.

Amplitude-modulated AC can be obtained by several electronic approaches. The most common electronic design is to mix two continuous AC sources that differ from each other in frequency. This electronic approach results in what is clinically known as **interferential current (IFC).** At present, there is no known physiologic or clinical advantage for amplitude-modulated AC over time-modulated AC or pulsed current.[94] Some manufacturers have used this modulation approach to create what they term **beat** (or **envelope**) frequency. Each beat seems to cause excitation of peripheral nerves much like a single pulse of a monophasic or a biphasic pulse[114–115] and therefore can also be termed a polyphasic pulse.[89] Amplitude-modulated AC is likely to remain an electronic concept without superior or unique clinical benefit over conventional pulsed stimulators[116–120] unless new data will prove otherwise in the future.

In continuous, unmodulated AC stimulators, the $RMS_A$ current (coulombs/sec) is always between 65 and 70 percent of the peak current. Modulation into **bursts** (Russian) or beats (interferential) reduce somewhat the $RMS_A$ current, but typically it remains unnecessarily high (50 to 100 mA) and may present undesired clinical responses.

## Pulsed Currents

A **pulsed current (PC)** is defined as an electrical current that is conducted as a signal (or signals) of short duration. Each pulse lasts for only a few msec or μsec followed by an interpulse interval. Different pulses may exhibit different shapes. Consequently, numerous names including but not limited to pulsating DC, spike, H-wave, square, faradic, exponential, and triangular, have appeared in the literature over the years. These names have led to enormous confusion regarding their common and unique association with physiologic responses and clinical benefits. Discriminating these pulses according to their waveforms (rather than names) drastically reduces the confusion. Once this is accomplished, the characteristics and properties of each pulse must be recognized. Two pulses of different shape but of the same waveform and similar characteristics are likely to elicit similar physiologic effects and clinical results.[94,120–122]

### Waveforms

Most, if not all, present and future PC stimulators can be classified under one of two waveform groups: monophasic or biphasic.

### MONOPHASIC

By definition, monophasic indicates that there is only one phase to each pulse. This type of waveform has also been called pulsating DC. Whether the shape of the pulse is square, triangular, twin peak, or half-way rectified sine wave, only one phase occurs in each case. In a monophasic pulse, current flow is still unidirectional, indicating that the polarity of one electrode is negative and of the other is positive.

### BIPHASIC

When two opposing phases are contained in a single pulse, the waveform is defined as a biphasic pulse. Shapes may include square, triangular, or sinusoidal, but they are all biphasic. Furthermore, biphasic pulses can be symmetric or asymmetric. Symmetric pulses with added interphase interval seem clinically preferred to asymmetric pulses, particularly if motor nerves are the target of excitation.[114,120,121] In the past, asymmetric pulses were more common (eg, faradic current and compensated monophasic). A major advantage of a symmetric biphasic pulse over an asymmetric pulse is that neither negative nor positive polarity requires any significant physiologic or clinical consideration. Illustrations of monophasic and biphasic waveforms are provided in Figure 3–7.

## Interpulse Interval

Irrespective of waveforms, all PC stimulators are characterized by a time separation between successive pulses. These temporal separations have been termed **interpulse intervals,** and each usually lasts from 10 to 999 msec. The exact time depends on the duration of each phase and pulse and the number of pulses per sec (Figure 3–8).

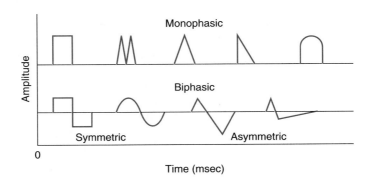

FIGURE 3–7. Basic pulsed-current wave forms.

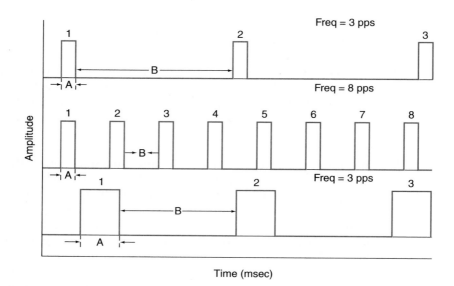

FIGURE 3–8. Frequency–pulse duration relationships of pulsed current. **(A)** Phase duration. **(B)** Interpulse interval. Note complete independence of duration and frequency.

### Interphase (Intrapulse) Interval

This time interval pertains only to biphasic waveform and is defined as a short, usually 50- to 100-μsec cessation of current flow between the two phases of each pulse (Figure 3–9). When added to a biphasic pulse, the interphase interval helps to reduce the peak current and phase charge neccessary to excite the peripheral nerve by 10 to 20 percent.[87,122]

### Pulse Characteristics and Properties

Regardless of waveform, pulsed currents exhibit some essential characteristics and properties that must be recognized. To account for all waveform classes, a single phase should be considered the basic, fundamental unit of description. The problem in choosing the phase is the traditional clinical preference of the term **pulse,** rather than the term **phase,** as the basic descriptive unit. To avoid misunderstanding, one must realize that, in a monophasic design, phase and pulse are synonymous. In biphasic pulses, each phase should be described. If symmetric, then the characteristics of both phases are identical, and the description of one phase should suffice. If asymmetric, the characteristics of both phases should be recognized.

An outstanding historical review by Geddes documented Fick as the first scholar to discuss the three important attributes of the phase (stimulus): **abruptness of onset** (rate of rise of phase ampli-

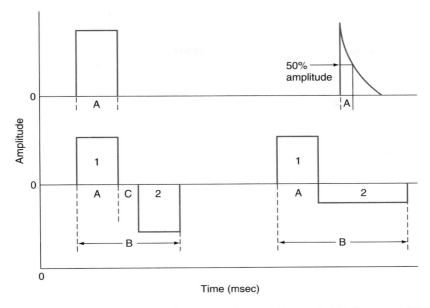

**FIGURE 3–9.** Phase and pulse duration. First phase = 1 and second phase = 2. **(A)** Phase time. **(B)** Pulse time. **(C)** Interphase interval time.

tude, also known as the *leading edge*), **amplitude,** and **duration.**[86,87] Other attributes, as well as additional characteristics, including phase and pulse duration, phase and pulse amplitude, phase and pulse charge, and pulse rate (frequency), must be described.

### Phase and Pulse Duration

The elapsed time from the initiation of the phase until its termination is defined as **phase duration.** The phase begins when the current departs from the zero line and ends as the current returns to the zero line. For the biphasic pulse, the pulse duration is determined by adding the two phase durations. Duration of the phases and pulses of monophasic and biphasic waveforms is illustrated in Figure 3–9.

### Phase and Pulse Amplitude

The highest instantaneous amplitude of the phase is defined as **peak phase,** or **peak current amplitude.** When monophasic pulses are used, the terms *peak phase current amplitude* and *peak pulse current amplitude* are synonymous. However, when symmetric or asymmetric biphasic pulses are considered, two peaks (one for each phase) can be recognized. Electronically, the amplitude refers to the magnitude differences between the peaks of the two phases and is measured P-P amplitude. Physiologically, investigators usually measure the peak amplitude from zero to one phase peak amplitude (Figure 3–10). Peak current amplitude must be distinguished from $RMS_A$ current amplitude.

### $RMS_A$ Current

One advantage of the pulsed current stimulators is the ability to keep the $RMS_A$ current (coulombs/sec) relatively low compared to the peak current amplitude. This low $RMS_A$ current is because pulsed currents contain relatively long interpulse intervals at which current amplitude is zero. Thus, the average amount of flow per sec is much lower than the peak current (Figure 3–11). The significance of relatively low $RMS_A$ current is in the safety of stimulation. Most PC clinical stimulators do not exceed 12 mA of $RMS_A$ current, and many are limited to only 2 to 5 mA. This limited $RMS_A$ current can be contrasted with the $RMS_A$ current of time- and amplitude-modulated AC stimulators where the currents usually reach 50 to 100 mA (see interferential and Russian current discussion on pages 82 and 85, respectively).

### Phase and Pulse Charge

**Phase charge** can be defined as the quantity of electricity that affects the biological medium with each phase of each pulse. Charge quantities of clinical stimulators are measured in microcoulombs (μC). In a monophasic pulse, phase and pulse charge are synonymous, and the total and net amounts of pulse charge are identical and are always greater than zero. In contrast, the charge contained in a biphasic pulse is the sum of charges of the two phases and thus contains a total amount of charge greater than the charge of each phase. The

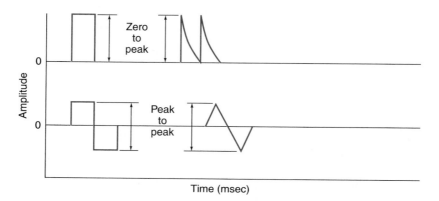

FIGURE 3–10. Peak current amplitude.

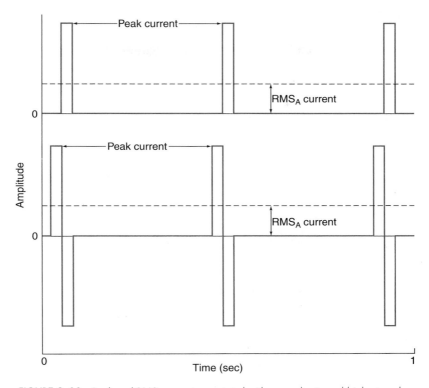

FIGURE 3–11. Peak and RMS$_A$ current associated with monophasic and biphasic pulses.

net amount may or may not equal zero. Symmetric biphasic pulses deliver twice the amount of charge contained in each phase to the tissues, while the net charge delivered remains zero (Figure 3–12).

When the net charge is different from zero, a DC component is recognized by electronic definition. Such a DC component provides a residue of electrical charges in the tissues. Only monophasic, and a few asymmetric biphasic pulses exhibit such residue, which may be of physiologic and clinical value.[3–5,8,9,15,18,25–28] Absence of a DC component refers to zero net charge (ZNC) and is characteristic of the symmetric biphasic pulses and most AC currents.

### *Pulse Rate (Frequency)*

The excitatory responses to the number of pulses of PC stimulators or the number of bursts (or "beat") of AC stimulators seem to be identical regardless of the number of phases contained in each

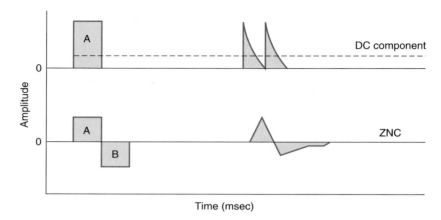

FIGURE 3–12. Phase and pulse charge. Note: In monophasic phase and pulse charge are synonymous = A. In biphasic phase charge = A (or B) and pulse charge = A + B (absolute value). ZNC = zero net charge.

pulse. For example, 50 monophasic, 50 biphasic, and 50 "bursts" or "beats" of AC currents all provide very similar tetanic contraction.[114,115] Thus, when the rate of pulsed current is considered, only the term *pulse* is used. The correct terminology should be **pulse frequency** (or **pulse repetition rate**), measured in pulses per second (pps). Alternating current frequency is usually expressed in Hertz (Hz) or the number of cycles per second (cps). Thus, Hz and pps represent the same property, that is, the number of pulses delivered each sec.

In the past, and based on the strict electronic definition, frequency has always been considered inversely proportional to pulse duration (also known as period). Stated another way, pulse frequency and phase or pulse duration always depend on each other when *continuous AC* is used. (See Figure 3–5.) In contrast, modern stimulators, particularly PC, are designed to produce short pulses with relatively long interpulse intervals (see next section). Such a design leads to complete independence of frequency and duration, at least from a physiologic perspective. Indeed, having an interpulse interval allows the therapist to change phase and pulse durations without affecting the pulse frequency, and vice versa. (See Figure 3–8.)

At present, a great deal of confusion seems to exist with regard to the recognition of "low-," "medium-," and "high"-frequency stimulators. By electronic standards, all PC and AC clinical stimulators are low frequency. However, some clinicians refer to 2 to 5 pps as low frequency and to 70 to 100 pps as high frequency. Others refer to 40 to 100 pps as low and 2500 to 4000 pps as medium frequency. The aforementioned adjectives, as used in the clinic, are probably relative adjectives and, more importantly, useless. In summary, all clinical stimulators, whether monophasic, biphasic, or medium frequency, effectively provide low-frequency pulses that range from 1 to several hundred pulses per second.

### Pulse and Current Modulation

When a PC is flowing continuously at a preset phase duration, peak amplitude, and pulse rate, there is no pulse or current modulation, and the setting is called **uninterrupted train of pulses,** or **continuous pulses.** Modulation of PC can be subdivided into two groups: phase/pulse modulation and current modulation. These two groups are not mutually exclusive and can occur simultaneously.

### Phase/Pulse Modulation

Phase/pulse modulation refers to an automatic increase and decrease of the phase/pulse characteristics. Usually, phase duration, phase peak amplitude, or pulse rate is programmed to increase and decrease (automatically) in preset ranges. This concept is illustrated in Figure 3–13.

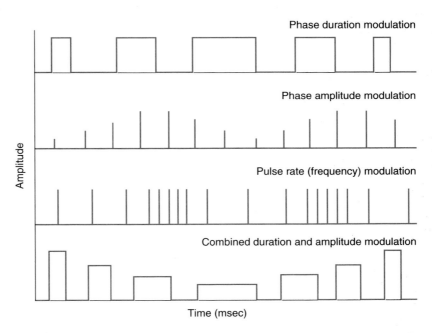

FIGURE 3–13. Modulation of phase/pulse characteristics. Note the so-called S-D modulation where, as amplitude decreases, duration increases.

Phase duration, peak amplitude, pulse rate modulation, or all of these are available in many clinical stimulators; they have, however, failed as yet to provide either physiologic or clinical advantages. The modulation of phase/pulse characteristics has been added to delay perceptual accommodation to current flow. Such a delay may prevail for several minutes, but in a 30- to 60-min treatment, a few minutes are insignificant. No greater pain suppression has yet been noted for automatically modulated pulse rates or durations than for nonmodulated pulses, thus contradicting promotional claims.[123-130]

### Current Modulation

**Current modulation** refers to the alteration of the pulsed current as a whole rather than to the properties of each pulse. One form of such modulation is bursts. Others are interruption (ON–OFF) and ramping of pulsed current flow.

#### BURSTS

Bursts are created when a pulsed current is permitted to flow for a few msec and then ceases to flow for a few msec in a repeated cycle. Much like the modulation of AC into bursts, such bursts can also occur with monophasic and biphasic pulses (Figure 3–14). Physiologically, individual pulses or bursts cause similar excitation thresh-

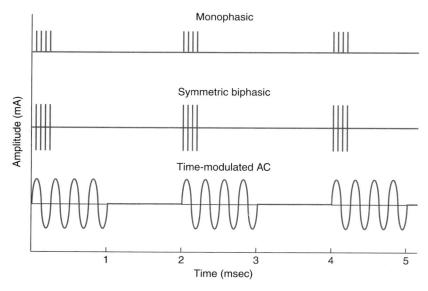

FIGURE 3–14. Bursts. Monophasic and biphasic pulsed bursts usually last only 1 msec while AC bursts last about 10 msec. (The limited space of the figure does not allow actual illustration of correct values.)

olds.[114,115,122] Five bursts or five pulses both cause twitch contractions, although the perception of the bursts is somewhat different from that of individual pulses. The number of bursts per sec, much like the number of pulses per sec, is predetermined by the physical therapist.

With one exception,[131,132] bursts have so far failed to add any advantage to clinical practice.[123–130,133–135] The clinician must recognize the fact that bursts and interburst intervals do not cause physiologically sufficient interruption of muscle contractions. Both bursts and interburst intervals are measured in milliseconds, intervals too short to permit relaxation during tetanic contraction. Thus, intervals should not be referred to as interruptions. Indeed, true interruption of pulsed current flow is a different category of current modulation.

### INTERRUPTED PULSES

True interruption modulation occurs when monophasic or biphasic pulses continue to flow for about 1 sec or longer and then cease to flow for 1 sec or longer. Clinically, many stimulators provide an interruption mode where the ON time can usually be varied between 1 and 60 sec and the OFF time between 1 and 120 sec. The interruption mode is of major clinical importance. Many clinical applications of electrical stimulation associated with the augmentation of muscle force, motor control, improved joint range of motion (ROM), and enhanced venous blood flow require such current modulation.[20,31–39,43–63,77–85]

### RAMPS

The last form of modulation to be considered is a ramp mode, also recognized by many clinicians as a surge mode. This modulation is associated with the ON portion of the interrupted mode. With a ramp, phase charge will increase gradually over a predetermined period, usually lasting from 1 to 5 sec, allowing for gradual increase of muscle contraction. Such modulation is called ramp-up. Many stimulators also provide ramp-down, resulting in a gradual decrease of phase charge toward the end of the ON time (Figure 3–15). Ramp-down is usually less effective in graduating muscle relaxation but is perceived by the subject as offering more comfortable stimulation than would be provided with only ramp-up mode.

Manual selection of the ramp-up and -down times, in which the physical therapist determines the times independently of the ON time, is clinically far superior to other options in which the ramp times are part of the ON time.

## Summary of Current Modulation

The practitioners must recognize that modulation of electrical currents can include both modulation of the individual phase/pulse characteristics and modulation of the pulsed current as a whole. At

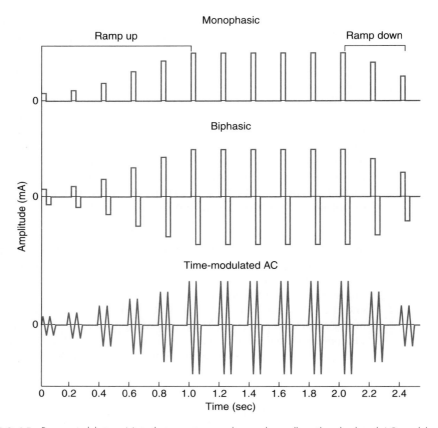

FIGURE 3–15. Ramp modulation. Note that ramping can be used equally with pulsed and AC modulated bursts.

present, automatic variation of individual pulse properties does not seem to have clinical value, whereas interrupted and ramping modulation of the pulsed current as a whole is of major importance for appropriate selection of different clinical protocols.

Finally, there seems to be considerable confusion regarding the differences between phase duration, interpulse interval, burst duration, interburst interval, ON duration, and OFF duration. These terms are differentiated in Table 3–1.

Figure 3–14 shows clearly that interburst intervals are not a physiologic interruption. Rather, they are an interval between successive bursts that parallels the interpulse interval of monophasic or biphasic pulses. It then follows that a nonmodulated PC having monophasic or biphasic pulses and a frequency of 50 pps should have an excitatory response very similar to that of an amplitude- or

## TABLE 3–1. CURRENT PULSE AND PHASE TERMINOLOGY

| Parameter | Synonyms | Measured Time |
|---|---|---|
| Phase duration | Pulse width, pulse time, pulse duration[a] | Microseconds[b] |
| Interpulse interval | Interpulse spacing, rest period | Milliseconds |
| Burst duration | Packets, beat, envelop | Milliseconds |
| Interburst interval | Interburst spacing, rest period | Milliseconds |
| Interrupted current | ON–OFF | Seconds |
| Ramp-up and -down | Surge up and down | Seconds |

[a] Phase duration and pulse duration are not necessarily synonyms.
[b] Can also be milliseconds.

time-modulated AC with 50 bps.[114] Interrupted mode can be added to monophasic and biphasic pulses, as well as to AC "bursting" current.

If interrupted, a ramp-up and ramp-down modulation should be added to both pulsed currents as well as to the interrupted or time- or amplitude-modulated AC, as illustrated in Figure 3–16.

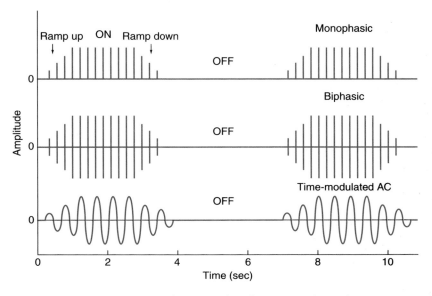

FIGURE 3–16. Interrupted current mode with ramp-up and ramp-down.

## Identification of Clinical Stimulators

As previously discussed, all noninvasive clinical stimulators are classified as transcutaneous electrical stimulators (TES). The majority of these are also TENS because they all conduct pulsed current through surface electrodes and cause excitation of peripheral nerves. Few of those TENS deliver bursts of time-modulated AC, the so-called Russian current, or "beats" of amplitude-modulated AC, the so-called interferential current. The different names for stimulators, such as low voltage, high voltage, interferential current (IFC), Russian, American, medium frequency, TENS, NMES, and EMS, help sales representatives and sales-oriented clinicians, but have little bearing on physiologic and objective clinical benefits or on the most effective use of these various devices.

In the last few years a new group of TES has been promoted in the clinic that may require a separate classification. Whereas these stimulators conduct their current through surface electrodes, they do not, in most instances, excite the peripheral nerves.[89] Thus, in generic terminology, they are not TENS but are classified as subliminal or nonperceived TES. The promoters of these devices seem to prefer meaningless names such as Microcurrent, MENS Therapy, Electro-Acuscope, Myopulse, Myomatic, MENS-O-MATIC, Alfastim, Pain Suppressor, Biopulse, and more. The list of names seems to keep growing and with it the confusion, misapplication, and false information to patient and clinician alike.

Evaluation of the various stimulators must not be based on *names*. The astute clinician should examine the pulse characteristics and determine whether these characteristics are in agreement with the appropriate stimulation protocols. An appropriate protocol is defined as that which is based on *objective* clinical results or presently valid physiologic rationale, or both. The purpose of this section is to examine briefly the most common groups of stimulators and evaluate them according to their pulse characteristics and current modulation, rather than according to their names and promotional misconcepts. Indeed, the more important characteristics that should be recognized by the astute clinician in each TES are waveform, phase duration, phase charge, pulse rate, $RMS_A$ current, and various options of current modulations.

This section should allow the physical therapist to recognize that clinical stimulators irrespective of name are not uniquely different, but simply represent different electronic designs that will achieve the same physiologic effects and clinical results. Some stimulators are clinically more versatile than others because they can be set to comply appropriately with more clinical protocols. No single stimulator is optimally designed to provide all clinical treatments.

## *Low-voltage Stimulators*

The term *low voltage* is a useless and misleading descriptor for a group of classic stimulators. Previous electrotherapy texts nevertheless identify low-voltage devices as a group of three different stimulators, including DC, the so-called galvanic, and two pulsed stimulators: faradic and diadynamic. A short description of each follows.

## *Direct Current (Galvanic) Stimulators*

The basic design of a galvanic stimulator incorporates a continuous direct current. Such a current flows unidirectionally for at least 1 sec, but can be reversed, interrupted, and ramped. By definition, the DC stimulator does not have pulses, thus no waveform or pulse parameters. In the simple DC stimulator, there is neither reversal of polarity nor ramp capability. Interruption is accomplished manually with a switch on the stimulating electrode. In more sophisticated units, the therapist can set the time intervals of interruption, ramping, and reversal of polarity prior to operation, and they are then automatically instituted during treatment.

The major *direct* physiologic responses to DC stimulation are the electrochemical changes that occur at the cellular and tissue levels. The change of skin pH under the electrodes causes a reflex vasodilation, thus indirectly increasing arterial blood flow to the skin.[96,97,136,137] Because of the prolonged flow of DC, current amplitude must be extremely low, and therefore the direct effect of such current is primarily limited to superficial tissues (such as skin). Excitatory responses can be elicited only if such DC is interrupted. The electrical excitation affects only very superficial nerve fibers and is usually painful. Discrimination among large sensory fibers, motor fibers, and pain-conducting fibers is difficult to obtain when current flow is of a duration greater than 500 μsec.

When a state of denervation prevails, the physical therapist can transcutaneously use interrupted DC to directly stimulate the denervated muscle fibers. The superficial effect of such stimulation, the inevitable elicitation of only twitch contractions, and the painful perception of the stimulation render a very limited clinical effectiveness to such DC (see Chapter 8).

The value of DC in alleviating pain, with or without iontophoresis, has been clinically tested[136–144] but may not be the treatment of first choice because of the unpleasant and potentially harmful stimulation.[136,137] Pulsed currents having a short phase duration are likely to be more effective and are much more comfortable to the patient.[145] As a last resort, and particularly when the pain is caused by superficial structures, DC should be considered. The physical therapist must be aware of the potential hazard of chemical skin burns with DC, because $RMS_A$ current, current density, and treatment time may all contribute to excessive stimulation. A major step toward minimizing the adverse chemical irritation may be achieved by automatic reversal of the polarity every 60 sec. With this approach Howard and coworkers[97] reported success when applying hydroxocobalamin (vitamin $B_{12}$) iontophoresis for 4 hours without any noticeable skin irritation. Use of such an approach may radically change the clinical efficacy of iontophoresis. In fact, iontophoresis may become even more effective if short-duration (μsec) monophasic pulsatile current is used.[145,146] In contrast to DC, monophasic pulses are associated with considerably lower electrode–skin interface impedance, much more comfortable perception of the stimulation, and less chance for irreversible skin irritation even with several hours of stimulation. Recent data documented effective transdermal delivery of insulin,[147] beta blockers,[148] and other therapeutic peptides/proteins.[149] Taken together, these data promise a marked revision in the theory and clinical practice of electrically mediated transdermal drug delivery.

### Faradic Current

Faradic current, whether implemented as general or localized faradism, has been used clinically since the late 19th century. The faradic pulse is an asymmetric biphasic pulse. From the early 1940s until the late 1960s, faradic current was considered more comfortable than DC. Most physical therapists mistakenly believed that the relative comfort of the faradic pulse derived from its being a form of AC. Current knowledge strongly indicates that the real reason for relative comfort was that the faradic pulse was simply of a shorter duration than the DC. The duration of the main phase of the faradic pulse is typically 1 msec (Figure 3–17). By today's standards, this pulse duration is much too long for optimizing comfort. Indeed, the phase duration of most modern pulses, whether monophasic or biphasic, is only between 5 and 300 μsec. Duration of the phase is one factor responsible for patient comfort irrespective of the type of current.

The asymmetric biphasic waveform of the faradic current renders such current less desirable than a symmetric biphasic waveform, even with a design of shorter pulses.[94] Today's knowledge suggests that well-designed stimulators should provide both monophasic (for polarity-dependent applications) and symmetric biphasic pulses for polarity-independent applications in which comfort is a priority.[94,114,120] Having an asymmetric waveform such as the faradic or the "H-wave" pulses is unlikely to offer any physiologic, clinical, or engineering advantage over either monophasic or symmetric biphasic waveforms.[150] Most clinical faradic stimulators have variable pulse rates, usually 1 to 60 pps, but not variable phase duration. Many other

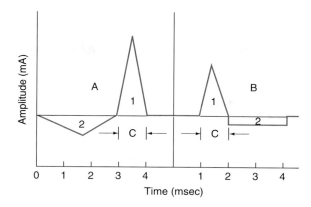

FIGURE 3–17. Faradic current. **(A)** Original wave shape. **(B)** Modified wave shape. Note that both waves are asymmetric biphasic. Phase 1 is the main phase for excitation, usually lasting 1 msec **(C)**. The amplitude of the second phase is too low to cause excitation.

stimulators have a ramp-up and ramp-down (surge) mode but no true interrupted pulses mode (Table 3–2). Lack of comfort and limited current modulation reduce the clinical versatility and number of treatment protocols that the classical faradic stimulator can provide.

### Diadynamic Current

Diadynamic current is actually a monophasic pulsed current developed in the early 1900s. Diadynamic current is usually a sine wave at a carrier frequency of 100 Hz, which is either half-wave or full-wave rectified. The result is a monophasic pulse of 5-msec phase duration. Half-wave rectification yields a pulse rate of 50 pps (also known as MF current). Full-wave rectification yields 100 pps (also known as DF current). The former has a 5-msec interpulse interval, whereas the latter has no such interval (Figure 3–18). Diadynamic current usually offers two modulation options. One is known as CP, in which the MF and DF are exchanged every 1 sec. The other modulation, LP, ramps up and down every other pulse over a period of 5 to 7 sec. These modulations are illustrated in Figure 3–19 but their clinical significance has not been objectively documented.

Diadynamic current, like other TENS devices, provides *direct* excitatory responses, but, because of its long pulse duration, it is very uncomfortable. The unidirectional current flow, long pulse duration, and relatively short (or absent) interpulse interval render cellular and tissue chemical changes similar to those of continuous DC. Early reports from Europe suggested many different excitatory responses and clinical procedures,[151] but all can be achieved with far greater comfort

## TABLE 3–2. TRAITS OF ELECTRICAL STIMULATORS

| Trait | Stimulator Commercial Name | | | | |
|---|---|---|---|---|---|
| | Low-volt Faradic | High Voltage | Russian Current | Interferential Current | Diadynamic Current |
| Channels | 1 | 1–2 | 2–4 | 2–4 | 1–4 |
| Modes | Continuous ramp only[a] | Continuous/ Interrupted | Continuous/ Interrupted[c] | Continuous | Continuous |
| Waveform | Asymmetric biphasic | Monophasic | Time-modulated AC | Amplitude-modulated AC | Monophasic |
| Phase duration | 1000 μsec (fixed) | 5–20 μsec (fixed) | 50–200 μsec (variable) | 125 μsec (fixed) | 5 msec (fixed) |
| Phase charge (max) | 60 μC | 12–14 μC | 30 μC | 20–25 μC | 50 μC? |
| Pulse rate | 1–60 pps | 1–200 pps | 1–100 pps | 1–200 pps | 50–100 pps |
| RMS$_A$ | 5–6 mA | 1.5 mA | 50–100 mA | 50–80 mA | 25–50 mA |
| Polarity | No[b] | Yes | No | No | Yes |

[a] There is ramp-up and -down but NOT interruption.
[b] May have polarity-like traits because of the asymmetric waveform.
[c] "Russian" can be ramped.

and ease using the microsecond pulses of modern TENS units. Diadynamic currents are likely to remain obsolete unless comparative data can be presented to demonstrate their superiority over modern TENS.

### TENS and NMES

Early in this chapter, the statement was made that most clinical stimulators are TENS (except true DC and subliminal stimulators). TENS includes diadynamic, faradic, H-wave, high-voltage, interferential, and Russian, or any other PC stimulator. Unfortunately, too many physical therapists differentiate TENS units from these other stimulators because they are small and battery powered. Others consider TENS units only when applied to modulate pain.[152] High-voltage and interferential stimulators can also be battery operated and can be equally effective in reducing pain.[153,154] Hopefully, this chapter has settled this issue by pointing out that *all pulsed current stimulators that are applied transcutaneously are TENS*. They may differ in their waveform, pulse characteristics, and the current modulations that they may or may not offer.

Some of these battery-powered TENS units offer monophasic pulses, whereas others offer symmetric or asymmetric biphasic pulses;

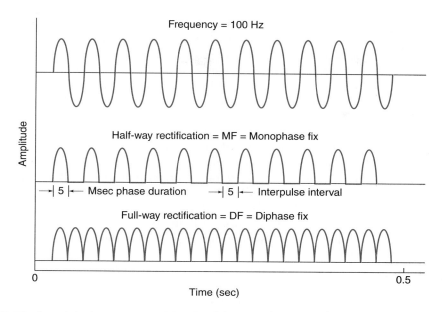

FIGURE 3–18. Typical diadynamic current. Note that if the original sine-wave frequency is 100 Hz, the phase (pulse) duration is 5 msec and the interpulse interval is also 5 msec (MF). In DF there is no interpulse interval.

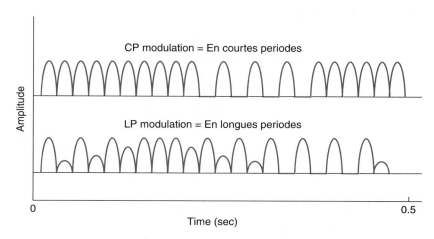

FIGURE 3–19. Modulations of diadynamic current. CP alternates the MF and DF every few seconds. LP alters the amplitude of every other pulse.

few offer time- or amplitude-modulated AC pulses. Phase duration usually ranges between 40 and 400 μsec. Maximal peak current amplitude reaches between 50 and 100 mA. In some units, pulse rate is variable, whereas in others it is fixed. Stimulators that are used for pain management provide phase charge limited to about 18 μC. They may or may not have automatic modulation of pulse characteristics and usually have no current modulation, so that pulses are delivered as a continuous train.

On the other hand, those TENS units that are used for neuromuscular training are commonly called NMES. Better designed units have a variable phase duration of between 20 and 300 μsec and maximum peak current amplitude of 100 to 150 mA. Their phase charge can reach 25 to 45 μC; thus, they are more powerful than the "pain" units. These stimulators are usually modulated to provide interrupted pulses, but the better NMES devices also offer continuous pulses.

The major and *direct* effect of all TENS units takes place at the cellular level. Indirectly, they also affect the biological system at the tissue, segmental, and systemic levels. The cellular level includes excitation of sensory, motor, and pain-conducting nerve fibers. Many of the pain management stimulators provide fairly comfortable sensory excitation but limited motor excitation. The neuromuscular TENS units are equally comfortable at lower level stimulation, but they also provide stronger motor excitation. The units that reach only 20 to 25 μC may not be sufficiently powerful for vigorous contraction of large muscle groups.[45]

### Interferential Current

Interferential current (IFC) has been available in Europe since the early 1950s. Popularity of IFC in the United States has become evident in the last 10 to 15 years, following a vigorous advertising campaign. The typical IFC stimulator utilizes two sinusoidal AC output circuits that differ somewhat in frequency. When these two outputs intersect, the frequency difference causes the sine waves' amplitudes to summate, resulting in the so-called "beat" or "envelope" (Figure 3–20). From an electrophysiological perspective, each "beat" represents a polyphasic pulse of varying amplitude, from which the term amplitude-modulated AC was derived.[89,91,114] The significance of such electronic explanation to the physiologic responses and clinical results is most likely negligible. The parameters that seem most relevant and meaningful to the clinicians and researchers are often not acknowledged by the manufacturers and users (Table 3–2). Current knowledge strongly suggests that IFC simply represents a different (and not the most effective) electronic approach to achieve the same basic physiologic and clinical responses achieved by other TENS devices.

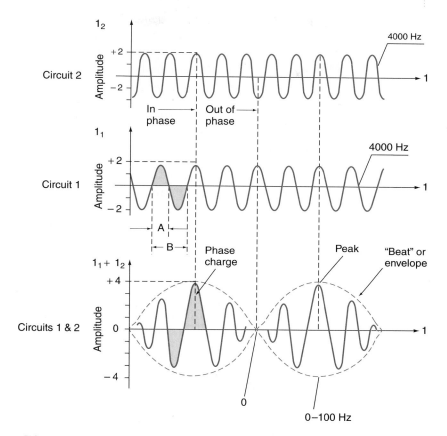

FIGURE 3–20. Generation of interference current. **(A)** Phase duration. **(B)** Pulse cycle duration. Note that, when two circuits are in phase, the amplitude of the envelope is twice as high, providing intensity adequate for excitation.

Objective testing of the many commercial claims used to promote IFC stimulation proved them false. Interferential stimulators do not offer less skin impedance,[120] cannot penetrate deeper, and are not more effective in pain or edema management compared with other TENS devices. In fact, several recent controlled clinical studies failed to show any advantage of true IFC over placebo IFC in reducing jaw pain or vertical jaw opening,[116] in enhancement of peripheral blood flow[117] in pain management of patients with osteoarthritis of the knee,[118] or swelling absorption following open reduction of ankle fractures.[119] Objective data also showed that interferential current is inferior to symmetric biphasic waveform when comfort of strong stimulation was the test objective during neuromotor excitation.[155–157] Recently, the conventional four-electrode (quadripolar) arrangement of the IFC stimulator was shown to be less effective in controlling urinary incontinence than the two-electrode (bipolar) system where the interference occurs inside the stimulator (premodulation).[82,83,85,158] These data not only further discredit the promotional claims for uniqueness of the true interferential concept,[159,160] but imply that setting up the patient with the premodulated (bipolar) IFC should allow one to direct the current much more precisely and effectively to the target area.[158,161] Furthermore, the premodulated IFC takes less time to set up and should become the preferred method in clinical application.

By adding a "vector" system, or claiming a three-dimensional current flow by adding a third output, a mathematical argument occurs.[89] To date, no in vitro, experimental, or clinical data have been found to support these concepts. In all likelihood, these electronic features have no clinical benefits. Interferential current, then, is simply a different electronic approach that achieves the same basic excitatory responses that monophasic and biphasic PC can achieve. Indeed, such an electronic approach is much less efficient and may be less effective than conventional TENS. Among the reasons for diminished efficiency are excessive (unnecessary) $RMS_A$ current as well as the false presumption that the quadripolar, four-electrode arrangement is better than the bipolar, two-electrode configuration.

The maximum $RMS_A$ current of most interferential stimulators can reach 50 to 90 mA. In comparison, most other biphasic PC units reach about 3 to 12 mA. Yet, biphasic pulses of appropriate phase parameters can provide all of the basic excitatory responses, much like IFC but with much less energy.[114]

The claim that automatic modulation of pulse frequency can facilitate superior clinical results has not been supported by the literature.[116–119] Because clinical testing has so far failed to support such a claim for conventional TENS,[123–129] it is unlikely that such support will be found when IFC is used.

From an electrophysiologic perspective, the main *direct* effect of interferential current occurs at the cellular level, much like other PC units. Indirect effects of IFC may involve the tissue, segmental, and systemic levels (see the previous section on TENS).

As clinical stimulators, IFCs in their present design are not versatile. They can elicit sensory stimulation, which should make them suitable to manage pain. They likewise should be effective, if used properly, in masking pain during mobilization or joint range exercises. If they offer interrupted mode—and only few IFC models offer it—they can be used for regaining muscle force, improving joint ROM, and reducing chronic edema, provided that the elicited motor stimulation and resultant muscle contraction are sufficiently strong.

The IFC stimulators are not suitable for curbing or absorbing acute edema because these protocols may depend on polarity.[3–5,8,9] The lack of polarity may also render them inadequate in the management of slow-to-heal wounds.[11,15,16,18,25–28] They may also be inadequate for use with small electrode sizes because the inherent high $RMS_A$ current may irritate or even burn the skin. (See the next section, Russian Current, for similar observations.)

Without available clinical data to support their superiority over conventional TENS, the IFC stimulators must be regarded as redundant. They are redundant because any electrophysiologic response or clinical results they provide can be achieved at least as effectively and usually at a lower cost by other conventional stimulators.

### Russian Current

The term *Russian current* applies to stimulators in which a continuous sine wave output of about 2500 to 5000 Hz is modulated to yield 50 bursts per second (bps). Each burst is actually a polyphasic pulse waveform.[89] From a strict electronic perspective, Russian current can be defined as time-modulated AC.[91,162] (The important characteristics of the Russian current are summarized in Table 3–2.) The generation of such current is illustrated in Figure 3–21. Contrary to promotional claims regarding the uniqueness and superiority of such a waveform for muscle activation,[155–157,163] electrophysiologic evaluation offers sound refutation of these claims. The reason for a carrier frequency of 2500 Hz is unlikely to be a unique medium-frequency effect on comfort of stimulation. Rather, and much as in the case of IFC, it was selected because the reciprocal of 2500-Hz frequency yields single pulse and phase durations of 400 and 200 μsec, respectively. Thus, the phase duration is narrowed to a range that correlates with relatively comfortable stimulation. Yet, in accordance with the strength–duration curve, one must compensate for the shorter duration by increasing the pulse amplitude in order to elicit excitation of peripheral nerves. The amount that the continuous sine wave peak current amplitude can be increased is limited, however, because under such conditions, $RMS_A$ current is always about 70 percent of the peak. To reduce the $RMS_A$ current output, the manufacturer of the Russian approach elected to time modulate the sine wave into 50 bps by creating an interburst interval of 10 msec (Figure 3–21). Such bursts reduce the $RMS_A$ current somewhat and allow peak current amplitude and thus phase charge to increase so that a very powerful motor stimulation can be achieved.

The inefficiency of such an approach is again related to an excessively high $RMS_A$ current (50 to 100 mA). Induced muscle contraction at 50 to 65 percent of maximal voluntary contraction (MVC) has been obtained with such current but also with symmetric bipha-

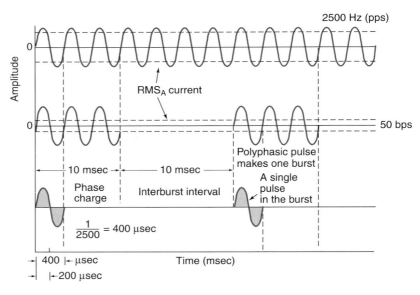

FIGURE 3–21. Russian current. Note that by providing interburst intervals, the $RMS_A$ current is reduced.

sic pulses.[34–37,39,44–46,49,161] The latter requires only about one tenth of the $RMS_A$ current of the former.[114] Other limitations of Russian current include less comfortable perception, fixed pulse rate in earlier units (that severely limited the number of clinical procedures it could offer), and a fixed phase duration (so that adjustments for individual patients' comfort are not possible).[163]

The main *direct* physiologic effect of Russian current is at the cellular level, but (indirectly) the tissue, segmental, and systemic levels may also be affected, as with other TENS stimulators.[31–49,114] Recent improvements in its design include variable phase duration and pulse rate, as well as options for both continuous and interrupted pulses.

Having a newer design of Russian current stimulator, the clinical uses may include management of pain, and, if used correctly, they can effectively mask pain during mobilization or joint ROM exercises. These applications depend on elicitation of sensory stimulation. The Russian current can be effectively used for regaining muscle force, improving joint ROM, and reducing chronic edema, provided that the elicited motor stimulation and resultant muscle contraction are sufficiently strong.

Like the IFC, Russian current stimulators are not suitable for curbing or absorbing of acute edema as these protocols may depend on polarity.[3–5,8,9] The lack of polarity may also render them inadequate in the management of slow-to-heal wounds.[11,15,16,18,25–28] They may likewise prove inadequate when small electrode sizes are used, because the inherent high $RMS_A$ current may irritate or even burn the skin. These latter problems have been minimized in the newer models by changing the stimulator design to function as a constant voltage generator. The observant reader probably noticed that the Russian current and IFC are different in electronic design, but in clinical efficacy and limitations they are very similar.

### "High-voltage" Stimulation

As in the case of all popular stimulators, many promotional claims regarding high voltage have caused tremendous confusion, misconception, and inappropriate use of these stimulators. A book by Alon and DeDomenico attempted to clarify many of these false claims.[153] This section reiterates the appropriate electrophysiologic and clinical attributes of the high-voltage units.

A high-voltage stimulator, also known as high-voltage pulsed current (HVPC), is *not* a galvanic stimulator. The typical twin-peak pulse of the HVPC stimulator has no known significant physiologic or clinical uniqueness, and a single peak is probably as effective for excitation as is the twin peak.[87,89,114] Thus, high-voltage units should simply be considered a monophasic pulsed current TENS, with very short phase duration (5 to 20 μsec) and very high peak current amplitude (2000 to 2500 mA). When phase duration is so short, peak current must be very high in order to excite peripheral nerves (S-D curve), and to generate such peak current, the voltage must also be high. This is the electrophysiologic reason for high voltage. The interpulse intervals are very long and constitute at least 99 percent of each second (Figure 3–22). Thus, $RMS_A$ current is very low, reaching a maximum of only 1.2 to 1.5 mA. The maximal phase charge is also limited to a maximum of 12 to14 μC. Such charge makes this group of stimulators one of the weakest on the market.

The combination of very short pulse duration and high peak current allows relatively comfortable stimulation. Furthermore, this combination provides an efficient means of exciting sensory, motor, and pain-conducting nerve fibers. Perceptual discrimination of those responses is relatively easy to achieve.[153]

The HVPC stimulators are TENS units. As such, they *directly* affect the cellular level. Indirect effects are at the tissue, segmental, and systemic levels, much as with other TENS units. Any attempt to attribute unique or different physiologic responses to the application of HVPC has yet to be demonstrated, and is unlikely to succeed. The usefulness of these stimulators is therefore in their clinical versatility and not because of physiologic uniqueness or superiority.

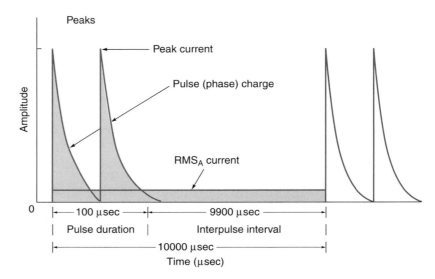

FIGURE 3–22. High-voltage monophasic pulsed current.

As clinical stimulators, HVPCs offer many clinical uses. Because these stimulators offer polarity (monophasic waveform), they may prove effective in curbing and absorbing acute edema,[1,3–5,8,9] as well as in the acceleration of dermal and subdermal tissue regeneration.[15,18,19,25–28,164] Their characteristics are adequate for pain management.[154,165,166–168] Recent models of the HVPC have the option of interrupted pulses mode, and thus management of disuse atrophy and motor control[169–172] and chronic edema[7,10] are claimed to be achieved by those stimulators.

Clinical versatility does not mean that the HVPC stimulators are without limitations. Indeed, they are not optimally designed. They are less than adequate for stimulation of large muscle groups,[173,174] and they are not suitable for stimulation of denervated muscles or in iontophoresis.[153] Their monophasic waveform and phase/pulse parameters make them less comfortable than time-modulated AC (Russian), amplitude-modulated AC (IFC), or symmetric biphasic PC.[94,120,156,157]

### Subliminal Stimulation

Subliminal or subsensory TES devices are a somewhat recent class of transcutaneous PC stimulators. Although specifications on these stimulators are not readily available through the manufacturers, Table 3–3 provides their general description. The distinction of this class of stimulators is their delivery of low peak and $RMS_A$ current that is designed not to cause peripheral nerve excitation, thus the term **subliminal** or **nonperceived stimulation.**

## TABLE 3–3.   CHARACTERISTICS OF THE SUBLIMINAL STIMULATORS

| Source | Characteristics |
| --- | --- |
| Waveform | From reversing DC to monophasic |
| Mode | Continuous |
| Phase duration[a] | Inverse of frequency (1.5–500 msec) |
| Phase charge (maximum)[b] | 0.9–300 μC |
| Pulse frequency | 0.3–320 pps (adjustable) |
| Polarity | Yes |
| Total current | 25–600 μA (adjustable) |
| Channels | One or two |

[a] Shorter duration, higher frequency.
[b] Depends on frequency: lower frequency, higher charge.
(Modified from Alon G: Electro-orthopedics: A review of present electrophysiologic responses and clinical efficiacy of transcutaneous stimulation. Adv Sports Med Fitness 2:295, 1989)

Several hypotheses have been offered in the attempt to describe the physiologic responses to subliminal stimulation. Manufacturers have claimed that such a device can detect abnormal distribution of the body's bioelectrical conductivity and that the stimulation can reestablish healthy conductive properties. The stimulation serves as a corrective measure at the cellular level, to promote healing of various cells and tissues with dysfunction. This correction arrests the progression of pathologic processes. Another hypothesis offered is that the servo-mechanisms built into the devices augment athletic performance by supplementing the electrical energy required for optimal muscle contraction.[175–177] Supportive data of claims and hypotheses for subliminal stimulation are scarce at best.[178] Promoters of subliminal stimulators frequently "borrow" from studies using conventional PC devices and use such data to propose that the subliminal stimulation resolves abnormal electrical steady state of various cells and promotes cell metabolism, adenosine triphosphate (ATP) synthesis, calcium ion concentration, and serotonergic response.[165,179–180]

Because subliminal stimulation is below sensory perception, controlled testing against a placebo seems mandatory. In one study, subjects were asked to state the weight that they could lift before and after receiving six 30-minute subliminal stimulation treatments. This study, however, was an uncontrolled and nonparametric approach to measure effects of subliminal stimulation.[181] Several independent, double-blind studies in which subliminal stimulation was compared with placebo stimulation in the management of delayed-onset muscle soreness (DOMS), have all resulted is statistically equal measures of muscle force, pain-free ROM, and postexercise soreness.[182–185] Other controlled animal and clinical trials have been reported in refereed journals. Whether wound healing,[11,186,187] elbow tendinitis,[188] or coracoacromial pain,[189] none have shown better than placebo results. Indeed, the only published, prospective, double-blind clinical study to show better than placebo effect on knee joint stiffness required an average of 9 hours of daily (nightly) stimulation over 4 consecutive weeks.[190] Future studies may prove that subliminal stimulation requires many hours of stimulation, a reasonable proposal for a home program.

### *Transcranial Electrical Stimulation*

The application of surface electrodes on two opposing sides of the head is one approach to transcranial electrical stimulation (TCES) that begins to show potential in the management of selected clinical conditions. To date, two distinctly different groups of stimulators have been used as TCES. One approach is to generate monophasic pulsed current at 15,000 Hz, which is then time modulated to 15 bursts (Figure 3–23). The polarity may or may not be reversed automatically every 5 sec. The second approach is to generate a continuous AC (sine or square waves) at frequencies ranging from 0.1 to 2000 Hz. (See Figure 3–5.) In most clinical applications, the frequency has been set at either 5 or 100 Hz. Common to both type of TCES

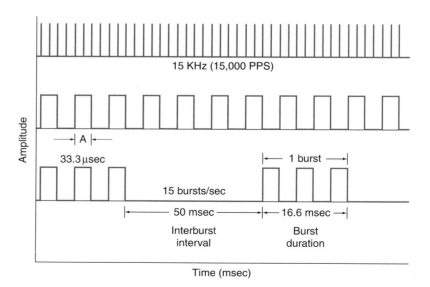

FIGURE 3–23. Phase duration (msec).

stimulators is the restriction that peak current must not exceed 4 mA. Higher peak amplitudes may cause seizures,[191] and thus all previously discussed TENS devices must not be used transcranially.

Transcranial stimulation has at least two possible ways to affect the central nervous system (CNS). One mode is the direct effect whereby the electrical current passes directly through the CNS. Dymond and Coger[192] stimulated patients transcranially with a monophasic pulsed current at 100 pps and peak current up to 1.5 mA. They recorded directly from hippocampal sites and measured potential differences in the range of 0.5 to 27 millivolts (mV). This range amounted to about 5 percent of the voltages applied transcranially. Other investigators have estimated that 45 percent of transcranially applied current passes directly through brain tissue.[193] These currents may modulate neural activity in the various centers in which their density is sufficient to alter nerve excitation and may affect the quantities of neurotransmitters, neuromodulators, and/or neurohormones.[103,104,106,194]

The second mode of action is indirect. Placement of the electrodes over the temple area may potentially affect the trigeminal, facial, and possibly the vagus and glossopharyngeal nerves whose cell bodies are located throughout the brain stem. Synaptic connections from there to other regions may modulate neural transmission through ortho- and antidromic modulation of local excitatory responses.[103] The influence on neuromodulators and neurohormones may be similar to that obtained by the direct effect.[104,111] Indeed, the direct and indirect effects of TCES need not be mutually exclusive, and may have simultaneous effects under appropriate stimulation conditions.

The clinical benefits of TCES cover a wide spectrum. Among the more successful reports are the management of migraine and tension headaches, provided that the patients perceived the electrical stimulation.[195,196] Other investigators report control of anxiety and insomnia, but not depression,[197] improvement of the profile of mood state in patients who survived head injury,[104,109] and management of children with cerebral palsy and delayed motor development.[107,108,110,198] A significant improvement was also reported in the revised Beta Examination intelligence quotient test of subjects who sustained brain dysfunction associated with addiction to alcohol or polydrugs,[195–202] and job-related stress.[203,204]

Acceptance of TCES by the mainstream medical community has not yet occurred. There is a clear need to explore the adequate stimulation characteristics, electrode placement, treatment time, and the clinical conditions that may benefit from this relatively new intervention. These issues are likely to be investigated in the next few years, as this form of electrotherapy could become an attractive alternative to other interventions.

# FUNDAMENTAL PHYSIOLOGIC RESPONSES

One of the most difficult tasks facing the clinician has been to organize, comprehend, and interpret electrophysiologic information into a functional, clinically practical, and integrated data base. Having no such system, much of the physiologic data cannot be systematically related to the pathologic processes that electrical stimulation may be capable of modifying. The purpose of this section is to offer a new framework that organizes the fundamental physiologic responses elicited by transcutaneous stimulation. Such clinically oriented organization can then be used to examine the physiologic correlates of either pulsed or nonpulsed currents and will enable the clinician to better integrate such knowledge with the clinical signs and symptoms that electrical stimulation attempts to resolve.

## Biological Effects

The flow of electrical current through a biological conductive medium results in three basic effects. These direct effects may be recognized as electrochemical, electrophysical, and electrothermal. Theoretically, every time electrical current flows through the body, all three effects occur. The magnitude of these effects can be identified and measured with appropriate equipment at the cellular level. Recognizing which of the three effects dominates during the stimulation is a prerequisite for the understanding of the physiologic responses to electrical stimulation.

### Electrochemical Effects

Electrochemical effects are recognized when the conducted current causes formation of new chemical compounds. The steady state of existing chemical compounds is being altered by the current flow, a phenomenon most recognized with the application of DC stimulation. The unidirectional flow of DC redistributes sodium and chlorine to form a new chemical compound in the tissue under the electrodes. These changes at the tissue level (see next section) can be summarized as follows:

$$2Na + 2H_2O \rightarrow 2NaOH + H_2 \uparrow (alkaline)$$
$$2Cl_2 + 2H_2O \rightarrow 4\,HCl + O_2 \uparrow (acid)$$

The alkaline and acid formation occurs under the negative and positive electrodes, respectively.[96] The liberation of hydrogen and oxygen ions may be involved in further chemical reactions, particularly at the cellular or even molecular level.

As long as these DC-induced chemical reactions are not excessive, the normal response of the intact body is to increase local blood flow in order to restore the normal pH of the tissue. Chemical changes that exceed the body's ability to reverse them and reestablish the steady state will result in blistering or even chemical burns of the stimulated tissue. Decreasing current amplitude, shortening treatment time, or reversing polarity every few seconds or minutes minimizes these hazards.[97]

Practical elimination of chemical change at the *tissue level* can be obtained if a very short-duration, pulsed rather than direct current is used. Absence of measurable chemical changes at the tissue level does not indicate that electrochemical changes do not take place at the cellular level. Indeed, the origin of the electrolytic process is in each cell. The changes, however, are so minute and transient that the clinical significance of such changes has only recently appeared in the literature. Specifically, it has been proposed that the electrochemical reaction occurs between the mitochondrial membrane-bound $H^+$ adenosine triphosphatase (ATPase) and adenosine diphosphate (ADP), which leads to the formation of ATP. Synthesis of DNA by electrical current has also been demonstrated at the molecular level, but the associated chemical reaction has not been elucidated.[179] Slowdown of microvessel leakage[8,9,205] and facilitation of enzymatic activity (such as citrate synthase, 3-hydroxyacyl-CoA dehydrogenase, cytochrome-c oxidase, and ATPase) has likewise been reported.[202–211] Whether these cellular responses are electrochemically mediated is not clear at the present time.

Two of Faraday's laws can be used to quantify the amount of chemical changes during an electrolytic reaction. One law indicates that the amount of chemical reaction is directly proportional to the quantity of electricity passing through the electrolytic solution. Quantities of the electrical energy are obtained by calculating the phase charge (Q), $RMS_A$ current, or both. The charge delivered by a clinical DC stimulator may reach 5000 to 60,000 $\mu$C. Because current equals coulombs/sec (the rate of flow of charges), this charge is equivalent to 5 to 60 mA of $RMS_A$ current. However, clinical monophasic PC stimulators usually reach only 12 to 20 $\mu$C and 1.5 to 2 mA of $RMS_A$ current. These amounts of $RMS_A$ current can explain why burns of the tissue can result from careless application of DC, whereas the chemical effects of a PC as used clinically do not present a known harmful chemical effect.

Faraday's second law states that the amount of various electrolytic substances liberated by a given amount of charge per phase is directly proportional to their chemical equivalent weights. Thus, at the cellular level, the electrolysis is likely to affect the calcium ions more than it affects the potassium or sodium ions. Calcium is highly associated with the cellular process of muscle contraction and relaxation as well as with the formation and remodeling of connective and osseous tissues.[212–217] In contrast to calcium, the lighter equivalent weighted potassium, chlorine, and sodium are all associated with the process of nerve excitation. The fact that one can observe nerve excitation long before the electrolytic effects on bone, connective tissue, or muscle may be related to the electrolytic quantities and concentration that are required to cause these different physiologic changes. To achieve the calcium-dependent electrophysiologic effects, a longer treatment time of several hours daily is probably indicated. In fact, the electrical effect on calcium, potassium, sodium, and other ions' concentration and their dynamics may not be electrochemical but rather electrophysical.

### Electrophysical Effects

Unlike the electrochemical effects, the electrophysical effects do not cause change in the molecular binding of ions. Rather, the electrical charge causes ionic movement, whether they are electrolytes or nondissociated molecules such as proteins or lipoproteins. The electrophysical effect has also been termed electrokinetic effect. The best-known physiologic consequences of such ionic movement include the excitation of peripheral nerves, where in the presence of adequate phase charge, the sodium and potassium ions move across the cell membrane. Such direct cellular effects may lead to many different indirect responses, including the contractions of skeletal or smooth muscles, activation of endogenous analgesic mechanisms, and various vascular responses, all of which are discussed in other chapters of this text.

Other direct cellular effects are associated with the electrophysical influence on ions and may not depend on nerve excitation. Electrolytes including calcium and magnesium and other ions such as free amino acids and proteins are also forced to move in the presence of electromotive force provided by the stimulator.[9] Such movement may lead to increase or decrease in ionic concentration and trigger a host of subsequent indirect physiologic responses.[3–6,8,11–29,190] In a broad sense, many of the direct effects that occur at the cellular level can be classified as excitatory and nonexcitatory responses.

### Electrothermal Effect

The mobility of charged particles in a conductive medium causes microvibration of these particles. This vibration and the associated frictional forces leads to the production of heat.[162] The amount of electrical-to-heat conversion is described by Joule's law: The amount of heat production (H) is proportional to the square of the $RMS_A$ current ($I^2$), the impedance (R), and the time (t) for which the current flows (ie, treatment time). The formula is expressed by the equation:

$$H = 0.24I^2Rt$$

The heat production is given in gram-calories. From a clinical perspective, high $RMS_A$ current, high skin impedance, and prolonged treatment time may all lead to a measurable thermal effect. If DC stimulation is used, skin impedance is usually very high, so both the amplitude and treatment time must be minimized to avoid excessive thermal effect. If a continuous AC is used, skin impedance decreases as frequency increases. As long as the $RMS_A$ current amplitude is low (up to a few milliamps), the thermal effect will decrease as frequency increases because the impedance decreases. However, with higher frequency, phase and pulse duration automatically become shorter, and there is usually a need to increase the AC current amplitude if nerve excitation is the stimulation objective[86,87,89,101,153]; consequently, an increase in thermal effect can be calculated. A pulsed current having a very short phase duration (5 to 300 µsec) and a pulse rate of up to 100 to 200 pps usually results in a much smaller $RMS_A$ current compared to AC. As a result, the thermal effect of pulsed current is usually dramatically lower than that provided by an AC stimulator.[153] Finally, it must be emphasized that the aforementioned differences in thermal effects between DC, AC, and PC stimulators are more theoretical than practical, because all three stimulator categories cause minimal heat production that may not be measured at the tissue level[153,162] and may not have known physiologic consequences even at the cellular level.

## Physiologic Model

Because electrical current is conducted through a conductive biologic medium, alteration in physiologic processes can occur at various levels of the total system. Functionally, four levels can be recognized: cellular, tissue, segmental, and systemic.

At each level, many different processes can be modified by the stimulation, which in turn may enhance or suppress the respective physiologic activities. Furthermore, the effect of the stimulation can be direct, indirect, or both.

The main effects of the stimulation at each of the four levels are listed in the following outline (D = direct; IND = indirect; UNKN = unknown):

1. Cellular level
   a. Excitation of peripheral nerves (D).
   b. Changes of membrane permeability of *none,* or less excitatory cells (calcium channels) (D or IND).
   c. Modification of fibroblast and fibroclast formation (D or IND).

    d. Modification of osteoblast and osteoclast formation (D or IND).

    e. Modification of microcirculation: arterial, venous, and lymphatic (capillary flow) (UNKN).

    f. Changes of protein and blood-cell concentration (UNKN).

    g. Alteration of enzymatic activity (D or IND).

    h. Enhancement of protein synthesis (D).

    i. Modification of mitochondrial size and concentration (D or IND).

2. Tissue level

    a. Skeletal muscle contraction and its effects on muscle force, contraction speed, reaction time, and fatigability (IND). (*Note:* For denervated muscle, the effect is direct.)

    b. Smooth muscle contraction or relaxation and its effect on arterial and venous blood flow (IND).

    c. Tissue regeneration, including bone, ligament, connective, and dermal tissues (D or IND).

    d. Tissue remodeling, including softening, stretching, decreasing viscosity, and fluid absorption from joint cavities and interstitial spaces (D or IND).

    e. Changes in tissue thermal and chemical balance (D or IND).

3. Segmental level

    a. Muscle group contraction and its effect on joint mobility and synergistic muscle activity (IND).

    b. Muscle pumping action effects on the lymphatic drainage, venous flow, and arterial blood flow of large circulatory and lymphatic vessels (macrocirculation) (IND).

    c. Alteration of lymphatic drainage and arterial blood flow not associated with skeletal muscle contraction (IND).

4. Systemic level

    a. Analgesic effects associated with endogenous polypeptides, such as beta-endorphins, dopamines, and dynorphins (IND).

    b. Analgesic effects associated with neurotransmitters, such as serotonin, enkephalins, and substance P (IND).

    c. Circulatory effects associated with polypeptides, such as vasoactive intestinal polypeptide (VIP) or calcitonin gene-related peptide (CGRP) (IND).

    d. Modulation of internal organ activity, such as kidney and heart functions (IND).

Regardless of the form of electrical current used, there is always a direct effect, usually electrochemical or electrophysical, or both, at the cellular level under the stimulating electrodes. This direct effect can also prevail at the tissue level if a DC or a PC having a very long phase duration (50 to 300 msec) and monophasic waveform are used. Provided that the pulse rate is very high (several hundred to several thousand pulses), even pulses of very short duration can induce direct tissue response, but such clinical stimulators are not commonly available. Direct effects at the tissue level (mostly electrophysical and possibly electrothermal) may also occur with a symmetric biphasic PC, time- or amplitude-modulated AC, or continuous AC, if the $RMS_A$ current per unit area (current density, phase charge density, or both) is excessively high.

Indirect effects of current flow are expected at all four levels. Indirect alterations of cellular, tissue, segmental, and systemic functions are defined as those physiologic reactions or responses that are triggered by the direct effects. They may occur at or remote from the actual area where the current flows.

The combination of direct and indirect effects results in physiologic responses to the application of surface stimulation. Depending on the electrical stimulation procedure, the relevant responses should be recognized and must be specified as the **physiologic targets** of the stimulation. Within the limits of current knowledge, the achievement of clinical results seems to be highly dependent on the establishment of appropriate physiologic responses.

The use of the aforementioned model can be demonstrated in the following example: When electrical stimulation is used to suppress pain, the direct effect occurs at the cellular level, where PC or AC currents cause excitation of peripheral nerve cells. The **indirect physiologic effects** predominate at the systemic or segmental levels, or both, as indicated by the release of endogenous analgesic substances, such as endorphins, enkephalins, serotonin, and the suppression of substance P. The physiologic target of the stimulation is therefore non-noxious sensory (or sometimes motor or painful) excitation **(direct effect),** and the clinical objective is a temporary reduction of pain perception.[129–135,218]

Another example is related to the use of stimulation to retard muscle atrophy associated with disuse, and to enhance a muscle's capacity to develop contractile force. Direct effect is obtained at the cellular level by the excitation of peripheral nerves. Unlike the previous example, however, where predominantly sensory fibers were excited, the motor fibers are excited as well. The indirect physiologic effect occurs at both tissue and segmental levels. The contraction of skeletal muscle fibers represents the tissue level. If sufficient numbers of motor units are activated, the whole muscle or muscle group will contract. This activity may be coupled with movement at the joint. If few muscle groups are stimulated, few segments are affected simultaneously. Additionally, indirect physiologic responses resulting from muscle contraction include cellular-level modification of capillary blood flow and enhancement of enzymatic activity.[43,206–211] Indirect segmental response includes large-vessel blood flow associated with the pumping action of the muscles.[10,63] The physiologic target is motor stimulation, and the clinical objective can be muscle force gain.[43–62]

A direct physiologic effect that simultaneously involves both cellular and tissue levels is usually associated with a DC stimulation. The unidirectional, continuous current flow alters the pH of the cells and tissue under the electrodes. The indirect physiologic response is vasodilation of arterial capillaries (cellular) and small arteries (tissue) in an attempt to restore the steady-state pH and temperature of the affected tissue.[136,137]

The foregoing discussion and examples may suffice to draw a conclusion. Knowledge of the electrical current and its waveform and characteristics, recognition of its direct and indirect effects, and understanding of the physiologic levels at which these effects take place can provide a systematic, clinically oriented framework. This model can then be used to select the treatment method needed to obtain the best clinical results. Furthermore, the model may serve to improve communication among the various professionals and eliminate the use of undefined, ambiguous terminology (eg, that TENS is used to "improve circulation," "heal tissue," or "balance the body's energy").

## Physiologic Correlates of Electrical Stimulation

Generally stated, transcutaneous stimulation can induce *direct* physiologic responses in both the excitatory and the nonexcitatory systems. A short summary of those responses follows.

### Nonexcitatory Responses

All living cells depend in part on various magnitudes of internally generated electrical potentials. The source of these potentials seems to be associated with the concentration gradient of ions across the cell membrane.[214,215,219] Changes in the concentration gradient may be linked with the opening of ion channels and lead to enhancement of DNA and protein synthesis.[179,180] One may hypothesize that such protein synthesis and the resultant enhanced formation of collagen fiber is clinically significant. Indeed, clinical evidence that resuscitation of dermal and subdermal connective tissues can be accelerated by externally applied electrical current is growing continuously.[11,15–28] Similarly, bone tissue (and possibly ligaments and cartilage) and scar tissue can also be remodeled if appropriate quantities of electrical energy are delivered at the right timing of the healing process.[22,98–100,165]

The exact mechanism by which transcutaneous stimulation influences the nonexcitatory cells in pathology and disease of human subjects is very complex and, at present, has not been adequately elucidated. First, whether the process is electrochemical, electrophysical, or both is not clear and is rarely identified in the literature. Second, different cells at different states (ie, pathologic or healthy) seem to respond differently to electrical energy. Proteins are an example of charged ions that, when abnormally present in the interstitial spaces or joint cavities, may be displaced into the lymphatic capillaries.[6,9] On the other hand, the proteins that are the building blocks of collagenous fibrous tissues seem to be synthesized rather than displaced by the stimulation.[14–18,24–28,98,165,179] Other ions (such as calcium, magnesium, potassium, and sodium) play a major role in the function of nonexcitatory cells. The mobility and concentration of these ions may also be modified in part by externally induced electrical energy. Consequently, cellular metabolism and nutrition may be enhanced.[100,219]

Hypothetically, any current flow through a conductive medium should have some *direct* influence on nonexcitatory cells. If the current source is DC, then a direct effect on the *tissue* level should also be realized, as pH and temperature changes can occur.[97,136,137] Modern pulsed currents and alternating currents *directly* affect only the cells.[89,220] The *indirect* effect of both current sources is typically associated with circulatory response. Pulsed current's effect on cell metabolism may lead to increased microcirculation, including arterial, venous, and lymphatic capillary exchange.[6,8,9] Experimental evidence supporting these effects on human subjects is limited,[67–70] and the most appropriate pulse characteristics and treatment procedures to achieve effective nonexcitatory cell response have not been determined. The reader, however, must realize that whether electrical stimulation is used for pain management, muscle force gain, inflammation control, or venous insufficiency, nonexcitatory cells and excitatory cells are both affected by the current flow.

### Excitatory Responses

Excitation of peripheral nerves by transcutaneous stimulation is a well-established phenomenon. Stimulation directly affects the nerve cells.[86,87,92,115,121,221] Strength–duration (S-D) curves have been established for each of the three main groups of fibers, including those that transmit tactile, proprioception, and pressure stimuli; motor impulses; and painful or noxious stimuli.[87,95,114,174,221,222] A typical response of these three excitatory categories is illustrated in Figure 3–24.

The oversimplified concept that larger-diameter nerve fibers are

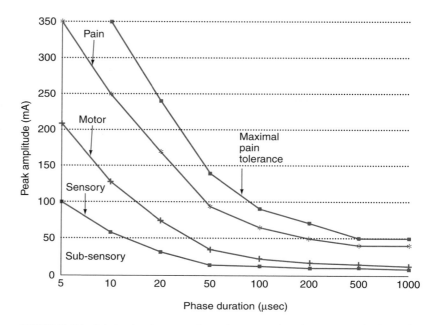

FIGURE 3–24. Relationship between phase duration and peak current amplitude as determinants of peripheral nerve excitation (so-called S-D curve). Note the sequential excitation irrespective of phase duration. Subsensory indicates that duration–amplitude combination is inconsequential.

excited before smaller-diameter nerve fibers are excited is based on the erroneous assumption that all nerve fibers are located at the same distance from the stimulating electrodes.[223] In reality, the exact diameter–distance combination relative to the stimulating electrode is rarely known, and thus the small or medium-sized nerve fibers are many times excited before large fibers. In fact, unlike the volitional contraction recruitment order of motor nerves from small to large, the electrically elicited excitation is probably random and includes a combination of large, small, and medium nerve fibers.[223,224]

A clinical, functional interpretation of these excitatory responses (and related literature) may warrant the following observations:

1. Sensory, motor, and painful stimulation are perceived as the three basic excitatory responses to transcutaneous stimulation.
2. Excitation proceeds in the order of sensory stimulation, motor stimulation, and painful stimulation. This order prevails regardless of phase duration, waveform, pulse rate, or electrode size, as long as all three nerve groups are at approximately the same distance from the stimulating electrode.[87,95,114,174,221–223]

3. Perceptual discrimination among the three responses is more easily achieved if pulse duration is set in the range of 20 to 200 μsec.[221] Electrode size also affects this perceptual discrimination.[95,174,222]

4. If optimal discriminatory perception or electronic efficiency are not considered, a simple physiologic statement can be made that any combination of phase duration (in microseconds or milliseconds) and amplitude (in milliamperes) can be used to achieve the excitation. Such duration–intensity (amplitude) combination in effect represents generation of sufficient phase charge to discharge the nerve.[86,87,114,121] Once excited, the nerve impulses will propagate and will provide the indirect physiologic responses.

5. Variations of pulse rate alter the frequency of firing of the excited nerves but do not alter the sequence of the three excitatory responses. Different firing rates affect some of the indirect physiologic responses; most notably the types of muscle contraction (twitch[38,40–42] or tetanic[32–37,39]), fatigability,[225–227] and (possibly) the endogenous analgesic mechanism.[123,129,132]

Whereas the direct excitatory effect of PC and AC is well understood and the limits are clearly drawn, the indirect effects are numerous, less well defined, and only partially established. The scope of indirect physiologic responses may be realized by recognizing that all body systems can be influenced by the afferent and efferent neurologic pathways. Thus, cardiac,[228–231] digestive,[232–233] endocrine,[234–235] limbic,[104,106] neuromuscular,[32–62] respiratory,[235–237] skeletal,[71–76] and vascular[7,10,63–70,238–240] functions can all be indirectly affected by PC and AC stimulation. Many of these indirect effects are discussed in the remaining chapters of this text, although at present many others have not been established.

The complexity of indirect physiologic responses is further magnified by their simultaneous interaction. For example, motor excitation causes muscle contraction, which may increase the muscle force and at the same time increase interstitial pressure and promote lymphatic and venous blood flow. Such motor excitation also results in production of waste products, and the lactic acid formation provides a chemical signal to increase blood flow so the waste products can be removed.[206,237–242] The complexity is extended further by the observation that nonpathologic and pathologic conditions respond differently to electrical stimulation. A case in point is the augmentation of peripheral blood flow by sensory stimulation repeatedly reported in clinical studies[14,68–70,228–231] and the failure to show such increase in healthy subjects.[159,160,238–239,241–242] Likewise, the results with twitch contractions for patients with compromised microcirculation[12,13,29] are contrasted with reduced peripheral blood flow in healthy volunteers.[240]

Clinically, the resolution of the complex pathologic processes may greatly depend on the use of proper stimulation procedures and clinical monitoring of the physiologic responses to the stimulation. The question is, how can this be done practically in the clinic?

Establishing specific values of current amplitude, in milliamperes or volts, for each clinical problem is unlikely to yield appropriate physiologic responses. Differences in body parts and pathologies, continuous changes in tissue conductivity, intersubject variations, and differences in stimulators and electrode size are just some of the uncontrolled variables that all but prevent the clinician from selecting standard machine settings based on measured current amplitude. A much better approach to providing standardized and systematic treatment techniques is offered on the basis of the direct excitatory responses perceived by the patient.

As discussed earlier, the three categories of perceived excitation are sensory, motor, and painful stimulation. Each of the three can be established despite the aforementioned uncontrolled variables. Once the prescribed excitatory level is achieved, the clinician can estimate (or measure, if possible) some of the indirect physiologic responses. For example, when motor excitation is indicated, the physical therapist can estimate both the vigor of muscle contraction and muscle fatigue. Such estimations should help to promote faster force development while eliminating muscle soreness. Similarly, neurovascular vasoconstriction usually requires only minimal sensory excitation. By setting current amplitude to such an excitatory level, the physical therapist can then assess skin temperature and color and can ascertain the changes of the indirect physiologic responses. Having established the resultant physiologic targets of the stimulation, clinical results can be predicted with much greater certainty.

The presented physiologic model is sufficiently functional to include most of the clinical situations but nevertheless has some limitations. The model does not include one additional dimension—the subliminal, nonperceived stimulation. Nonperceived stimulation is excluded because most clinical problems seem to respond better to perceived excitation. Another difficulty may arise when stimulation is provided to patients with sensory loss, as sensory excitation may not be perceived by the subject. The astute physical therapist, however, can find several procedures that will overcome such difficulties.

In summary, physiologic responses to DC, PC, and AC occur at four levels of the biologic system (cellular, tissue, segmental, and systemic). The effects can be direct or indirect, and they may involve simple, well-established physiologic responses as well as a very complex, largely unknown chain of interactive physiologic process. In daily practice, the clinician must recognize the currently known responses, establish the appropriate treatment procedure, and set the stimulation characteristics to achieve the sensory, motor, or painful perception indicated by treatment goals. Adequate excitatory responses, and evaluation of clinically measurable indirect responses, are likely to provide the physical therapist with systematic, reproducible, and clinically successful utilization of electrical stimulation.

### Relevant Laws and Calculation

There are many laws and equations associated with both the electrical and physiologic aspects of electrotherapy. Knowledge of some of them may help the clinician to better understand the interrelationships among the various stimulation characteristics and their influence on the clinical application of electrotherapy.

The law of excitation expresses the interaction of voltage, current, charge, and energy required to excite peripheral nerves.[87] Two of these characteristics, phase charge and $RMS_A$ current, may have immediate clinical relevance. Skin impedance is an additional factor of clinical concern. *Phase charge* is a term with which most clinicians are not familiar, yet it is the phase charge that determines whether or not a nerve will be excited.[114,115] Phase charge is a term that defines the quantity of electricity that affects the biological system with each phase of each pulse. Insufficient charge will fail to excite the nerve, whereas excessive charge may harm the tissue.[243]

### Phase Charge

For a constant-current stimulator having a monophasic square-wave pulse (Figure 3–25), phase charge (q) is represented by the area under the curve and is expressed as the product of phase duration (t) and peak current amplitude (I).

$$q = I \times t \qquad (1)$$

A symmetric biphasic square-wave pulse having two equal phases can be expressed as

$$q = 2 (I \times t) \qquad (2)$$

A symmetric sine-wave pulse (Figure 3–25) is expressed as

$$I (t) = I \sin \varpi T \qquad (3)$$

where

$$I(t) = \text{current amplitude in amperes as a function}$$
$$\text{of time (t) in seconds}$$
$$I = \text{peak current amplitude (amperes)}$$

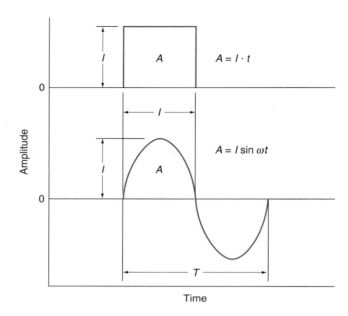

FIGURE 3–25. Monophasic square wave and symmetric biphasic sine wave.

$\varpi$ = angular velocity (radians/sec)
T = period of one cycle (sec)

Angular velocity ($\varpi$) is related to the frequency (f) and the period (T) by

$$f = \varpi/2\pi \text{ and } T = 2\pi/\varpi \text{ or } T/2 = \pi/\varpi \qquad (4)$$

One phase duration is defined by the interval between t = 0 and t. Because t = T/2 and T/2 = $\pi/\varpi$, each phase charge (q) is given by the integral over this time interval $t_0$ and t, yielding

$$q = I\,\varpi\,(\cos 0 - \cos \pi/\varpi) = 2I/\varpi \qquad (5)$$

Because $\varpi = 2\pi f$, the phase charge equation can be written as

$$q = I/\pi f \qquad (6)$$

Equations 1 and 6 are used to calculate the phase charge of a monophasic pulse and a burst modulated AC sine wave, respectively. Assuming that peak current amplitude I = 200 mA and that phase duration t = $200 \times 10^{-3}$ msec (200 $\mu$sec), then

1. Monophasic square pulse:

$$q = I \times t = 200 \times 10^{-3} \times 200 = 40\ \mu C$$

2. One phase of a 2500-Hz burst-modulated AC sine wave (eg, of the Russian current):

$$q = \frac{I}{\pi f} = \frac{200 \times 10^{-3}}{3.14 \times 2500} = \frac{200 \times 10^{-3}}{7.850 \times 10^{-3}} = 25.4 \times 10^{-6} = 25.4 \ \mu C$$

The following conclusions can be drawn:

1. The charge delivered by a square wave is significantly greater than that of the sine wave.
2. Comparison of a symmetric biphasic square-wave pulse with a symmetric biphasic sine wave is accomplished by doubling the charge delivered by one phase. In the example, the results are 80 versus 50.8 $\mu C$ for the square and sine waves, respectively.
3. The calculations demonstrate that for equal phase durations, one needs significantly less amplitude to excite the nerve with square waves than with sine waves. Thus, sine wave is a less efficient waveform for excitation.
4. Any change in phase duration must require a concomitant adjustment of pulse amplitude in order to provide the same charge.

Stimulators known as HVPC stimulators are designed as constant-voltage, rather than constant-current, stimulators. To calculate phase charge for this monophasic, twin-peak pulse, the following equation is used:

$$q = cv \tag{7}$$

where

$$C = \text{capacitance of output capacitors } (\mu F)$$
$$V = \text{voltage amplitude (volts)}$$

Typically, there are two output capacitors, one ($q_1$) of 0.010 $\mu F$ and a second ($q_2$) of 0.015 $\mu F$, representing the first and second peaks of the pulse, respectively. Assuming the maximal voltage output V = 500 volts, the phase charge of the first spike is

$$q_1 = 0.010 \times 10^{-6} \times 500 = 5 \times 10^{-6} = 5 \ \mu C$$

The phase charge of the second spike is

$$q_2 = 0.015 \times 10^{-6} \times 500 = 7.5 \times 10^{-6} = 7.5 \ \mu C$$

Summing the two peaks of the pulse:

$$q_p = q_1 + q_2 = 5 \ \mu C + 7.5 \ \mu C = 12.5 \ \mu C$$

Additional observations can now be made regarding the clinical aspects of phase charge:

1. Compared with other TENS units, which can deliver 20 to 40 μC of charge per phase, the presently available HVPC stimulators may only reach 12.5 μC. Yet, the HVPC stimulators can effectively cause excitation of sensory, motor, and pain-conducting fibers. The reason for this effectiveness is explained by the law of excitation, which states that at shorter phase durations, less charge is needed to cause threshold excitation.[41,132]

2. Despite being called high voltage, these stimulators are not powerful. Indeed, one of their deficiencies is phase charge insufficient to strongly activate large muscle groups, such as the quadriceps femoris muscle.[108,111]

3. Whether one uses high voltage or low voltage; or whether the pulse is monophasic, biphasic, or AC time- or amplitude-modulated makes no difference. As long as there is sufficient phase charge for a given phase duration, excitation of the nerve will occur. This statement holds true whether the charge is negative or positive.[56,139,142]

### RMS$_A$ Current Determination

RMS$_A$ current can be defined as the absolute value sum of all phase charges averaged over one second (coulombs/sec). Because most modern clinical stimulators deliver pulsed currents, peak current amplitude is always significantly higher than is RMS$_A$ current. Determination of the RMS$_A$ current of a pulsed-current stimulator can be obtained using the following equation:

$$I_{RMS_A} = q/t \qquad (8)$$

where

$$q = \text{phase charge (C), and}$$
$$t = \text{pulse (period) duration (sec)}$$

Using the relationships $f = 1/t$, equation (8) can be written as

$$I_{RMS_A} = q \times f \qquad (9)$$

where

$$f = \text{frequency of applied current (Hz)}$$

Knowing the waveform and the number of pulses per second, one can calculate the RMS$_A$ current. For example, having a phase charge $q = 20$ μC, the following calculations are made for monophasic and biphasic pulses and burst modulated AC:

1. Monophasic pulses at 50 pps will yield

$$I_{RMS_A} = 20 \times 10^{-6} \times 50 = 1 \times 10^{-3} = 1 \text{ mA}$$

2. Symmetric biphasic pulses at 50 pps contain 100 phases. The $RMS_A$ current is

$$I_{RMS_A} = 20 \times 10^{-6} \times 100 = 2 \times 10^{-3} = 2 \text{ mA}$$

3. A burst-modulated AC such as the one used by the Russian current occurs in bursts, each containing 25 sine-wave pulses, or 50 phases. Using 50 bps means that 2500 phases are delivered each second. Thus,

$$I_{RMS_A} = 20 \times 10^{-6} \times 2500 = 50 \times 10^{-3} = 50 \text{ mA}$$

Knowing the $RMS_A$ current is of major importance to the clinician, because excessive $RMS_A$ current (called average current by many clinicians) may be harmful to the tissue. If electrode size is known, $RMS_A$ current density is determined through division of the $RMS_A$ current by electrode area. The preceding calculations provide the following observations:

1. In PC stimulators, the number of pulses per second directly affects the $RMS_A$ current. Even if peak current amplitude reaches 1000 to 2000 mA, the $RMS_A$ current may be only 1 mA if phase duration is short and pulse rate is low.
2. Monophasic and biphasic waveforms deliver dramatically less $RMS_A$ current than burst-modulated AC such as Russian current if the number of pulses is equivalent.
3. A monophasic and biphasic pulse is far more efficient than the AC stimulators such as the Russian or IFC stimulators if the objective is to induce the desired physiologic responses with the minimum necessary $RMS_A$ current. The efficiency reflects both physiologic and electronic design criteria. If $RMS_A$ current is low, then small electrodes can be used, because density will remain within tolerable and safe limits. The PC stimulators are a good example because of their very low $RMS_A$ current. Consequently, both large and small electrodes are used clinically with low probability of causing harm. Most AC stimulators should not be used with very small electrodes, because their $RMS_A$ current may reach 80 to 100 mA and may cause skin irritation or burn.

$RMS_A$ current is proportionate to the amount of heat production in the tissue. The equation to express electrical-to-thermal energy conversion is

$$H = 0.24 \text{ I}^2Rt \tag{10}$$

where

$$H = \text{heat generation (gram-calories or g-cal)}$$
$$I = RMS_A \text{ current (A)}$$

$$R = \text{tissue impedence (ohms)}$$
$$t = \text{treatment time (sec)}$$
$$0.24 \text{ is a constant}$$

Let us use the $\text{RMS}_A$ current values of 1, 2, and 50 mA, calculated previously for monophasic, biphasic, and bursts of AC pulses, respectively. Let us assume electrode–skin impedance of 500 $\Omega$ and treatment time of 30 min. The thermal effects are summarized in Table 3–4. Let us assume the following changes: smaller electrode size so that skin impedance is increased to 800 $\Omega$ and pulse rate is 100 pps instead of 50 pps. Thus, $\text{RMS}_A$ current is now 2, 4, and 100 mA for monophasic waveforms, biphasic waveforms, and burst-modulated AC, respectively. The new calculation yields the following results: monophasic, 1.29 g-cal; biphasic, 5.47 g-cal; and burst-modulated AC, 3456.00 g-cal. The preceding calculations clearly indicate the substantial thermal effect of burst-modulated AC, but not PC on the skin.

### Skin Impedance

Skin impedance is one major obstacle to current penetration into the deeper tissues, and it should be minimized by proper stimulator design and good treatment technique. The equation denoting impedance (Z) is:

$$Z = \sqrt{R^2 + (X_L - X_c)^2} \tag{11}$$

where

$$R = \text{static resistance } (\Omega)$$
$$X_L = \text{inductive reactance } (\Omega)$$
$$X_C = \text{capacitative reactance } (\Omega)$$

Inductive reactance ($X_L$) is negligible in a biologic medium, and resistance (R) is not altered by pulsed current. Thus, only capacitative reactance ($X_C$) can be reduced by proper stimulation characteristics. The equation denoting $X_C$ is

$$X_C = \frac{1}{2\pi f C} \tag{12}$$

### TABLE 3–4. THERMAL EFFECT OF ELECTRICAL STIMULATION

| Waveform | Calculation | Results (g-cal) |
|---|---|---|
| Monophasic | $0.24 \times (1.0 \times 10^3)^2 \times 500 \times 1800$ | 0.18 |
| Biphasic | $0.24 \times (2.0 \times 10^3)^2 \times 500 \times 1800$ | 0.81 |
| Polyphasic | $0.24 \times (50 \times 10^3)^2 \times 500 \times 1800$ | 540.00 |

where

$$\pi = \text{constant (3.14)}$$
$$f = \text{frequency of applied voltage (Hz)}$$
$$C = \text{capacitance of tissue (farads)}$$

Equation (12) indicates that the higher the frequency, the lower the capacitative resistance. This outcome is the basis for the claims that IFC at frequencies of 4000 to 5000 Hz reduces skin impedance and therefore penetrates better than other PC stimulators. Frequency, however, is related to phase duration (t) by the equations:

$$f = 1/T \qquad\qquad (13a)$$
$$t = T/2 \qquad\qquad (13b)$$

We can then rewrite

$$f = 1/2t \qquad\qquad (13c)$$

where

$$f = \text{frequency of applied voltage (Hz)}$$
$$T = \text{pulse duration also known as period (sec)}$$
$$t = \text{phase duration (sec)}$$

Equation (13c) clearly shows that the higher the frequency, the shorter the phase duration. Remembering that frequency is also inversely proportional to impedance, one can assert that phase duration is proportional to skin impedance. Stated differently, the shorter the phase duration, the lower the skin impedance. This statement is true even if the number of pulses per second of a PC stimulator is low. The clinical implications are as follows:

1. IFC does not reduce skin resistance and does not penetrate deeper than other TENS.[120]
2. The phase duration of present IFC units (4000 Hz) is 125 µsec. Any monophasic or biphasic waveform having a 125-µsec phase duration will have the same skin impedance as an IFC.
3. Electrode size and voltage also affect skin impedance. Therefore, claiming that "medium" frequency is the major factor in reducing skin impedance is misleading and is ignored by the astute clinician.

## SURFACE ELECTRODES

Surface electrodes serve as the interface between the stimulator and human conductive tissues. They are an integral part of the complete stimulation system and play a critical role in whether the desired physiologic response is achieved when applied to the patient. Of great importance in understanding surface electrodes is recognizing lead arrangements, electrode material, selecting adequate size, and appropriately placing the electrodes. The absence of consistent and appropriate terminology has resulted in the misuse of electrodes in clinical practice and has caused clinical efforts to fail. The purpose of this section is to provide functionally appropriate definitions and explanations of the aforementioned concepts.

## The Leads

Regardless of the stimulator name, manufacturer, or waveform, there is always a pair of leads emerging from its panel. Contrary to widespread belief, neither lead is a ground. The two leads simply represent the two segments of a circuit that, when connected to the body part, will provide a conductive path for electrical current flow. If not connected to the body, a potential difference (voltage generated by the stimulator) will exist between the leads, but current will not flow because the circuit is not closed.

If either a DC or a monophasic PC stimulator is considered, then one lead, and the electrode(s) connected to it, will be positive with respect to the second lead. This is equivalent to saying that the second lead is negative relative to the first lead. This factor does not mean, however, that one of the leads is a ground. It is correct to say that there is a polarity designation of the two leads. The recognition of lead polarity is important in those few cases in which a treatment procedure requires specific polarity.

The application of DC stimulation includes a well-established polarity selection, particularly when iontophoresis is used.[136–144] If a monophasic PC is used, stimulation polarity may be important when applied to slow-to-heal ulcers and wounds.[11,15,16,18,25–28] Polarity may also be important in the attempt to curb acute edema associated with inflammatory reaction.[3–5,8,9] When treating pain, muscle disuse atrophy, chronic edema, neurovascular disorders, protective muscle spasm, or joint ROM, there do not seem to be any data to support polarity consideration.

If symmetric biphasic PC or AC stimulators are used, the polarity of the leads alternates so rapidly that, practically speaking, there is no polarity to consider. Thus, all of the aforementioned clinical problems that do not depend on polarity can be treated with such waveforms, as well as by the monophasic pulses.

The major problem that many clinicians seem to face is recognizing which are the two essential leads that complete the circuit. This challenge results from the fact that in some stimulators, the two leads emerge from the same socket, whereas in others (mostly the classical high voltage PC), one essential lead emerges from the center of the panel and the other extends from the side (Figure 3–26). In many HVPC units, the side lead actually appears as two leads. This dual lead results because the lead is bifurcated inside the stimulators. The physical therapist must recognize that this is only one (bifurcated) lead and not the two essential leads that complete the circuit. In fact, bifurcations of either of the two essential leads can take many configurations (Figure 3–26); but regardless of how many bifurcations are present, they represent only branching out of the two essential leads.

The major advantage of a bifurcation is to stimulate more than one area concurrently. The disadvantage results from the fact that different areas may have different skin impedances. Although the amount of current and charge per phase that passes through the bifurcated leads is identical, the physiologic responses may vary significantly, and may be subliminal, nonperceived stimulation under one electrode and sensory, perceived stimulation under the other.

Another disadvantage results from the fact that the total surface area of the electrodes connected to one essential lead is the sum of the areas of all of the electrodes connected at the end of the bifurcation (Figure 3–27). If the total area is larger than the areas of the electrode(s) connected to the other essential lead, then the stimulation is likely to be stronger under the latter electrode because of the greater current density. The clinician must recognize these potential problems and correct them in order to provide the desired physiologic responses in the appropriate areas of the body.

## Electrode Material

The essential requirements of all surface electrodes are summarized in Table 3–5. The most used materials in clinics today are carbon im-

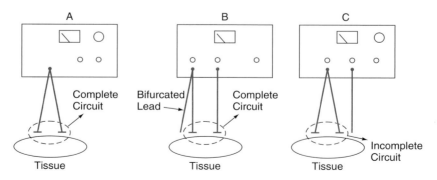

FIGURE 3–26. Electrode lead connections. **(A)** is complete circuit. In **(B),** the bifurcated lead and the center lead can make a complete circuit. In **(C),** the circuit is not complete because the "two" leads are actually one lead that has been bifurcated.

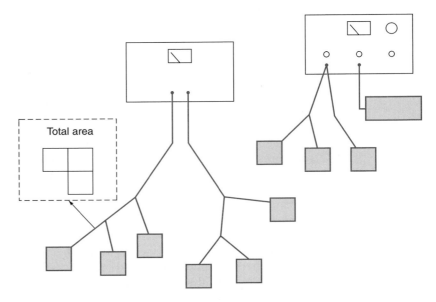

FIGURE 3–27. Multiple bifurcation of both essential electrode leads.

## TABLE 3–5. SURFACE ELECTRODES DESCRIPTION

**Requirements**

- High and uniform conductive characteristics
- Flexibility to contour various body parts
- Durability and resistance to breakdown by mechanical or electrical energies
- Uniform pressure of application whether secured by self-adhesive material or external straps
- All electrodes lose conductivity over time, particularly self-adhesive, so their uniformity of conduction must be checked frequently
- The perimeters do not necessarily indicate the effective electrode size

**Deficiencies**

*Carbon-silicon*

- Time-consuming application
- May be displaced during movement
- Wet sponges dry over short time, thus losing conductivity and conductance uniformity
- Difficult to secure over shoulders, neck, back, and pelvis
- Nonuniform pressure over irregular surfaces

*Self-adhesive*

- Less conductive than carbon–silicon application
- Rapid loss of conduction and conductance uniformity
- May be unpleasant to remove
- Individual patient use
- Relatively expensive
- More likely to cause skin irritation and/or discomfort

pregnated silicon composites and self-adhesive polymer material over (usually) a conductive metallic or nonmetallic base. The nonadhering electrodes require the addition of a conductive medium, usually water-soaked sponges or nonallergenic water-based gel. Irrespective of the conductive medium, these electrodes must be secured to the body part with one or several optional elastic straps or tape. The self-adhering electrodes require no straps, which makes their application much easier and faster. However, they quickly lose adhesiveness and uniformity of conduction, making their life cycle relatively short.

Despite the less-than-perfect uniformity of conduction and considerable difference in overall conductance (Figure 3–28), both groups of electrodes conduct current very adequately into the body.[222] Their major deficiencies are also summarized in Table 3–5. The clinician must pay particular attention to the fact that when a self-adhesive electrode loses adherence or uniformity of conductivity, or both, the effective electrode size may be dramatically smaller than the electrode's perimeter. Such reduction of effective electrode size may lead to skin irritation and even burn due to high $RMS_A$ current density. Thus, frequent inspection of the adherence and conduction of these electrodes is an essential measure to prevent adverse reaction of the patient. Any area of skin redness that is smaller than the electrode size itself (or the patient's perception that the stimulation is smaller than the electrode size) is a warning sign of inadequate electrode conduction that must be addressed immediately.

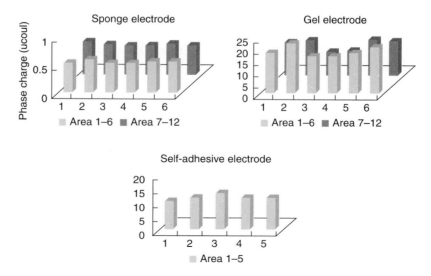

FIGURE 3–28. Distribution of conductance over the surface of 3 types of electrode materials. The distribution is not always equal.

## Electrode Size

The size of surface electrodes is associated with skin impedance, $RMS_A$ current density, perceptual discrimination of the excitatory responses, and specificity of stimulation. In general, the larger the electrode size, the smaller the skin impedance. A 100 cm$^2$ electrode may offer only 100 to 1000 $\Omega$ of impedance,[244] whereas a 2-mm (tip) electrode may reach 50,000 to 100,000 $\Omega$ of impedance. The relationship of size to impedance is likely nonlinear and in fact has not been adequately described in clinical publications.[95,174] Clinically, the physical therapist must first decide how large or small the target area is that should be stimulated. Only then can the electrode size be selected. Using an electrode that is smaller than the target area creates unnecessarily high electrode–skin interface impedance, a practice that frequently occurs when large joints (such as the knee or hip) are stimulated with 5 × 5-cm (2 × 2-inch) electrodes. Similar statements can be extended to large muscles such as the quadriceps femoris that usually require 200- to 250-cm$^2$ electrode size.[60,245] The higher the skin impedance, the less the penetration of the current. Using large electrodes may help to minimize this problem.

The effect of electrode size on $RMS_A$ current density is obvious; there are several clinical implications. First, current density should not exceed safety limits; therefore, small electrodes should not be used if $RMS_A$ current is high. Second, the electrodes connected to the two essential leads may be identical in size and yet the patient will report more stimulation under one electrode: This is because factors other than size can also affect skin impedance. Increasing the size of this one electrode will decrease current density and should resolve the problem. Third, if the stimulator output is limited, then the use of large electrodes may not provide sufficient $RMS_A$ current density for the physiologic response to be achieved. Bifurcation of leads may cause the same problem. Reduction of electrode size may restore sufficient $RMS_A$ current density but may provide less-than-optimal stimulation. Stronger stimulators, which have a higher phase charge, may offer a better solution.

The effect of electrode size on perceptual discrimination between sensory, motor, and pain-fiber excitation was explored by Alon[174] and Alon and coworkers.[95] In essence, larger electrodes produce stronger motor response without pain, whereas smaller electrodes elicit painful stimulation soon after the motor excitation. The most likely explanation of the phenomenon is that by increasing the electrode size, more motor units are being placed immediately under the electrodes and therefore recruited simultaneously.[60,245,246] Furthermore, larger electrodes exhibit considerably less electrode–skin interface impedance.[95,174,222] Thus, more muscle contraction is being generated at lower phase charge, making the stimulation more comfortable.

Sometimes, the effective electrode size is smaller than the overall electrode size, one reason being that the electrode does not conduct uniformly. This effective reduction in electrode size may result in less comfortable stimulation.[95] The clinical implications relate to the stimulation procedures. If vigorous muscle contraction is the objective, electrode size should be large. Size, however, is relative to the muscle mass[60,95,245]; therefore, the electrode size appropriate for wrist or elbow extensor groups is much too small when the quadriceps femoris, erector spinae, or abdominal muscles are the targets of stimulation.[247–249] Likewise, patients of different body sizes may require different-sized electrodes.

If treatment methods involve stimulation of trigger or acupuncture points, very small electrodes are likely to minimize motor stimulation, because motor fibers are usually deeper than sensory and pain-conducting fibers.[87,224] Coupled with very high skin impedance and current density, sensory and pain-conducting fibers are usually excited before motors fibers.

Although large electrodes minimize painful stimulation, they disperse current flow through the tissue, thereby making the stimulation less specific. The clinical consequence is that muscles that are not the target of stimulation may also contract. If this is undesirable, then using smaller electrodes, a bipolar electrode technique, or both (see the following section), should eliminate the problem. Smaller electrodes may isolate the individual muscle from the rest of the group, but the stimulation may prove painful before sufficient contraction can be achieved.[162] The clinician must therefore change electrode size in accordance with treatment objectives and patient response.[250]

## Electrode Placement Techniques

One of the most confusing aspects of clinical electrical stimulation has been the selection and administration of appropriate electrode placement. Again, misleading and inconsistent terminology seems to be a major source of confusion. In fact, there are only two basic techniques of electrode placement: **monopolar** and **bipolar.** These two techniques prevail regardless of whether DC, PC, or AC stimulators are used.

Monopolar and bipolar techniques have nothing to do with the polarity of the current, and either technique can be used with any stimulator on the market. The terms monopolar and bipolar simply indicate whether only one essential lead and its electrode(s) are placed over the areas to be stimulated, or both essential leads and their electrodes are placed over the target area(s).

## *Monopolar Technique*

In the monopolar technique, only one of the two essential leads, and the electrode(s) connected to it, are placed over the target area to be affected by the stimulation. This electrode has been called the **treatment** or **stimulating electrode.** The other lead and its electrode(s) are placed over an area that is not to be affected by the stimulation and can be called the **nontreatment, dispersive,** or **return electrode.** The target area is where the basic excitatory response should be perceived. Contrary to what is reported in most electrotherapy texts, this area is not only a muscle. Bursae, dermal ulcers, hematomas, joints, and trigger and acupuncture points are also included in the list of target areas, depending on the clinical problem and its appropriate treatment procedure.

The nontreatment electrode is commonly known as the dispersive electrode because it is usually, though not always, a large electrode. Its large size minimizes current density, preventing current from being perceived under it. Thus, any size will suffice, and this electrode can be placed over various body parts, as long as no excitatory response is perceived under it. If the treatment electrode is very small, then the nontreatment electrode need be only somewhat larger. The exact size is therefore relative and is determined by the clinician, based on the response of the patient. A perception of sensory stimulation under the nontreatment electrode is not contraindicated but is unnecessary and should be avoided.

The treatment electrode can be a single electrode or several. The latter arrangement is obtained by bifurcation of the lead. Multiple electrodes are usually justified if the stimulator provides only one channel and if there is more than one target area requiring stimulation (an example would be two wounds/ulcers at different sites of the lower limb). A schematic illustration of a monopolar technique with and without bifurcation is provided in Figure 3–29. It is important that the sum of the areas of the electrodes in a bifurcated lead be less than the area of the nontreatment, dispersive electrode, in order to avoid perception of current under the latter.

At present, the only two clinical problems that may mandate the use of a monopolar technique are one protocol for treatment of dermal ulcers and wounds,[11,15,16,18,19,25–28] and one protocol if the clinical objective is to curb edema.[3–5,8,9] Using a monophasic PC, or DC stimulation and a monopolar technique, allows the physical therapist to treat the ulcer with positive or negative electrical charges. The same is true for curbing and absorbing of acute edema with monophasic PC. Unfortunately, the question of which polarity of the treatment electrode should yield the best results remains controversial and must await further study.[10]

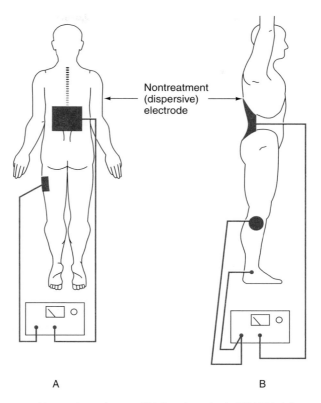

Nontreatment
(dispersive)
electrode

A                                    B

FIGURE 3–29. Monopolar technique. **(A)** Simple method. **(B)** With bifurcated lead so that both knee and ankle can be treated simultaneously.

Iontophoresis using DC requires monopolar technique so the treatment electrode can be of the correct polarity to drive the medication into the body.[143,144] Trigger and acupuncture point stimulation are more conveniently obtained with the monopolar technique because the stimulation target areas are very small.

### Bipolar Technique

As defined, the bipolar technique requires that both the essential leads and the electrodes connected to them be placed over the target area in order for the area to be affected by the stimulation. It follows that both the complete conductive circuit and the current flow through the tissue should be confined to the area where the clinical problem is present. Unlike the monopolar technique, the excitatory responses are now perceived under both electrodes of the circuit.

Obviously, the two electrodes are usually, but not necessarily, of the same size and material, and the nontreatment, dispersive electrode is not used.

Bipolar placement of the electrodes can be used with any stimulator, including HVPC stimulation. Some clinicians have been misled to believe that a dispersive electrode must be used with HVPC. Use of a dispersive pad is absolutely false. Indeed, one of the essential leads of many old HVPC stimulators is customarily connected to a large dispersive electrode, but this electrode can be easily replaced with a smaller electrode if a bipolar technique is indicated.[153]

As in the monopolar placement, bifurcation of the leads may be accomplished with a bipolar technique. Indications for bifurcation of electrode leads include a situation in which the target area is large but the available electrodes are too small. (An example could be a radiating pain that covers a large part of dermatomal distribution, or a protective muscle spasm across the whole lower back.) Figure 3–30 illustrates bipolar and bifurcated bipolar techniques.

Like the monopolar technique, the bipolar technique is used regardless of whether the PC is monophasic or biphasic or whether an AC stimulator is used. The symmetric biphasic PC and AC do not present a polarity factor; thus, it makes no difference which of the two electrodes is placed proximally and distally on the skin over the target area. If monophasic pulses or some of the asymmetric bipha-

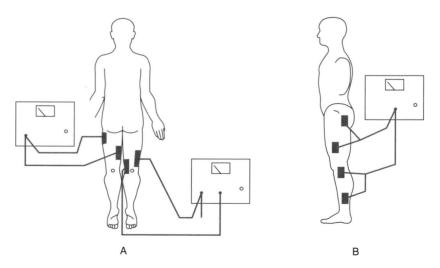

A                                        B

FIGURE 3–30. Bipolar techniques. **(A)** Simple method over a joint or muscle. **(B)** Bifurcated along dermatomal distribution.

sic pulses are used, polarity may affect the excitatory response. Classically, the assumption has been made that excitation occurs only under the negative electrode.[96] This assumption must be seriously questioned, as it is very easy to demonstrate excitation under the positive electrode.[87] Thus, when the two electrodes of a monophasic PC stimulator are placed on the skin over the target muscle, the selection of which electrode should be negative and which should be positive is based simply on strength and comfort of contraction.

Many of today's stimulators offer two or more channels. When two or more channels are used simultaneously over the same target area, each channel is still arranged as a bipolar placement technique. The dual channel arrangement, however, can take several configurations, as illustrated in Figure 3–31. Using different configurations to improve pain relief has been advocated.[152] However, no objective clinical data have been found to support such a contention.

Bipolar placement should be selected over monopolar placement if the presented clinical impairments are muscle disuse atrophy, neuromuscular facilitation, ROM limitation, protective muscle spasm, or most circulatory disorders. Particularly when the clinical problem requires motor stimulation, the bipolar technique should be less time consuming, should provide more specific excitation of the target muscles, and elicit stronger contraction.[95,250] If only sensory excitation is indicated, then either bipolar or monopolar placement techniques can be equally effective.

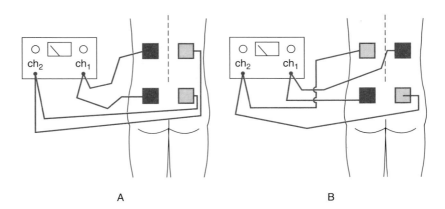

A                                                    B

FIGURE 3–31. Bipolar placement using two-channel stimulation. **(A)** Longitudinal paravertebral configuration. **(B)** Crossed pattern arrangement.

## PRINCIPLES OF CLINICAL DECISION MAKING

The decisions regarding when, why, and how to use electrical stimulation require a system that embodies several constituents. First and foremost is the identification of the patient problem for which electrical stimulation should be indicated. From a clinical electrotherapy perspective, these problems are usually a host of physical impairments or symptoms, or both, which affect physical performance. Next is the recognition of the physiologic rationale (mode of action) by which the electrical energy may help to resolve the impairment or symptom. The physiologic mechanism should describe how the stimulation affects molecular, cellular, tissue, and systemic responses that may explain the clinical results. Selection of stimulation characteristics, appropriate electrode sizes, and electrode placement follows. The stimulation characteristics should be set based on objective clinical trials where the efficacy of the intervention has been demonstrated and reported in refereed publications. If such clinical data are not available, the characteristics should be based on the ability to elicit the mode of action by which the stimulation is presumed to help alleviate the clinical impairment.

Stimulation time within a session, as well as the number of sessions, must not be based on an arbitrary decision (most clinicians stimulate for 20 to 30 minutes without knowing why!). Rather, the decision regarding how long to stimulate should be based on the ability to achieve the clinical objective(s). In many cases, this means many hours of daily stimulation. The decision to modify or to discontinue stimulation should likewise be based on the inability to achieve the physiologic and particularly the clinical objectives. Termination of the treatment is also indicated when the clinical objective is reached. Depending on the nature of the problem and the diagnosis, the clinical objective(s) can be met after one treatment or after many months of treatment. Setting an arbitrary number of treatments as dictated by insurance guidelines is a common practice, but it contradicts sound knowledge of effective intervention.

## CLINICAL PROCEDURES

To illustrate the process of making clinical decisions, several examples are presented:

1. A patient sustained a strain injury to the medial aspect of the knee 2 hours ago. The strain caused an inflammatory reaction with the clinical signs/symptoms of pain, redness, ecchymosis,

swelling, warmth, and limited ROM. The problem to be treated by electrical stimulation is to curb and absorb the swelling. The reason for selecting management of swelling rather than pain is the hypothesis that resolving the inflammation by elimination of the swelling is a more direct approach to the pathology, and its resolution will inevitably also eliminate the pain and ROM limitation. The mode of action is based on animal experiments showing that electrical stimulation can minimize leakage of proteins and blood cells and accelerate their removal from the interstitial spaces.[3–5,8,9] Not having objective clinical data, the treatment protocol (Table 3–6) is based on the physiologic rationale and animal data. Note the importance of having a monophasic waveform, monopolar technique, and treatment time of "many hours" daily, because curbing occurs only during stimulation.[3,4] Clinical improvement is expected within 24 to 48 hours, and complete resolution of the swelling is expected to be achieved within 3 to 6 days. Thus, if there is no improvement within 48 hours, or if the inflammation is worse, the protocol should be discontinued.

2. A person underwent limb amputation below the knee 2 months ago. About 3 cm of the incision has not healed despite  good wound management. Objective clinical data favor the use of electrical stimulation as a means of accelerating wound healing. At least three different clinical protocols have been described in published literature. Of the three, stimulating directly into the wound has the best objective clinical data[11,14,15,18,21,25–28] and reasonably sound physiologic rationale, and therefore is selected as the first-choice protocol. The rationale is possibly a combination of several modes of action including the delivery of missing positive potentials,[11,15,25–28] enhancement of DNA and protein synthesis leading to collagen fiber regeneration,[175,176,216,217] bactericidal effect,[251–259] and promotion of microcirculation.[12–14,29,68–70] The characteristics of stimulation are summarized in Table 3–6. Note the possible importance of having a monophasic waveform and monopolar technique where the stimulating electrode must be sterile and made of nonadhering, biocompatible material. Optimal treatment time has not been established and varies from 30 minutes twice daily[14,15,25–28] to 3 hours daily.[30] The beginning of observable improvement is expected within 2 to 3 days. If there is no detectable improvement after 3 to 4 weeks of daily stimulation, the protocol is probably ineffective and should be terminated. If the first protocol failed to promote healing, the other two protocols should be attempted. They must be considered as trial and error because only one controlled clinical study of each approach has been published,[20,29] and the physiologic rationale is

## TABLE 3–6. PARAMETER SETTINGS FOR THE THREE CASE STUDIES

| Clinical Condition | Wave Form | Mode | Phase Duration | Pulse Rate | Polarity | Intensity | Treatment Time |
|---|---|---|---|---|---|---|---|
| **Case 1** | | | | | | | |
| Acute edema (References 5, 8, 9) | Monophasic | Continuous pulses | 5–100 μsec | 100–125 pps | Negative covers edematous area | Sensory stimulation | 2–8 hrs daily |
| **Case 2** | | | | | | | |
| Wound/ulcer first choice (References 11, 14, 15, 18, 25–28) | Monophasic | Continuous pulses | 5–140 μsec | 80–125 pps | Positive (healing) Negative (bactericidal) | Sensory stimulation | 30–60 min 2× daily |
| Wound/ulcer second choice (Reference 29) | Mono- or biphasic | Continuous pulses | 20–200 μsec | 2–5 pps | Not applicable | Motor stimulation | 30–45 min 2× daily |
| Wound/ulcer third choice (Reference 20) | Asymmetric biphasic | Interrupted ON 4 sec OFF 4 sec Ramps 0 sec | 250 μsec | 40 pps | Not applicable | Motor stimulation | 2 hrs daily |
| **Case 3** | | | | | | | |
| Shoulder subluxation CNS (References 53, 54) | Symmetric biphasic | Interrupted ON 10–30 sec OFF 12–2 sec Ramps 2 sec | 50–300 μsec | 35 pps | Not applicable | Motor stimulation | 1.5–6 hrs daily |

not well established. Thus, prediction of success and failure are not available at this writing.

3. A survivor of a cerebrovascular accident (CVA) with onset one week ago is referred for physical rehabilitation. Among many impairments and functional deficits, the patient has a subluxation of the hemiplegic shoulder and is unable to volitionally activate the muscles around the shoulder complex. The clinical objectives of using electrical stimulation include reducing the shoulder subluxation, increasing force of the shoulder musculature, and facilitating recovery of active motions and possibly selected functions of the upper extremity. Preferably, the stimulation should be provided simultaneously with the performance of these functions.

Incorporation of electrical stimulation with the management of shoulder subluxation is supported by the rationale that electrical stimulation facilitates metabolic actions, including activation of selected enzymes, ions, and proteins that are essential for muscle contraction.[43,60,206–211,245] The stimulation causes excitation of the motor nerves, promotes force gain, and retards disuse atrophy.[50–55,57–62] Through its sensory components and repetitive stimulation, the electrical intervention may facilitate synaptic associations that may lead to partial recovery of meaningful neural control.[55,58] In the presence of CNS damage, only limited improvement of these cellular and tissue responses can be obtained by exercises alone. Setting up the stimulation characteristics (Table 3–6) is based on objective clinical studies.[53,54] Electrode size and placements depend on the clinical presentation of the patient but are likely to include one channel over the deltoid and additional channels over other muscle groups. Note that symmetric biphasic waveform may be preferred because of comfort, that the ON and OFF times are gradually modified, and that treatment time is gradually increased to 6 hours daily, 7 days each week. Improvement of subluxation, muscle force, and passive and active ROM are expected within 6 weeks. Stimulation should continue as long as upper extremity function is improving and should be terminated if muscle contraction cannot be elicited within five to six sessions, if patient's pain increases as a result of the stimulation, or if vital signs become unstable.

# Summary

Mastering the knowledge and skills required for effective use of electrical stimulation in the clinic is highly dependent on successful integration of the ever-changing information from the fields of electronics, electrophysiology, electropathology, and medical practice. The most essential domains of knowledge include the following:

1. The ability to evaluate, select, and operate the various stimulators and differentiate the types of currents, characteristics, and modulations most appropriate for treatment of any given clinical condition.
2. The ability of the clinician or student to establish the pathophysiologic framework, processes, and interactions among the various body systems that combine together as the clinical presentation of patient performance. The synthesis of these domains should enable the clinician to incorporate the electrical stimulation into the most effective and efficient management program to help resolve patients' impairments and functional deficiencies.

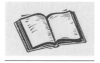

## REVIEW QUESTIONS

1. What electrical parameters and electrode characteristics must be considered to ascertain the effectiveness and safety of stimulation?
2. Compare and contrast all common and unique properties and modulations of DC, AC, and PC stimulators.
3. Describe the physiologic model and how electrical stimulation operates within this general framework.
4. What will be your selection of characters, modulations, and electrode sizes and positions if a given patient presents with disuse atrophy of the abdominal musculature? What is the reason for each of your selections?
5. What are the most important features, properties, and modulations that will ascertain the most versatile, yet not redundant, stimulator? Versatility pertains to being able to use the stimulator for all clinical conditions in which electrical stimulation has shown clinical (or at least animal) efficacy.

## References

1. Crisler GR. Sprains and strains treated with the ultra faradic M-4 impulse generator. J Flo Med Assoc, 11:32, 1953.
2. Michlovitz S, Smith W, Watkins M. Ice and high voltage pulsed stimulation in treatment of acute lateral ankle sprains. J Orthop Sports Phys Ther, 9:301–304, 1988.
3. Bettany JA, Fish DR, Mendel FC. Influence of high voltage pulsed direct current on edema formation following impact injury. Phys Ther, 70:219–224, 1990.

4. Bettany JA, Fish DR, Mendel FC. Influence of cathodal high voltage pulsed current on acute edema. J Clin Electrophysiol, 2:5–8, 1990.

5. Taylor K, Fish DR, Mendel FC, Burton HW. Effect of a single 30-minute treatment of high voltage pulsed current on edema formation in frog hind limbs. Phys Ther, 72:63–68, 1992.

6. Levy A, Dalith M, Abramovici A et al. Transcutaneous electrical stimulation in experimental acute arthritis. Arch Phys Med Rehabil, 68:75–78, 1987.

7. Griffin JW, Newsome LS, Stralka SW, Wright PE. Reduction of chronic posttraumatic hand edema: A comparison of high voltage pulsed current, intermittent pneumatic compression, and placebo treatments. Phys Ther, 70:279–286, 1990.

8. Karnes JL, Mendel FC, Fish DR, Burton HW. High-voltage pulsed current: Its influence on diameters of histamine-dilated arterioles in hamster cheek pouches. Arch Phys Med Rehabil, 76:381–386, 1995.

9. Cook HA. Morales M, La Rosa EM et al. Effects of electrical stimulation on lymphatic flow and limb volume in the rat. Phys Ther, 74:1040–1046, 1994.

10. Faghri PD. The effects of neuromuscular stimulation-induced muscle contraction versus elevation on hand edema in CVA patient. J Hand Surg, 10:29–34, 1997.

11. Baker LL, Chambers R, DeMuth SK, Villar F. Effects of electrical stimulation on wound healing in patients with diabetic ulcers. Diabetes Care, 20:405–412, 1997.

12. Kaada B. Promoted healing of chronic ulceration by transcutaneous nerve stimulation (TMS). VASA, 12:262, 1983.

13. Kaada B, Emru M. Promoted healing of leprous ulcers by transcutaneous nerve stimulation. Acupunct Electrother Res, 13:165–170, 1988.

14. Lundeberg TC, Eriksson SV, Malm M. Electrical nerve stimulation improves healing of diabetic ulcers. Ann Plast Surg, 29:328–331, 1992.

15. Kloth LC, Feedar JA. Acceleration of wound healing with high voltage, monophasic, pulsed current. Phys Ther, 68:503–508, 1988.

16. Carley PJ, Wainapel SF: Electrotherapy for acceleration of wound healing: Low intensity direct current. Arch Phys Med Rehabil, 66:443, 1985.

17. Karba R, Vodovnik L, Presern-Strukelj M, Klesnik M. Promoted healing of chronic wounds due to electrical stimulation. Wounds, 3:16–23, 1991.

18. Griffin JW, Tooms RE, Mendius RA et al. Efficacy of high voltage pulsed current for healing of pressure ulcers in patients with spinal cord injury. Phys Ther, 71:433–444, 1991.

19. Gogia PP, Marques RR, Minerbo GM. Effects of high voltage galvanic stimulation on wound healing. An adjunct modality used to enhance wound healing. Ostomy/Wound Management, 38(1):29–35, 1992.

20. Jercinovic A, Karba R, Vodovnik L et al. Low frequency pulsed current and pressure ulcer healing. IEEE Trans Rehabil Eng, 2:225–232, 1994.

21. Wood JM, Jacobson WE, Schallreuter KU et al. Pulsed low-intensity direct current (PLIDC) is effective in healing chronic decubitus ulcers in stage II and III. J Invest Dermatol 98:574, 1992.

22. Weiss DE, Eaglstein WH, Falanga V. Exogenous electric current can reduce the formation of hypertrophic scars. J Dermatol Surg Oncol, 15:1272–1275, 1989.

23. Stromberg BV. Effects of electrical currents on wound contraction. Ann Plast Surg, 21:121–123, 1988.

24. Reich JD, Tarjan PP. Electrical stimulation of the skin. Int J Dermatol, 29:395–400, 1990.

25. Gentzkow GD, Pollack SV, Koth LC, Stubbs HA. Improved healing of pressure ulcers using Dermapulse, a new electrical stimulation device. Wounds, 3(5):158–170, 1991.

26. Gentzkow GO, Alon G, Taler GA, Eltoral IM, Montroy RE. Healing of refractory stage III and IV pressure ulcers by a new electrical stimulation device. Wounds, 5:160–172, 1993.

27. Alon G, Azaria M, Stein H. Diabetic ulcer healing using high voltage TENS. Phys Ther, 66:775, 1986.

28. Alon G, Desales-Schroen, Conner PG. The effects of monophasic pulsatile current on pressure ulcers healing process. Proceedings. IEEE Eng Med Biol Soc, XIII:602–604, 1991.

29. Finsen V, Persen L, Lovlien M et al. Transcutaneous electrical nerve stimulation after major amputation. J Bone Joint Surg (Br), 70-B: 109–112, 1988.

30. Frantz R. The effect of TENS on healing of pressure ulcers. Wound Repair and Regeneration, 2:65, 1995.

31. Williams JGP, Street M: Sequential faradism in quadriceps rehabilitation. Physiotherapy, 62:252–254, 1976.

32. Eriksson E, Haggmark T. Comparison of isometric muscle training and electrical stimulation supplementing isometric muscle training in the recovery after major knee ligament surgery: A preliminary report. Am J Sports Med, 7:169–171, 1979.

33. Gould M, Donnermeyer D, Gammon GG et al. Transcutaneous muscle stimulation to retard disuse atrophy after open meniscectomy. Clinical Orth Rel Res, 178:190–197, 1983.

34. Wigersstad-Lossing I, Grimby G, Jonsson T et al. Effects of electrical muscle stimulation combined with voluntary contraction after knee ligament surgery. Med Sci Sports Exerc, 20:93–98, 1988.

35. Arvidsson I, Arviddson H, Eriksson E et al. Prevention of quadriceps wasting after immobilization—An evaluation of the effect of electrical stimulation. Orthopaedics, 9:1519–1528, 1986.

36. Delitto A, McKowen JM, McCarthy JA et al. Electrically elicited co-contraction of thigh musculature after anterior cruciate ligament surgery. Phys Ther, 68:45–50, 1988.

37. Delitto A, Rose SJ, McKowen JM et al. Electrical stimulation versus voluntary exercise in strengthening thigh musculature after anterior cruciate ligament surgery. Phys Ther, 68:660–663, 1988.

38. Kidd GL, Oldham JA, Stanley JK. A comparison of uniform patterned and eutrophic electrotherapies in a clinical procedure of rehabilitation of some movements in the arthritic hand. Clin Rehabil, 3:27–39, 1989.

39. Snyder-Mackler L, Ladin Z, Schepsis AA et al. Electrical stimulation of the thigh muscles after reconstruction of the anterior cruciate ligament. J Bone Joint Surg, 73-A:1025–1036, 1991.

40. Oldham JA, Stanley JK. Rehabilitation of atrophied muscle in the rheumatoid arthritic hand. A comparison of two methods of electrical stimulation. J Hand Surg, 14B:294–297, 1989.

41. Petterson T, Smith G, Oldham JA, Home TE, Tallis RC. The use of patterned neuromuscular stimulation to improve hand function following surgery for ulnar neuropathy. J Hand Surg, 19B:430–433, 1994.

42. Oldham JA, Howe TE, Petterson T, Smith G, Tallis RC. Electrotherapeutic rehabilitation of the quadriceps in elderly osteoarthritis patients: A double blind assessment of patterned neuromuscular stimulation. Clin Rehabil, 9:10–20, 1995.

43. Gibson JNA, Smith K, Rennie MJ. Prevention of disuse muscle atrophy by means of electrical stimulation: Maintenance of protein synthesis. Lancet, Oct 1:767–770, 1988.

44. Caggiano E, Emrey T, Shirley S, Craik RL. Effects of electrical stimulation or voluntary contraction for strengthening the quadriceps femoris muscles in an aged male population. J Orthop Sports Phys Ther, 20:22–28, 1994.

45. Synder-Macklar L, Delitto A, Stralka SW, Bailey SL. Use of electrical stimulation to enhance recovery of quadriceps femoris muscle force production in patients following anterior cruciate ligament reconstruction. Phys Ther, 74:901–907, 1994.

46. Morrissey MC, Brewster CE, Shields CL et al. The effects of electrical stimulation on the quadriceps during postoperative knee immobilization. Am J Sports Med, 13:40–45, 1985.

47. Abdel-Moty E, Fishbain DA, Goldberg M et al. Functional electrical stimulation treatment of postradiculopathy associated muscle weakness. Arch Phys Med Rehabil, 75:680–686, 1994.

48. Abdel-Moty E, Khalil TM, Rosomoff RS, Rosomoff HL. Functional electrical stimulation in low back pain patients. Pain Management, 1: 258–263, 1988.

49. Lieber RL, Silva PD, Daniel DM. Equal effectiveness of electrical and volitional strength training for quadriceps femoris muscles after anterior cruciate ligament surgery. J Orthop Res, 14:131–138, 1996.

50. Kraft GH, Fitts SS, Hammond MC. Techniques to improve function of the arm and hand in chronic hemiplegia. Arch Phys Med Rehabil, 73:220–227, 1992.

51. Glanz M, Klawansky S, Stason W, Berkey C, Chalmers TC. Functional electrostimulation in poststroke rehabilitation: A meta-analysis of the randomized controlled trials. Arch Phys Med Rehabil, 77:549–553, 1996.

52. Baker LL, Parker K, Sanderson D. Neuromuscular electrical stimulation for the head-injured patient. Phys Ther, 63:1967–1974, 1983.

53. Baker LL, Parker K. Neuromuscular electrical stimulation of the muscles surrounding the shoulder. Phys Ther, 66:1930–1937, 1986.

54. Faghri PD, Rodgers MM, Glaser RM et al. The effects of functional electrical stimulation on shoulder subluxation, arm function recovery, and shoulder pain in hemiplegic patients. Arch Phys Med Rehabil, 75:73–79, 1994.

55. Burridge J, Taylor P, Hagan S, Swain I. Experience of clinical use of the Odstock dropped foot stimulator. Artificial Organs, 21:254–260, 1997.

56. Petajan JH. Sural nerve stimulation and motor control of tibialis anterior muscle in spastic paresis. Neurology, 37:47–53, 1987.

57. Merletti R, Andina A, Galante M et al. Clinical experience of electronic peroneal stimulators in 50 hemiparetic patients. Scand J Rehabil Med, 11:111–118, 1979.

58. Bogataj U, Gros N, Kljajic M et al. The rehabilitation of gait in patients with hemiplegia: A comparison between conventional therapy and multichannel functional electrical stimulation therapy. Phys Ther, 75:490–502, 1995.

59. Waters RL, McNeal DR, Clifford B, Faloon W. Functional electrical stimulation of the peroneal nerve for hemiplegia long-term clinical follow-up. J Bone Joint Surg, 67A:792–793, 1985.

60. Kern H. Functional electrical stimulation in paraplegic spastic patients. Artificial Organs, 21:195–196, 1997.

61. Bowman BR, Baker LL, Waters RL. Positional feedback and electrical stimulation: An automated treatment for the hemiplegic wrist. Arch Phys Med Rehabil, 60:497–502, 1979.

62. Baker LL, Yeh C, Wilson D et al. Electrical stimulation of wrist and fingers for hemiplegic patients. Phys Ther, 59:1495–1499, 1979.

63. Faghri PD, Van Meerdervort HF, Glaser RM, Figoni SF. Electrical stimulation-induced contraction to reduce blood stasis during arthroplasty. IEEE Trans Rehabil Eng, 5:62–69, 1997.

64. Tichy VL, Zankel HT. Prevention of venous thrombosis and embolism by electrical stimulation of calf muscles. Arch Phys Med Rehabil, 30:711–715, 1949.

65. Doran FSA, White M, Frury M. A clinical trial designed to test the relative value of two simple methods of reducing the risk of venous statis in the lower limbs during surgical operations, the danger of thrombosis, and a subsequent pulmonary embolus, with a survey of the problem. Br J Surg, 57:20–30, 1970.

66. Bodenheim R, Bennett H. Reversal of Sudeck's atrophy by the adjunctive use of transcutaneous electrical nerve stimulation. Phys Ther, 63:1287–1288, 1983.

67. Kaada B. Vasodilation induced by transcutaneous nerve in peripheral ischemia (Raynaud's phenomenon and diabetic polyneuropathy). Euro Heart J, 3:303–314, 1982.

68. Lundeberg T, Kjartansson J, Samuelsson UE. Effect of electric nerve stimulation on healing of ischemic skin flaps. Lancet, Sept 24:712–714, 1988.

69. Kjartansson J, Lundeberg T, Samuelsson UE et al. Transcutaneous electrical nerve stimulation (TENS) increases survival of ischemic musculocutaneous flaps. Acta Physiol Scand, 134:95–99, 1988.

70. Kjartansson J, Lundeberg T, Samuelsson UE et al. Calcitonin gene related peptide (CGRP) and transcutaneous electrical nerve stimulation (TENS) increase cutaneous blood flow in a musculocutaneous flap in the rat. Acta Physiol Scand, 134:95–99, 1988.

71. Gotlin RS, Hershkowitz S, Juris PM et al. Electrical stimulation effect on extensor lag and length of hospital stay after total knee arthroplasty. Arch Phys Med Rehabil, 75:957–959, 1994.

72. Melzak R, Vetere P, Finch L. A comparison of TENS and massage for pain and range of motion. Phys Ther, 63:489–493, 1983.
73. Jensen JE, Conn RR, Hazelrigg G, Newett JE. The use of transcutaneous neural stimulation and isokinetic testing in arthroscopic knee surgery. Am J Sports Med, 13:27–203, 1985.
74. Morgan B, Jones AR, Mulcahy KA et al. Transcutaneous electric nerve stimulation (TENS) during distension shoulder arthrography: A controlled trial. Pain, 64:265–267, 1995.
75. Walker RH, Morris BA, Angulo DL et al. Postoperative use of continuous passive motion, transcutaneous electrical nerve stimulation, and continuous cooling pad following total knee arthroplasty. J Arthroplasty, 6:151–156, 1991.
76. Rizk TE, Christopher RP, Pinals RS, Higgins AC, Frix R. Adhesive capsulitis (frozen shoulder): A new approach to its management. Arch Phys Med Rehabil, 64:29–33, 1983.
77. Axelgaard J, Brown JC. Lateral electrical surface stimulation for the treatment of progressive idiopathic scoliosis. Spine, 8:242–260, 1983.
78. Sullivan JA, Davidson R, Renshaw TS et al. Further evaluation of the scoliotron treatment of idiopathic adolescent scoliosis. Spine, 11:903–906, 1986.
79. Eckerson LF, Axelgaard J. Lateral electrical stimulation as an alternative to bracing in the treatment of idiopathic scoliosis. Phys Ther, 64:483–490, 1984.
80. El-Sayyad M, Conine TA. Effect of exercise, bracing and electrical surface stimulation on idiopathic scoliosis: A preliminary study. Int J Rehabil Res, 17:70–74, 1994.
81. Sand PK. Pelvic floor stimulation in the treatment of mixed incontinence complicated by a low pressure urethra. Obstet Gynecol, 88:757–760, 1996.
82. Dumoulin C, Seaborne D, Quirion-DeGirardi C, Sullivan SJ. Pelvic-floor rehabilitation, part 1: Comparison of two surface electrode placement during stimulation of the pelvic-floor musculature in women who are continent using bipolar interferential currents. Phys Ther, 75: 1067–1074, 1995.
83. Dumoulin C, Seaborne D, Quirion-DeGirardi C, Sullivan SJ. Pelvic-floor rehabilitation, part 2: Pelvic-floor reeducation with interferential currents and exercise in the treatment of genuine stress incontinence in postpartum women—A cohort study. Phys Ther, 75:1075–1081, 1995.
84. Richardson DA, Miller KL, Siegel SW et al. Pelvic floor electrical stimulation: A comparison of daily and every-other-day therapy for genuine stress incontinence. Urology, 48:110–118, 1996.
85. Laycock J, Jerwood D. Does pre-modulated interferential therapy cure genuine stress incontinence? Physiotherapy, 79:553–559, 1993.
86. Geddes LA. A short history of the electrical stimulation of excitable tissue. Physiologist, 27(suppl):1, 1984.
87. Reilly JP. Electrical Stimulation and Electropathology. New York, NY, Cambridge University Press, pp 95–132, 1992.

88. Robinson AJ. Transcutaneous electrical nerve stimulation for the control of pain in musculoskeletal disorders. J Orthop Sports Phys Ther, 24:208–226, 1996.

89. Alon G. (guest ed) Electrotherapy. Physical Therapy Practice, Vol 1, No 2, Andover Publication, pp 1–71, 1992.

90. Rush PJ, Shore A. Physician perception of the value of physical modalities in the treatment of musculoskeletal disease. Br J Rheumatol, 33:566–568, 1994.

91. Section on Clinical Electrophysiology. Electrotherapeutic Terminology in Physical Therapy. Alexandria, VA, American Physical Therapy Association, 1990.

92. Hultman E, Sjoholm H, Jaderholm-Ek I, Krynicki J. Evaluation of methods for electrical stimulation of human skeletal muscle in situ. Pfluegers Arch, 398:139–141, 1983.

93. Petrofsky JS, Petrofsky S. A wide-pulse-width electrical stimulator for use on denervated muscles. J Clin Eng, 17:331–338, 1992.

94. Bowman BR, Baker LL. Effects of wave form parameters on comfort during transcutaneous neuromuscular electrical stimulation. Ann Biomed Eng, 13:58–66, 1985.

95. Alon G, Kantor G, Ho HS. Effects of electrode size on basic excitatory responses and on selected stimulus parameters. J Orth Sports Phys Ther, 20:29–35, 1994.

96. Kovacs R. Electrotherapy and Light Therapy (5th ed). Philadelphia, PA, Lea & Febiger, p 88, 1947.

97. Howard JP, Drake TR, Kellog DL Jr. Effects of alternating current iontophoresis on drug delivery. Arch Phys Med Rehabil, 76:463–466, 1995.

98. McLeod KJ, Rubin CT. The effect of low-frequency electrical fields on osteogenesis. J Bone Joint Surg, 74-A:920–929, 1992.

99. Lavine LS, Grodzinsky AJ. Current concepts review. Electrical stimultion of repair of bone. J Bone Joint Surg, 69-A:626–630, 1987.

100. Sisken BF, Walker J, Orgel M. Prospects on clinical applications of electrical stimulation for nerve regeneration. J Cell Biochem, 51:404–409, 1993.

101. Katims JJ, Long D, Ng LKY. Transcutaneous nerve stimulation: Frequency and waveform specificity in humans. Appl Neurophysiol, 49:86–91, 1986.

102. Taylor DN, Lee CT. Frequency-dependent effects of sine-wave cranial transcutaneous electrical nerve stimulation in human subjects. Acupuncture & Electro-Therapeutics Research, 17:221–227, 1992.

103. Taylor DN, Lee CT, Katims JJ, Ng LKY. Effects of cranial transcutaneous electrical nerve stimulation on measures of autonomic, somatic and cognitive activity. Acupuncture & Electro-Therapeutics Research, 14:29–42, 1989.

104. Shealy CN, Cady RK, Wilkie RG, Cox R, Liss S, Clossen W. Depression a diagnostic neurochemical profile and therapy with cranial electrical stimulation (CES). J Neurol Orthop Med Surg, 10:319–321, 1989.

105. Cassuto J, Liss S, Bennett A. The use of modulated energy carried on a high frequency wave for the relief of intractable pain. Int J Clin Pharm Res, 113:239–241, 1993.

106. Pickworth WB, Fant RV, Butschky MF et al. Evaluation of cranial elec-
     trostimulation therapy on short-term smoking cessation. Biol Psychia-
     try, 42:116–121, 1977.
107. Malden JW, Charash LI. Transcranial stimulation for inhibition of prim-
     itive reflexes in children with cerebral palsy. Neurol Rep, 9:33–38, 1985.
108. Okoye R, Malden JW. Use of neurotransmitter modulation to facilitate
     sensory integration. Neurol Rep, 10:67–72, 1986.
109. Smith RB, Tiberi A, Marshall J. The use of cranial electrotherapy stim-
     ultion in the treatment of closed-head-injured patients. Brain Injury,
     8:357–361, 1994.
110. Childs A, Crimson ML. The use of cranial electrotherapy stimulation
     in post-tranumatic amnesia: A report of two cases. Brain Injury, 2:
     243–247, 1988.
111. Childs A. Fifteen-cycle cranial electrotherapy stimulation for spasticity.
     Brain Injury, 7:179–181, 1993.
112. Mann TI, Silverstone LM. Clinical use of a new electronic dental anes-
     thesia device. J Dental Research, 68:1027–1029, 1989.
113. Clark MS, Silverstone LM, Lindenmuth J et al. An evaluation of the
     clinical analgesia/anthesia efficacy on acute pain using the high fre-
     quency neural modulator in various dental settings. Oral Surg Oral
     Med Oral Pathol, 63:501–505, 1987.
114. Kantor G, Alon G, Ho HS. The effects of selected stimulus waveforms
     on pulse and phase characteristics at sensory and motor thresholds.
     Phys Ther, 74:951–962, 1994.
115. Johnson RM, Kasper S. Compound nerve action potentials produced
     by signals from clinical stimulators. Phys Ther, 66:85, 1986.
116. Taylor K, Newton RA, Personius W et al. Effects of interferential cur-
     rent stimultion for treatment of subjects with recurrent jaw pain. Phys
     Ther, 67:346–350; 1987.
117. Nussbaum E, Rush P, Disenhaus L. The effects of interferential therapy
     on peripheral blood flow. Physiotherapy (Canada), 76:803–807, 1990.
118. Young SL, Woodbury MG, Fryday-Field K et al. Efficacy of interferential
     current stimulation alone for pain reduction in patients with os-
     teoarthritis of the knee: A randomized placebo centrol clinical trial.
     Phys Ther, 71(suppl):252, 1991.
119. Christie AD, Willoughby GL. The effect of interferential therapy on
     swelling following open reduction and internal fixation of ankle frac-
     tures. Physiother Theory Pract, 6:3–7, 1990.
120. Plevney BL, Nutter PB. Comparison of subject comfort using three elec-
     trical stimulation systems. Research project submitted to the depart-
     ment of physical therapy in partial fulfillment of the requirements for
     the master of science degree, University of Southern California, 1981.
121. Gorman PH, Mortimer JT. The effect of stimulus parameters on the re-
     cruitment characteristics of direct nerve stimulation. IEEE Bio Med
     Eng, 30:407–414, 1983.
122. Butikofer R, Lawrence PD. Electrocutaneous nerve stimulation—I:
     Model and experiment. IEEE Bio Med Eng, 26:69–77, 1979.
123. Leo K. Perceived comfort levels of modulated versus conventional
     TENS current. Phys Ther, 64:745, 1984.

124. Barr JO, Weissenbuehler SA, Bandstra EJ et al. Effectiveness and comfort level of transcutaneous electrical nerve stimulation (TENS) for elderly with chronic pain. Phys Ther, 67:775, 1987.

125. Barr JO, Nielsen DH, Soderberg GL. Transcutaneous electrical nerve stimulation characteristics for altering pain perception. Phys Ther, 66:1515–1521, 1986.

126. Leo KC, Dostal WF, Bossen DG et al. Effect of transcutaneous electrical nerve stimulation characteristics on clinical pain. Phys Ther, 66:200–205, 1986.

127. Jette DU. Effect of different forms of transcutaneous electrical nerve stimulation on experimental pain. Phys Ther, 66:187–190, 1986.

128. Meyler WJ, de Jongste MJL, Rolf CAM. Clinical evaluation of pain treatment with electrostimulation: A study on TENS in patients with different pain syndromes. Clin J Pain, 10:22–27, 1994.

129. Mannheimer C, Carlsson CA. The analgesic effect of transcutaneous electrical nerve stimulation (TENS) in patients with rheumatoid arthritis: A comparative study of different pulse patterns. Pain, 6:329–334, 1979.

130. Barr JO, Forrest SE, Potratz PE et al. Effectiveness of transcutaneous electrical nerve stimulation (TENS) in the elderly with chronic pain. Phys Ther, 69:396, 1989.

131. Tulgar M, McGlone F, Bowsher D, Miles JB. Comparative effectiveness of different stimulation modes in relieving pain. Part I. A pilot study. Pain, 47:151–155, 1991.

132. Tulgar M, McGlone F, Bowsher D, Miles JB. Comparative effectiveness of different stimulation modes in relieving pain. Part II. A double-blind controlled long-term clinical trial. Pain, 47:157–162, 1991.

133. Ordog GJ. Transcutaneous electrical nerve stimulation versus oral analgesic: A randomized double-blind controlled study in acute traumatic pain. Am J Emer Med, 5:6–8, 1987.

134. Moystad A, Krogstad BS, Larheim TA. Transcutaneous nerve stimulation in a group of patients with rheumatic disease involving the temporomandibular joint. J Prosth Dent, 64:596–600, 1990.

135. Marchand S, Charest J, Li J, Chenard J-R, Lavignolle B, Laurencelle L. Is TENS purely a placebo effect? A controlled study on chronic low back pain. Pain, 54:99–106, 1993.

136. Ciccone CD. Iontophoresis. In Robinson AJ, Snyder-Mackler L (eds). Clinical Electrophysiology. Baltimore, MD, Williams & Wilkins, pp 347–354, 1995.

137. Costello CT, Jeske AH. Iontophoresis: Applications in transdermal medication delivery. Phys Ther, 75:554–563, 1995.

138. Chantraine A, Ludy JP, Berger D. Is cortisone iontophoresis possible? Arch Phys Med Rehabil, 67:38–40, 1986.

139. Reid KI, Dionne RA, Sicard-Rosenbaum L, Lord D, Dubner RA. Evaluation of iontophoretically applied dexamethasone for painful pathologic temporomandibular joints. Oral Surg Oral Med Oral Pathol, 77:605–609, 1994.

140. Glass JM, Stephen RL, Jacobson SC. The quality and distribution of radiolabeled dexamethasone delivered to tissue by iontophoresis. Int J Dermatol, 19:519–525, 1980.

141. Perron M, Malouin F. Acetic acid iontophoresis and ultrasound for the treatment of calcifying tendinitis of the shoulder: A randomized control trial. Arch Phys Med Rehabil, 78:379–384, 1997.
142. Bertolucci LE. Introduction of anti-inflammatory drugs by iontophoresis: Double blind study. J Orthop Sports Phys Ther, 4:103–108, 1982.
143. Hasson SH, Henderson GH, Daniels JC, Schieb DA. Exercise training and dexamethasone iontophoresis in rheumatoid arthritis: A case study. Physiother Can, 43(2):11–14, 1991.
144. Hasson SM, English SE, Daniels JC, Reich M. Effect of iontophoretically delivered dexamethasone on muscle performance in rheumatoid arthritic joint. Arthritis Care Res, 1(3):177–182, 1988.
145. Bagniefski T, Burnette RR. A comparison of pulsed and continuous current iontophoresis. J Controlled Release, 11:113–122, 1990.
146. Reinauer S, Neusser A, Schauf G, Holzle E. Iontophoresis with alternating current and direct current offset (AC/DC iontophoresis): A new approach for the treatment of hyperhidrosis. Br J Dermatol, 129:166–169, 1993.
147. Siddiqui O, Sun Y, Liu J-C, Chien JW. Facilitated transdermal transport of insulin. J Pharm Sci, 76:341–345, 1987.
148. Okabe K, Yamaguchi H, Kawai Y. New iontophoretic transdermal administration of the beta blocker metoprolol. J Controlled Release, 4:79–85, 1986.
149. Chien YW, Siddiqui Y, Shi WM, Liu JC. Transdermal iontophoretic delivery of therapeutic peptides/proteins. Ann NY Acad Sci, 507:32–51, 1987.
150. McDowell BC, Lowe AS, Walsh DM, Baxter GD, Allen JM. The lack of hypoalgesic efficacy of H-wave therapy on experimental ischemic pain. Pain, 61:27–32, 1995.
151. Pabst HW. Treatment of peripheral circulatory disorders with frequency modulated impulse currents. Arch Phys Ther, Balneologie, 12:230–234, 1960.
152. Mannheimer JS, Lampe GN. Clinical Transcutaneous Electrial Nerve Stimulation. Philadelphia, PA, FA Davis, pp 199–218, 1984.
153. Alon G, DeDomenico G. High Voltage Stimulation: An Integrated Approach to Clinical Electrotherapy. Chattanooga, TN, Chattanooga Corporation, 1987.
154. Oliver GC, Rubin RJ, Salvati EP et al. Electrogalvanic stimulation in the treatment of levator syndrome. Dis Colon Rectum, 28:662–663, 1985.
155. Snyder-Mackler L, Garrett M, Roberts M. A comparison of torque generating capabilities of three different electrical stimulating currents. J Orthop Sport Phys Ther, 11:297–301, 1989.
156. McNeal DR, Baker LL. Effects of joint angle, electrodes and waveform on electrical stimulation of the quadriceps and hamstrings. Ann Biomed Eng, 16:299–310, 1988.
157. Baker LL, Bowman BR, McNeal DR. Effects of waveform on comfort during neuromuscular electrical stimulton. Clin Orthop, 233:75–85, 1988.
158. Laycock J, Green R. Interferential therapy in the treatment of incontinence. Physiotherapy, 74:161–168, 1988.
159. Indergand HJ, Morgan BJ. Effect of interferential current on forearm vascular resistance in asymptomatic humans. Phys Ther, 75:306–312, 1995.

160. Bergslien O, Thoreson M, Odemark H. The effects of three electrotherapeutic methods on blood velocities in human peripheral arteries. Scand J Rehabil Med, 20:29–33, 1988.

161. Sander TC, Schrank EC, Kelln BM, Quillen WS, Sellin R, Underwood FB, Finstuen K. Differences in torque generation by trial and three different waveforms. J Clin Electrophysiol, 6:10–13, 1994.

162. Ward AR. Electricity Fields and Waves in Therapy. Marickville, Australia Science Press, pp 17–33, 1980.

163. Protas EG, Dupny T, Gardea R. Electrical stimulation for strength training. Phys Ther, 64:751–752, 1984.

164. Owoeye I, Spielholz NI, Fetto J et al. Low intensity pulsed galvanic current and the healing of tenotomized rat achilles tendons: Preliminary report using load-to-breaking measurements. Arch Phys Med Rehabil, 68:415–419, 1987.

165. Morris L, Newton RA. Use of high voltage pulsed galvanic stimulation for patient with levator ani syndrome. Phys Ther, 67:1522–1525, 1987.

166. Sohn N, Weinstein MA, Robbins RD. The levator syndrome and its treatment with high voltage electrogalvanic stimulation. Am J Surg, 144:580–582, 1982.

167. Nicosia JF, Abcarian H. Levator syndrome: A treatment that works. Dis Colon Rectum, 28:406–408, 1985.

168. DeGirardi CQ, Seaborne D, Goulet FS et al. The analgesic effect of high voltage galvanic stimulation combined with ultrasound in the treatment of low back pain: A one-group pre-test/post-test study. Physiother Can, 36:327–333, 1984.

169. Balogun JA, Onilari OO, Akeju OA, Marzouk DK. High voltage electrical stimulation in the augmentation of muscle strength: Effects of pulse frequency. Arch Phys Med Rehabil, 74:910–916, 1993.

170. Balogun JA. Pain complaint and muscle soreness associated with high-voltage electrical stimulation: Effect of ramp time. Percep Motor Skills, 62:799–810, 1986.

171. Wong RA. High voltage versus low voltage electrical stimulation: Force of induced muscle contraction and perceived discomfort in healthy subjects. Phys Ther, 66:1209–1214, 1986.

172. LeDoux J, Quinones MA. An investigation of the use of percutaneous electrical stimulation in muscle re-education. Phys Ther, 61:678, 1981.

173. Mohr T, Carlson B, Sulentic C et al. Comparison of isometric experience and high volt galvanic stimultion on quadriceps femoris muscle strength. Phys Ther, 65:606–612, 1985.

174. Alon G. High voltage stimulation: Effects of electrode size on basic excitatory responses. Phys Ther, 65:890–895, 1985.

175. Matteson JH. Cybernetic technology and high-performance athletic training. Nat Strength Condit Assoc J, 6:32–33, 1984.

176. Picker RI. Current trends: Low-volt pulsed microamp stimulation, parts I and II. Clin Management, 9:10–21, 1990.

177. Royal FF. Cybernetics and electro-medicine. J Ultramolec Med, 2:41–44, 1984.

178. Barron JJ, Jacobson WE, Tidd G. Treatment of decubitus ulcers—A new approach. Minn Med, 68:103–106, 1985.

179. Bourguignon GJ, Bourguignon LYW. Electric stimulation of protein and DNA synthesis in human fibroblasts. FASEB J, 1:398–401, 1987.
180. Biedebach MC: Accelerated healing of skin ulcers by electrical stimulation and the intracellular physiological mechanisms involved. Acupunct Electrother Res, 14:43–59, 1989.
181. Lerner FN, Kirsch DL. Microstimulation and placebo effect. J Chiropr, 15:101–106, 1981.
182. Alon G, Fink AM, Anderson PA et al. The effect of subliminal stimulation on elbow flexors strength, fatigue and soreness. Phys Ther, 68:789, 1988.
183. Kulig K, DeYoung L, Maurer C et al. Comparison of the effects high-velocity exercises and microcurrent neuromuscular stimulation on delayed onset muscle soreness. Phys Ther, 71:S115, 1991.
184. Kulig K, Jarski R, Drewek E et al. The effects of microcurrent stimulation on CPK and delayed onset muscle soreness. Phys Ther, 71:S115–116, 1991.
185. Rapaski D, Isles S, Kulig K et al. Microcurrent electrical stimulation: Comparison of two protocols in reducing delayed onset muscle soreness. Phys Ther, 71:S116, 1991.
186. Leffmann DJ, Arnall DA, Holmgren PR, Cornwall MW. Effect of microamperage stimulation on the rate of wound healing in rats: A histological study. Phys Ther, 74:195–200, 1994.
187. Byl NN, McKenzie AL, West JM, Whitney JD, Hunt TK et al. Pulsed microamperage stimulation: A controlled study of healing of surgically induced wounds in Yucatan pigs. Phys Ther, 74:201–219, 1994.
188. Rolle WC, Alon G, Mirschel RP, Sobel J. Comparison of subliminal and placebo stimulation in the management of elbow tendinitis. J Clin Electrophysiol 6:4–9, 1994.
189. Sinnreich MJ, Davis CM, DiSipio LJ et al. Microelectric nerve stimulation (MENS) and coracoacromial arch pain: The effects after one treatment. Phys Ther, 72:S68, 1992.
190. Zizic TM, Hoffman KC, Holt PA et al. The treatment of osteoarthritis of the knee with pulsed electrical stimulation. J Rheumatol, 22:1757–1761, 1995.
191. Wassermann EM. Risk and safety of repetitive transcranial magnetic stimulation: Report and suggested guidelines from the international workshop on the safety of repetitive transcranial magnetic stimulation, June 5–7, 1996. Electroencephalogr Clin Neurophysiol, 108:1–16, 1998.
192. Dymond AM, Coger RW, Serafetinides EA. Intracerebral current levels in man during electrosleep therapy. Biol Psychiatry, 10:101–104, 1975.
193. Rush S, Driscoll DA. Current distribution in the brain from surface electrodes. Anesth Analg, 47:717–723, 1968.
194. Rosenthal SH. Alteration in serum thyroxine with cerebral electrotherapy (electrosleep). Arch Gen Psychiatry, 28:28–29, 1973.
195. Solomon S, Guglielmo KM. Treatment of headache by transcutaneous electrical stimulation. Headache, 25:12–15, 1985.
196. Solomon S, Elkind A, Freitag F et al. Safety and effectiveness of cranial electrotherapy in the treatment of tension headache. Headache, 29:445–450, 1989.

197. Philip P, Demotes-Mainard J, Bourgeois M, Vincent JD. Efficiency of transcranial electrostimulation on anxiety and insomnia symptoms during a washout period in depressed patients; a double-blind study. Biol Psychiatry, 29:451–456, 1991.

198. Syron SC, Alon G. The effects of transcranial electrical stimulation on the functional performance of children with cerebral palsy. Phys Ther, 74(suppl):515, 1994.

199. Schmitt R, Capo T, Boyd E. Cranial electrotherapy stimulation as a treatment for anxiety in chemically dependent persons. Alcoholism: Clin Exper Res, 10:158–160, 1986.

200. Schmitt R, Capo T, Frazier H et al. Cranial electotherapy stimulation treatment of cognitive brain dysfunction in chemical dependence. J Clin Psych, 45:60–63, 1984.

201. Smith RB. Confirming evidence of an effective treatment for brain dysfunction in alcoholic patients. J Nervous Mental Dis, 170:275–278, 1982.

202. Patterson MA, Firth J, Gardiner R. Treatment of drug, alcohol and nicotine addiction by neuroelectric therapy: Analysis of results over 7 years. J Bioelect, 3:193–221, 1984.

203. Matteson MT, Ivancevich JM. An exploratory investigation of CES as an employee stress management technique. J Health Hum Res Admin, 9:93–109, 1986.

204. Gibson TH, O'Hair DE. Cranial application of low level transcranial electrotherapy vs relaxation instruction in anxious patients. Am J Electromed, 1:1821–1825, 1987.

205. Reed BV. Effect of high voltage pulsed electrical stimulation on microvascular permeability to plasma proteins. Phys Ther, 68:491–497, 1988.

206. Stanish WD, Valiant GA, Bonen A et al. The effects of immobilization and electrical stimulation on muscle glycogen and myofibrillar ATPase. Can J Appl Sport Sci, 7:267–271, 1982.

207. Theriault R, Theriault G, Simoneau J-A. Human skeletal muscle adapatation in response to chronic low-frequency electrical stimulation. J Appl Physiol, 77:1885–1889, 1994.

208. Gauthier JM, Theriault R, Theriault G, Gelinas Y, Simoneau J-A. Electrical stimulation-induced changes in skeletal muscle enzymes of men and women. Med Sci Sports Exer, 24:1252–1256, 1992.

209. Martin TP, Stein RB, Hoeppner PH, Reid DC. Influence of electrical stimulation on the morphological and metabolic properties of paralyzed muscle. J Appl Physiol, 72:1401–1406, 1992.

210. Kim CK, Bangsbo J, Strange S, Karpakka J, Saltin B. Metabolic response and muscle glycogen depletion pattern during prolonged electrically induced dynamic exercise in man. Scand J Rehabil Med, 27:51–58, 1995.

211. Soderlund K, Greenhaff PL, Hultman E. Energy metabolism in type I and type II human muscle fibres during short term electrical stimulation at different frequencies. Acta Physiol Scand, 144:15–22, 1992.

212. Jehle H. Charge fluctuation forces in biological systems. Ann NY Acad Sci, 158:240–246, 1969.

213. Wang Q, Zhong S, Ouyang J et al. Osteogenesis of electrically stimulated bone cells mediated in part by calcium ions. Clin Orthop, 348:259–268, 1998.

214. Brighton CT, Shaman P, Heppenstall RB et al. Tibial nonunion treated with direct current, capacitative coupling, or bone graft. Clin Orthop, 321:223–234, 1995.

215. Nogami H, Aoki H, Okagawa T et al. Effects of electric current on chrondrogenesis in vitro. Clin Orthop Relat Res, 163:243–245, 1982.

216. Franke A, Reding R, Tessmann D. Electrostimulation of healing abdoinal incisional hernias by low frequency, bipolar, symmetrical rectangular pulses. Acta Chir Scand 156:701–705, 1990.

217. Fujita M, Hukuda S, Doida Y. The effect of constant direct electrical current on intrinsic healing in the flexor tendon in vitro. J Hand Surg, 17B:94–98, 1992.

218. Wang B, Tang J, White PF et al. Effect of the intensity of transcutaneous acupoint electrical stimulation on the postoperative analgesic requirement. Anesth Analg, 85:406–413, 1997.

219. Al-Mohanna FA, Caddy KWT, Bolsover SR. The nucleus is insolated from large cytosolic calcium ion changes. Nature, 367:745–750, 1994.

220. Newton RA, Karselis TC. Skin pH following high voltage pulsed galvanic stimulation. Phys Ther, 63:1593–1596, 1983.

221. Alon G, Allin J, Inbar GE. Optimization of pulse charge during transcutaneous electrical stimulation. Aust J Physiother, 29:195–201, 1983.

222. Alon G, Kantor G, Ho HS. The effect of three types of surface electrodes on threshold excitation of human motor nerve. J Clin Electrophysiol, 8:2–8, 1996.

223. Knaflitz M, Merletti R, De Luca CJ. Inference of motor unit recruitment order in voluntary and electrically elicited contractions. J Appl Physiol, 68:1657–1667, 1990.

224. Grill WM, Mortimer JT. Stimulus waveforms for selective neural stimulation. IEEE Eng Med Biol, 14:375–385, 1995.

225. Grimby G, Wigerstad-Lossing I. Comparison of high- and low-frequency muscle stimulators. Arch Phys Med Rehabil, 70:835–838, 1989.

226. Synder-Mackler L, Binder-Macleod SA, Williams P. Fatigability of the human quadriceps femoris muscle following anterior cruciate ligament reconstruction. Med Sci Sport Exer, 25:783–789, 1993.

227. Binder-Macleod SA, Synder-Mackler L. Muscle fatigue: Clinical implication for fatigue assessment and neuromuscular electrical stimulation. Phys Ther, 73:902–910, 1993.

228. Mannheimer C, Carlsson CA, Emanuelsson H et al. The effects of transcutaneous electrical nerve stimulation in patients with severe angina pectoris. Circulation, 71:308–316, 1985.

229. Mannheimer C, Carlsson CA, Vedin A, Wilhelmsson C. Transcutaneous electrical nerve stimultion (TENS) in angina pectoris. Pain, 26:291–300, 1986.

230. Nitz J, Cheras F. Transcutaneous electrical nerve stimulation for angina pectoris. Aust J Physiother, 39:109–113, 1993.

231. Rasmussen MB, Andersen C, Andersen P, Frandsen F. Cost-benefit analysis of electric stimulation of the spinal cord in the treatment of angina pectoris. Ugeskrift For Laeger, 154:1180–1184, 1992.

232. Vulpio C. Transcutaneous electrical nerve stimulation in the prevention of postoperative ileus and pain. Chir Patol Sper (Italy), 36:3–13, 1988.

233. Akyuz G, Kayhan O, Babacan A, Gener FA. Transcutaneous electrical nerve stimulation (TENS) in the treatment of postoperative pain and prevention of paralytic ileus. Clin Rehabil, 7:218–221, 1993.

234. Twist DJ, Culpepper-Morgan JA, Ragnarsson KT et al. Neuroendocrine changes during functional electrical stimulation. Am J Phys Med Rehabil, 71:156–163, 1992.

235. Pandit JJ, Bergstrom E, Frankel HL, Robbins PA. Increased hypoxic ventilatory sensitivity during exercise in man: Are neural afferents necessary? J Physiol, 477:169–175, 1994.

236. Pandit JJ, Robbins PA. Acute ventilatory responses to hypoxia during voluntary and electrically induced leg exercise in man. J Physiol, 477:161–168, 1994.

237. Phillips CA. Functional electrical stimulation and lower extremity bracing for ambulation exercises of spinal cord injured individual: A medically prescribed system. Phys Ther, 69:842–850, 1989.

238. Hecker B, Carron H, Schwartz DP. Pulsed galvanic stimulation: Effects of current frequency and polarity on blood flow in healthy subjects. Arch Phys Med Rehabil, 66:369–374, 1986.

239. Walker DC, Currier DP, Threlkeld AJ. Effects of high voltage pulsed electrical stimulation on blood flow. Phys Ther, 68:481–485, 1988.

240. Wong RA, Jette DV. Changes in sympathetic tone associated with different forms of transcutaneous electrical nerve stimultion in healthy subjects. Phys Ther, 64:478–482, 1984.

241. Balogun JA, Tang S, He Y et al. Effects of high-voltage galvanic stimulation of ST36 and ST37 acupuncture points on peripheral blood flow and skin temperature. Disabil Rehabil, 18:523–528, 1996.

242. Indergand HJ, Morgan BJ. Effects of high-frequency transcutaneous electrical nerve stimulation on limb blood flow in healthy humans. Phys Ther, 74:361–367, 1994.

243. Shannon RV. A model of safe levels for electrical stimulation. IEEE Bio Med Eng, 39:424–426, 1992.

244. Lambert HL. Influence of skin resistance and current distribution on tolerance during galvanic therapy. Eur J Phys Med Rehabil, 4:186–189, 1994.

245. Neumayer C, Happak W, Kern H, Gruber H. Hypertrophy and transformation of muscle fibers in paraplegic patients. Artificial Organs, 21:188–190, 1997.

246. Adams GR, Harris RT, Woodard D, Dudley GA. Mapping of electrical muscle stimulation using MRI. J Appl Physiol, 74:532–537, 1993.

247. Alon G, McCombe SA, Koutsantonis S et al. Comparison of the effects of electical stimulation and exercise on the abdominal musculature. J Orthop Sports Phys Ther, 8:567–573, 1987.

248. Alon G, Frederickson R, Gallager L et al. Electrical stimulation of the abdominals: The effects of three versus five weekly treatments. J Clin Electrophysiol, 4:5–11, 1992.

249. Alon G, Taylor DJ. Electrically elicited minimal visible tetanic contraction and its effect on abdominal muscles strength and endurance. Eur J Phys Med Rehabil, 7:2–6, 1997.

250. Ferguson JP, Blackley MW. Knight RD et al. Effects of varying electrode site placements on the torque output of an electrically stimulated invol-

untary quadriceps femoris msucle contraction. J Orthop Sports Phys Ther, 9:24–29, 1989.

251. Pareilleux A, Sicard N. Lethal effects of electrical current on *Escherichia coli.* Appl Microbiol, 19:421–424, 1970.

252. Spadaro JA, Berges TJ, Barranco SD et al. Antibacterial effects of silver electrodes with weak direct current. Antimicrob Agents Chemother, 6:637–642, 1974.

253. Bolton L, Foleno B, Means B et al. Direct current bactericidal effect on intact skin. Antimicrob Agents Chemother, 18:137–141, 1980.

254. Rowley BA, McKenna JM, Chase GR. The influence of electrical current on an infecting micro-organism in wounds. Ann NY Acad Sci, 238:543–551, 1974.

255. Barranco SD, Spadaro JA, Berger TJ et al. In vitro effect of weak direct current on *Staphylococcus aureus.* Clin Orthop, 100:250–255, 1974.

256. Kincaid CB, Llavoie KH. Inhibition of bacterial growth in vitro following stimulation with high voltage, monophasic, pulse current. Phys Ther, 69:651–655, 1989.

257. Szuminsky NJ, Albers AC, Unger P, Eddy JG. Effect of narrow, pulsed high voltages on bacterial viability. Phys Ther, 74:660–667, 1994.

258. Guffy JS, Asmussen MD. In vitro bactericidal effects of high voltage pulsed current versus direct current against *Staphylococcus aureus.* J Clin Electrophysiol, 1:5–9, 1989.

259. Laatsch LJ, Ong PC, Kloth LC. In vitro effects of two silver electrodes on select wound pathogens. J Clin Electrophysiol, 7:10–15, 1995.

# Section Two

## Clinical Applications of Electrotherapy

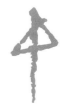

# Electrical Stimulation for Improving Muscle Performance

Jessie Van Swearingen

## Introduction

C linical electrotherapy refers to the application of electricity directly to the body to produce a desired therapeutic goal or outcome—in this case, enhanced muscle performance. The best chance of ensuring the desired outcome of intervention (improved muscle performance) will be achieved requires that the clinician first be able to (1) accurately define the impaired characteristics of muscle performance, and (2) identify the disability associated with the muscular impairment. Specifics of the electrical stimulation applied to improve muscle performance vary with the aspect of muscle performance that is the target of intervention. For example, the characteristics of **neuromuscular electrical stimulation (NMES)** that would enhance maximal muscle force production are different from the characteristics for improving muscle relaxation.

Furthermore, the efficacy of NMES as an intervention for individuals with impairments of muscle performance is best demonstrated in the alleviation of problems at the level of the person, or disability as defined by the World Health Organization's International Classification of Impairments, Disability, and Handicaps (ICIDH).[1] Little has been done to document the relationship be-

143

tween impairments and disability, leaving the practicing clinician the challenge of validating practice with every intervention.

## THE PATIENT'S PROBLEM AND EXPECTATIONS

Consider the patient with unilateral facial paresis stemming from the onset of Bell's palsy three months previous to the start of care in physical therapy. The physical therapist uses NMES to facilitate facial neuromuscular recovery, and the force of the facial muscles improves (reduction of the impairment), but the patient is unable to produce the patterned muscle activity of the facial expression of a smile recognized by others as an indication of the patient's joy or happiness (persisting disability). If the use of NMES has helped the patient raise the corner of the mouth toward the ear (a component movement of a smile) twice as far as before intervention but the patient's problem—inability to communicate joy through facial expressions—persists, then the use of NMES in rehabilitation for facial paresis associated with Bell's palsy is of questionable value.

## EVALUATION

To achieve the intended therapeutic outcome, the therapist must have at least (1) a picture in his or her mind of what must occur at the tissue level as a result of the application of NMES, (2) a means of measuring the effect on muscle performance of the electrically elicited tissue response, and (3) some measure of the impact on the patient's problems. Given the above process, the physical therapist would know if the objectives of intervention using NMES were met at the impairment level (eg, change in muscle strength) or the disability level (eg, recognizable smile). In addition, if the facial muscle force improved (eg, as measured by the increased excursion of facial movements) to match the movement excursion of the uninvolved side of the face and the facial expressions of emotion remained distorted, the clinician has the information to determine that NMES for increasing facial muscle force is not an appropriate intervention for the treatment of unilateral facial paresis.

Differentially, if the NMES applied to facilitate facial muscle force results in no improvement in the excursion of facial movements, then an appropriate process of clinical decision making might be to first question whether the characteristics of the applied electrical stimulation elicited the intended neuromuscular tissue response. Could the characteristics of NMES be adjusted to achieve the desired tissue and performance outcomes? If the desired muscle performance and disability outcomes are not achieved, then the continued application of NMES is a means of keeping the patient busy, not an intervention.

Electrotherapy in the clinical practice of enhancing neuromuscular performance has exploded over the last 20 years in the United States. Prior to the mid-1970s, electrical stimulation was used primarily to treat denervation atrophy in skeletal muscles.[2,3] The tremendous proliferation of equipment with a broad array of stimulating current characteristics places the clinician in the role of "designer." The days of one machine and one treatment should be gone. The equipment of today affords the clinician the option to design waveforms of the stimulating current best suited to produce the tissue effects associated with the desired treatment outcomes. Knowing characteristics of muscle and nerve cell responses to an electrical impulse and principles of neurophysiologic function, the physical therapist can apply a systematic process to the task of choosing the characteristics of electrical stimulation to match the desired outcome of intervention.

# DIAGNOSIS: THE PHYSIOLOGIC BASIS FOR NMES

## Review of Peripheral Neuromuscular Physiology

Electrical impulses in the nerve fiber travel as action potentials from the site of generation to the axon terminal at the synapse with the target muscle or neuron. For the motor nerve, the action potential generated in the membrane of the initial segment or axon hillock of the axon by a change in the electrical potential of the membrane is sufficient to bring the membrane potential to threshold for generating one or a number of action potentials. The action potential is continuously self-regenerated along the length of the axon, leaving a momentary wave of hyperpolarization (decreased electrical excitability) behind as the impulse travels to the axon terminal. Neurotransmitter is released from the axon terminal in response to the change in the terminal calcium concentration, resulting from the action potential–mediated depolarization of the terminal membrane. Neurotransmitter diffuses across the synaptic cleft and binds to a receptor on the muscle cell membrane of the motor endplate. If the depolarization of the endplate resulting from neurotransmitter-receptor binding is adequate, one or a number of muscle action potentials are generated in the muscle membrane (sarcolemma). Excitation–contraction coupling of muscle (muscle contraction) occurs if the muscle action potential change is conducted to the interior of the muscle fiber by the transverse tubule system, and calcium stored in the terminal cisternae is released into the sarcoplasm of the muscle cell surrounding the myofibril (the ordered array of muscle contractile proteins).[4,5]

## Physiology of Electrically Elicited Responses

Electrical stimulation applied across the surface of the skin over a portion of the intact peripheral neuromuscular system can evoke an action potential in a muscle or nerve fiber identical to the physiologically generated potentials. The evoked potential is identical, and the action potential is conducted in the same manner except the evoked potential travels in both directions along the nerve fiber from the initial stimulation site. The electrically elicited potential generated at a point along the peripheral nerve fiber does not have a wave of hyperpolarization "behind" to prevent the bidirectional spread of the current. Consequently, stimulation of a peripheral motor nerve fiber results in orthodromic (physiologic direction of spread of the potential change) conduction of the impulse toward the neuromuscular junction and antidromic conduction (impulse travel opposite physiologic direction) toward the ventral horn, motor neuron cell body.

The evoked action potential in the peripheral alpha motor axon results in a muscle contraction that also appears to be the same as a voluntary physiologic muscle contraction. However, the order of recruitment of motor units differs for electrically elicited contractions[6–8]; thus, the type and number of motor units active and the fatigability of the evoked muscle contraction will differ from voluntary muscle contractions.[9]

Because NMES often involves stimulating peripheral nerves with a mixture of motor and sensory axons or stimulation of muscle nerves anatomically close to sensory nerve branches, mention of the sensory nerve response to electrical stimulation is appropriate. Stimulation of sensory nerve fibers elicits action potentials identical to action potentials generated by stimulation of other nerve fibers and by the physiologic activation. However, the physiologic pattern of activation differs, as stimulating the sensory nerve fiber bypasses the encoding of the stimulus by the sensory receptor.

In addition to differences in motor unit recruitment and patterns of activation, electrical stimulation over a peripheral nerve evokes action potentials in all axons within the peripheral nerve: autonomic, motor nerve, and sensory fibers. Therefore, the electrically elicited intense muscle contraction is frequently accompanied by an intense sensory perception such as pain.[10] Thoughtful selection and subtle adjustments of the characteristics of the stimulating current can result in some degree of biased recruitment of specific nerve fibers, reducing the discomfort while still achieving components of the desired motor response. However, studies of subjects' reports of discomfort with various current waveforms suggests that individuals differ in their perception of comfort with each waveform.[10,11] Delitto et al[12] studied the influence of individual behavioral factors and current factors, finding the individual's coping style, perception of amplitude, or unpleasantness of the stimulation, as well as whether the stimulation evoked a muscle contraction, to be important factors in determining the individual's discomfort with NMES.

## PROGNOSIS: RECRUITMENT OF NERVE AND MUSCLE

For the excitable cells of the neuromuscular system, some combination of stimulus amplitude and duration will depolarize the cell membrane to threshold for action potential generation. Both large-amplitude, short-duration electrical stimuli and small-amplitude, long-duration stimuli can excite the neuromuscular system. The activation of peripheral nerve fibers is orders of magnitude easier than activating isolated (denervated) muscle fibers.[13] Electrical stimulation applied across the skin of a person with a neuromuscular system intact from the motor neuron to the muscle elicits the muscle contraction via the nerve to the muscle. The placement of the stimulating electrodes directly over the muscle does not alter the sequence of tissue excitability. The muscle response occurs by excitation of the muscle nerve to the muscle fibers because of the much greater ease of excitability of neural tissue.

Theoretically, nerve fibers also differ in their ease of activation. When an electrical stimulus of a given pulse duration and frequency is used, as the amplitude of the stimulus is increased, axons within a nerve are progressively recruited by size of the fiber. The axons of largest diameter are the easiest to activate and are recruited before axons of smaller diameter. The recruitment of motor units by electrical stimulation progresses from large to smaller nerve fibers,[6–8] the reverse of the order of voluntary contractions governed by Heneman's Size Principle (small to large motor units).[14] Physiologically, the reverse order means the fast fatigue (FF) units are recruited before fast fatigue resistant (FR), which are recruited before the slow (S) motor units. However, Sinacore et al[15] demonstrated preferential activation of fast-twitch fibers of the FR motor unit, over activation of muscle fibers of the FF or S motor units, following 50 electrically elicited isometric muscle contractions at 80 percent of the individual's maximal voluntary isometric contraction (MVIC) peak torque (previously determined). The investigators suggested the electrical stimulation may activate some superficial, small flexion reflex afferent fibers, which have a biased input to the FR motoneurons in the spinal cord.[15]

The reversal of recruitment order for electrically elicited contractions has several implications for designing interventions to facilitate neuromuscular performance. Electrical stimulation potentially provides a means of preferentially recruiting more fast motor units than would usually be activated for a voluntary contraction. Thus, use of NMES may be possible to bias exercise training toward a specific motor unit, particularly the larger motor units. Also, fatigue may occur more rapidly as a greater proportion of the fatigable motor units are recruited for a given level of motor unit recruitment.[16] The ability to bias an exercise intervention toward recruitment of more fast motor units may be a clinical advantage in treating individuals with disorders known to have a preferential impairment of fast-twitch muscle fibers. For example, a disproportionate impairment of fast-twitch muscle fibers has been recognized in aged individuals,[17] individuals exposed to high or sustained steroid drug therapy, individuals with a history of alcohol abuse, and individuals with end-stage renal disease and rheumatoid arthritis, to name a few.[18]

Finally, clinicians might consider whether the combination of electrical stimulation and voluntary muscle contraction produces greater muscle force than either electrical stimulation or voluntary contraction alone. Theoretically, the electrical stimulation should be recruiting some different motor units not activated at a given moment by voluntary recruitment[6,15,19–21] (see Summary).

The nature of the response to NMES will be different depending on the type of nerve fibers recruited. If fast motor units are preferentially recruited more often than for voluntary contractions, then the rate of rise and fall of tension of the twitch response of the muscle will be more rapid than for the voluntary contraction.[22] Voluntary contractions involve more slow motor units for which the rate of rise and fall of twitch tension is more gradual.[23] Clinically, electrically elicited whole muscle contractions may lack the smooth, graded onset of voluntary contractions, reflecting not only the biased motor unit recruitment, but also the synchronous recruitment of motor units.[23–25] Voluntary contractions involve asynchronous activation brought about by segmental reflexes, allowing for a smooth switching between active and inactive motor units to maintain the muscle activity, while allowing recovery time for individual motor units that were previously activated.[26] Electrically stimulated contractions activate motor units by size of the axon and proximity to the stimulating electrode. Thus, all axons of the same size and relative distance from electrode are activated synchronously.[24,25] Muscle fatigue occurs rapidly with electrically stimulated contractions involving preferential and synchronous activation of the more readily fatigable fibers.[16,23,24] In certain clinical conditions, such as the individual with marked muscle spasm that is limiting movement and producing discomfort, the fatiguing effects of NMES may be useful in reducing the impairment, not a detriment to the outcome of the intervention.

Modulating the rate of activation by adjusting pulses per second (pps) or frequency in cycles per second (cps) can be helpful in avoiding early or excessive fatigue, while optimizing electrically elicited muscle performance. Twitch contractions of muscle fibers produced at rates of activation of 1 to 5 pps become tetanic (like voluntary contractions) with higher stimulation rates of 25 to 30 pps. Certainly, the higher the frequency of stimulation, the greater the frequency of activation of active motor units, and the greater the force production.[27] Burke et al[28] demonstrated a marked facilitation of the force output of muscle following the second of two closely spaced stimuli, a phenomenon of muscle known as the *catch-like property*. Specific variations of the rate of activation of motor units hold promise for optimizing electrically elicited muscle perfomance.[16,27,29]

## INTERVENTION: CLINICAL DECISION MAKING

### Choosing the Current Waveform for NMES

In today's market, the variety of currents with subtly different characteristics illustrated by the current time plots of the waveforms enables the physical therapist a great degree of flexibility in selecting the stimulus characteristics to achieve the desired therapeutic response. Choosing wisely from the options, the therapist can theoretically enhance effectiveness by customizing characteristics of the stimulating current to optimize the therapeutic outcome and enhance patient comfort and satisfaction (Table 4–1). The following discussion and scenarios demonstrate some of the clinical decision making that may be involved.

First, if the intent is to stimulate innervated muscle, as in NMES to facilitate muscle performance, then the potentially useful waveforms should have (1) a rapid rate of change and (2) a short pulse duration to target primarily the muscle nerve fibers. The next stage of decision making depends on the targeted therapeutic outcome, and what type of muscle contraction of innervated muscle is congruent ("fits") with the goals for the outcome of intervention.

### NMES to Reduce Impairment of Muscle Force

Increased muscle force or tension production is best achieved with intense tetanic contractions of muscle. The greatest force of muscle contraction is produced with the maximum number of motor units

| TABLE 4-1. | BRIEF SUMMARY OF EFFECTS OF INCREASING SPECIFIC CHARACTERISTICS OF NMES | |
|---|---|---|
| **Characteristics of NMES Increased** | **Effect on Neuromuscular Tissues[a]** | **Change in Performance** |
| Amplitude | 1. Stimulate nerve fibers and recruit motor units at a greater depth from the surface of the skin<br>2. Stimulate nerve fibers of progressively smaller diameter (ie, A-alpha, A-beta, B, C, A-delta)<br>3. Recruit motor units of progressively smaller size (ie, FF, FR, S) | 1. Increased force production, increased fatigue<br>2. Increased force production, increased sensory perception of the stimulus<br>3. Increased force production, increased time to peak tension |
| Pulse duration | 1. Stimulate nerve fibers of progressively smaller diameter, at a given amplitude<br>2. Recruit motor units of progressively smaller size<br>3. Increased magnitude of tissue reactions (ie, polar effects) to stimulating currents delivering a net charge | 1. Increased force production, increased sensory perception of the stimulus<br>2. Increased force production, increased time to peak tension, little or no change in fatigue |
| Rate of activation (frequency) | 1. Progressive increase in the firing rate of stimulated nerve fibers<br>2. For motor axons: progressive change of muscle response from twitch to unfused tetany to fused tetany<br>3. Slight decrease in threshold for activation of impulse in the nerve fiber | 1. Increased force production, increased rate of fatigue with high-intensity stimulation<br>2. Increased force production, smoothing of muscle contraction from brief twitch to sustained contraction<br>3. Increased force production (at a given intensity and rate) |
| Peak current[b] | Evoke the neuromuscular tissue effects of the current at greater depths of the tissue | Increased magnitude of the evoked response |
| Average current[b] | Usually little or no change in neuromuscular tissue effects | Increased thermal and physiochemical (polar) effects |

[a] Numbers in this column correspond to numbers in the column to the right.
[b] Given characteristics of the chosen current; not characteristics directly increased or decreased using the machine controls.

responding and motor units firing at their highest rate of activation.[23] A current waveform with a high peak current enables a greater depth of stimulation, increasing the potential number of motor units responding, and a high pulse rate or frequency maximizes firing rate of recruited motor units.[30,31] The pulse duration should be short, because the target fibers are motor axons with the lowest threshold for activation (members of the A-alpha, largest size class). The higher the amplitude tolerated, the greater will be the number of responding motor units, usually at increasing depths from the surface electrode. The short duration pulse, particularly if less than 200 μsec, is unlikely to evoke impulses in the smaller C and A-delta pain fibers that may reduce the patient's tolerance for increasing stimulus amplitude.[32] The shortest pulse duration that activates motor nerve fibers might seem ideal, but at least in theory, the shortest duration may selectively activate only the largest of the motor axons (FF only), thus leaving many motor units of the generally mixed motor unit composition of human muscle inactive. Therefore, pulse durations greater than the shortest that evokes a response are used in NMES for increasing muscle force.

The biphasic triangular (sawtooth) waveform, delivered in 300 msec bursts, with an intraburst frequency of 2500 Hz and a rate of activation of 50 bursts per second (bps), fits the criteria for increasing muscle force with NMES. The sawtooth waveform has a high peak current and a low average current, enhancing tolerance for high-amplitude stimulation. The biphasic pulses of the sawtooth waveform meet the nervous system's desire for a rapid rate of change, and the high frequency of the pulses within each burst reduces the risk of accommodation of the axons. The short duration of each pulse explains why the total amount of current delivered to the tissue remains low, while still achieving the high rate of activation of active motor units. Furthermore, the symmetric, balanced biphasic pulses of the sawtooth bursts result in no net current charge (ie, polar or DC effects) delivered to the tissues. The polar effects of a current can result in tissue reactions, limiting repeated use of electrical stimulation (eg, skin irritation) or contraindications for the use of NMES in some patients (eg, electrolyte imbalance). Because of the characteristics of the sawtooth waveform current, commonly known as *Russian current* or medium frequency stimulation, the outcome of NMES appropriately applied with this current type is primarily used for increasing muscle force.[19,33]

Other pulsed current waveforms, although perhaps not as ideal, would be applicable for NMES for increasing muscle force. The symmetric, biphasic rectangular waveform delivered at a high rate and high amplitude, should recruit very similar motor units and produce a similar muscle contraction. The pulse duration of the peak current is the same as for the average current of the pulse and greater than the pulse duration at peak current for the sawtooth waveform of the same average current. The greater pulse duration for any given peak current level means more total current (the characteristic the patient feels) delivered at any one moment using the biphasic rectangular, and perhaps more discomfort at the same amplitude. Therefore, at tolerable amplitudes, the peak current of the biphasic rectangular waveform is likely to be less, and thus the depth of stimulation less, and the number of motor units recruited fewer. The lack of within burst, high-frequency modulation (characteristic of the pulsed sawtooth waveform) may allow some motor units to accommodate to the biphasic rectangular pulse, resulting in a decrease in number of or firing rate of the electrically recruited motor units. The symmetric, biphasic rectangular waveform, like the sawtooth, delivers no net charge to the tissues beneath the electrodes, and thus NMES using these waveforms could be considered the most efficient form of NMES, specifically eliciting a response of neuromuscular tissues.

Improving muscle force through recruiting many motor units, at maximal or near-maximal firing rates, is also possible with the twin-peak, paired-pulse waveform typically used for high-voltage, pulsed-current stimulation in wound healing. In general, the rapid rate of change and short pulse durations, combined with customized settings for a high rate of activation, are desirable for NMES. The high peak current and low average current of the twin-peak, paired-pulse waveform enables the increased depth of stimulation at higher amplitudes to still be tolerable for the patient. The range of pulse durations for the paired pulse may be restricted to durations too short to recruit a quorum of motor units of varying sizes, activating only those with the lowest threshold and limiting maximal recruitment for increasing muscle force.[34] As a unidirectional current, the paired pulse does produce polar effects, and the potential for tissue effects other than NMES exists. Although the polar effects may be a disadvantage if the tissue reactions are not tolerated by the patient, unidirectional current has been shown to alter tissue permeability (electro-osmosis), facilitating absorption of inflammation or blocking the formation of edema.[35] For certain subacute conditions, such as postsurgical ligament repairs, arthrotomy, or muscle strain, the dual facilitation of increasing muscle force and control of inflammation possible through NMES using a pulsed, unidirectional current may be desirable.

The symmetric and asymmetric current waveforms typical of traditional alternating current (AC) clinical generators and the battery-powered, portable home units should be capable (given selection of appropriate pulse durations and rates of activation) of eliciting neuromuscular responses and related outcomes of intervention equivalent to the responses and outcomes achieved with present-day, standard clinical generators delivering the bursting, 2500 Hz, biphasic triangular waveform. However, results of a randomized, controlled clinical trial of increasing quadriceps femoris muscle force for functional recovery after reconstruction of the anterior cruciate ligament (ACL) indicated that NMES of the quadriceps using the battery-powered home unit was less effective than NMES using the current waveform produced by the clinical generators.[36] Several features of

NMES using the low-amplitude stimulators are important in understanding the reduced impact on the impairment of (quadriceps) muscle force and consequently disability (difficulty walking) described for the patients in rehabilitation following ACL reconstruction. First, consider whether the outcomes the investigators reported are directly related to the equipment used and the specific stimulation waveform, or more directly associated with the differences in the exercise intervention electrically elicited, or a combination of stimulator and the evoked exercise.

The stimulation characteristics for the clinical generator and battery-powered units were different in the study of functional recovery following ACL reconstruction.[36] Consequently, the pattern of recruitment of motor units would also have been different for the two treatment groups. For example, the high peak current and low average current of the clinical generator enabled a high-amplitude stimulation, whereas the equivalent peak and average current of the battery-powered unit enabled low-amplitude stimulation. The higher peak current and low average current of the clinical generator stimulation would be expected to result in a greater depth of stimulation and better tolerance for increasing the amplitude of the stimulus. The increased depth and amplitude of the high-amplitude stimulation enables the recruitment of more motor units, preferentially of the largest, FF motor unit type. The high-amplitude stimulation was also delivered at a higher frequency (75 bps) than the low-amplitude (55 pps), implying a greater rate of activation of the activated motor units for the high-amplitude than for the low-amplitude condition.[36]

The characteristics of the electrical stimulation applied in the two conditions would have been expected to result in a greater number of motor units, particularly of the largest type, firing at a greater rate in the high-amplitude condition compared to the low-amplitude, battery-powered home unit treatment condition. The expected outcome of performing muscle contractions at higher levels of motor unit recruitment is greater force production, as demonstrated by the quadriceps femoris recovery (70 percent of uninvolved for the high-amplitude NMES group versus 51 percent for the low-amplitude NMES group).

Clearly, the investigators determined the effectiveness of the high-amplitude NMES compared with the commonly practiced low-amplitude home NMES protocol for post-ACL reconstruction rehabilitation,[36] not the efficacy of NMES using the battery-powered generators. To determine the efficacy of the battery-powered equipment for use in post-ACL reconstruction rehabilitation would require that an equivalent amplitude of neuromuscular performance be produced by use of the clinical and battery-powered home generators, regardless of the current waveforms delivered.

Before dismissing home NMES, consider whether an equivalent intensity neuromuscular contraction can be elicited by battery-powered home NMES units. The manner by which amplitude of the stimulus is increased for many of the portable units may prohibit equivalent intensity of the neuromuscular response or at least the clinician's ability to know that equivalent characteristics have indeed been delivered. Increasing the amplitude on the unit is often electronically achieved within the unit by some combination of increasing the amplitude of the stimulus and the pulse duration. Thus, the delivered waveform may be delivering more current, but of characteristics that recruit more motor units (and likely smaller pain and other sensory fibers, as well) at the same depth of stimulation, not more motor units at greater depths of the muscle. For bulky muscles or muscles with multiple compartments at various depths from the surface of the skin, such as the quadriceps femoris, the depth of stimulation may be important for maximal recruitment. In addition, as hinted above, the increase in pulse duration increases the potential for recruitment of the smaller pain fibers, thereby reducing the patient's tolerance for subsequent increases in intensity.

The typical pulse duration available on the battery-powered home units (300 μsec and greater) is in a range adequate for stimulating the smaller pain fibers, and may be a reason individuals using the units do not tolerate as high an amplitude of stimulation as may be necessary to elicit the intensity of neuromuscular response required for the better quadriceps femoris recovery demonstrated for individuals receiving high-amplitude NMES.

Many of the presently available battery-powered home units provide pulsed, symmetric biphasic or asymmetric-balanced biphasic waveforms, but with a large phase charge (secondary to the relatively long pulse durations) or inaccurate balancing of the negative and positive phases, resulting in the delivery of a net charge to the tissues. Skin irritation and unpleasant sensations seem more common with the use of the portable units and particularly at higher amplitudes of NMES, further limiting the ability to implement the equivalent dosage of the high-amplitude NMES produced by the clinical generators.

The limitations of the characteristics of NMES, desired for the high-intensity exercise training necessary for maximizing the recovery of muscle force production and the rate of recovery of force in the rehabilitation of individuals with muscle force deficits, may have been appropriately designed for the portable home stimulation units. Manufacturers (and clinicians if the option was available in the home units recommended) who are aware of the potential for tissue effects and the force of muscle contractions elicited by NMES might be understandably reluctant to enable individuals with muscle force deficits (eg, post–reconstructive surgery for repair of musculoskeletal tissues) to perform this aspect of the rehabilitation unsupervised.

To summarize briefly, NMES appears to be an effective component of a clinical intervention for the impairment of weakness, given that the characteristics of the electrical stimulation are chosen to produce high-intensity muscle activation. An increase in the ability of the activated muscle unit to produce force occurs when the muscle is consistently activated above the usual level of activation for that muscle (principle of overload).[37] Voluntary muscle contractions producing force output in the range of 60 to 70 percent of the MVIC force have been demonstrated to produce increases in muscle force[37,38] that would be expected to be clinically meaningful (eg, a level of increasing muscle force associated with a reduction of disability). Therapeutic electrical currents that recruit many motor units (and particularly the largest) at a high rate of activation are most effective for NMES for improving muscle force.[19,30] The so-called Russian current is an example of the characteristics of stimulation effective in improving muscle force; other current waveforms with appropriately selected characteristics may be shown to be equally or more effective.

One characteristic of the high-amplitude NMES for improving muscle force, which may be a limiting factor in the amount of force gain possible or the rate of muscle force increases, is the high pulse or bursting rate. The high rate of activation of an electrically elicited contraction, which preferentially involves the more rapidly fatiging motor units, leads to rapid and marked neuromuscular fatigue. Recently Binder-Macleod et al[16] demonstrated greater force production over a series of 30 electrically elicited, intense muscle contractions by progressively reducing the rate of stimulation during the session. A few commercially available electrical simulators (certainly more will soon be on the market) offer variable-frequency current options. Varying the rate of activation over a session, the clinician may be able to further improve outcomes of high-amplitude NMES applications for improving muscle force.

## NMES to Reduce Impairment of Local Muscle Endurance

The usefulness of NMES in enhancing the endurance aspect of muscle performance, or the ability of the neuromuscular system to produce force over a prolonged period of time, is less well documented.[39,40] Little evidence exists to suggest that NMES provides any more benefit than endurance exercise alone; however, the clinical investigations are lacking. Selectively enhancing the endurance performance of the fast-twitch muscle fibers may be a possibility. Using histochemical staining of vastus lateralis muscle biopsy samples, Sinacore et al[15] demonstrated differential activation of the FR motor units following a brief (5-minute) bout of electrically evoked, intense muscle contractions. The investigators suggested that the electrical stimulation may have activated smaller, more superficial sensory afferent nerve fibers in the skin and subcutaneous tissues. This small fiber or flexion reflex afferent sensory input preferentially targets the FR motoneuron.[26] Biased activation of the FR motor units might be the effect of electrically evoked flexion reflex afferent input not usually a part of voluntary muscle activation.[23]

Given the impairment of decreased muscle endurance, NMES applied to facilitate muscle contractions of relatively low to moderate force (submaximal), repeated without fatigue over a prolonged period of time, is indicated. Physiologically, the NMES would be most effective if the stimulation activated the small, or S, and intermediate, FR, motor units, at a tetanic but moderate rate of activation. Pulsed-current waveforms with a pulse duration intermediate on the spectrum between activating the largest A fibers (eg, pulse duration = 20 to 50 μsec), and the smaller C and A-delta fibers (eg, pulse duration > 250 μsec), a rate of activation slightly greater than just producing tetany (eg, 30 to 40 pps) and amplitude adjusted to produce a well-tolerated, submaximal muscle contraction is desired. A peak current equivalent to the average current, as for the biphasic rectangular waveform, may be indicated to recruit the smaller (S) as well as the larger FR motor units at all depths of the stimulus. A symmetric, or well-balanced asymmetric, waveform is desired to avoid the potential effects of accumulated net charge in the tissues because the duration of stimulation for each session will characteristically be long. The symmetric, biphasic-current waveform, with a pulse duration of 100 to 150 μsec, delivered at 35 pps, and amplitude adjusted to a level evoking a submaximal contraction fits the criteria for NMES for increasing local muscle endurance well.

## NMES to Reduce Impairment of Range of Motion

Neuromuscular electrical stimulation has also been used in the treatment of limited joint range of motion (ROM) due to soft tissue restrictions or weakness. Muscle performance is facilitated by NMES to move the joint through the ROM or through an increased ROM. When voluntary movement is lacking, NMES can activate the muscles to passively move the joint through the full excursion of joint motion. Activation of the antagonist muscle group by NMES can be used to "actively stretch" contractures of the agonist muscle group. For example, NMES of the wrist and finger extensor muscle group has been applied to elongate contracted finger flexors of the individual with resting hand postural deformities secondary to hemiparesis. To effectively use NMES to actively stretch soft tissues, limiting joint motion requires extensive periods of stimulation consistently applied, often 7 days a week.[41,42] Submaximal, sustained muscle contractions with a gradual rise and fall of force simulate a slow, passive stretch. Characteristics of stimulation similar to those for endurance exercise with perhaps a more gradual ramp of the amplitude to peak is indicated, attempting to avoid fatigue,[28] avoid eliciting a stretch reflex, and avoid tissue irritation.

When voluntary movement sufficiently moves the joint partially through the ROM, NMES can be added to facilitate completion of the ROM. The NMES not only facilitates the movement but also provides a form of feedback, reinforcing the motor recruitment necessary to complete the ROM (ie, knowledge of results).[43]

## NMES to Reduce Impairment of Resting Muscle Tension

The application of NMES to reduce the impairment of neuromuscular performance (spasticity) has a sound physiologic rationale. Few reports of the impact of NMES to reduce spasticity on alleviating the associated disability (ie, difficulty walking, difficulty eating) exist in refereed literature.[44–48] Essentially three ways of applying NMES to reduce spasticity can be identified based on the neurophysiology of motor units and spinal networks: (1) Stimulate the antagonist of the spastic muscle,[44–46] (2) stimulate the spastic muscle (agonist),[47] and (3) alternately stimulate the spastic agonist and antagonist muscles.[48] Each of the methods relies in part on activating segmental neuromuscular reflexes to reduce the overactivity of the spastic muscle. Stimulating the antagonist to the spastic muscle activates the Ia afferent of the antagonist, which activates the Ia interneuron and reciprocally inhibits the spastic (agonist) alpha motoneuron of the muscle, reducing the activity of the spastic muscle.

Using NMES to stimulate the spastic (agonist) muscle results in antidromic conduction of the evoked action potential along the agonist motor axon toward the alpha motoneuron in the ventral horn of the spinal cord segment. The antidromic conduction along the motor axon presumably also travels along the axon collateral branch to the Renshaw cell. The activated Renshaw cell recurrently inhibits the agonist and synergist motoneuron of the segmental motor center.

The NMES of the spastic muscle also activates the Ib afferent, mediating autogenic inhibition of the agonist via the Ib interneuron. If the NMES characteristics produce maximal or near maximal activation of the spastic muscle, muscle fatigue occurs, reducing the spasticity because the fatigued muscle fibers are unable to respond. Applying NMES alternately to the spastic agonist muscle and the antagonist of the muscle theoretically evokes the combined effects of reciprocal inhibition, recurrent inhibition, autogenic inhibition, and, given the appropriate characteristics, muscle fatigue, to reduce the spasticity.

## NMES to Reduce Impairment of Movement Control

Neuromuscular electrical stimulation can be used to reeducate muscles that were temporarily paralyzed or reduced to minimal voluntary activation,[49,50] or muscles assuming performance of a new role, because of a functional or surgically created substitution.[51] For example, NMES may be useful in neuromuscular reeducation following the surgical transposition of a hypothenar muscle for an irreparably damaged thenar neuromuscular unit. Or NMES may be useful in neuromuscular reeducation of a wrist flexor muscle group, inactive because of a neurological insult. The initial recovery from the neurological insult results in a predominant extensor limb pattern of activation, inactivating the wrist flexor muscle group and prohibiting writing in any usual posture of the wrist and hand. When the individual cannot voluntarily activate the quadriceps femoris muscle group to lift the extended leg following knee surgery, NMES may again be useful for neuromuscular reeducation. (Many of the applications of NMES to reduce the impairment of movement control use characteristics of stimulation similar to those used for increasing muscle force but with lower-amplitude training stimuli, and may produce improvement in muscle force production by providing neuromuscular reeducation.)

A basic premise of neuromuscular reeducation is that the activation of most skeletal muscles results in feedback to the central nervous system about the muscle activated. For muscles that have not been activated for a period of time, the feedback provides a sensory awareness of the muscle and the associated action (if movement occurs) for the nervous system. Following NMES of a muscle, voluntary activation improves, much like the improvement in muscle performance following voluntary muscle contraction exercise. Thus, for the patient who is unable to activate a specific muscle but for whom the innervation of the muscle is intact, NMES effectively activates the muscle, enabling the process of muscle reeducation. Reports of clinical experiences indicate that not only do increases in motor recruitment occur with voluntary activity following NMES, but performance time may also decrease, with muscle activity occurring more rapidly after the nervous system recognizes the need to act.

## EFICACY AND EFFICIENCY OF NMES

The clinical indications for NMES are numerous for individuals with intact motor units but with impaired performance. For any condition in which the necessary muscle performance to reduce the impairment cannot be voluntarily produced or produced adequately to accomplish the desired outcome of intervention, NMES may be a useful adjunct to the therapeutic process. If NMES and the specific characteristics of the NMES are appropriately selected, based on a careful assessment of the impairment of neuromuscular performance, then the application of NMES should be an efficacious component of the intervention. However, applying NMES for neuromuscular reeducation of the dorsiflexor muscle group to reduce foot drop in gait for a person with a severed common peroneal nerve is not efficacious. Motor units must be intact for NMES to be useful. Using NMES to facilitate muscle force but with stimulation characteristics that produce muscle contractions generating less than 60 percent of the MVIC force of the muscle is also not an efficacious intervention.

Problems with effectiveness of interventions using NMES arise when the equipment available for the patient to use (eg, home electrical stimulation units) cannot reproduce the stimulating current, or the patient using the equipment cannot reproduce the same stimulating current that produced the neuromuscular response necessary to achieve the desired outcome in the supervised clinical setting.

## COST BENEFIT

If the intervention with NMES is efficacious, effective, or both, reimbursement should not be in question. However, global statements that NMES is or is not efficacious or effective as an adjunct to treatment for specific neuromuscular impairments clearly cannot be made. The only indication of efficacy and effectiveness is if the observed or measured neuromuscular response evoked by NMES matches the impairment targeted for treatment. With little clinical research documenting efficacy or effectiveness of NMES for specific impairments and disability, the physical therapist has only two options for documenting the use of NMES for reimbursement: (1) Document the relationship between the neuromuscular response to the NMES and the targeted impairment and show progressive reduction of impairment with treatment, and (2) document progressive reduction of the associated disability with the change in impairment.

The clinician may do well, in terms of both reimbursement and in developing the plan of care for physical therapy, to recognize NMES as an adjunct to the intervention, but not the intervention. As described, NMES is a procedure usually most appropriate for reducing impairments of muscle performance. Reduction in the patient's disability is not a reasonable expectation of NMES alone, and only in the context of comprehensive rehabilitation program has NMES been demonstrated to have an impact on disability.[36,52–55] The benefit of NMES for the clinician and the patient is if NMES enables a greater degree of recovery, or improves the efficiency of the process of recovery (eg, faster rate of improvement,[56,57] reduced resources for recovery). Much like the skilled hands of the master clinician, NMES may be a valuable asset to the intervention, but it is not of itself the intervention. Used in this way, therapists may accurately consider NMES a component of therapeutic exercise or neuromuscular reeducation and request reimbursement for the intervention as a whole, not for an NMES procedure.

## ANALYSIS AND SYNTHESIS OF REPORTED RESEARCH

Does NMES work? Related to improving muscle force, the answer appears to be twofold. Investigations applying NMES for improving healthy muscle force in healthy persons in North America have rarely demonstrated force outcomes greater than performance using volitional exercise, from the use of NMES or NMES superimposed on voluntary contractions. According to reports of the Russian scientist Yakov Kots' work,[33] muscle force gains in healthy muscle are possible with the application of NMES. Either Kots misrepresented data on muscle force after high-amplitude training, or studies in this country have not replicated Kots' "Russian technique" for NMES.

Kots[33] reported that certain requirements of NMES for improving healthy muscle force were necessary to attain the 10 to 30 percent gains in adults and 30 to 40 percent gains in muscle force of highly trained, elite athletes: (1) NMES amplitude to a level recruiting all muscle fibers and (2) recruitment of muscle fibers at maximal tetany (ie, maximal rate of activation). Kots[33] reportedly stated that the Russian technique used for NMES produced a relative blockade of sensory afferent fibers, allowing for sufficient stimulation of motor axons to activate all fibers at the maximal firing rate while eliciting little or no sensation of pain. In addition, some of the subjects of Kots' studies of NMES for improving muscle force were elite athletes, likely accustomed to routinely tolerating a degree of discomfort with training, and probably highly motivated to withstand "whatever it takes" to be the best in the world. Similar results of NMES for improving muscle force were attained in a lesser-known, single case study in which the subject and the characteristics of stimulation, particularly the amplitude, were very similar to Kots' work with athletes. A world-class weight lifter, training for the Olympics, trained to his voluntary maximal muscle performance and then used NMES, with the characteristics adjusted to mimic the Russian technique, including extremely high-amplitude levels of stimulus. Force gains beyond those achieved with maximal volitional exercise training occurred for the elite athlete using extremely high-amplitude NMES.[50]

The evidence for a benefit in using NMES over volitional exercise for improving muscle force in individuals with muscle force deficits, though not conclusive, deserves attention. All comparative studies demonstrate that the higher the intensity of exercise, the greater the changes in the impairment of muscle force production (usually isometric torque production).[36,53,58] The inconsistency in the outcomes of the studies arises from the inability to know when the "maximally tolerated" NMES or the voluntary "maximal" contraction is truly maximally recruiting all muscle fibers. Ensuring maximal recruitment is a problem for both the measurement of outcomes and the exercise training. The burst superimposition technique used in one study for measuring the outcome of training, using high- and low-amplitude NMES quadriceps femoris muscle exercise and high-intensity volitional quadriceps femoris muscle exercise, is one way of determining maximal recruitment,[36] but this has not been routinely done as a component of measurement or training. (Anyone who has experienced the burst superimposition technique might argue that any manner of providing the threat of experiencing the technique while the individual exercises will increase the likelihood of voluntary maximal recruitment for each repetition.) The following review of a representative sample of studies using NMES for improving force of the muscles of individuals with and without deficits in muscle performance is presented to define what is known about the efficacy of NMES. In the process, what is needed to be known becomes more clear.

## Outcomes of NMES for Improving Muscle Force in Rehabilitation

All of the studies reviewed involving individuals with muscle force deficits indicated some improvements in muscle performance for individuals receiving NMES during rehabilitation (Table 4–2). Though the literature is growing with reports of positive outcomes of NMES in rehabilitation, the definitive evidence of muscle force is scarce. Of the 17 studies reviewed, 4 [52,59–61] lack any comparison group (either a nonintervention control group or a group receiving an intervention

**TABLE 4–2. STUDIES REPORTING OUTCOMES OF NMES FOR INCREASING MUSCLE FORCE**

| Author(s) | Subjects | Electrical Stimulation | Comparison Group | Measures: Impairment (I)/Disability (D) | Results |
|---|---|---|---|---|---|
| **In Rehabilitation** | | | | | |
| Snyder-Mackler et al, 1995 | 110 subjects after ACL reconstruction | **Three Groups** High-amplitude NMES* Low-amplitude NMES** Combined high and low NMES* *Pulsed, 2500 Hz, sawtooth wave, 75 bps; max tolerated amplitude ** Pulsed, biphasic, rectangular waves, 300 μsec, 55 pps; max tolerated amplitude > 55 mA | Volitional exercise, maximal voluntary isometric contraction (MVIC) with monitoring and visual feedback provided | I: Quadriceps femoris MVIC (measured torques with burst superimposition technique) D: Knee flexion during stance phase of gait (measured using a 2-dimensional motion analysis) 4 weeks | Differences between two groups receiving high-amplitude NMES and the two groups that did not (low-amplitude NMES and volitional exercise groups) favoring high-amplitude NMES in: • Recovery of the quadriceps femoris • Flexion excursion of the knee in gait |
| Currier et al, 1993 | 17 subjects after ACL reconstruction | **Two groups** High-amplitude pulsed, sinusoidal waves, 50 bps; max tolerated high-amplitude NMES with pulsed electromagnetic frequencies (PEMF) and volitional exercise; max tolerated | Control group | I: Quadriceps femoris MVIC torque Thigh girth 6 weeks | In the first 6 weeks following surgery: • No difference between groups for muscle strength decrease • NMES and NMES and PEMF groups had less decrease in thigh girth than controls |
| Karmel-Ross et al, 1992 | 5 children with spina bifida | Low-amplitude pulsed, symmetric, biphasic, rectangular wave, 347 μsec, 35 pps; max tolerated amplitude | None | I: Quadriceps femoris MVIC torque D: Timed tasks: • Walking • Stair climbing ascent and descent | Improved muscle force for two subjects; improved function for four subjects |
| Snyder-Mackler et al, 1991 | 10 subjects after ACL reconstruction | High-amplitude pulsed, 2500 Hz, sawtooth wave, 75 bps | Volitional, high-amplitude cocontractions: quadricep and hamstrings | I: Quadricep and hamstrings: isokinetic average and peak | Difference favoring NMES group for: • Quadricep muscle force |

| Study | Subjects | Electrical stimulation | Comparison | Outcome measures | Results |
|---|---|---|---|---|---|
| | | Cocontraction: quadricep and hamstrings; max tolerated amplitude | | torque at 90 and 210 degrees/sec; D: Gait characteristics: • Walking speed • Stance time • Cadence • Flexion/extension excursion of the knee during gait; 4 weeks | • All gait characteristics • Flexion excursion during stance |
| Draper et al, 1991 | 30 subjects after ACL reconstruction | Low-amplitude pulsed, biphasic rectangular wave, 35 pps max tolerated amplitude with volitional exercise | Surface electromyographic (sEMG) biofeedback assisted volitional exercise | I: Quadriceps femoris MVIC torque | Difference between groups favoring sEMG biofeedback for quadriceps muscle force recovery |
| Wigerstad-Lossing et al, 1988 | 23 subjects after ACL reconstruction | Low-amplitude NMES with volitional pulsed, asymmetric-balanced, rectangular biphasic wave, 300 $\mu$sec; 30 pps; max tolerated amplitude within 65–100 mA range | Volitional, isometric | I: Quadricep femoris: • MVIC torque • Isokinetic peak torque at 30 degrees/sec Cross-sectional area Fiber type area Muscle enzyme activity (glycolytic and oxidative) 6 weeks | Differences between groups favoring the NMES group for: • Less reduction in MVIC torque • Less reduction in cross-sectional area • No reduction (less than control) in muscle enzyme activity • Increase in ratio of FF to S fiber area |
| Delitto et al, 1988 | Single subject after ACL reconstruction | High-amplitude pulsed, 2500 Hz, sawtooth wave, 50 bps; co-contraction: quadriceps and hamstrings; max tolerated amplitude | None | I: Bilateral quadriceps femoris and hamstring MVIC torque at 65 degrees of flexion Thigh girth Serial measures across phases: baseline, NMES, withdrawal of NMES, NMES (7 weeks) | Increased muscle force of involved extremity muscles and girth measures for all intervention phases, maintenance of change during withdrawal of NMES |

**TABLE 4–2. STUDIES REPORTING OUTCOMES OF NMES FOR INCREASING MUSCLE FORCE (CONTINUED)**

| Author(s) | Subjects | Electrical Stimulation | Comparison Group | Measures: Impairment (I)/Disability (D) | Results |
|---|---|---|---|---|---|
| Kahanovitz et al, 1987 | 117 subjects with low back pain | **Two Groups** High-amplitude pulsed, monophasic modified spike wave, 400 μsec, 300 pps; Low-amplitude pulsed, symmetric, biphasic rectangular wave, 300 μsec, 35 pps; max tolerated amplitude | Volitional exercises control group | I: Flexor and extensor muscle groups MVIC isometric and isokinetic MVIC torque 4 weeks | Differences between group favoring low amplitude NMES and exercise groups over high amplitude and control for muscle force increases |
| Sisk et al, 1987 | 22 subjects after ACL reconstruction, knee immobilized | Low-amplitude: NMES with volitional exercise pulsed, biphasic rectangular wave, 300 μsec, 40 pps; max tolerated amplitude | Volitional, MVIC | I: Quadriceps femoris, MVIC torque 6 weeks | No difference in muscle force between groups |
| Morrissey et al, 1985 | 15 subjects after ACL reconstruction, immobilized 6 weeks | Low-amplitude: pulsed, asymmetric-balanced, rectangular biphasic; 50 pps; max tolerated amplitude 8+ hours/day | Control group | I: Quadricep femoris MVIC torque at −60 and −45 degrees of extension Thigh girth 6, 9, 12 weeks | At 6 weeks, decline in muscle force production less for the NMES group No differences between groups at 9 and 12 weeks in muscle torque; or in girth measures at 6, 9, and 12 weeks |
| Gould et al, 1983 | 20 subjects after open meniscectomy | Low-amplitude: pulsed, monophasic square wave, 100 μsec, 35 pps; max tolerated amplitude | Volitional, MVIC | I: Quadriceps femoris, hamstrings, dorsiflexors, plantarflexors, MVIC torque, muscle leg volumes (atrophy) 2 weeks | Difference between groups favoring NMES for percent recovery of torque compared to the unoperated limb and less atrophy |

| Study | Subjects | NMES Parameters | Comparison | Measures | Results |
|---|---|---|---|---|---|
| Grove-Lainey et al, 1983 | Subjects after knee surgery | High-amplitude: NMES with volitional exercise; pulsed, alternating current, 250 microseconds, 100 bps; max tolerated amplitude | Volitional, MVIC | I: Quadriceps femoris, MVIC torque 6 weeks | No difference between groups |
| Singer et al, 1983 | 15 subjects with chronic knee pathology; quadriceps atrophy | High-amplitude: pulsed, 75–350 μsec, 50–100 pps; max tolerated amplitude | None | I: Quadriceps femoris, MVIC torque 4 weeks | Muscle force increased; sum of increases for all subjects = 22 percent increase over initial |
| Curwin et al, 1980 | Subjects after knee ligament surgery, knee immobilized in a cast | High-amplitude: attempt to duplicate "Russian" current | Control group | I: Quadricep femoris Biochemical measures: • Muscle glycogen • Myofibrillar ATPase | No difference in muscle glycogen between groups Myofibrillar adenosine triphosphatase (ATPase) increase in NMES group compared to control |
| Godfrey et al, 1979 | Subjects in knee rehabilitation | High-amplitude: pulsed, asymmetric biphasic (faradic) waves 60 pps; max tolerated amplitude | Volitional, isometric exercise at 75 percent MVIC | I: Quadricep femoris isokinetic peak torque at 3, 10, and 25 deg/sec | Differences between group in favor of NMES for total quadriceps torque for all angular velocities |
| Eriksson and Haggmark, 1979 | 8 subjects, after knee ligament surgery, knee immobilized in a cast | Low-amplitude: pulsed current, 200 pps; amplitude under subject's pain perception; [on: 5 sec/off: 5 sec; for one hour] | Volitional, isometric contractions | I: Clinical rating of quadriceps femoris function and atrophy Enzyme activity of the quadriceps femoris 5 weeks | NMES group demonstrated better quadricep function and greater oxidative enzyme (SDH) activity than the volitional exercise only group |
| Johnson et al, 1977 | Subjects with chondromalacia of the patella | High-amplitude: pulsed, asymmetrical, biphasic rectangular wave (faradic), 65 pps; max tolerated amplitude | None | I: Quadricep femoris force Thigh girth | Increase in quadriceps force (related to the amplitude of NMES tolerated) Slight increase in thigh girth |

## TABLE 4-2. STUDIES REPORTING OUTCOMES OF NMES FOR INCREASING MUSCLE FORCE (CONTINUED)

| Author(s) | Subjects | Electrical Stimulation | Comparison Group | Measures: Impairment (I)/Disability (D) | Results |
|---|---|---|---|---|---|
| **In Healthy Muscle** | | | | | |
| Duchateau and Hainaut, 1988 | 11 healthy subjects | Submaximal: pulsed current, 200 μsec pulse, 100 pps; amplitude to produce 60–65 percent of MVIC torque | Volitional, submaximal isotonic; with monitoring feedback of contraction force aiming for 60–65 percent of MVIC | I: Adductor pollicis muscle:<br>• MVIC<br>• Electrically evoked MVIC<br>• Electrically evoked fatigue test<br>Muscle electrical activity (subcutaneous electrodes)<br>2 weeks | Difference between groups favoring voluntary exercise group in:<br>• Increased muscle force production<br>• Accelerated tetanus time course<br>• Increased resistance to fatigue |
| Soo et al, 1988 | 15 healthy subjects (9 men, 6 women) | Low-amplitude: pulsed, 2500 Hz sinusoidal wave, 50 bps; amplitude to produce 50 percent of MVIC torque | None | I: Bilateral quadricep femoris MVIC torque<br>5 weeks | Difference between NMES trained and "control" leg muscle force for the men only |
| Alon et al, 1987 | 32 healthy subjects | **Two Groups**<br>Low-amplitude: NMES* with volitional exercise; NMES* alone; * pulsed, symmetric, biphasic, rectangular wave, 400 μsec, 50 pps; max tolerated amplitude; 5 sec on; 5 sec off | Volitional exercise control group | I: Abdominal muscle force<br>• Percent change per week<br>D: Time to maintain a curl sit up<br>4 weeks | NMES combined with exercise increased muscle force more than NMES alone; both stimulation groups greater than others<br>No change in endurance |
| Wolf et al, 1986 | 27 healthy subjects/athletes | High-amplitude: pulsed, monophasic rectangular wave, 300 μsec, 75 pps; max tolerated amplitude superimposed on volitional exercise | Volitional exercise, full body squat control group | I: Force output of squat<br>D: 25-yard dash time vertical jump<br>6 weeks | No difference between NMES with exercise, and exercise alone training groups; both training groups better than the control group on all measures |

| Study | Subjects | NMES parameters | Comparison | Outcome measure | Results |
|---|---|---|---|---|---|
| Mohr et al, 1985 | 17 healthy subjects | Low-amplitude: pulsed, monophasic, paired-pulse wave, 20 μsec, 50 pps; max tolerated amplitude | Volitional, MVIC exercise | I: Quadriceps femoris, MVIC torque 3 weeks | Volitional greater than NMES and control group in muscle torque |
| Selkowitz, 1985 | 24 healthy subjects | High-amplitude: pulsed, 2200 Hz sawtooth wave, 50 bps; max tolerated amplitude | Control group | I: Quadriceps femoris MVIC torque at 60 degrees of flexion 4 weeks | Difference between groups in favor of greater quadriceps torque for the NMES group |
| Stefanoska and Vodovnik, 1985 | 13 healthy subjects | Two groups 1. Pulsed, 2500 Hz alternating sinusoidal wave, 25 bps 2. Pulsed, monophasic, rectangular wave, 300 μsec, 25 pps; max tolerated amplitude, as monitored = 5 percent of MVIC torque | Control group | I: Quadriceps femoris muscle MVIC torque 3 weeks | Both NMES groups increased muscle force compared to controls; increases were small |
| Currier and Mann, 1983 | 35 healthy subjects | Two groups High-amplitude NMES* High-amplitude NMES* with volitional exercise; *Pulsed, 2500 Hz, sawtooth wave, 50 bps; max tolerated amplitude | Volitional, MVICs Control group | I: Quadriceps femoris muscle: • Isometric (MVIC) torque • Isokinetic peak torque at 100, 200, and 300 degrees/sec Thigh girth 5 weeks | Both NMES groups and the volitional exercise group greater than control for quadriceps femoris: • Isometric torque No difference between groups for: • Isokinetic torque No changes in any group for thigh girth |
| Laughman et al, 1983 | 58 healthy subjects | High-amplitude: pulsed, 2500 Hz, sawtooth wave, 50 bps, 70 mA amplitude | Volitional, high-amplitude, isometric exercise (mean: 78 percent of MVIC) Control group | I: Quadricep femoris muscle MVIC torque at 60 degrees of flexion 5 weeks | High amplitude NMES and volitional exercise groups greater than control for quadricep muscle torque No difference between NMES and volitional exercise groups |

**TABLE 4–2.** STUDIES REPORTING OUTCOMES OF NMES FOR INCREASING MUSCLE FORCE (CONTINUED)

| Author(s) | Subjects | Electrical Stimulation | Comparison Group | Measures: Impairment (I)/Disability (D) | Results |
|---|---|---|---|---|---|
| McMiken et al, 1983 | 16 healthy subjects | High-amplitude: pulsed, monophasic square wave, 75 pps; max tolerated up to 80 percent of MVIC torque | Volitional, isometric, with monitoring and feedback aiming for up to 80 percent MVIC troque | I: Quadriceps femoris muscle MVIC torque at 30 degrees of flexion 3 weeks | No difference between NMES and volitional groups in muscle torque |
| Romero et al, 1982 | 18 healthy subjects | High-amplitude: pulsed, biphasic (faradic) wave, 500 μsec, 2500 Hz, max tolerated amplitude; bilateral | Control group | I: Quadriceps femoris muscle, MVIC torque and peak isokinetic torque at 30 and 60 degrees/sec Thigh girth 5 weeks | Difference between groups favoring NMES for isometric muscle torque and isokinetic at 30 degrees/sec only No difference in girth |
| Halbach and Straus, 1980 | 6 healthy subjects | High-amplitude: halben-wellen-strom wave, 50 Hz (selected to mimic "Russian" tech-nique); max tolerated amplitude | Volitional, high-speed, isokinetic exercise: velocity spectrum | I: Quadriceps femoris muscle, isokinetic peak torque at 120 degrees/sec Thigh girth | Increase favoring the voli-tional exercise group for peak isokinetic torque (Largest one-week in-crease in isokinetic torque was for subject tolerating the greatest amplitude of NMES) No changes in thigh girth |
| Garrett et al 1980 | 30 healthy subjects | High-amplitude: pulsed, high-frequency, sinuso-idal, 50 bps (attempted "Russian" technique); max tolerated amplitude | Volitional, MVIC Control group | I: Quadriceps femoris muscle MVIC torque 5 weeks | NMES and volitional exer-cise groups both greater muscle torque than control group No difference between NMES and volitional groups |

| Study | Subjects | Stimulation parameters | Comparison | Outcome measures | Results |
|---|---|---|---|---|---|
| Currier et al, 1979 | 37 healthy subjects | Low-amplitude: pulsed, asymmetric, biphasic rectangular wave, 25 pps superimposed on MVIC; max tolerated amplitude | Volitional, MVIC | I: Quadriceps femoris muscle MVIC torque 2 weeks | No difference in the increases in MVIC torque between groups |
| Kots, 1977 (as reported by Kramer JF et al, 1980) | Healthy adults; highly trained athletes | High-amplitude: burst 1600–2500 Hz, sinusoidal wave, 50 bps (ie, the "Russian technique"); amplitude to recruit all muscle fibers | None | I (shoulder muscles, gastronemius, quadriceps): Muscle force contraction velocity of muscle Local muscle endurance 2 to 7+ weeks | Increases in force (4–5 weeks): 10–30 percent increases in healthy adults 30–40 percent increases in athletes Improved contraction velocity (2–3 weeks) Increases in muscle endurance (7+ weeks) |
| Massey et al, 1965 | | High-amplitude, pulsed, monophasic square wave, 1000 pps; max tolerated amplitude | Volitional, progressive resistive exercise (PRE) Volitional, MVIC Control group | I: 10 upper extremity muscles: MVIC torque of specific muscle groups | Exercise and NMES groups all better than control and: PRE group > MVIC group > NMES |

different than NMES—usually the standard therapy), 3[57,62,63] compare NMES with a control group (ie, a comparison group not receiving any rehabilitation intervention), and 10[21,36,39,53,58,64–68] compare NMES-assisted exercise and volitional exercise comparison groups. The investigations of NMES with volitional exercise comparison groups shed light on whether muscle force improvements with NMES are the result of the intensity of training with NMES or characteristics of NMES evoked contractions. Six of the studies comparing NMES and volitional exercise training indicated better outcome measures with NMES[21,36,39,53,58,67]; in two of the studies the outcome favored the volitional exercise group[64,65]; and the outcome of two studies indicated that NMES and volitional training were equivalent.[66,68]

The intensity of exercise training induced by NMES or voluntary effort during rehabilitation is critical to determine the role of NMES in the recovery of muscle force. Of the six studies demonstrating a difference in favor of NMES, only Godfrey et al[58] indicated the level of intensity of the volitional exercise during rehabilitation. After ACL reconstruction surgery, the volitional exercise group performed voluntary isometric contractions at 75 percent of MVIC torque (high intensity) while the NMES group received high-amplitude NMES. The results indicate better muscle performance following NMES exercise training based on the sum of the peak torques of testing at multiple angular velocities. The low number of subjects and the use of summary scores for torque weaken any argument for the superiority of NMES over volitional exercise for improving the force of weakened muscle.

Feedback about absolute or relative force output during volitional exercise would be useful in encouraging the individual to produce a maximal effort for each contraction. The investigations by Snyder-Mackler et al[36,53] and Draper et al,[64] using surface electromyographic (sEMG) biofeedback to assist volitional contractions, indicate that subjects received feedback about the intensity of the volitional muscle contractions during the exercise training; evidence of feedback was not reported for any of the other intervention studies. One of the studies providing feedback[53] involved cocontractions of the quadriceps and hamstring muscles, a difficult activity for the individual following surgical reconstruction of the ACL and apprehensive about the imbalanced production of force resulting in knee movement and possibly more pain and injury. For individuals receiving NMES, the NMES may have served as a wise "cocontraction coordinator," removing the difficulty of producing matched quadriceps and hamstring contraction, and thus enabling the patient to tolerate increasing intensity of the evoked muscle contractions.

Comparative studies of the effectiveness of sEMG biofeedback-assisted voluntary exercise and NMES in rehabilitation, such as the study by Draper et al,[64] may be helpful in understanding the role of NMES in improving force of weakened muscles. If the effectiveness of NMES for improving muscle force is through evoking high-intensity exercise for the weakened muscle, then the use of sEMG biofeedback may be effective in setting a goal for the intensity of voluntary contractions. Biofeedback also provides necessary information for muscle reeducation to enable the maximal or near maximal voluntary recruitment of the recovering muscle associated with improvements in force.

## NMES and Healthy Muscle

Among studies using NMES for enhancing performance of healthy muscle (Table 4–2), 11 of the 16 reviewed demonstrated equivalent outcomes,[55,69–74] or outcomes favoring volitional exercise for increasing muscle force.[34,56,75–76] Of the 5 studies demonstrating greater muscle force with NMES,[33,77–80] the results of 2 are difficult to interpret because no comparison or control group was included,[33,77] and 2 compared force training with NMES to a nonexercising control group only.[79–80]

The intensity of the training with NMES and volitional exercise was indicated in 3 [70–71, 75] of the 11 studies reviewed. Of these studies, Laughman et al,[70] and McMiken et al,[71] both indicated equivalent muscle force outcomes of quadriceps femoris training with NMES and volitional modes of exercise. Duchateau et al,[75] studying the improvement of adductor pollicis muscle force with NMES and volitional exercise and measuring outcomes by voluntary and evoked testing protocols, indicated better muscle performance after volitional exercise. The difference in outcome of Duchateau et al's[75] investigation and the others that also controlled for the intensity of training could be related to the muscle group studied. The adductor pollicis has been described as having a greater proportion of S motor units than the majority of human skeletal muscles.[22,31] In contrast, the quadriceps femoris muscle (frequently the muscle group studied) is composed of a relatively even distribution of slow and fast motor units. Further investigation of the response to NMES of different muscle groups is important, lest the assumption that all skeletal muscles are equal continues erroneously.

# Summary

An interpretation of the role of NMES for improving muscle force based on the reported literature is that NMES applied to assist the performance of high-intensity muscle contractions can be effective in increasing muscle force and function. The results of investigations of the use of NMES do not conclusively indicate a unique benefit of NMES beyond the benefits of high-intensity exercise training on improving muscle force. However, the point should be emphasized that NMES may have a very important role in assisting the patient who for some reason (eg, hesitancy, inadequate neuromotor control, and pain) cannot voluntarily perform high-intensity exercise training to effectively accomplish improving muscle force.

However, the results reported for Kots'[33] work, some of the findings of histochemical changes in muscle after NMES,[15,20] and the physiologic basis of NMES[23] should not be ignored. The apparent benefit of NMES shown in the studies of strengthening individuals with muscle force deficits can be explained by the consistent activation of the same motor units—a condition which is highly favorable for muscle force training. If the electrodes are applied to the same location, preparation of the skin is similar, and the characteristics of stimulation are similar, the same motor units will be activated for every contraction during every exercise session. The higher the ampitude, the greater the depth of stimulation, and the greater the opportunity to recruit all motor units. Using NMES to maximize recruitment consistently recruits the same motor units every training session, whereas voluntary maximal activation may result in greater variability in the activation of motor units in different training sessions.

Although preferential activation of the largest axons (those with the lowest threshold) means for any level of contraction force, more fast motor units are active than for a voluntary contraction, the NMES pattern of activation does not exclude activation of slow motor units. The fact that the size difference in axons of the large versus small motor units is minimal, and that large and variable tissue restraints to current flow exist between the surface of the skin and the muscle nerve, likely limits marked differences in activation of specific motor units. However, the potential to activate a different population of motor units with NMES than the motor units voluntarily activated can be supported. Under carefully controlled conditions, Trimble and Enoka[23] demonstrated changes in muscle twitch responses elicited by Hoffmann reflexes (H-reflexes) and direct motor responses (M-responses), and changes in submotor NMES twitch force related to H-reflexes consistent with activating a faster-contracting population of motor units by NMES applied over the muscle.

Sinacore et al[15] demonstrated preferential activation of fast-twitch fibers, particularly the FR, following 50 electrically elicited isometric muscle contractions at 80 percent of the individual's MVIC peak torque (previously determined). The activation of the fast-twitch muscle fibers by the electrical stimulation of human skeletal muscle is compelling evidence of selective fast motor unit activation by NMES. A word of caution: The evidence comes from analysis of muscle biopsy samples. Muscle biopsy samples, usually 10 by 5 mm in size, are a minute representation of a muscle group the size of the quadriceps femoris muscle. The sample was drawn from the vastus lateralis portion of the quadriceps femoris muscle group, a region the investigators describe as remote from the area of the stimulating electrodes. As current dissipates in areas remote from the stimulating electrodes, the largest of the nerve fibers (eg, fast motor unit axons) with the lowest threshold are the most likely to respond. The fact that not all of the fast-twitch fibers in the sample of the vastus lateralis were activated suggests that the site is not representative of the entire muscle. At near maximal recruitment of the quadriceps femoris muscle group, the complete absence of activation of S motor units seems unlikely. However, in a sample of muscle the authors considered representative, no evidence of slow-twitch fiber activation was shown. Interpretations about an entire muscle group from observations of muscle biopsy samples must be considered cautiously.

Similar caution should be exercised in accepting interpretations of the potential for higher-frequency activation of selected motor units. At higher levels of force output, the rate of activation of motor units is the predominant mechanism of increasing force, whereas motor unit recruitment becomes less of a contributing factor.[30–31,81] The rate of firing of active motor units rises steeply at higher levels of force output, with firing rates reportedly as high as 50 Hz with voluntary contractions and discharge rates as high as 200 Hz reported in some muscles. Some investigators suggest that the extremely high firing rates of particularly the fast motor units are an indication of the untapped potential of the largest motor units that may be captured or targeted for capture by high-amplitude NMES.[30–31] Studies recording or stimulating motor units to such firing rates primarily involved intraneuronal recording and activation of single motor units. Again, the discharge rates of motor units activated by NMES applied at the skin surface may be a very different situation.

In addition to the alteration of the applied current rate of activation by the intervening tissues, NMES will simultaneously activate nerve fibers other than the fast motor unit axons, altering segmental motor center activity and the subsequent response of the motor unit. For example, Renshaw cells known to limit discharge rates of motor units may be activated by the antidromic conduction of NMES-elicited nerve action potentials.[22–23] Physiologic mechanisms of fatigue, believed to be mediated by muscle membrane responses, and intracellular chemical changes (eg, calcium concentration) and membrane responses of organelles may block high rates of activation.[82]

Physiologically, the motor unit appears to be designed to optimize muscle performance while minimizing fatigue.[23,82] The identification of new modes of applying NMES to optimize motor unit performance appear to be on the horizon. For example, Binder-Macleod and Guerin[16] demonstrated the progressive reduction of rate coding preserving force output over a greater number of repetitions of exercise. This mode of NMES and other methods of applying NMES efficiently enhance the force of muscle contraction by evoking phenomena such as the "catch-like" property of muscle.[28] Adaptions in the electrical generators, methods of applying NMES in rehabilitation, and selection of patients may converge to expose a unique use of NMES in improving the force of muscles too impaired to perform their functional role. Understanding the physiologic effects of NMES on muscle tissue and recognizing the limitations of methods of investigations of the peripheral neuromuscular system and application of NMES are essential to maximizing the ability to facilitate optimal muscle performance with NMES, reduce impairment, and lessen disability.

## CASE STUDY

A 34-year-old man was referred to physical therapy for rehabilitation following a motor vehicle accident. The diagnosis provided was multiple lower extremity fractures and soft tissue injuries, including a comminuted fracture of the pelvis with dislocation of the left hip, and internal derangement of the right knee with a tear of the posterior cruciate ligament (PCL). The young man had undergone an open reduction, bone graft, ligament graft, and microvascular surgical procedures, as well as approximately 5 months of bedrest and varying degrees of immobilization of the pelvis, hip, and right knee. Prior to the accident, he was a semiprofessional soccer player, earning his living playing for a national indoor soccer league team. The goal of rehabilitation is recovery of lower extremity movement and function, and return to playing form by the beginning of the winter indoor soccer season in 8 months.

The physical therapy plan of care includes exercises and stretching to increase joint ROM; force and endurance of the lower extremity musculature; and progressive ambulation, partial weight bearing, to advance to full weight bearing and functional activities of running, cutting, sidestepping, kicking, and jumping, with improved muscle force. Initially, NMES was applied to the quadriceps femoris muscles bilaterally, using a symmetric, biphasic rectangular wave, with a pulse duration of 150 μsec, a rate of 35 pps, a duty cycle of 6 sec on and 12 sec off, and the amplitude set to produce a submaximal tetanic isometric contraction of the muscle groups for 20 min, increasing the duration up to 60 min as tolerated, twice a day. A high-voltage, monophasic, paired-pulse wave or an asymmetric-unbalanced, biphasic wave was considered for the stimulating current to promote the reabsorption of inflammation or edema likely present after prolonged immobilization, while producing submaximal contractions, but with a net charge. Polar effects were decided against because of the risk of current damage to the tissues. (Much of the skin of the thighs had been covered by a cast for several months and was fragile, and the competency of the vascular status raised concern for the ability of the tissues to tolerate and restore any microscopic changes in tissue or extracellular fluid composition the polar current might create.) The patient was also working on stretching and ROM exercises, ambulation with crutches, aerobic exercise in the pool (primarily arms, but increasing use of lower extremities), and a progressive weight training program for the upper extremities and trunk musculature.

The intent of using NMES in the manner described initially was to increase the local muscle endurance capacity of the quadriceps femoris muscle group, emphasizing training of the oxidative muscle fibers (S and FR motor units). Because of the history of microvascular surgery (ie, impairment of circulation) and the prolonged immobilization (a greater detriment to the slow motor units, which are deprived of frequent activation, than to the fast motor units, which are accustomed to only occasional activation, thus less deprived by immobilization), NMES was used to increase the oxidative muscle function. To prepare for the high-amplitude NMES to increase muscle force, the aerobic or oxidative training of the muscle is important to enable the muscle to recover after the high-intensity training, which preferentially activates the fast motor units and activates motor units at higher rates of activation. Adaptations of two fatigue tests were used to measure the endurance performance of the quadriceps femoris muscle group before and after NMES: (1) number of MVICs to 50 percent of the initial MVIC torque produced, up to 50, and a comparison of the work done in the first five compared to the last five MVICs of the series[83]; and (2) recovery MVIC torque 30 sec after a 1-min fatigue test, consisting of 50 MVICs.[84] Only the measure of impairment (muscle endurance) was used to monitor outcome at this stage of rehabilitation, because restricted lower extremity ROM and ambulatory status limited the use of disability measures, such as cadence, cycling time, distance, or walking speed.

After 5 weeks of physical therapy, lower extremity ROM had increased; the patient was independently ambulating with crutches on

## CASE STUDY *continued*

all surfaces, performing the pool aerobic exercise for 40 min continuously twice a day, and had sufficient lower extremity ROM to begin to use an exercise bicycle (seat adjusted) for aerobic training as well. The upper body resistive exercise program progressed without difficulty. The NMES for the quadriceps femoris muscle groups bilaterally was changed, applying a 2500-Hz sawtooth wave, 50 bps, 10 sec on, 50 sec off, for 10 contractions; amplitude gradually increased to achieve an MVIC torque 75 to 80 percent of the voluntary MVIC.

Before and every 2 weeks after the initiation of the high-amplitude NMES for improving the quadriceps femoris muscle force program, MVIC torque was measured at 60 degrees of knee flexion. Physical performance measures of disability, such as walking, running, and vertical jump, were not recorded until the patient could ambulate with a straight cane or without assistive devices.

The patient's self-report of physical performance and psychosocial status were monitored using the Functional Status Questionnaire, a health-related quality of life (HRQL) measure[85] beginning at the time of discharge from the institution to outpatient care), and at 3-month intervals continuing through the rehabilitation. (The Medical Outcomes Survey, Short-Form 36[86] would have been equally suitable, depending on the patterns of use of HRQL instruments of a facility.)

## REVIEW QUESTIONS

1. An otherwise healthy professional football player suffers a deep bruise to the thigh and presents with swelling of the thigh and weakness of the knee extensors (decreased maximal voluntary contraction [MVC] torque of the involved compared to the uninvolved quadriceps femoris muscle group). The goal of treatment is reduction of intramuscular inflammation and recovery of muscle force, with a rapid return to "playing shape."
   a. Of a given stimulating current, what characteristic would you change to primarily increase the depth of stimulation?
   b. The stimulus rate coding (frequency) should be selected to produce what type of muscle contraction?
   c. What rate of activation (pps) would you choose to achieve the type of muscle contraction described in part b?
2. To increase the types of motor units recruited as well as the number, which of the following characteristics of NMES would you change?

    a. Amplitude
    b. Pulse duration
    c. Rate (frequency)

3. A patient is recovering from a torn gastrocnemius–soleus muscle tendon, surgically repaired, with healing sufficient for MVCs. You choose to use NMES to reduce the impairment of muscle force. Identify an impairment and a disability measure appropriate for determining outcomes of the intervention

4. The patient in question 3 was taking high doses of oral steroids prior to the tendon rupture, secondary to receiving a kidney transplant 6 months earlier. What muscle fiber type might be expected to have undergone substantial atrophy in this patient? Identify the goal to accomplish and specific target of NMES, and the characteristics of NMES (amplitude, pulse duration, rate, waveform) reasonable for improving muscle force to reduce this individual's impairment of gastrocnemius–soleus muscle performance.

5. What might be the effect on the neuromuscular response of the target muscle of NMES by the NMES-evoked antidromic stimulation of Ia afferents of the muscle? Describe the physiologic basis for the effect.

6. For individuals with impaired muscle force performance, has NMES been shown to be the most effective procedure for recovery from the force deficit? What information would convince you that NMES is better than other mechanisms for increasing force in individuals with impaired muscle force performance?

# References

1. International Classification of Impairments, Disabilities, and Handicaps. Geneva, Switzerland, World Health Organization, 1980.

2. Delitto A, Snyder-Mackler L, Robinson AJ. Electrical stimulation of muscle: Techniques and applications. In Robinson AJ, Snyder-Mackler L (eds), Clinical Electrophysiology: Electrotherapy and Electrophysiologic Testing. Baltimore, MD, Williams & Wilkins, pp 121–154, 1995.

3. Kramer JF, Mendryk SW. Electrical stimulation as a strength improvement technique: A review. J Ortho Sports Phys Ther, 4:91–98, 1982.

4. Kandel ER, Siegelbaum A, Schwartz JH. Nerve cells and behavior, synaptic transmission, directly gated transmission at the nerve–muscle synapse. In Kandel ER, Schwartz JH, Jessell TM (eds), Principles of Neural Science (3rd ed). New York, NY, Elsevier, pp 18–32, 123–134, 135–152, 1991.

5. Guyton AC. Membrane physiology, nerve, and muscle. In Guyton AC (ed), Textbook of Medical Physiology (7th ed). Philadelphia, PA, WB Saunders, pp 88–134, 1986.

6. Garnett R, Stephens JA. Changes in the recruitment threshold of motor units produced by cutaneous stimulation in man. J Physiol (Lond), 311:463–473, 1981.

7. Hultman E, Sjoholm H. Energy metabolism and contraction force of human skeletal muscle *in situ* during electrical stimulation. J Physiol (Lond), 354:525–532, 1983.

8. Stephens JA, Garnett R, Bulli NP. Reversal of recruitment order of single motor units produced by cutaneous stimulation during voluntary contraction in man. Nature, 272:362–364, 1978.

9. Luscher HR, Ruenzel P, Henneman E. How the size of motoneurons determines their susceptibility to discharge. Nature, 282:859–861, 1979.

10. Delitto A, Rose SJ. Comparative comfort of three waveforms used in electrically eliciting quadriceps femoris contractions. Phys Ther, 66:1704–1707, 1986.

11. Bowman BR, Baker LL. Effects of waveform parameters on comfort during transcutaneous neuromuscular electrical stimulation. Ann Biomed Eng, 13:59–74, 1985.

12. Delitto AA, Strube MJ, Shulman AD, Minor SD. A study of discomfort with electrical stimulation. Phys Ther, 72:410–421, 1992.

13. Goodgold J, Eberstein A. A review of nerve and muscle physiology. In Goodgold J, Eberstein A (eds), Electrodiagnosis of Neuromuscular Diseases. Baltimore, MD, Williams & Wilkins, pp 18–31, 1972.

14. Henneman E, Somjen G, Carpenter DO. Functional significance of cell size in spinal motoneurons. J Neurophysiol, 28:560–580, 1965.

15. Sinacore DR, Delitto A, King DS, Rose SJ. Type II fiber activation with electrical stimulation: A preliminary report. Phys Ther, 70:416–422, 1990.

16. Binder-Macleod SA, Guerin T. Preservation of force output through progressive reduction of stimulation frequency in humans. Phys Ther, 70:619–625, 1990.

17. Brooks SV, Faulkner JA. Skeletal muscle weakness in old age: underlying mechanisms. Med Sci Sports Exer, 26:432–439, 1994.

18. Rose SJ, Rothstein JM. Muscle mutability: Part I. General concepts and adaptions to altered patterns of use. Phys Ther, 62:1773–1787, 1982.

19. Delitto A, Snyder-Mackler L. Two theories of muscle strength augmentation using percutaneous electrical stimulation. Phys Ther, 70:158–164, 1990.

20. Kabric M, Appel HJ, Resic A. Fine structural changes in electrostimulated human skeletal muscle. Eur J Appl Physiol, 57:1–5, 1988.

21. Wigerstad-Lossing I, Grimby G, Jonsson T et al. Effects of electrical muscle stimulation combined with voluntary contractions after knee ligament surgery. Med Sci Sports Exer, 20:93–98, 1988.

22. Kukulka CG, Clamann PH. Comparison of recruitment and discharge properties of motor units in human brachial biceps and adductor pollicis during isometric contractions. Brain Res, 219:45–55, 1981.

23. Trimble MH, Enoka RM. Mechanisms underlying the training effects associated with neuromuscular electrical stimulation. Phys Ther, 71:273–282, 1991.

24. Clamann HP, Gillies JD, Skinner RD, Henneman E. Quantitative measures of output of a motoneuron pool during monosynaptic reflexes. J Neurophysiol, 37:1328–1337, 1974.

25. Gorman PH, Mortimer JT. The effect of stimulus parameters on the recruitment characteristics of direct nerve stimulation. IEEE Trans Biomed Eng, 30:407–414, 1983.

26. Gordon J. Spinal mechanisms of motor coordination. In Kandel ER, Schwartz JH, Jessell TM (eds). Principles of Neural Science (3rd ed). New York, NY, Elsevier, pp 581–595, 1991.

27. Kernell D. Neuromuscular frequency-coding and fatigue. In Gandevia SC, Enoka RM et al (eds). Fatigue: Neural and Muscular Mechanisms. New York, NY, Plenum Press, pp 135–145, 1995.

28. Burke RE, Nelson PG. Accommodation to current ramps in motoneurons of fast and slow twitch motor units. Intl J Neurosci, 1:347–356, 1971.

29. Burke RE, Rudomin P, Zajac FE. The effect of activation history on tension production by individual muscle units. Brain Res, 109:515–529, 1976.

30. Kanosue K, Yoshida M, Akazawa K et al. The number of active motor units and their firing rates in voluntary contractions of the human brachialis muscle. Jpn J Physiol, 29:427–433, 1979.

31. DeLuca CJ, LeFever RS, McCue et al. Behavior of human motor units in different muscles during linearly varying contractions. J Physiol (Lond), 329:113–128, 1982.

32. Li CL, Bak A. Excitability characteristics of the A and C fibers in a peripheral nerve. Exp Neurol, 50:67–79, 1976.

33. Kots Y. Electrostimulation. Babkin I, Timentsko N (tr). Paper presented at Symposium on Electrostimulation of Skeletal Muscles, Canadian Soviet Exchange Symposium, Concordia University, December 6–10, 1977, as reported in Kramer JF, Mendryk SW. Electrical stimulation as a strength improvement technique: a review. J Ortho Sports Phys Ther, 4:91–98, 1982.

34. Mohr T, Carlson B, Sulentic C, Landry R. Comparison of isometric exercise and high volt galvanic stimulation on quadriceps femoris muscle strength. Phys Ther, 65:606–612, 1985.

35. Reed BV. Effect of high voltage pulsed electrical stimulation on microvascular permeability to plasma proteins. Phys Ther, 68:491–495, 1988.

36. Snyder-Mackler L, Delitto A, Bailey S, Stralka SW. Strength of the quadriceps femoris muscle and functional recovery after reconstruction of the anterior cruciate ligament. J Bone Joint Surg, 77-A:1166–1173, 1995.

37. Astrand P, Rodahl K. Textbook of Work Physiology (2nd ed.). New York, NY, McGraw-Hill, 1977.

38. McDonagh MJN, Davies CTM. Adaptive responses of mammalian skeletal muscle to exercise with high loads. Eur J Appl Physiol, 52:139–155, 1984.

39. Eriksson E, Haggmark T. Comparison of isometric muscle training and electrical stimulation supplementing isometric muscle training in the recover after major knee ligament surgery. Am J Sports Med, 7:169–171, 1979.

40. Hartsell HD. Electrical stimulation and isometric exercise effects on selected quadriceps parameters. J Ortho Sports Phys Ther, 8:203–209, 1986.

41. Bowman BR, Baker LL, Waters RL. Positional feedback and electrical stimulation: an automated treatment for the hemiplegic wrist. Arch Phys Med Rehabil, 60:497–501, 1979.

42. Winchester P, Montgomery J, Bowman B, Hislop H. Effects of feedback stimulation training and cyclical electrical stimulation on knee extension in hemiparetic patients. Phys Ther, 63:1096–1103, 1983.

43. Brooks VB. The Neural Basis of Motor Control. New York, NY, Oxford University Press, 1986.

44. Carnstam B, Larsson LE, Prevec TS. Improvement in gait following functional electrical stimulation. I. Investigations on changes in voluntary strength and proprioceptive reflexes. Scand J Rehab Med, 9:7–13, 1977.

45. Petersen T, Klemar KB. Electrical stimulation as a treatment of lower limb spasticity. J Neuro Rehab, 2:103–108, 1988.

46. Apkarian JA, Naumann S. Stretch reflex inhibition using electrical stimulation in normal subjects and subjects with spasticity. J Biomed Eng, 13:67–73, 1991.

47. Robinson CJ, Kett NA, Bolam JM. Spasticity in spinal cord injured patients. I. Short-term effects of surface electrical stimulation. Arch Phys Med Rehabil, 69:598–604, 1988.

48. Vodovnik L, Bowman BR, Hufford P. Effects of electrical stimulation on spinal spasticity. Scand J Rehab Med, 16:29–34, 1984.

49. Howson DC. Peripheral neural excitability: Implications for transcutaneous electrical nerve stimulation. Phys Ther, 58:1467–1473, 1984.

50. Baker LL, Parker K. Neuromuscular electrical stimulation for muscles surrounding the shoulder. Phys Ther, 6:1930–1937, 1986.

51. Craik RL. Clinical correlates of neural plasticity. Phys Ther, 62:1452–1462, 1982.

52. Karmel-Ross K, Cooperman D, Van Doren C. The effect of electrical stimulation on quadriceps femoris muscle torque in children with spina bifida. Phys Ther, 72:723–730, 1992.

53. Snyder-Mackler L, Ladin Z, Schepsis AA, Young JC. Electrical stimulation of the thigh muscles after reconstruction of the anterior cruciate ligament. J Bone Joint Surg, 73A:1025–1036, 1991.

54. Delitto A, Brown M, Strube MJ et al. Electrical stimulation of quadriceps femoris in an elite weight lifter: a single subject experiment. Intl J Sports Med, 10:187–191, 1989.

55. Wolf SL, Gideon BA, Saar et al. The effect of muscle stimulation during resistive training on performance parameters. Am J Sports Med, 14:18–23, 1986.

56. Halbach JW, Straus D. Comparison of electro-myostimulation to isokinetic training in increasing power knee extensor mechanism. J Orthop Sports Phys Ther, 2:20–24, 1980.

57. Morrissey MC, Brewster CE, Shields CL et al. The effects of electrical stimulation on the quadriceps during postoperative knee immobilization. Am J Sports Med, 13:40–45, 1985.

58. Godfrey CM, Jayawardena H, Quance TA, et al. Comparison of electrostimulation and isometric exercise in strengthening the quadriceps muscle. Physiotherapy Canada, 31:265–267, 1979.

59. Delitto A, Rose SJ, McKowen JM et al. Electrical stimulation versus voluntary exercise in strengthening thigh musculature after anterior cruciate ligament surgery. Phys Ther, 68:660–663, 1988.

60. Singer KP, Gow PJ, Otway WF, Williams M. A comparison of electrical stimulation, isometric and isokinetic strength training programmes. New Zealand J Sports Med, 11:61–63, 1983.

61. Johnson DH, Thruston P, Ashcroft PJ. The Russian technique in the treatment of chondromalacia patellae. Physiotherapy Canada, 29:266–268, 1977.

62. Currier D, Ray JM, Nyland J et al. Effects of electrical and electromagnetic stimulation after anterior cruciate ligament reconstruction. J Orthop Sports Phys Ther, 17:177–184, 1993.

63. Curwin S, Stanish WD, Valiant G. Clinical applications and biochemical effects of high frequency electrical stimulation. Can Athl Ther Assoc J, 7:15–16, 1980.

64. Draper V, Balard L. Electrical stimulation versus electromyographic biofeedback in the recovery of quadriceps femoris muscle function following anterior cruciate ligament surgery. Phys Ther, 20:93–98, 1991.

65. Kahanovitz N, Nordin M, Verdame R et al. Normal trunk muscle strength and endurance in women and the effect of exercises and electrical stimulation, Part 2: Comparative analysis of electrical stimulation and exercises to increase trunk muscle strength and endurance. Spine, 12:112–118, 1987.

66. Sisk TD, Stralka Sw, Deering MB, Griffin JW. Effects of electrical stimulation on quadriceps strength after reconstructive surgery of the anterior cruciate ligament. Am J Sports Med, 15:215–219, 1987.

67. Gould N, Donnermeyer D, Gammon GG et al. Transcutaneous muscle stimulation to retard disuse atrophy after open meniscectomy. Clin Orthop Rel Res 178:190–197, 1983.

68. Grove-Lainey C, Walmsley RP, Andrew GM. Effectiveness of exercise alone versus exercise plus electrical stimulation in strengthening the quadriceps muscle. Physiother Can, 35:5–11, 1983.

69. Currier DP, Mann R. Muscular strength development by electrical stimulation in healthy individuals. Phys Ther, 63:915–921, 1983.

70. Laughman RK, Youdas JW, Garrett TR. Strength changes in the normal quadriceps femoris muscle as a result of electrical stimulation. Phys Ther, 63:494–499, 1983.

71. McMiken DF, Todd-Smith M, Thompson C. Strengthening of human quadriceps muscles by cutaneous electrical stimulation. Scand J Rehab Med, 15:25–28, 1983.

72. Romero JA, Sanford TL, Schroeder RV et al. The effects of electrical stimulation of the normal quadriceps on strength and girth. Med Sci Sports Exer, 14:194–197, 1982.

73. Garrett TR, Laughman RK, Youdas JW. Strengthening brought about by a new Canadian muscle stimulator: A preliminary study. Phys Ther, 60:616, 1980.

74. Currier DP, Lehman J, Lightfoot P. Electrical stimulation in exercise of the quadriceps femoris muscle. Phys Ther, 59:1508–1512, 1979.

75. Duchateau F, Hainaut K. Training effects of submaximal electrostimulation in a human muscle. Med Sci Sports Exer, 20:99–104, 1988.

76. Massey BH, Nelson RC, Sharkey BC, Comden T. Effects of high frequency electrical stimulation on the size and strength of skeletal muscle. J Sports Med Phys Fit, 5:136–144, 1965.

77. Soo C-L, Currier DP, Threlkeld AJ. Augmenting voluntary torque of healthy muscle by optimization of electrical stimulation. Phys Ther, 68:333–337, 1988.

78. Alon G, McCombe SA, Koutsantonis S et al. Comparison of effects of electrical stimulation and exercise on abdominal musculature. J Orthop Sports Phys Ther, 8:567–573, 1987.

79. Selkowitz DM. Improvement in isometric strength if the quadriceps femoris muscle after training with electrical stimulation. Phys Ther, 65:186–196, 1985.

80. Stefanoska A, Vodovnik L. Change in muscle force following electrical stimulation. Scand J Rehab Med, 17:141–146, 1985.

81. Milner-Brown HS, Stein RB, Yemm R. Mechanisms for increased force during voluntary contractions. J Physiol (Lond), 226:18–19, 1972.

82. Enoka RM, Stuart DG. Neurobiology of muscle fatigue. J Appl Physiol, 72:1631–1648, 1992.

83. Thorstensson A, Karlsson J. Fatigability and fibre composition of human skeletal muscle. Acta Physiol Scand, 98:318–322, 1976.

84. Sinacore DR, Coyle EF, Hagberg JM, Holloszy JO. Histochemical and physiological correlates of training- and detraining-induced changes in the recovery from a fatigue test. Phys Ther, 73:661–667, 1993.

85. Jette AM, Davies AR, Cleary PD, et al. The functional status questionnaire: Reliability and validity when used in primary care. J Gen Intern Med, 1:143–149, 1986.

86. Ware JE, Sherbourne CD. The MOS 36-item short-form health survey (SF-36). Medical Care, 30:473–483, 1992.

# 5

# Electrical Stimulation for Tissue Repair: Basic Information

Nancy N. Byl

## Introduction

ost textbooks on wound healing and tissue repair fail to discuss either the physiology of natural endogenous electrical currents and wound healing or the benefit of externally applied (exogenous) electrical currents for accelerating wound healing and repair.[1] However, textbooks written for professionals in rehabilitation place emphasis on the application of physical agents and electrotherapeutic modalities for wound healing.[2]

Some clinicians believe there are insufficient controlled basic science and clinical research studies that confirm the effectiveness and appropriateness of applying exogenous electrical currents to accelerate healing, whereas others claim the research is inconclusive and some types of current (eg, direct electrical current) could potentially injure compromised tissue. Unfortunately, the disbelievers ignore early controlled clinical trials carried out with animals like salamanders and amphibians as well as those in rats, pigs, and dogs whose size, skin, or regenerative properties limit full extrapolation to humans. For example, a wound representing 25 percent of the body surface of a rat can completely heal spontaneously in 30 days, whereas a full-thickness skin lesion representing 25 percent of the human body can never heal spontaneously.[3]

This chapter summarizes the physiologic principles of wound healing with a special emphasis on the role of electrical fields in healthy and injured tissues. The purpose of this chapter is to review (1) the natural phenomenon of self-repair; (2) the phases of wound healing; (3) the environment conducive to repair; (4) the specificity of electric fields in healing; and (5) clinical implications. This chapter serves as the theoretical foundation for applied clinical decision making for electrical stimulation and wound healing.

# THE MOST BASIC PRINCIPLE OF HEALING: SELF-REPAIR

**Self-repair** is one of the most important attributes of living organisms. Self-repair, in its most ubiquitous form, represents the body's effort to maintain a steady state. Tissue growth is a balance of turnover, compensatory growth, epimorphic regeneration, wound healing, and atrophy.

Ideally, repair must lead to morphologic structures that can carry on the same physiologic activities as performed by the original structures.[4–14] In the embryo, structure precedes physiologic competence, but in regeneration, the distinction between morphology and physiology is not as well defined. Unfortunately, the phenomenon for repair and regeneration is not a perfect process. For example, even if an organism is starving to death, it will still repair injuries or regenerate lost appendages.[9] If motor and sensory nerves remain intact but the spinal cord is severed anteriorly, the appendage will be paralyzed but will still regenerate. If an animal is chronically anesthetized, it will still replace missing appendages.[13]

## Turnover

**Turnover** is fundamental to all repair and regenerative mechanisms. At the molecular level, all compounds are constantly replaced in accordance with their individual half-lives. At the cellular level, renewing tissues such as epidermis and blood cells maintain homeostasis as their proliferation in the germinative compartments make up for the equal and opposite loss of cells in the differentiated compartment.[9] Organs that do not normally express mitotic activity are nevertheless capable of doing so following reduction in mass or increased functional demand. Nerves and muscle also tend to be mitotically static and must therefore maintain themselves by turnover limited to the subcellular levels of organization. Whether occurring at the molecular, cellular, or histologic level of organization, in all types of turnover, it is important for synthesis and degradation to stay in equilibrium.

## Compensatory Growth (Hypertrophy)

Organs and tissues adjust their dimensions to the physiologic needs impinging on them: Overuse promotes hypertrophy; disuse leads to atrophy.[9] When part of an organ is removed, there is a subsequent enlargement in mass of the remaining parts, triggered either by the reduction in the total mass per se or by the concomitant increase in functional demand. For example, the achievement of compensatory renal growth following removal of one kidney occurs by a combination of cellular hyperplasia and hypertrophy accompanied by usual increases in ribonucleic acid (RNA), deoxyribonucleic acid (DNA), and protein synthesis. Although the remaining kidney does not completely double its mass, it increases its excretory and resorptive activities to meet normal needs of the body.

In other nonsurgically deleted organs, functional overload leads to appropriate compensatory growth. For example, in the heart, relieving the right ventricle of its task at the expense of the left ventricle results in an accelerated, compensatory growth of the left ventricle until it is twice the size of its counterpart.[9,13] For example, the left ventricle will increase in size as a consequence of aortic stenosis; in addition, the right ventricle will increase in size as a consequence of pulmonary arterial constriction or hypoxia from increased exercise.[12]

## Atrophy

Organs that can hypertrophy can also atrophy. **Atrophy** is seen in several different tissues. For example, red blood cells represent a renewing population (erythropoiesis) dependent on proliferation and differentiation of precursor cells in the bone marrow. Normally, the rate of production equals the rate of destruction, resulting in a stable blood count. However, under conditions of low oxygen tension, the rate of erythropoiesis increases until the number of circulating red cells is sufficient to supply the oxygen needs of the body. When exposed to high levels of oxygen or increased atmospheric pressure, the body finds itself with a superabundance of red cells and decelerates the rate of erythropoiesis until the natural demise of circulating cells restores the balance.[9]

The morphologic maintenance of muscle depends on adequate exercise. Cutting a nerve leads to muscle atrophy from disuse.[9,10] The entire organ diminishes in size, and there is a decrease in the number of myofibrils and filaments in the sarcoplasm. Subsequent reinnervation restores muscle mass similar to the hypertrophy of muscle fibers following increased exercise.

Atrophy can be induced in virtually all organs and tissues of the body, wherever one can experimentally reduce or eliminate functional demand. However, the organ never disappears altogether. This failure of total atrophy under conditions of complete disuse argues against the theory of growth regulation by functional demand. We generally have more tissue of each organ in the body than we need. One can surmise only that this represents an adaptation to the need for a margin of safety such that physiology can adapt readily to the vicissitudes of the environmental demands.

## Epimorphic Regeneration

The replacement of an amputated appendage by a direct outgrowth from the severed cross-section is called **epimorphic regeneration.**[12] In the newt, limb regeneration may give rise to a functional replacement within a few months, but only when a remnant of the amputated appendage is left behind. Regeneration territories are capable of participating in their own regeneration, but the territories of different types of appendages do not overlap.

Another prerequisite for epimorphic regeneration is the infliction of a wound. Without epidermis, and the healing of this epidermis, epimorphic regeneration cannot take place. The wound must include a sufficient cross-section of the appendage itself, and there must be a loss of continuity of the epidermis. The overlying wound epidermis interacts with the subjacent mesodermal tissues.[10] The cells of the mesodermal tissue lose their specialized characteristics and migrate distally to contribute to the formation of the blastema that develops between the wound epidermis and the amputated mesodermal tissue, the same location where a scar forms in a nonregenerating appendage.

The regenerating events at the cell and tissue level are associated with an increase in the rate of DNA synthesis and protein synthesis. Also, postamputation vascular interruption and attendant depletion of oxygen in the stump are correlated with prevailing anaerobic metabolism. The pH declines with increased autolytic activity. Skeletal muscle fibers become depleted of their glycogen as the anaerobic catabolism gives rise to lactic acid. Once the blastema forms, metabolic pathways become aerobic again, lactate dehydrogenase declines, and the Krebs cycle is restored.

## Differences in Epimorphic Regeneration and Tissue Repair

The question is whether epimorphic regeneration is an exaggerated version of tissue repair or a qualitatively distinct developmental process.[10–14] While there are a number of similarities, both processes are initiated by trauma. Epimorphic regeneration and tissue repair cannot take place unless appropriate tissues remain from which renewal can proceed. Both processes are achieved by a combination of cell migration, proliferation, and redifferentiation. They both produce developmentally potent cells from which the new parts will differentiate.

The differences, however, are striking. Internal tissues of the body can repair injuries in the absence of epidermal participation while amputated appendages can regenerate only when epidermal wound healing occurs. In tissue repair, there is a loss of cellular specialization, but the cells can redifferentiate into something entirely different. However, in regenerating appendages, the degree of dedifferentiation must be more or less the same type of tissues from which they came. Occasionally, under unusual circumstances, a cell can change into another histologic type (metaplasia). Epimorphic regeneration always occurs in a proximal–distal direction, but in tissue repair, differentiation proceeds as well distally as it does proximally, and commonly differentiates simultaneously in all locations.

In regeneration, entirely new structures are formed, and new bones and muscles develop as the limb itself is replaced. In tissue repair, there is a completion of the continuity of interrupted parts, but nothing more. The extent to which tissue repair can do this is not unlimited. Nerves are required for epimorphic regeneration as a means to ensure the functional competence of the new structure, but in tissue repair, denervated limbs can still heal their fractures, reunite their severed tendons, and heal integumental lesions. Even skeletal muscles can repair themselves while undergoing denervation atrophy.

Probably, and most importantly, tissue repair is universal. The ubiquity of the skin reflects the essential nature of wound healing in all organs and organisms. Epimorphic regeneration, in contrast, is a luxury with spotty distribution in the animal kingdom, reflecting the adaptive nature of the phenomenon. Animals can live without epimorphic regeneration but not without tissue repair. Regeneration cannot be regarded as an exaggerated sample of tissue repair. Although regeneration is capable of achieving far more spectacular feats of development, tissue repair is actually the most essential for function.

Regeneration is common in cold-blooded vertebrates, but mammals, which are warm blooded, do not regenerate. Adaptation to the land environment has been correlated with a decline in regenerative abilities. For example, fish and aquatic amphibians regenerate most limbs. Lizards can replace lost tails but not lost legs.[10] However, water does not appear to be the only important element. Terrestrial vertebrates walk on land, where their limbs are more vulnerable to mechanical abuse than their aquatic ancestors. A regenerating leg, subject to repeated trauma, would not regenerate normally, if at all. In addition, the granulation tissue forecasts the repair of the interrupted dermal tissues and produces a scar. Scars provide tensile strength, but they also interfere with inductive interactions between wound epidermis and underlying mesoderm, which would be required for regeneration. Regenerative ability may also have disappeared because of metabolic reasons. For example, warm-blooded animals have high metabolic rates and require frequent feedings. Thus, they are not only in danger of starving to death within days or weeks, but they are also at risk of dying from dehydration. Warm-blooded animals also have warm body fluids, which are optimal for growing bacteria. As a consequence, wounds must heal quickly to reduce the risk of infection.

## INJURED TISSUES: THE BASIC PRINCIPLES OF WOUND HEALING

Wound healing in higher mammals is a relatively complex but straightforward process. All tissues and organs of the body, with the exception of the teeth, are capable of repairing injuries.[9] An injury is an interruption in the continuity of tissues. Proliferation, migration, and differentiation of involved cells repair the injured tissue by reestablishing continuity. Each cell gives rise to its own kind of repair process (Figure 5–1).

Epithelial tissue heals primarily by **cellular migration.**[7,8] Mesodermal tissues have a different mode of repair. Aggregates of cells migrate into the lesion where they eventually redifferentiate into the tissue in question. This repair may take the form of granulation tissue as in the case of dermis, fracture callus in the case of broken bones, or comparable accumulations of collagen between the cut ends of a severed tendon. Repair cells originate from local sources adjacent to the lesion, and redifferentiate into the same tissue from which they originated. The tendons and bones reconstitute along their longitudinal axis. Dermis repairs as a sheet of scar tissue without significant polarity. The gap traversed by this mechanism is very limited because tissue forms only between the severed parts, without differentiating totally new elements.

A mild injury heals rapidly. A severe injury that damages a large area of tissue, penetrates all depths, and involves all phases of healing requires a long time to heal and accumulates significant scarring. Also, there are circumstances when wound healing does not occur properly, particularly in patients with systemic disease, those with

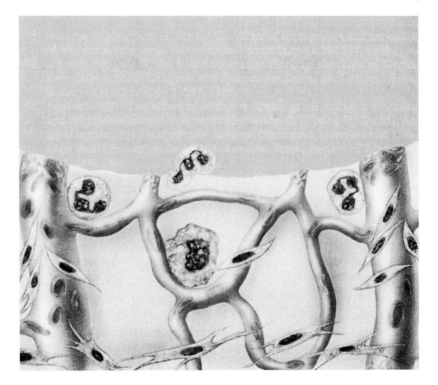

FIGURE 5–1. A schematic representation of the edge of the wound just after injury. Vessels have thrombosed and an inflammatory exudate, mostly polymorphonuclears, is appearing. Serum covers or fills the wound, and serum contains stimulators of cell replication at least partly made by platelets.

denervation (eg, paraplegics), and patients in whom pressure of the skeleton consistently pushes on the skin and causes ischemia and ultimate skin breakdown.

## Initial Response to Injury

Injury initiates bleeding, coagulation, inflammation, cell replication, angiogenesis, epithelialization, and matrix synthesis.[15–19] Rapid constriction of blood vessels immediately occurs postinjury. Coagulation limits blood loss and releases biological products that convert fibroblasts and endothelial cells into a reparative mode.

The repair process occurs in an orderly fashion, but some overlap occurs between the different phases of healing and repair. Following blood vessel damage from injury, plasma platelet cells extravasate to initiate coagulation and to form a fibrin clot to stop the bleeding. This coagulation also acts as an attractant and a temporary matrix for inflammatory cells and fibroblasts. The fibrin forms an environment for cellular movement initiated by thromboblasts, endothelial cells, or injured tissue products of coagulation that regulate the cells in the injured area. Intact thrombin serves as a growth factor that degrades thrombin and stimulates platelets and monocytes.[15,18,20,21]

Thrombin activates platelets and leads to **mast cell degranulation.** Thrombin also provides the environment for the binding of vitamin K to calcium. In addition, thrombosis activates the formation of kinins and releases cytokinins, which transform growth factors and attract and activate fibroblasts. Over time, fibrin clots gradually lyse and convert into collagen matrix to complete the repair. This provisional fibrin allows macrophages, fibroblasts, and capillaries to infiltrate granulation tissue. The fibrin gel degrades in about 3 weeks.[22]

Coagulation also releases platelets. The platelets serve to attract granulocytes and macrophages. Later, the monocytes replace the granulocytes and differentiate into macrophages to continue the debridement and initiate the laying down of granulation tissue. Wound fibroblasts migrate into the wound, proliferate, and secrete extracellular matrix. Cell growth and migration require new blood vessels.

## Phases of Healing: *Inflammation*

### Early Inflammatory Phase
A **molecular cascade** activates inflammation leading to infiltration of granulocytes that consume bacteria and debris. In the first 24 hours, there is an infiltration of granulocytes to debride necrotic debris and foreign material. The granulocytes move to the injury site as a result of chemical properties associated with the wounded tissue. This chemotaxis directs cellular movement. Matrix degradation products from elastin, collagen, and plasma fibronectin also attract granulocytes. The chemoattraction may increase oxidative metabolism of the granulocytes. The granulocytes (mature granular leukocytes including basophils, eosinophils, and neutrophils) prevent infection and debride the wound.

### Late Inflammatory Phase
The critical controlling cells in wound healing are the **macrophages.** They secrete a variety of important growth factors (eg, epidermal, fibroblast, insulin, platelets).[23–27] (See Figure 5–2). Competence growth factors move the cell from the resting state into the cell cycle, and progression factors stimulate mitogenesis (induction of cell mi-

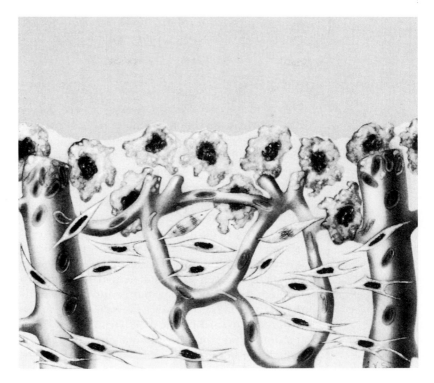

FIGURE 5–2. The developing "granulation tissue" now shows a more orderly arrangement of inflammatory response which is now predominantly macrophagic. Fibroblasts have appeared mostly from perivascular cells. Their mitoses are seen near the most distal functioning vessels. Endothelial capillary buds are appearing in the center of the preexisting capillary arcade. Macrophages are now in a position to stimulate angiogenesis and fibroplasia.

tosis) and DNA synthesis. The growth factors also stimulate the proliferation of matrix production by fibroblasts, including proliferation of smooth muscle and endothelial cells, leading to angiogenesis. Circulating monocytes are also actively recruited into the tissue and converted to macrophages.

The growth of endothelial cells occurs simultaneously with fibroplasia by macrophage products. Granulation tissue composed of collagen, fibronectin, and hyaluronic acid is then laid down. Exposure to the external environment leads to wound reepithelialization, with the epithelial cells moving into the defect. New cells proliferate at the wound edge in 1 to 2 days and migrate under the necrotic tissue or foreign bodies along the undisrupted basement membrane or provisional matrix of fibrin and fibronectin. Hemidesmosomes reform and attach to the basement membrane. Remodeling requires months for completion, removing loose extracellular matrix material and slowly depositing type I collagen. The end result is scar formation.

## Phases of Healing: *Repair*

### *Parenchymal Migration*

**Parenchymal migration** is critical to healing and repair. The infiltration of these cells requires cellular guidance. There are four types of directed cell motility: chemotaxis, haptotaxis, contact guidance, and the edge effect.[28,29] **Chemotaxis** involves movement up a concentration gradient of a soluble chemoattractant. Parenchymal cells can also respond to chemotactic signals, but adherence to the matrix and surrounding cells usually prevents them from moving. **Haptotaxis** involves movement of a concentration gradient of substrate-bound adhesion elements. As the cell moves, it pulls its trailing edge along and a new membrane is inserted into the leading edge. **Contact guidance** occurs as the cell is forced to move along paths of least resistance through the extracellular matrix and results in the cell aligning along the matrix. Two groups of cells, placed at opposite edges of a plasma clot, move toward each other. This may be the effect of cellular contraction acting on the plasma clot to cause the fibrin strands to stretch out between the two groups, providing the path of least resistance between the strands. The fourth type of cell motility includes the **edge effects.** Cells must polarize to form a leading edge that attaches to the matrix and a trailing edge that is pulled along.

### *Angiogenesis*

**Angiogenesis** is the process of formation of new blood vessels by directed endothelial cell migration and growth.[21,24] Platelets arrive very early in the process of wound healing and are involved in this angiogenic cascade. They release an enzyme that degrades the heparin and heparin sulfate components of basement membrane and endothelial cell surface. (See Figures 5–3 and 5–4.) Macrophages also play a role in angiogenesis.[30,31] A number of factors facilitate angiogenesis when macrophages are active, including the accumulation of lactate. The intrinsic lactate production and the oxidation-reduction potential of the cell influence angiogenesis. Local hypoxia also causes a shift to anaerobic glycolysis with increased lactate production and an activation of both angiogenesis and collagen synthesis.[32] As the blood vessels mature, they carry more oxygen.

### *Reepithelization*

When the epidermis is compromised, the natural separation between the organism and the environment is lost and body fluids es-

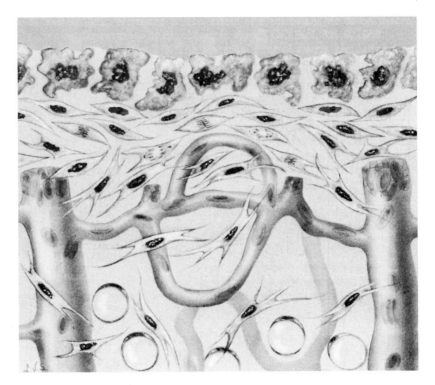

FIGURE 5–3. A new functioning capillary loop has been formed. The "wound module" is complete. Some of the old vasculature, now being in an area of lessened metabolic demand, is dropping out. Compare this idealized version with the photomicrographs in Figures 5–1 and 5–2.

cape. In superficial wounds, epithelium arises from the cells at the wound edge as well as from the dermal appendages, such as hair follicles. In deep wounds, the migrating epithelium arises only from the cells at the wound edge. Epithelium moves across the defect as an advancing front (**free edge effect**) where the cells facing a defect in a sheet of cells move out to cover the defect.[32–34] Hemidesmosomes attach the epithelial cells to their substratum. These cells seal together to prevent leakage through the epithelial sheet. The leading edge cells also become phagocytic, clearing debris and plasma clot from their path. The peripheral cells surrounding the epithelial defect are involved in the movement across the defects, and the cells close to the area of injury are actively dividing to provide new cells. The rate of epithelial coverage will increase in the wound, and the wound does not need to be debrided if the basal lamina is intact or if the wound is kept moist.[1]

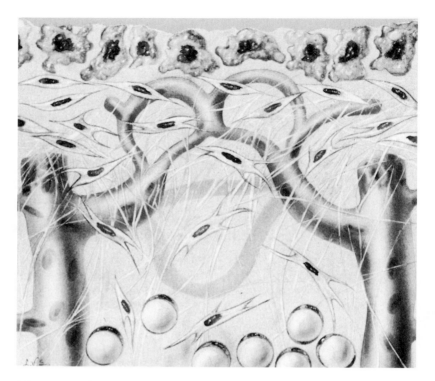

FIGURE 5–4. The edge of the wound has advanced, more new capillary loops have formed while those behind have dropped out. The supplying artery and vein are getting larger and larger. Compare this with Figure 5–2, which is an actual photograph of new vasculature advanced to about the same degree.

## Matrix Formation and Collagen Deposition

**Fibronectins** appear early in the coagulation phase and are involved in wound contraction, cell migration, collagen matrix deposition, and reepithelialization. Fibroblasts, endothelial cells, epithelial cells, and macrophages normally produce fibronectins,[35–38] and they can be found in the tissue stroma and the basal lamina.[31,38–42] They are among the first proteins laid down in a wound and form part of the preliminary matrix. Fibronectin binds with a wide variety of molecules involved in wound healing, particularly collagen (types I–IV). Fibronectin also binds with actin, cell surface receptors on fibroblasts, dermatan, fibrin, heparin sulfates, and hyaluronic acid (HA). Fibronectin appears to function as a linkage between the collagen matrix and the cell's cytoskeleton through specific receptors. Initially, fibronectin provides cell attachments for the fibroblasts. Later, fibronectin is secreted as part of the matrix in close association with collagen, decreasing as the wound matures and type I collagen replaces type III. Granulation tissue fibroblasts coat with a layer of fibronectin matrix, acting as the scaffold for collagen deposition.[35,39,42,43]

There are four major types of mucopolysaccharides participating in tissue structure and repair:

1. **Chondroitin sulfate** impairs the adhesion of cells to fibronectin and collagen, possibly promoting cell mobility.
2. **Heparin sulfate** adheres to the cell surface and basement membranes and may be involved with cell adhesion.
3. **Hyaluronic acid** facilitates cell mobility.
4. **Keratin sulfate** is not understood in terms of its role in wound healing.

In addition, **glucosamine sulfate** is viewed as the building block of the ground substance of the articular cartilage, the **proteoglycans.** Glucosamine sulfate is thought to be a stimulant of proteoglycan biosynthesis, an inhibitor of proteoglycan degradation, and a rebuilder of damaged cartilage.[44] Although the role of proteoglycans is poorly understood in wound repair, they appear to create a charged, hydrated environment that facilitates cell mobility.

Collagen gives connective tissue strength. Type I is the major structure of bones, skin, and tendons. Type II is found mostly in cartilage and is usually found in association with type I. Type III is an immature collagen that is elevated for 3 to 4 days postinjury before the levels of type I collagen increase. Type IV is found in the basement membranes, and type V is found in the cornea in association with type III. Normal dermis contains about 80 percent type I and 20 percent type III collagen. Fibroblasts synthesize and secrete types I and III to form the neomatrix as early as 24 hours after injury.[45–48] Granulation tissue has higher levels of type II than most normal tissues, even though type I is still the major component.[32,45,46,48]

Very little is known about the control of collagen synthesis. Growth factors, nutritional elements, the partial pressure of oxygen, and lactate concentrations influence collagen synthesis. What is known is that collagen synthesis is not necessarily proportional to the number of fibroblasts. Lactate may induce both fibroblasts and macrophages, which release ascorbate, growth factors, and oxygen to allow collagen biosynthesis and deposition to proceed at a higher rate. As angiogenesis proceeds, the metabolites release in increasing amounts and accelerate collagen matrix synthesis. Accumulation of collagen in the wound area is dependent on the ratio of collagen synthesis to collagen degradation by local enzymes. Collagen degradation increases as the wound matures.

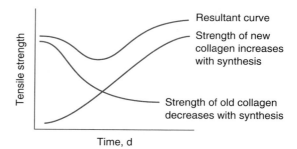

FIGURE 5–5. Concept of wound strength that is expressed as a balance between lysis of the old collagen, which holds the sutures, and the new collagen, which welds the wound edges. Any deficit of synthesis or exaggeration of lysis makes the wound's weak point even weaker for a longer time. *(Redrawn from Hunt TK, Dunphy JE: Fundamentals of Wound Mangement. New York, Appleton-Century-Crofts, 1979, p 33.)*

## Wound Contraction

The tissue edges are slowly brought closer to each other by the process of wound contraction. Wound contraction reduces the size of the tissue defect. If wound contraction continues too far, it can inhibit function and cause disfigurement and excessive scarring.[32,42,47–49] The myofibroblast may be responsible for wound contraction. **Myofibroblasts** contain an actin–myosin contractile system similar to the actin microfilaments found in smooth muscle cells. Myofibroblasts are also called stress fibers and are contractile fibers containing actin, alpha-actin, filamin, myosin, and tropomyosin. The

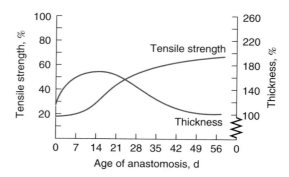

FIGURE 5–6. Tensile strength development in the wound. Note the rapid increase of strength after the initial "lag phase." The initial peak in thickness is clinically defined as the *healing ridge.* The late, slow increase in strength despite loss of thickness reflects collagen turnover and remodeling. *(Redrawn from Lange Medical Publications in Dunphy JE, Way LW [eds]: Current Surgical Diagnosis and Treatment, 3rd ed. New York, Appleton-Century-Crofts, 1977, p 113.)*

filaments align along the long axis of the fibroblasts and provide the attachment for the surrounding extracellular matrix.[48] The unresolved issue continues to be whether myofibroblasts are important, necessary, or irrelevant to the process of wound contraction.

## Phases of Healing: *Remodeling*

For up to a year, the scar tissue remodels according to areas of stress and function. **Remodeling** is the process of restoring the tissue back to normal function without excessive collagen that would interfere with normal use. This process of remodeling also goes on throughout life to some extent as discussed under "Turnover" on page 184. (See Figures 5–5 and 5–6.)

# AN ENVIRONMENT CONDUCIVE FOR HEALING

Although wounds will naturally try to heal themselves, the speed and quality of healing is best in a healthy environment. The application of the right therapeutic treatment in an unhealthy environment may lead to nonhealing. Thus, controlling the internal and external environment as much as possible is important.

## Proper Acute Management of a Wound

The proper acute management of a wound can significantly influence healing. One of the most important procedures in emergency care management of a wound is proper cleansing. Control the bleeding with pressure,[50] which usually takes 15 to 20 minutes. When there is access to water or saline, high-pressure irrigation is better for removing bacteria and foreign material from wounds than low-pressure irrigation. Irrigation with normal saline is the fluid of choice and alcohol should be avoided. This irrigation can be done with a 35-cc syringe, or an 18- or 19-gauge needle for a contaminated wound and an 18-gauge needle for a noncontaminated wound. If the wound is not contaminated, use of low-pressure irrigation or surgical debridement with a sharp knife is proper.

Apply topical agents to facilitate cleansing, but avoid topical agents that are toxic. Alcohol is the most damaging, followed by detergents. PhisoHex and Betadine are commonly used detergents in the operating room. Today, topical povidone–iodine solution can decrease the rate of wound infection without causing tissue necrosis.[51] The 1 percent solution is as effective as a 10 percent solution,[52] and delayed infection is uncommon.[53] Some claim that povidone–iodine disrupts the healing process; however, animal studies do not confirm a decrease in tensile strength.[54]

Detergent agents raise the rate of wound sepsis and cause focal tissue necrosis. Topical antibiotics, especially ampicillin and kanamycin, effectively decrease infection rates in operative wounds.[55] Topical antibiotics may be useful for contaminated wounds, especially if povidone–iodine is contraindicated.

The care of the patient as a whole takes precedence over treatment of a local wound. Be sure that the airway is secure and that there are no cervical spine injuries. Check circulation and then control bleeding with local pressure over the wound. Direct pressure is superior to tourniquets, which can cut off blood flow to noninjured tissue. At the same time, elevate the part. Apply cold packs intermittently (15 to 20 minutes on and 30 minutes off). Maintained ice should be avoided because it could cause excessive edema. Check to see whether serious medical or psychological disorders are associated with the wound. Inquire about conditions, such as chronic use of corticosteroids, diabetes, or peripheral vascular disease, all of which could interfere with healing.

**Closure by primary intent** is the treatment of choice for repairing uninfected or grossly contaminated wounds. Closure by primary intent occurs when the wound is repaired without delay following the injury, prior to the formation of granulation tissue. This approach includes closure with skin tape, sutures, staples, or tissue adhesives. Primary closure yields the fastest healing. Most lacerations can be closed up to 8 hours from the time of injury. However, a clean shear laceration to the face can be closed safely up to 24 hours. In the case of a debilitated host, poor regional perfusion, lacerations resulting from a crush injury, or grossly contaminated wounds, the maximum time for primary repair is reduced by half.

**Healing by secondary intent** occurs when the wound is allowed to granulate on its own, without surgical closure. In this case, clean the wound as usual and then prepare and cover with a sterile dressing. Secondary intent is the procedure of choice for closing certain defects, like fingertip amputations. **Healing by tertiary intent** means the wound is initially cleaned and dressed as with secondary intent, but the patient returns in 3 to 4 days for definitive closure **(delayed primary closure).** This is the choice method for repairing contaminated lacerations that would lead to unacceptable scars if not closed.

Ideally, knowledge of the body's normal skin tension lines (natural creases in the skin when the skin is gathered) is important in the management of lacerations. Lacerations running parallel to skin tension lines leave less noticeable scars that those running perpendicular. When debriding, try to excise in such a manner as to make the final scar line up with the natural skin creases.

The edge of the sutured wound is also important. Ideally, the edges should be slightly turned out. Now epithelialization occurs twice as rapidly compared to inverted edges. The increased rate of epithelial barrier reduces wound infection and the final scar tends to be flatter and less noticeable. In addition, when suturing the wound, the wound edges should be approximated but not strangled. There should be minimal space between the approximate tissues and minimal pulling tension of the suture on the skin. The intrinsic tension equals the pressure with which the tissues within the suture loop are squeezed together. In the first 48 hours of healing, the intrinsic pressure within a suture loop tends to increase as a result of edema.

In summary, appropriate management of an acute wound can have a significant effect on healing. Using pressure and intermittent ice acutely will stop the bleeding and prevent unnecessary swelling. Then, the wound should be cleaned properly, wound edges approximated, and covered to maintain a moist environment. The patient should be educated about protecting the wound area until healing is secure and maintaining a high level of hydration during the healing process.

## Topical Agents That Can Facilitate Healing and Modulate Scarring

Fetal wound healing studies have helped us understand more about the environment which can modulate scar-free healing.[56–60] Both intrinsic and extrinsic differences exist between the fetus and the adult that may dramatically influence healing and scarring.[59–60]

One major extrinsic advantage of healing fetal skin wounds is that it is continually bathed in warm, sterile amniotic fluid rich in growth factors. Amniotic fluid provides a rich source of the extracellular matrix components which facilitate repair (eg, fibronectin and HA).[57] Hyaluronic acid is a key structural and functional component of the extracellular matrix whenever there is rapid tissue proliferation, regeneration, and repair. Hyaluronic acid fosters a permissive environment that promotes cell proliferation.[61] It lays down early in the matrix of both fetal and adult wounds, but its sustained availability is unique to fetal wound healing.[62–66]

Topically applied amniotic fluid and HA can enhance the quality of healing in adult wounds.[67,68] In randomized clinical trials in miniature Yucatan pigs, amniotic fluid, HA, or sterile saline was applied to induced incisional wounds. The surgeons were blinded to the fluids applied. The incisions treated with HA or amniotic fluid healed more quickly and with higher quality than the saline-treated lesions. Although the quality of the incisions treated with amniotic fluid were rated slightly higher than those treated with HA, the differences were not significant. After the first week posthealing, those treated with HA or amniotic fluid were slightly weaker than those treated with saline. However, after 2 weeks of healing, there were no differences in tensile breaking strength between the groups. Thus, amniotic fluid, HA, or fibronectin could be applied directly onto adult wounds to provide the growth factors and the wound matrix to simulate what occurs in fetal wound healing.

Explosive fetal growth combined with the prominent role of growth factors in both development[69,70] and adult wound repair[71,72] suggest that peptide growth factors may play an important regulatory role in fetal wound healing. In adults with diabetes, research is currently underway to determine whether the external application of growth factors can aid healing in difficult, nonhealing diabetic wounds, as well as improve the quality of healing in normal wounds.

In summary, recent research suggests that modifying the external environment of an adult healing wound with topically applied amniotic fluid, HA, and growth factors may enhance the quality of healing.

## The Role of Occlusion in Improving the Environment for Healing

In recent years, occlusive dressings have been used to control the environment of repair.[73] An occlusive dressing helps keep the tissues moist. These dressings can speed epithelialization in acute wounds, as well as induce granulation tissue and healing in chronic wounds, and they can also reduce pain. If one intends to take advantage of the benefits of applying exogenous electrical fields for wound healing, then the wound must be kept moist and covered. When dry, the scab interferes with the lateral voltage gradient.[74,75]

Occlusively dressed wounds do not frequently become infected. Some dressings are able to prevent pathogens from reaching the wound. The occlusive dressings increase the rate of epidermal resurfacing by approximately 40 percent. Moistness may make the migration route easier for the epithelium. Occlusive dressings may possibly increase the partial pressure of oxygen at the wound surface. The occlusive dressing may also possibly increase the activity of growth factors. Winter found that mononuclear cells, fibroblasts, and collagenous material appeared earlier in the dermis of occlusively dressed open wounds.[76] There was also decreased inflammatory infiltrate, decreased fibroblasts, and reduced breaking strength, but less scarring in the occlusively dressed wounds compared to open wounds.

The mitotic rate of regenerating epidermal cells is increased if the surface of a wound is covered with a moisture-retaining but oxygen-permeable "occlusive" dressing. However, the maximal effects are seen only when the oxygen tension of the wound surface raises by application of pure oxygen to the outside of the dressing. The rapidly regenerating epithelial cells migrate along the surface of the exudate that might be covering the wound rather than attach to the surface of the exposed dermis. This epidermal cell movement is a very energy-dependent process. Epidermal cells near a wound edge accumulate glycogen stores before they start moving from the site of attachment.

In venous stasis ulcers, there is commonly gross bacterial contamination and large amounts of exudate. Almost all oxygen disappears whether or not the dressing is permeable, and is probably the result of the oxygen uptake by the bacteria and the inflammatory cells. This event prevents the oxygen from reaching the wound surface. The rate of uptake is so great that even the most $O_2$ permeable dressings are not able to transmit enough gas to penetrate to the epidermis. Rather, it would be more important to select a dressing that favors or inhibits a particular bacterial flora. Under hyperbaric oxygenation, epidermis grows faster with increasing $PO_2$.

## Enhancing Oxygen for Tissue Repair

Oxygen plays a critical role in tissue healing.[77] Well-perfused, noninfected wounds heal in an orderly and predictable sequence. Although the clinical importance of oxygen in wound healing is well established, it is not universally recognized despite the fact that essential elements in tissue repair are oxygen dependent. Wounds heal poorly at high altitudes where the oxygen levels are low.

An immediate natural consequence of injury is **hypoxia.**[77] Hypoxia results from intravascular thromboses that block the main outflow of vessels and stop the bleeding. Circulation that was once adequate to meet the needs is diminished when the demands on the circulatory system for healing are increased. Thus, the wound becomes an energy sink,[78] leading to lactate accumulation, local acidosis, and tissue hypoxia. The measurement of 30 mm of $O_2$ in injured tissue is not uncommon.[79] Although this tissue hypoxia serves as a stimulus to repair, it also places the tissue at risk for infection because it impairs the function of the neutrophils, lymphocytes, macrophages, and fibroblasts. Systemic and environmental insults that are innately associated with poor vascularization (eg, diabetes, peripheral vascular disease) increase the risk for infection. Hypoperfused regions become hypoanoxic ($PO_2$, 0 to 10 mm Hg), hyperbaric ($PCO_2$, 50 to 60 mm Hg), and acidotic (pH, 6.5 to 6.9), with lactate levels up to 15 nmol. Such conditions can interfere with defenses and collagen deposition. Macrophages in a hypoxic, high-lactate environment also produce an angiogenic factor that stimulates angiogenesis in adjacent, better-oxygenated tissue.[77,80-83]

Phagocytic leukocytes are the most important line of defense against infection. However, the effect of leukocytosis is only as good as the degree of oxygen available. (See Figure 5–7.) Oxidative killing is most effective and efficient.[83] Cells also increase their respiration in the presence of oxygen. Oxygen is equivalent to an antibiotic and oxygenates leukocytes, which are critical to fighting infection.[84-86]

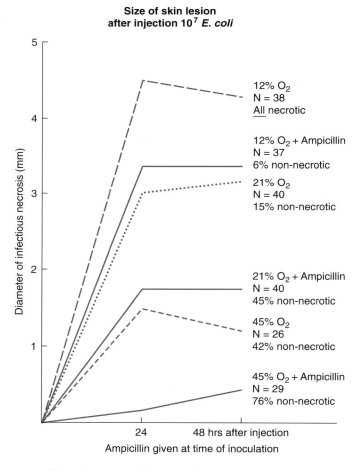

**Size of skin lesion
after injection $10^7$ *E. coli***

12% $O_2$
N = 38
All necrotic

12% $O_2$ + Ampicillin
N = 37
6% non-necrotic

21% $O_2$
N = 40
15% non-necrotic

21% $O_2$ + Ampicillin
N = 40
45% non-necrotic

45% $O_2$
N = 26
42% non-necrotic

45% $O_2$ + Ampicillin
N = 29
76% non-necrotic

Diameter of infectious necrosis (mm)

24    48 hrs after injection

Ampicillin given at time of inoculation

FIGURE 5–7. Effect of oxygen, antibiotics, or both, on lesion diameter after intradermal injection of bacteria into guinea pigs. Note that, at every level, oxygen adds to the effect of antibiotics and that raising $O_2$ in the breathing mixture from 12 to 20 percent or from 20 to 45 percent exerts an effect comparable to that of appropriately timed doses of antibiotics.

Fibroblasts are aerobic cells and require oxygen for both division and collagen synthesis. The hydroxylation of proline and lysine requires oxygen. These fibroblasts are precursors to the release of collagen from the cells. In vitro and in vivo studies show that collagen hydroxylation, cross-linking, and deposition are proportional to the partial pressure of oxygen ($PO_2$). Procollagen, which undergoes posttranslational modification in the cytoplasm, consists largely of hydroxylation of proline and lysine residues, allowing the cross-linking within and between collagen strands that provide tensile strength.[87] The amount of hydroxyproline is reported to more than double when arterial oxygen tension is increased from 40 to 200 mm Hg. Hunt and Pai found that in a 70 percent enriched oxygen experimental group, twice as much hydroxyproline was developed in sponge implants in rats as compared to rats in an 18 percent oxygen-enriched environment.[84] In another study,[88] patients with chronic, indolent, nonhealing soft tissue wounds were found to be hypoxic, with $PO_2$ values ranging from 5 to 20 mm Hg compared to 30 to 50 mm in controls. Goodson[89] and Rabkin and Hunt[90] showed that the measurement of collagen in growth can be made using subcutaneously implanted expanded polytetrafluoroethylene (ePTFE) tubes. Hydroxyproline deposition is proportional to wound tensile strength in rats, and this deposition is in proportion to arterial $PO_2$.

In the growth phase or in a hostile hypoxic microenvironment, fibroblasts may be easily damaged by a hostile, hypoxic microenvironment. Cell growth and proliferation of collagen deposition can be retarded by too much oxygen. The cell cycle for human fibroblasts is approximately 24 hours, and mitosis occurs in about 1 hour. Thus, rather than being continuously delivered, an oxygen dose of 1 to 2 hours every 24 hours is probably appropriate.[90]

The formation and extension of new blood vessels into the wound space (angiogenesis) is essential to the growth of new granulation tissue. New blood vessels appear to follow a gradient of angiogenic factors produced by hypoxic macrophages and not the oxygen gradient itself. If the normal gradient of oxygen tension is eliminated artificially or if a macrophage-free tissue space is created, angiogenesis may be inhibited either temporarily or permanently.

Macrophages are the primary agents in debridement. Their microbactericidal activity depends on both oxidative and nonoxidative systems. A supply of oxygen to macrophages ensures their maximal efficiency. Well-perfused tissues also increase the mobilization of leukocytes as well.[91]

Dehydration seriously depresses tissue $PO_2$[81] and seriously reduces the oxygen available for healing. Dehydration is common in older patients and in patients undergoing renal transplants. Increasing fluid consumption is probably one of the most important practices in wound healing. Breathing oxygen can also increase oxygen tension (eg, breathing 100 percent oxygen at sea level is associated with an increase of 1 to 2 percent of dissolved oxygen). Oxygen to the tissue can also be increased when delivered under pressure (hyperbaric oxygen). Quantification of a patient's $PO_2$ saturation level is good, particularly in someone who is ill or a person who has a non-healing wound. Ideally, $PO_2$ saturation should be 100 percent.

Physical therapists can enhance $PO_2$ by encouraging patients to drink a lot of water (eg, in one case, the $PO_2$ increased from 4 mm to 40 mm after four glasses of water).[92] Therapists can also heat compromised tissues slowly or raise the patient's body temperature to assist in the delivery of oxygen to the tissues.[91,92] However, heating is not recommended for acute wounds, ischemic tissue, or fibromyotic tissue.[93–95]

Electrical currents can also be applied to increase $PO_2$ in subcutaneous tissues and wounds. A steady current enhances the oxygen gradient (drawing oxygen molecules to an area) by the chemical action of the current-carrying ion (eg, a calcium gradient could attract oxygen). Another possibility is that the current creates an intracellular ionic gradient (eg, the larger pH gradients in the cytoplasm) or the exogenous current might polarize cells by the generation of the transcytoplasmic field (eg, the plasma membrane proteins). Mobile membrane proteins redistribute within the surface of the membrane by electrical fields as small as 1 mV per cell diameter.[96]

Only a few studies have focused specifically on the measurement of oxygen with electrical stimulation. The lateral voltage gradient at the wound edge creates a positive state in the middle of the wound and can attract oxygen. Gagnier and colleagues treated wounds in paraplegic patients using three waveforms (monophasic paired spike, positive biphasic, and alternating current [AC]). Transcutaneous oxygen tension measured for 1.5 hours showed significant increases in oxygen after 30 minutes of stimulation with the monophasic current and the biphasic current but not the alternating current. However, at the end of 30 minutes, the oxygen was increased in the AC-treated wounds as well.[97] Baker and colleagues studied 20 diabetic patients and age-matched controls with monophasic paired spikes with negative current. Transcutaneous oxygen levels were measured for 30 minutes during and after stimulation. Increased transcutaneous oxygen occurred 30 minutes after stimulation whether a contraction was facilitated or not.[98] Dodgens and colleagues studied another group of diabetic patients with treatment with monophasic (positive and negative) and a symmetric biphasic current. Transcutaneous oxygen doubled from 4.9 to 5.8 mm Hg.[99]

Byl and Hoft[92] measured subcutaneous oxygen in miniature Yucatan pigs and human subjects when being treated with electrical current and breathing oxygen-enriched air. Significant increases in subcutaneous oxygen were not measured following anodal microamperage stimulation (0.3 Hz, 0.5 µA) in miniature Yucatan pigs or human subjects breathing room air. However, when patients were breathing supplemental oxygen, a significant increase in $PsqO_2$ was measured during and after anodal stimulation, but not after cathodal stimulation. However, the flow index increased approximately 200 percent following cathodal stimulation. This increased flow index suggests that tissue oxygen tension ($PO_2$) can increase even when no significant changes are measured in $PsqO_2$.[92]

In summary, wound healing can be enhanced by appropriately treating a wound in the acute phase, applying substances that would enhance the early covering of a wound (eg, HA, amniotic fluid, or growth factors), using an occlusive dressing, and facilitating the delivery of oxygen to the wound with heating, hydration, or electrical stimulation.

# THE ROLE OF ELECTRICAL FIELDS AND THE REPAIR PROCESS

All types of injured cells (bone, muscle, nerve) possess their own injury currents. A rupture in the membrane permits a steady current to leak into the injured cell.[100,101] The role of epidermally generated electrical potentials in the healing of vertebrate skin is both a physiologic event in healing and a topic of interest to health professionals in rehabilitation. These electrical potentials may be critical to the healing of wounds.

Much of what we know about endogenous electrical currents has been learned from studies on regeneration. More than 20 years ago, 1 µA of current was measured leaving a wound in human skin immersed in saline.[102] In 1980, Illingworth and Barker[103] measured currents with densities of 10 to 30 µA/cm² at the stump surface of children's fingers whose tips had been amputated accidentally. The stump tip was positive with respect to the undamaged, proximal forelimb. The electrical potential steadily declined with time after the amputation. When comparing the currents in an amputated leg of a frog that did not regenerate, the currents leaving the tissue averaged about 7 µA/cm². In salamanders (capable of limb regeneration), the steady level of current ranges from a density of 20 to over 100 µA/cm². However, with $Na^+$ blocked, altering the current, one third of the salamander limbs did not regenerate.

The electrical currents are thought to exert their influence on the neural tissue, the wound epidermis (in regenerating limbs), and the migratory mesenchyme cells. In nerve repair, current densities are immediately very large (in lamprey, 10 to 100 $\mu A/cm^2$), but they rapidly fall to a stable level of 5 $\mu A/cm^2$. The **transepithelial potential (TEP)** actively maintained by the epidermis across itself serves as the electromotive force, driving currents from wounds in the skin.

The **epidermal battery** is best understood in the amphibian, in which there are $Na^+$ channels embedded in the outer membrane of the outer living layer of epidermal cells.[104–106] These are radically different from the $Na^+$ channels found in the plasma membrane of most other cell types. The $Na^+$ channels of the apical membrane of the skin's mucosal surface allows $Na^+$ to diffuse from outside to inside the cell. This diffusion occurs because the cells maintain a very low internal concentration of $Na^+$ by the active outward transport of $Na^+$ by the basal and lateral membranes, and by the entire membrane of the other epidermal cells below the mucosal layer. This outward active transport keeps the internal concentration of $Na^+$ in the epidermal cells low, providing a chemical gradient for the external $Na^+$ to diffuse into the epidermal cells.[107–108] This diffusion results in a net transport of $Na^+$ from the water in which the animal is immersed into its internal body fluids, with the body fluids positive with respect to the outside of the skin. The potential across the amphibian skin varies with the species and depends a good deal on the composition of the water in which the animal is immersed.

In human skin, blocking the sodium channels of the outer membranes disrupts the transport of major cations. This disruption reduces, abolishes, or reverses the transepithelial potential across the skin. The application of amiloride to a slit of the tarsal skin pad reduces the transepithelial potential at the slit by about one half, confirming that mammalian skin has an $Na^+$-dependent battery similar to that found in amphibians.

## Lateral Fields in the Vicinity of Wounds

An electrical leak is produced when a wound is made in the skin. This leak short circuits the epidermal battery, allowing the current to flow out of the wound (as long as the wound is not allowed to dry). At the wound, the potential drop from outside the skin to inside is relatively low. As the distance from the center of the wound increases, the electrical potential across the skin is found to be greater and greater. Finally, a point is reached, a few millimeters from the cavity of the wound, where the potential across the skin is the full value normally found in unwounded regions of that skin. In the cavity, most of this increase occurs in the first 0.5 mm of skin bordering the wound.[102] (See Figure 5–8.) In skin with a TEP of 40 to 80 mV, there is a steep lateral voltage gradient in the vicinity of the wound. The average lateral voltage gradient is 140 mV/mm. If the wound is

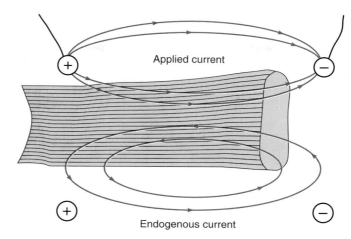

FIGURE 5–8. Polarity of endogenous and applied voltage gradients (and current flow) at the tip of a severed axon. The endogenous injury current (lower portion of the axon) shows that current enters the cut tip and flows in a distal-proximal direction inside the axon. As shown in the upper part of the drawing, an applied extracellular voltage (from a distally negative electrode pair) is of the same polarity as the extracellular component of the endogenous current; however, the applied current would penetrate the axon (because of its lowered input impedance near the cut tip), producing current flow in the reverse direction (proximal-distal) inside the axoplasm. *(Redrawn from Borgens RB, Robinson KK, Vanable JW, McGinnis ME: Electric Fields in Vertebrate Repair: Natural and Applied Voltages in Vertebrate Regeneration and Healing.* New York, Alan R. Liss, 1990, p 93; *reprinted by permission of Wiley–Liss, a division of John Wiley and Sons, Inc.)*

allowed to dry, the wound resistance increases and blocks the flow of current so that there is no lateral potential drop at the edge of wound[102] and the wound resistance increases.

As the wounds heal by migration of cells from the epidermis, the currents escaping through them are reduced. Thus, the lateral voltage gradients in the the vicinity of the wound also diminish. The decrease in wound current that occurs with healing provides a convenient, indirect way of monitoring healing.

## In Vitro Effect of Electrical Fields on Cells

With mammalian wounds, the electrical fields in the epidermis close to the edge of the wounds exceed 100 mV/mm (compared to amphibians, with 50 mV/mm). The effect of such large electrical fields on cell behavior is unclear. Robinson reviewed the research and noted that modest electrical fields across a wound control the migration and orientation of cells.[96]

Perpendicular cell orientation and directional migration have been measured in amphibian neurocrest cells in a direct current

(DC) electrical field.[109] Changes in cell shape and action distribution have also been induced by constant electrical fields.[109–111] This cell mobility is referred to as **galvanotaxis,** electrically guided cell loco-motion—the attraction of cells to the anode or cathode.[112,113] Apparently, the cells can be stimulated to migrate directionally without habituation.

This electrically facilitated mobility has been established in a variety of cells such as leukocytes, neutrophils,[114–116] macrophages,[117] fibroblasts, neural crest cells, and epithelial cells.[109–110,118] The neutrophils retract to the anode and then the cathode, facing margins and becoming perpendicularly aligned to the applied DC field. Fibroblasts migrate to the cathode in fields with modest strengths.[119–120] The movement is clearly defined at 50 to 100 mV/mm and just barely detectable at 1 mV/mm. At 100 to 150 mV/mm, the fibroblasts align perpendicularly to the field. Epidermal cells in fish scales also migrate toward the cathode when placed in fields of from 50 to 1500 maximum voltage potential (MVP)/mm.[121] The behavior of macrophages in an electrical field is incompletely understood and appears less responsive to electrical fields. Macrophages possibly migrate to either the anode or the cathode depending on the field strength. Using the mouse as a model, after 30 minutes in electrical fields ranging from 390 to 1500 MVP/mm, macrophages migrated toward the anode.[117] At low field strengths, activated macrophages migrate to the cathode. Leukocytes and macrophages moved toward the anode in currents as low as 15 mV.[114–116]

At greater than 20 to 40 $\mu$A, galvanotaxis increases to 95 to 97 percent, with the leukocytes proceeding best toward the positive pole at 60 $\mu$A. Fukushima et al studied this phenomenon by placing human leukocytes in 60 $\mu$A of current (with an estimated field strength of 10 to 20 mV/mm).[121] In frogs and mice, the leukocytes also aggregate around the anode. However, when an inflammatory reaction is elicited, the cells aggregated preferentially to the cathode. At 80 to 90 $\mu$A, there is a decrease in galvanotaxis. High-density or high-amplitude low-voltage microcurrent can be used to destroy tissues and must be avoided in wound healing.

## Effect of Electrical Fields on Capillary Permeability

Passing 5, 10, or 50 $\mu$A of DC current or 20 $\mu$A of AC current between electrodes placed in contact with a hamster cheek pouch increased the permeability to macromolecules, and marked extravasation of white blood cells occurred from the capillaries without any preference for the anode or cathode. There were no changes in blood flow rate and no changes occurred in macromolecular leakage or white blood cell extravasation in nonstimulated controls.[120,122–125] Sawyer found that small currents (20 μA) occasionally produce thromboses in small arteries and veins in a rat when the anode is directly contacting the bleeding vessels.[125] A current between 5 μA and 50 μA is estimated to promote the inflammatory response.[123] Yet, clinically, external electrical stimulation may frequently be above 50 μA.

## Specific Aspects of Wound Healing Impacted by Electrical Fields

There is strong evidence that confirms the migration of epidermal cells, fibroblasts, leukocytes, and macrophages by electrical fields of the same magnitude that exist in the epidermis at the margin of wounds. (See Figure 5–9.) Lateral fields at the edge of a wound conceivably could directly promote the inflammatory response, epithelialization, and fibrogenesis associated with wound healing. However, recall that epithelialization sets up a resistive barrier to wound currents that must flow in order to have lateral electrical fields in the epidermis.[119]

Thus, only the events of wound healing that precede complete epithelialization can be seriously considered as processes susceptible to a direct influence by epidermally generated lateral electrical fields. Consequently, collagen remodeling must be ignored, and wound contraction probably cannot be directly affected except as fibroblast immigration might be fostered by the lateral fields. This elimination of possibilities leaves the inflammatory response, epithelialization, fibrogenesis, and angiogenesis as the wound healing events that could be most influenced by lateral electrical fields.[100]

The lateral fields measured in epidermis are those in the narrow space between the upper living layer of the epidermis and the outer, cornified layer of the skin.[102] The regions close to the wound edge are more positive (or less negative) than those farther away from the wound because these fields exist in the return path of the wound current. The fields measured in the amphibian epidermis are of the opposite polarity because these are measured where the wound current flows from the inner surface of the epidermal battery to the wound. Similar subepidermal fields must also exist in mammalian skin, but this has not been measured. Practically, in water, the resistance of this path is too low. However, mammalian skin kept moist by an occlusive dressing might possibly create a circuitry that is more like that of amphibians. Movement of mammalian leukocytes and macrophages into the wound could be promoted during normal wound healing by epidermally generated fields.[96] If such fields exist in subepidermal regions of the skin, the negative end of the field is closer to the wound. Apparently, monocytes and macrophages must be activated in order to migrate toward the negative pole in fields of

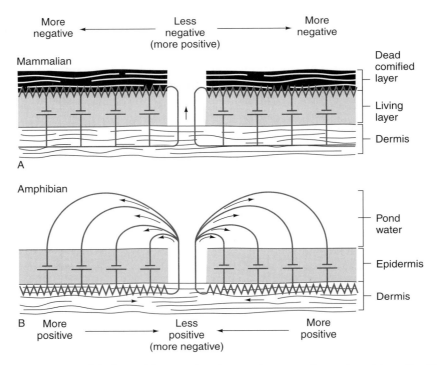

FIGURE 5–9. Comparison of the locus of the major lateral potential in mammalian and amphibian skin. **(A)** Mammalian skin. A steep lateral potential develops in the high-resistance space between the living and dead cornified layers of the epidermis. The space is on the return path of the current from the wound to the epidermal battery, in which the current (positive charge) is moving as it must, from more positive to less positive regions. In this path, then, points close to the wound are more positive than points away from the wound. **(B)** Amphibian skin (and possibly mammalian cornea and oral epithelium as well as skin that is kept moist by an occlusive dressing). The dead cornified layer is thin and moist (and is ignored in the diagram) and is not a significant barrier to the movement of sodium ions into the epidermal cells. The water bathing the outer surface of the epithelium provides a low-resistance path for the return of the wound current to the epidermal battery. Here, the significant locus of lateral potential drop is subepidermal, where the current flows from the epidermal battery toward the wound, again from more positive to less positive regions. In this path, the points close to the wound are less positive (more negative) than points at a distance from the wound. *(Panels A and B redrawn from Borgens RB, Robinson KK, Vanable JW, McGinnis ME: Electric Fields in Vertebrate Repair: Natural and Applied Voltages in Vertebrate Regeneration and Healing. New York, Alan R. Liss, 1990, p 193; reprinted by permission of Wiley–Liss, a division of John Wiley and Sons, Inc.)*

low strength. Their migration to the wound site could be promoted by subepidermal fields in the mammal if they were of sufficient magnitude. There are no data on the movement of capillary endothelial cells in imposed fields, but possibly capillary permeability could be increased by in vivo fields.

In summary, in mammalian skin, cells of the upper epidermal layers at the edge of a wound would be subjected to strong electrical fields. If these cells are so constituted that they migrate toward the anode, it would seem likely that lateral fields at the wound's edge would be a positive factor in wound epithelialization. Cells of the lower layer of mammalian epidermis and the monocytes and fibroblasts from the subepidermal layer might be subject to weaker fields whose polarity is opposite of those along the surface of the outer living layer of the epidermis. Therefore, migration of epidermal cells whose characteristic behavior would be to move toward the cathode in a field would be promoted, as would fibroblasts and possibly macrophages. That fields could cause an increase in capillary permeability, be responsible for augmenting the supply of white blood cells for debriding the wound, and provide chemotactic actors to stimulate neoangiogenesis and the immigration of fibroblasts are also remotely possible.

Immigration of monocytes (transforming into macrophages) appears to be independent of such an influence of electrical fields by the neutrophils that precede their arrival in the wound.[126] Stimulation of monocyte and macrophage immigration by subepidermal electrical fields could be important. We need these cells to debride the wound and to serve as a means, via macrophage-derived factors, of promoting the immigration of fibroblasts and in growth of capillaries.

The fact that fibroblast immigration is facilitated by macrophage-derived factors should not obscure the possibility that subepidermal fields could also have a role in promoting their migration into the wound. In a wound in which macrophages are severely depleted, fibroblast immigration was delayed. This delay of fibroblast migration implies that chemotaxis, a significant factor in promoting fibroblast immigration, is not the only means by which fibroblast migration is influenced.

## Electrical Fields Affect Wound Healing: Circumstantial Evidence

There is increasing research on the role of electrical fields and wound healing that will continue to validate the use of exogenous currents, but there is also circumstantial evidence that reinforces the benefit of these currents.

In healing of mammalian wounds, the outer layer of epidermal cells is the first to migrate during healing. These cells would be exposed to the strongest field existing at the edge of a wound. However, drying shuts off the electrical currents and the lateral fields[103] and may explain why dry wounds do not heal as rapidly as wounds that are not allowed to dry. Keeping both the epidermis around the wound moist as well as the wound itself raises an interesting issue: If the stratum corneum is kept wet enough for it to be conductive, the circuitry could be converted to one resembling the amphibian model in which the significant potential drop is subepidermal. Thus, in this case, migration of cells during wound healing would be exclusively toward the negative pole.

A third observation that suggests that lateral electrical fields might promote wound healing is found by interrelating the body of literature that describes the use of **diphenylhydantoin (DPH)** for epilepsy and its positive effects on wound healing related to the drug's effect on sodium transport in the epidermis.[102–131] The tensile strength of wounds in DPH-treated rats was stronger than normal and both epithelialization and fibrogenesis were accelerated.[132–134] Kellin and Gorlin repeated the experiment and found the same results.[135] Simpson et al gave DPH to patients with chronic leg ulcers. After 13 weeks, the ulcers in the control subjects worsened, while the DPH-treated lesions remained essentially the same or improved.[136]

This increased strength of wound healing with DPH is consistent with the gingival hyperplasia that is seen in approximately 40 to 50 percent of the patients taking DPH medications.[131] DPH produces an increase in the $Na^+$ conductance of the outer membrane of the outer living layer of the epidermis.[134] DPH is likely to have an effect on existing $Na^+$ channels. When these sodium channels are blocked by amiloride, the effect of DPH is abolished.

Lateral electrical fields can also be manipulated by (1) imposing fields via an external battery; (2) interfering with the epidermal battery; and (3) a combination of (1) and (2). When wound currents are reduced by blocking $Na^+$ channels, then wound healing is impaired. Also, if the wound currents are turned from inward to outward, then wounds also do not heal.[96] When the inward currents are restored, healing is not only restored, but in some cases enhanced.[110]

## Endogenous and Exogenous Electrical Currents for Healing Bone

Electrical fields have also been shown to be important in healing bone. As early as 1957, Fukada and Yasuda showed that bone had piezoelectric properties and generated electrical potentials in response to mechanical stress.[137] This piezoelectricity was later reported by Bassett and Becker. These authors hypothesized that collagen was the source of the potentials generated. The electrical potential which develops in bone is negative in the area of compression and positive in the area of tension.[138] In 1968, Cochran reported no significant difference in the response to stress between the potential patterns of dead and living bone.[139]

According to Wolff's law, living bone consistently adapts its structure to meet mechanical stress in an optimal way.[140] The question is whether it is possible to simulate this mechanical stress by creating an electrical stress to the bone. Since the 1960s, many experiments have been carried out to test this hypothesis. However, the outcomes of these studies have been difficult to compare because of the variation in evaluation methods, stimulation methods, and surgical techniques.

In normal resting bone, the epiphysis is electropositive in relation to the subepiphyseal area, with the metaphysis the most electronegative and the diaphysis the most electropositive in relation to the metaphysis. The polarity changes after a diaphyseal fracture, with the area of the diaphysis near the fracture becoming more electronegative than the metaphysis. When bone is stressed, the concavity is electronegative and the convexity is electropositive.

Bone stimulation is carried out using a variety of externally applied electrical currents: direct constant current, direct pulsed current, alternating current, or electromagnetic current. For direct constant current, the optimal current is within the range of 5 to 20 µA.[141] When currents were larger than 10 µA, some necrosis was observed. Actual tissue destruction was noted around the cathode when currents greater than 100 µA were applied.

Most of the bone healing experiments have been carried out in animals where stimulating electrodes were put into holes drilled in the cortex of the femur or tibia (usually the bone of a rabbit or dog). New bone formation around the electrodes was studied. In these experiments, new bone developed around the cathode.[142–146] In some cases, bone destruction was noted around the anode.[146–149] Only one group of researchers reported negative results and this research involved studying fracture healing using internal fixation with the osteosynthesis plate used as the cathode.

The best results have been associated with the cathode actually in the fracture gap and the anode some distance from the fracture (either in the bone or in the soft tissue).[150] Richez et al induced osteogenesis around the cathode and the anode when either 50 µA or 250 µA continuous galvanic current was delivered for at least 1 sec. However, the greatest reaction was around the cathode. Some hemorrhagic necrosis occurred in the bone marrow in the vicinity of the anode. Stimulation with 50 µA pulses (frequency of 0.5 Hz) induced more efficient osteogenesis than stimulation with 250 µA pulses with 0.1 Hz, but the differences were not significant. Dwyer and Wickham applied 5 µA of DC current for 5 to 16 weeks to cathodes inserted in the superior articular processes following spine fusion.[151] Total fusion was measured in 50% of the cases. Lavine et al found significant collagen formation in bone defects of fractures under the cathode with 15 µA of DC current.[152,153]

Ionic migration in the presence of an external current is thought to be one biochemical explanation for the success of electrical stimulation on bone healing.[154] Wollast found that $Ca^{++}$, $H_2PO_4^-$ and $HPO_4^{2-}$ accumulate at the cathode while $Na^+$ and $Cl^-$ accumulate at the anode because of undersaturation. If the surface under consideration is at right angles to the field, the faster ions will be driven either directly toward or directly away from the surface, depending on the orientation, with a net effect of zero.[155]

Bone has a large capacitative impedance at the interface of the electrode. Sansen et al measured about 5 $\mu A/mm^2$.[156] Consequently, an efficient stimulator will have to consist of a constant current source that is pulsed at frequencies that are sufficiently high to short-circuit the interface capacitance but avoid saturation at the battery voltage. In vitro, Durand et al found a linear variation of bone impedance as a function of the inter electrode distance. The cortex of the bone is 3 to 5 times more resistant than the marrow.[154]

In a study using mice, Borgens measured the current density in undamaged bone to be 0.5 to 12 $\mu A/cm^2$. The current was greatest at the epiphysis. In damaged bone, currents up to 100 $\mu A/cm^2$ were occasionally measured immediately after damage. These currents were reduced to 4.9 $\mu A/cm^2$ after several hours post fracture.[157]

There have been many controlled studies on the use of electrical stimulation and bone healing. Today, exogenous electrical currents are used in clinical practice to facilitate the healing of bone fusions and nonhealing fractures. The most commonly used currents have been direct, constant current or pulsed direct current. Currents in the range of 5 to 60 $\mu A$ have been most effective. Current was applied continuously, 8 to 24 hours a day for 1 to 6 weeks with enhanced repair measured compared to controls.[141,146,150–153,158,159,160,161–165] Exogenous electrical currents have also have been used to maintain mineralization.[165] In addition to electrical current, electromagnetic field stimulation has also been found to facilitate bone healing.[163–172] Both electrical stimulation and electromagnetic stimulation are reimburseable therapies for patients with nonhealing fractures or those who need reinforcement for a bone fusion.

## Need for Research: Electrical Fields and Healing

Further research is needed to study the physiology of the electrical fields. In particular, more information is needed about the following:

1. The steep lateral field between living and dead layers of the skin, including the study of the subepidermal lateral fields corresponding to the one measured in amphibian distal limb stumps

2. The effect of reducing the epidermal battery by blocking $Na^+$ channels and by reducing the $Ca^{++}$ content of the water in which the skin is bathed
3. The effect of increasing the epidermal battery
4. The effect of imposed electrical fields on cells in culture, particularly to determine whether mammalian epidermal cells migrate to the anode or to the cathode end of an imposed field

More studies are also needed regarding the physiologic effects of electrode placement. For example, when the whole wound bed is occupied by the electrode, the promotion of epithelialization is probably not as effective as it would be with an electrode that occupies a relatively small fraction of the wound bed and is placed in the center of a wound. More specifically, to maximize the benefits of exogenously applied currents, it is necessary to learn more about the following:

1. Endogenous fields during normal wound healing, particularly at the subepidermal level, corresponding to the lateral fields
2. Wound healing when the epidermal battery is modulated by increasing the potential, decreasing the potential or changing the direction of the electrical fields
3. The effects of channel blockers on electrical fields
4. The effects of imposed fields on cells in culture to determine whether mammalian epidermal cells, leukocytes, and macrophages migrate to the anode or cathode
5. The effects of the instrumentation used to impose electrical fields (eg, effects of electrodes on ions, geometry, metal electrodes)

# Summary

The body attempts to maintain a steady state through self-repair. The cells of some tissues turn over on a regular basis (eg, the outer layer of the skin). Some tissues constantly produce new cells (eg, red blood cells) and some tissues change as a result of functional use (eg, increasing bone deposition as a result of stress, Wolff's law). Most tissues shrink and atrophy as a result of disuse, and healing is a natural response to injury. The body has built-in mechanisms for wound healing which are based on the interaction and balance of endogenous and exogenous processes. Good circulation, cleanliness, exercise, hydration, nutrition, and oxygenation facilitate normal healing.

Endogenous electrical currents are present in normal, healthy soft tissue. Wounding can change the direction and intensity of the endogenous electrical fields. Further, exogenous electrical currents can be used to enhance or alter these endogenous currents. Electrical stimulation may be used to decrease the time required to heal, to minimize the disability associated with healing, or to activate the healing process when it has slowed or stopped. Thus, historically, exogenous, therapeutic electrical currents have been reserved for treating conditions of nonhealing such as those associated with compound fractures, contamination, disease, compromised circulation, absent sensation, or chronic pain. Each of these conditions must be carefully evaluated and the protocol for treatment appropriately matched to the condition.

However, there are times when even exogenous currents are not effective in achieving repair. In these cases, the physical therapist must work with the team to be sure the patient is not self-manipulating the wound for secondary gain or that the chronicity of the wound has not seriously degraded the cortical representation of the injured part, reinforcing the state of nonhealing.[173-177] The therapist must carefully assess the whole patient to recognize these conditions. The therapist should also be prepared to address issues of reeducation as well as recommend treatment beyond local wound care.

## REVIEW QUESTIONS

1. What are the four different processes of self-repair?
2. What are the critical differences between regeneration and tissue repair?
3. What is the initial response to injury?
4. What are the three phases of healing?
5. What are the basic elements of the repair phase of healing?
6. What should be done to maximize the environment for healing?
7. What do we know about the fetal wound environment that could be translated to adult wound healing?
8. What is an injury current?
9. How are the lateral electrical fields created about a healing wound?
10. In what ways do the electrical fields influence healing?
11. What is Wolff's Law and how does this law relate to healing?
12. How are exogenous electrical fields used in healing?
13. What research is still needed relative to electrical fields and wound healing?

# References

## *Introduction*

1. Hunt TK, Dunphy JE (eds), Fundamentals of Wound Management. New York, Appleton-Century-Crofts, 1979.
2. Kloth LC, Feedar JA (eds), Wound healing alternatives in management. Contemporary Perspectives in Rehabilitation, 2nd ed. Philadelphia, PA, FA Davis, 1995.
3. Moserova, J, Houskova, E. The Healing and Treatment of Skin Defects, Basel, Switzerland, S. Karger, 1989.

## *Self-Repair*

4. Borgens RB. Natural and applied currents in limb regeneration and development. In Borgens RB, Robinson KR, Vanable JW, McGinnis ME, McCaig CD (eds), Electric Fields in Vertebrae Repair: Natural and Applied Voltages in Vertebrate Regeneration and Healing. New York, Alan R. Liss, pp 27–75, 1989.
5. Borgens RB, McCaig CD. Endogenous currents in nerve repair, regeneration and development. In Borgens RB, Robinson KR, Vanable JW, McGinnis ME, McCaig CD (eds), Electric Fields in Vertebrate Repair: Natural and Applied Voltages in Vertebrate Regeneration and Healing. New York, Alan R. Liss, pp 77–116, 1989.
6. Goss RJ. Principles of Regeneration. New York, Academic Press, 1969.
7. Goss RJ, Grimes LN. Tissue interactions in the regeneration of rabbit ear holes. Am Zool, 12:151–157, 1972.
8. Goss RJ, Grimes LN. Epidermal downgrowths in regenerating rabbit ear holes. J Morphol, 146:533–542, 1975.
9. Goss RJ. The Physiology of Growth. New York, Academic Press, 1978.
10. Goss RJ. Prospects for regeneration in man. Clin Orthop, 151:270–282, 1980.
11. Goss RJ: Deer antlers: Regeneration, Function and Evolution. New York, NY, Academic Press, 1983.
12. Goss RJ. Epimorphic Regeneration in Mammals. In Hunt TK, Heppenstall RB, Pines E, et al: Soft and Hard Tissue Repair. New York, Praeger, 554–573, 1984.
13. Goss, RJ. Why mammals don't regenerate—or do they? News Physiol Sci, 2:112–115, 1987.
14. Goss RJ. Regeneration versus repair. In Cohen IK, Diegelmann RF, Lindblad WJ (eds), Wound Healing: Biochemical and Clinical Aspects. Philadelphia, PA, WB Saunders, 1992.

## *Principles of Wound Healing*

15. McMinn RMH. Tissue Repair. New York, Academic Press, 1969.
16. Hunt TK, Van Winkle W. Normal Repair. In Hunt TK, Dunphy JE (eds), Fundamentals of Wound Management, New York, Appleton-Century-Crofts, 1979.
17. Jennings, RW, Hunt, TK. Overview of postnatal wound healing. In Adzick, NS, Longaker, MT (eds), Fetal Wound Healing. New York, Elsevier, 1992.

18. Hunt TK (ed). Wound healing and Wound Infection. New York, NY, Appleton-Century-Crofts, 1980.

19. Peacock EE, VanWinkle W. Wound Repair. Philadelphia, PA, WB Saunders, 1976.

20. Henson PM and Johnston RB. Tissue injury in inflammation: Oxidants, proteinases and cationic proteins. J Clin Invest, 79:669–674, 1987.

21. Hunt TK, Knighton Dr, Thakral KK et al. Studies on inflammation and wound healing: Angiogenesis and collagen synthesis stimulated in vivo by resident and activated macrophages. Surgery, 96:48–54. 1984.

22. Gerden B, Saldeen T. Effect of fibrin degradation products on microvascular permeability. Throm Res, 13:995–1006, 1978.

23. Carpenter G. Epidermal growth factor: Biology and receptor metabolism. J Cell Sci, 3(suppl):1–9, 1985.

24. Assoian RK, Komoriya A, Meyers CA et al. Transforming growth factor-beta in human platelets: Identification of a major storage site, purification and characterization. J Biol Chem, 258:7155–7160, 1983.

25. Sporn MB, Roberts AB, Wakefield LM, et al. Transforming growth factor-beta: Biological function and chemical structure. Science, 233: 532–534, 1986.

26. Knighton DR, Phillips GD, Fiegel VD. Wound healing angiogenesis: Indirect stimulation by basic fibroblast growth factor. J Trauma, 30(12 suppl):134–144, 1990.

27. Baird A, Ling N. Fibroblast growth factors are present in the extracellular matrix produced by endothelial cells in vibro: Implications for a role of heparinase-like enzymes in the neovascular response. Biochem Biophys Res Commun, 142:428–435, 1987.

28. Bergmann KA, Singer SJ. Membrane insertion at the leading edge of motile fibroblasts. Proc Natl Acad Sci USA, 80:1367–1371, 1983.

29. Singer SJ, Kupfer A. The directed migration of eukaryotic cells. Ann Rev Cell Biol, 2:337–365, 1986.

30. Riches DW. The multiple roles of macrophages in wound healing. In Clark RAF, Henson PM (eds), The Molecular and Cellular Biology of Wound Healing, New York, Plenum Press, p 218, 1988.

31. Alitalo K, Hovi T, Vaheri A. Fibronectin is produced by human macrophages. J Exp Med, 151:602–613, 1980.

32. Erlich HP, Rajaratnam JB. Cell locomotion forces versus cell contractile forces for collagen lattice contraction: An in vitro model of wound contraction. Tissue Cell, 22:407–417, 1990.

33. Gibbons JR. Epithelial migration in organ culture: A morphological and time-lapse cinematographic analysis of migrating stratified squamous epithelium. Pathology, 10:207–218, 1978.

34. Miller TA. The healing of partial thickness skin injuries. In Hunt TK (ed), Wound Healing and Wound Infection. New York, Appleton-Century-Crofts, pp 81–96, 1980.

35. Williams IF, McCullagh KG, Silver IA. The distribution of types I and III collagen and fibronectin in the healing equine tendon. Connect Tissue Res, 12:211–227, 1984.

36. Grinnell F, Bennett MH. Fibroblast adhesion on collagen substrata in the presence and absence of plasma fibronectin. J Cell Sci, 48:19–34, 1981.

37. Horwitz A, Duggan K, Buck C et al. Interaction of plasma fibronectin with talin-A transmembrane linkage. Nature, 320:531–533, l986.

38. Irish PS, Hasty DL. Immocytochemical localization of fibronectin in human fibroblast cultures using a cell surface replica technique. J Histochem Cytochem, 31:69–77, l983.

39. Doillon CJ, Hembry RM, Ehrlich HP et al. Actin filaments in normal dermis and during wound healing. Am J Pathol, 126:164–170, l987.

40. Grinnell F, Bennett MH. Fibroblast adhesion on collagen substrata in the presence and absence of plasma fibronectin. J Cell Sci, 48:19–34, l981.

41. McDonald JA, Kelley DG, Broekelmann TJ. Role of fibronectin in collagen deposition: "Fab" to the gelatin-binding domain of fibronectin inhibits both fibronectin and collagen organization in fibroblast extracellular matrix. J Cell Biol, 92:485–492, l982.

42. Singer SJ. The fibronexus: A transmembrane association of fibronectin-containing fibers and bundles of 5 mm microfilaments in hamster and human fibroblasts. Cell, 16:675–685, l979.

43. Hynes RO, Yamada KM. Fibronectins: Multifunctional modular glycoproteins. J Cell Biol, 95:369–377, l982.

44. Crolle G, E'Este R. Glucosamine sulphate for the management of arthrosis: A controlled clinical investigation. Curr Med Res Opin, 7: 104–109, 1980.

45. Gabbiani G, Hirschel BJ, Ryan GB et al. Granulation tissues as a contractile organ. A study of structure and function. J Exp Med, 135: 719–734, l972.

46. Bailey AJ, Robins SP, Balian G. Biological significance of the intermolecular crosslinks of collagen. Nature (Lond), 251:105–109, l974.

47. Rudolph R, Woodward M. Spatial orientation of microtubules in contractile fibroblasts in vivo. Anat Rec, 191:169–181, l978.

48. Ryan GB, Cliff WJ, Gabbiani GB et al. Myofibroblasts in human granulation tissue. Hum Pathol, 5:55–67, l974.

49. Gabbiani G, Ryan GB, Majne G. Presence of modified fibroblasts in granulation tissue and their possible role in wound contraction. Experentia, 27:549–550, l971.

### *Proper Acute Management of a Wound*

50. Zukin, DD, Simon RR. Emergency Wound Care: Principles and Practice. Rockville, MD, Aspen, 1987.

51. Faddis D, Daniel D, Boyer J. Tissue toxicity of antiseptic solutions: A study of rabbit articular and periarticular tissues. J Trauma, 17: 895–897, 1977.

52. Berkelman RL, Holland BW, Anderson RL. Increased bacteriocidal activity of dilute preparations of povidone–iodine solutions. Clin Micro, 16:635–637, 1982.

53. Houang ET, Gilmore OJ, Reid C et al. Absence of bacterial resistance to povidone iodine. J Clin Pathol, 29:752–755, 1976.

54. Gilmore OJ, Reid C, Strokon A. A study of the effect of povidone–iodine on wound healing. Postgrad Med J, 53:122–125, 1977.

55. Glotzer DJ, Goodman WS, Lippman HG et al. Topical antibiotic prophylaxis in contaminated wounds. Arch Surg, 100:589–593, 1970.

## *Application of Topical Agents to Facilitate Healing*

56. Adzick NS, Harrison MR, Glick PL et al. Comparison of fetal, newborn and adult wound healing by histologic, enzyme-histochemical and hydroxyproline determination. J Pediatr Surg, 20:315–319, 1985.
57. Adzick NS, Longaker MT. Fetal Wound Healing. New York, Elsevier, 1992.
58. Harrison MR, Golbus MS, Filly RA (eds). The Unborn Patient. Philadelphia, PA, WB Saunders, 1990.
59. Longaker MT, Adzick NS et al. Studies in fetal wound healing. VII: Fetal wound healing may be modulated by elevated hyaluronic acid stimulating activity in amniotic fluid. J Pediatr Surg, 25:430–433, 1990.
60. Longaker MT, Whitby DJ, Adzick NS et al. Studies in fetal wound healing. VI: Second and early third trimester fetal wounds demonstrate rapid collagen deposition without scar formation. J Pediatr Surg, 25: 63–68, 1990.
61. Harris MC, Mennuti MT, Kline JA et al. Amniotic fluid fibronectin concentrations with advancing gestational age. Ob Gyn, 72:593–595, 1988.
62. Dahl L, Hopwood JJ, Laurent GB et al. The concentration of hyaluronate in amniotic fluid. Biochem Med, 30:280–283, 1983.
63. Longaker MT, Crombleholme TM, Langer JC et al. Studies in fetal wound healing. I: A fetal factor modulates extracellular matrix synthesis. J Pediatr Surg, 24:789–792, 1989.
64. Longaker MT, Chiu ES, Harrison MR et al. Studies in fetal wound healing. IV: Hyaluronic acid stimulating activity of fetal versus adult wound fluid. Ann Surg, 210:667–672, 1989.
65. Weigel PH, Fuller GM, LeBoeuf RD. A model for the role of hyaluronic acid and fibrin in the early events during the inflammatory response and wound healing. J Theor Biol, 119:219–234, 1986.
66. Williams SI, Longaker MT, Harrison MR, Stern R. Hyaluronic acid stimulating factor: Fetal urine is the source for this trophic factor in amniotic fluid. J Cell Biol, 107:593, 1988.
67. Byl NN, McKenzie A, West J, Stern R, Longaker MM. Amniotic fluid modulates wound healing. Eur J Rehab Med, 2:184, 1993.
68. Byl NN, McKenzie A, Longacker MM, Stern R, Hunt TK. HA modulates scar formation: Three week follow up. Eur J Rehab Med, 3:10, 1993.
69. Chang B, Longaker MT, Tuchler RE et al. Do human fetal wounds contract: Presented at the 35th Annual Meeting of the Plastic Surgery Research Council, Washington DC, April 1990.
70. Heine UI, Munoz EF, Flanders KC et al. Role of transforming growth factor-b in the development of the mouse embryo. J Cell Biol, 105:2861–2876, 1987.
71. Barbul A, Pines E, Caldwell M, Hunt TK (eds). Progress in Clinical and Biologic Research Growth Factors and Other Aspects of Wound Healing. New York, Alan R. Liss, 266:243–258, 1988.
72. Pessa ME, Bland, KI, Copeland EM. Growth factors and the determinants of wound repair. J Surg Res, 42:207–217, 1987.

## The Role of Occlusion

73. Hinmna CC, Maibach H, Winter GD. Effect of air exposure and occlusion on experimental human skin wounds. Nature (Lond), 200:377, 1963.

74. L'Etang, HJCJ (ed). An Environment for Healing: the Role of Occlusion: International Congress and Symposium Series, 88. London, Royal Society of Medicine, pp 1–157, 1985.

75. Eaglstein WH. The effect of occlusive dressings on collagen synthesis and reepithelialization in superficial wounds. In L'Etang HJCJ (ed), An Environment for Healing: the Role of Occlusion: International Congress and Symposium Series, 88. London, Royal Society of Medicine, pp 31–38, 1985.

76. Winter GD. Formation of the scab and the rate of epithelization of superficial wounds in the skin of the young domestic pig. Nature (Lond), 193:293, 1962.

## The Role of Oxygen

77. Silver IA. Oxygen and tissue repair. In L'Etang HJCJ (ed), An Environment for Healing: the Role of Occlusion: International Congress and Symposium Series, 88. London, Royal Society of Medicine, pp 6–25, 1985.

78. Niinikoski J, Hunt TK, Dunphy JE. Oxygen supply in healing tissue. Am J Surg, 123:247–252, 1972.

79. Silver IA. Measurement of oxygen tension in healing tissue. In Kreuzer F (ed). Progress in Respiratory Research III, International Symposium on Oxygen Pressure Recording, New York: S. Karger, Basel, Switzerland, pp 124–135, 1968.

80. Knighton, DR and Hunt TK. The Defenses of the Wound. In Howard RJ, Simmons RL (eds), Surgical Infectious Diseases, 2nd ed. Norwalk, CT, Appleton & Lange, pp 188–193, 1988.

81. Hunt TK, Pai MP. Effect of varying ambient oxygen tensions on wound metabolism and collagen synthesis. Surg Gynecol Obstet, 135:561–567, 1972.

82. Hunt TK. Physiology of Wound Healing. In Clowes CHA (ed). Trauma, Sepsis and Shock: The Physiological Basis of Therapy. New York, Marcel Dekker, pp 443–471, 1988.

83. Beaman L, Beaman BL: The role of oxygen and its derivatives in microbial pathogenesis and host defense. Ann Rev Microbiol, 38:27–48, 1984.

84. Hunt TK, Heppenstall RB, Pines E, et al (eds), Soft and Hard Tissue Repair, Biological and Clinical Aspects. New York, Praeger, p 455, 1984.

85. Knighton DR, Halliday B, Hunt TK. Oxygen as an antibiototic: a comparison of inspired oxygen concentration and antibiotic administration on in vivo bacterial clearance. Arch Surg, 121:191–195, 1986.

86. Niinikoski J. Oxygen and wound healing. Clin Plast Surg, 4: 361, 1977.

87. Niinikoski J. Effect of oxygen supply on wound healing and formation of experimental granulation tissue. Acta Physiol Scand (suppl), 334: 1–72, 1969.

88. Wallyn RJ, Gumbiner SH, Goldfien S et al. Treatment of anaerobic infections with hyperbaric oxygen. Surg Clin North Am, 44:107, 1964.

89. Goodson WH, Hunt TK. Development of a new miniature method for the study of wound healing in human subjects. Surg Forum, 37:592, 1986.

90. Rabkin J, Hunt TK. Local heat increases blood flow and oxygen tension in wounds. Arch Surg, 122:221, 1987.

91. Feng LJ, Price D, Hohn D et al. Blood flow changes and leukocyte mobilization in infection: A comparison between ischemia and well-perfused skin. Surg Forum, 34:603, 1983.

92. Byl NN, Hopf H. The use of oxygen in wound healing. In McCulloch JM, Kloth LC, Feedar JA (eds), Wound Healing Alternatives in Management. Contemporary Perspectives in Rehabilitation. Philadelphia, PA, FA Davis, pp 365–404, 1995.

93. Rubin MJ et al. Acute effects of ultrasound on skeletal muscle oxygen tension, blood flow and capillary density. Ultrasound Med Biol, 26: 271–277, 1990.

94. Hogan RD, Burke KM, Franklin TD. The effect of ultrasound on microvascular hemodynamics in skeletal muscle: Effects during ischemia. Microvasc Res, 23:370–379, 1982.

95. Klemp P et al. Reduced blood flow in fibromyotic muscles during ultrasound. Scand J Rehabil Med, 215:21–23, 1983.

96. Robinson KR. The responses of cells to electrical fields: A review. J Cell Biol, 101:2023–2027, 1985.

97. Gagnier KA, Manix NL, Baker LL, Rubayl S. The effects of electrical stimulation on cutaneous oxygen supply in paraplegics. Abstract and podium presentation. Annual Conference, APTA. Phys Ther, 68:835, 1988.

98. Baker L et al. The effects of electrical stimulation on cutaneous oxygen supply in normal older adults and diabetic patients. Phys Ther 66:749, 1986.

99. Dodgen PW et al. The effects of electrical stimulation on cutaneous oxygen supply in diabetic older adults. Phys Ther, 67:793, 1987.

### The Role of Electrical Fields in Healing

100. Borgens RB, Vanable JW, Jaffe LF. Bioelectricty and regeneration. Large currents leave the stumps of regenerating newt limbs. Proc Natl Acad Sci USA, 74:4528–4532, 1977.

101. Borgens RB. Chapter 5: Integumentary Potentials and Wound Healing in Electric Fields in Vertebrate Repair: Natural and Applied Voltages in Vertebrate Regeneration and Healing. Borgens RB, Robinson KR, Vanable JW, McGinis ME, McCaig CD (eds). New York, NY, Alan R. Liss, pp 171–224, 1989.

102. Barker AT, Kaffe F, Vanable JW. The glabrous epidermis of cavies contains a powerful battery. Am J Physiol, 242:358–366, 1982.

103. Illingworth CM, Barker AT. Measurement of electrical currents emerging during the regeneration of amputated finger tips in children. Clin Phys Physiol Meas, 1:87, 1980.

104. Kirshner LB. Electroylyte transport across the body surface of freshwa-

ter fish and amphibia. In Ussing HH and Thorn NA (eds), Transport Mechanisms in Epithelia. Copenhagen, Munksgaard, p 447, 1983.

105. Sariban-Sohraby S, Benos DJ. The amiloride-sensitive sodium channel. Am J Physiol, 250:175–190, 1986.

106. Van Driessche W, Zeiske W. Ionic channels in epithelial cell membranes. Physiol Rev, 65:833–903, 1985.

107. DiBona DR, Mills JW. Distribution of Na$^+$ pump sites in transporting epithelia. Fed Proc, 38:134–143, 1979.

108. Robinson DH, Mills JW. Quabain binding in tadpole ventral skin. II. Localization of Na$^+$ pump sites. Am J Physiol, 253:R410–R417, 1987.

109. Luther PW, Peng HB, Lin JC. Changes in cell shape and action distribution induced by constant electrical fields. Nature, 303:61–64, 1985.

110. Stump RF, Robinson KR. Ionic current in Xenopus embryos during neurulation and wound healing. In Nucciteli R (ed), Ionic Currents in Development. New York, Alan R. Liss, p 223, 1986.

111. Cooper MS, Keller RE. Perpendicular orientation and directional migration of amphibian neural crest cells in DC electric fields. Proc Natl Acad Sci USA, 81:160–164, l985.

112. Monguio J. Uber die polare wirkung des galvarischen stromes and leukozyten. Biology 93:553, 1933.

113. Cooper MS, Schliwa M. Electrical and ionic controls of tissue cell locomotion in DC electric fields. J Neurosci Res, 13:223–244, l985.

114. Dineur E. Note sur la sensibilite des leucocytes a l electricite. Bull Seances Soc Belge Micros (Bruxelles), 18:113, 1892.

115. Monguio J. Uberie polare wirkung des galvanischen Stromes auf Leukozyten. Z Biol, 93:553, 1933.

116. Fukushima K, Senda N, Inui H, Miura H, Tamai Y, Murakamo, Y. Studies in galvanotaxis of leucocytes. Med J Osaka Univ, 4:195, 1953.

117. Orida N, Feldman JD. Directional protrusive pseudopodial activity and motility in macrophages induced by extracellular electric fields. Cell Motility, 2:243–255, 1982.

118. Nucatelli R and Erickson CA. Embryonic cell motility can be guided by physiological electrical fields. Exp Cell Res, 147:l95–201, 1983.

119. Erickson CA, Nuccitelli RL. Embryonic fibroblast motility and orientation can be influenced by physiological electric fields. J Cell Biol, 98:296–307, 1984.

120. Cooper MS, Schliwa M. Electrical and ionic controls of tissue cell locomotion in DC electric fields. J Neurosci Res, 13:223–244, 1985.

121. Fukushima K, Sanda N, Inui H et al. 1953 studies on galvanotaxis of leukocytes. I. Galvanotaxis of human neutrophilic leukocytes and methods of measurement. Med J Osaka Univ, 4:195, 1953.

122. Mitchell P. Keilin's respiratory chain concept and its chemosmotic consequences. Science 206:1148–1159, 1979.

123. Nannmark U, Buch F, Albrektsson T. Vascular reactions during electrical stimulation. Vital microscopy of the hamster cheek pouch and the rabbit tibia. Acta Orthop Scand, 56:52–56, 1985.

124. Sawyer PN, Suckling EE, Wesolowski SA. Effect of small electric cur-

rents on intravascular thrombosis in the visualized rat mesentery. Am J Physiol, 198:1006–1010, 1960.

125. Sawyer PN, Wesolowski SA. Electrical hemeostasis. Ann NY Acad Sci, 115:455, 1964.

126. Simpson DM, Ross R. The neutrophilic leucocyte in wound repair: A study with antineutrophil serum. J Clin Invest, 51:2009–2023, 1972.

127. McGinnis ME, Vanable JW. Wound epithelium controls stump currents. Dev Biol, 116:174, 1986.

128. McGinnis ME, Vanable JW. Electrical fields in *Notophthalmus viridescens* limb stumps. Dev Biol, 116:184-193, 1986.

129. Houck JC, Cheng RF, Waters MD. Diphenylhydantoin: Effects on connective tissue and wound repair. In Woodberry DM, Penry JK, Schmidt RP (eds). Antiepileptic Drugs. New York, Raven Press, pp 267–281, 1972.

130. Pollack SV. Systemic medications and wound healing. Int J Dermatol, 21:489–496, 1982.

131. Shapiro M. Acceleration of gingival wound healing in non-epileptic patients receiving diphenylhydantoin sodium (Dilantin). Exp Med Surg, 16:41, 1958.

132. Shafer WG, Beatty RE, Davis WB. Effect of dilantin sodium on tensile strength of healing wounds. Proc Soc Exp Biol Med, 98:348, 1958.

133. Shafer WG. Effect of dilantin sodium on growth of human fibroblast-cell cultures. Proc Soc Exp Biol Med, 104:198, 1960.

134. Watson EL, Woodbury DM. Effects of diphenylhydantoin on active sodium transport in frog skin. J Pharmacol, 180:767–776, 1972.

135. Kellin EE, Gorlin RJ. Healing qualities of an epilepsy drug. Dent Prog, 1:26, 1961.

136. Simpson GM, Kuntz E, Slafta J. Use of sodium diphenylhydantoin in treatment of leg ulcers. NY State J Med, 65:886, 1965.

## *Electricity and Bone Healing*

137. Fukada E, Yasuda I. On the piezoelectric effect on bone. J Physiol Soc Jpn, 12:1158, 1957.

138. Bassett CAL, Becker RO. Generation of electric potentials by bone in response to mechanical stress. Science, 137:1063, 1962.

139. Cochran GV, Pawluk RJ, Bassett CAL. Electromechanical characteristics of bone under physiologic moisture conditions. Clin Orthop, 58:249–270, 1968.

140. Burny F, Herbst E, Hinsenkamp M. Electric Stimulation of Bone Growth and Repair. New York, NY, Springer-Verlag, 1978.

141. Friedenberg ZB, Roberts PG, Didizian NH, Brighton CT. Stimulation of fracture healing by direct current in the rabbit fibula. J Bone Joint Surg, 53A:1400–1408, 1971.

142. Bassett CAL. Electromechanical factors regulating bone architecture. In Fleish R, Backwood HJJ, Owen M (eds), Third European Symposium on Calcified Tissues. New York; Berlin, Springer-Verlag, p 78, 1966.

143. Bassett CAL, Hermann I. The effect of electrostatic fields on macro-molecular synthesis by fibroblasts in vitro. J Cell Biol, 329:9, 1968.

144. Becker RO, Murray DG. The electrical control system regulating fracture healing in amphibian. Clin Orthop, 73:169–198, 1970.

145. Becker RO, Bassett CAL, Bachman CH. Bioelectrical factors controlling bone structure. In Frosh H (ed), Bone Biodynamics. Boston, MA, Little, Brown and Co, 1964.

146. Von Satzger G, Herbst E. Electrical stimulation of osteogenesis. I. Pseudarthrosis of the tibia: Experimental study of bone healing in the rabbit tibia. II. A clinical study of two cases of congenital pseudarthrosis of the tibia. In Burny F, Herbst E, Hinsenkamp M (eds), Electric Stimulation of Bone Growth and Repair. New York, NY, Springer-Verlag, 55, 1978.

147. Bassett CAL, Pawluk RJ, Becker RO. Effects of electric currents on bone in vivo. Nature, 204:652–654, 1964.

148. Friedenberg, ZB, Kohanim M. The effect of direct current on bone. Surg Gynecol Obstet, 127:97–102, 1968.

149. Friedenberg ZB, Andrews ET, Smolenski BI et al. Bone reaction to varying amounts of direct current. Surg Gynecol Obstet, 131:894–899, 1970.

150. Freidenberg ZB, Harlow MC, Brighton CT. Healing of nonunion of the medial malleolus by means of direct current: a case report. J Trauma, 11:883–885, 1971.

151. Dwyer AF, Wickham GG. Direct current stimulation in spinal fusion. Med J Aust, 1:73–75, 1974.

152. Lavine LS, Lustrin I, Shamos MH, Moss ML. The influence of electric current on bone regeneration in vivo. Acta Orthop Scand, 42:305–314, 1971.

153. Lavine LS, Lustrin I, Rinaldi R, Shamos M. Clinical and ultrastructural investigations of electrical enhancement of bone healing. Ann NY Acad Sci, 238:552, 1974.

154. Durand B, Christel P, Assailly R. In vitro study of electric impedance of bone. In Burny F, Herbst E, Hinsenkamp M (eds), Electric Stimulation of Bone Growth and Repair. New York, NY, Springer-Verlag, p 19, 1978.

155. Wollast R, Hinsenkamp M, Burny F. Physiocochemical effect of an electric potential on bone growth. In Burny F, Herbst E, Hinsenkamp M (eds), Electric Stimulation of Bone Growth and Repair. New York, NY, Springer-Verlag, pp 29–33, 1978.

156. Sansen W, DeDijcker F, Stan S, Mulier JC. Four-point measurement of the impedance of bone in vivo. In Burny F, Herbst E, Hinsenkamp M (eds), Electric Stimulation of Bone Growth and Repair. New York, NY, Springer-Verlag, pp 15–18, 1978.

157. Borgens RB. Endogenous ionic current transverse intact and damaged bone. Science, 225:478–482, 1984.

158. Richez J, Chamay A, Bieler L. Bone changes due to pulses of direct. Virchows Arch (Pathol Anat), 357:11–18, 1972.

159. Brighton CT. Current concepts review: The treatment of nonunions with electricity. J Bone Joint Surg, 63-A:847–851, 1981.

160. Goh JCH, Bose K, Kang YK, Nugroho B. Effects of electrical stimula-

tion on biomechanical properties of fracture healing in rabbits. Clin Orthop, 233:268–273, 1988.

161. Herbst E, Josefsson M, Bjorkman JA et al. Electrical stimulation of fracture healing. Part II: Experimental study. Technical Report, 13:74, 1974.

162. Kleczynski S. Electrical stimulation to promote the union of fractures. Intl Orthop, 12:83–87, 1988.

163. Stan S, Mulier JC, Sansen W, DeWaele P. Effect of direct current on the healing of fractures. In Burny F, Herbst E, Hinsenkamp M (eds), Electric Stimulation of Bone Growth and Repair. New York, NY, Springer-Verlag, 147–153, 1978.

164. Treharne RW, Brighton CJ, Korostoff I, Dolland SR. Application of direct, pulsed SGP-shaped current to in vitro fetal rat tibia. In Brighton CT, Black J, Palar SR (eds), Electrical Prospectives of Bone and Cartilage. New York, NY, Grune and Stratton, 1979.

165. Skerry TM, Pead MJ, Lanyon LE. Modulation of bone loss during disuse by pulsed electromagnetic fields. J Ortho Res, 7:600–608, 1991.

166. Blumlein H, McDaniel J. Effect of the magnetic field component of the Kraus–Lechner method on the healing of experimental nonunion in dogs. In Burny F, Herbst E, Hinsenkamp M (eds), Electric Stimulation of Bone Growth and Repair. New York, NY, Springer-Verlag, pp 35–46, 1978.

167. Herber H, Cordey J, Perren SM. Influence of magnetic fields on growth and regeneration in organ culture. In Burny F, Herbst E, Hinsenkamp M (eds), Electric Stimulation of Bone Growth and Repair. New York, NY, Springer-Verlag, pp 35–40, 1978.

168. Kraus W, Lechner F. Die Heilung von pseudarthrosen and spontanfrakturen durch strukturbildende elektrodynamische potentiale. Much Med Wochenschr, 114:1814–1819, 1972.

169. Mammi GI, Rocchi R, Cadossi R, Assari L, Traina GC. The electrical stimulation of tibial osteotomies: Double-blind study. Clin Orthop Rel Res, 288:246–253, 1993.

170. Mooney V. A randomized double-blind prospective study of efficacy of pulsed electromagnetic fields for interbody lumbar fusion. Spine, 15:708–712, 1990.

171. Sharrard WJ. Double blind trials of pulsed electromagnetic fields of delayed union of tibial fractures. J Bone Joint Surg, 72-B:347–355, 1990.

172. Skerry TM, Pead MJ, Lanyon LE. Modulation of bone loss during disuse by pulsed electromagnetic fields. J Orthop Res, 9:600–608, 1991.

173. Byl N, Merzenich MM, Cheung S et al. A primate model for studying focal dystonia and repetitive strain injury: Effects on the primary somatosensory cortex. Phys Ther, 77:269–284, 1997.

174. Byl NN, Merzenich MM, Jenkins WM. A primate genesis model of focal dystonia and repetitive strain injury. I: Learning-induced dedifferentiation of the representation of the hand in the primary somatosensory cortex in adult monkeys. Neurology, 47:508–520, 1996.

175. Flor H, Braun C, Elbert T, Birbaumer N. Extensive reorganization of the primary somatosensory cortex in chronic back pain patients. Neurosci Lett, 224:5–8, 1997.
176. Merzenich MM, Kaas JH, Wall J et al. Topographic reorganization of somatosensory cortical areas 3b and 1 in adult monkeys following restricted de-differentiation. Neuroscience, 8:33–55, 1983.
177. Moyers B. Healing and the Mind. New York, NY, Main Street Books, Doubleday, p 152, 1995.

# Externally Applied Electric Current for Tissue Repair[*]

Carrie Sussman and Nancy N. Byl

## Introduction

n the healthy state, the epidermis maintains a consistent electrical potential in the skin. When a wound is made in the skin, as long as the wound is not allowed to dry, an electrical leak short-circuits this **epidermal battery,** allowing current to flow out of the wound.[1,2,3] At the center of the wound site, the potential drop from outside to inside the skin is relatively low. However, as the distance from the wound increases, the potential across the skin returns to the full value normally found in unwounded regions of that skin.[4,5,6] Over the years, researchers have tried to accentuate healing and repair by applying **external electrical** currents to accentuate this **injury** current. As basic and clinical science studies demonstrated the efficacy of these externally applied currents, physical therapists began applying different types of electrical currents to facilitate healing in clinical practice.

Patient referrals for electrical stimulation (ES) treatment are usually made when a wound has not responded to other treatment interventions. Thus, the most common referral is a patient with a chronic wound such as a **neuropathic ulcer,** or a **pressure ulcer.** Patients with

[*] Portions of this chapter are reprinted with permission from C. Sussman and N. Byl, Electrical Stimulation for Wound Healing, in *Wound Care: A Collaborative Practice Manual for Physical Therapists and Nurses.* C Sussman and BM Bates-Jensen (eds). Gaithersberg, MD, Aspen, 1998.

"**healthy wounds**" are usually referred only for purposes of accelerating healing to enable early return to work, sports, and activities of daily living. The referral initiates the diagnostic process by determining candidacy for ES treatment. The physical therapist is responsible for determining the candidacy of each patient for physical therapy.

The **diagnostic process** includes four steps.[7] The first step is assessment, or data gathering. Data gathering begins with the reason for the referral, the history, and a systems review. Step two is to review the information to determine the candidacy for physical therapy (PT) intervention and which specific examinations need to be performed. Step three is to evaluate the data collected to determine the wound healing diagnoses, prognoses, and expected outcomes. After this process is complete, the physical therapist goes to step four: the clinical decision that PT intervention, including electrical stimulation, is an appropriate intervention.

Once appropriate candidacy is determined, the physical therapist proceeds to the decision-making process related to the intervention with ES. First, the therapist must determine the specific treatment protocol that is appropriate for the **biological phase** of wound healing. Then, the therapist must select the measurement tools that will be employed to evaluate the effectiveness of the treatment and define the periodicity of follow-up to ensure that the goals are being met. Reassessment must be done at regular intervals (usually weekly or at most biweekly), to modify the treatment protocol. If there is immediate evidence of deterioration in either the wound or the patient, then the overall management should immediately be reevaluated.[8] Whenever possible, patients would be encouraged to self-manage their electrical stimulation program at home. Although ES protocols for wound healing will be the focal point of this chapter, in all cases, ES would supplement exercise, positioning, education, and the standard wound management strategies (eg, dressing, medications, hydration, and nutrition).

## ASSESSMENT

### Reason for Referral

The patient referred for physical therapy to facilitate wound healing is usually a patient who does not show signs of normal wound repair. Either the patient has a severe wound or a nonhealing wound, or the environment for healing is compromised. This wound is usually a soft tissue lesion, but occasionally the patient may have a nonhealing fracture or a surgical wound that fails to close. Although the purpose of the referral for ES is to maximize repair, the referral may also accomplish other objectives. Thus, the patient may be referred for physical therapy to:

- Clean up a necrotic wound that has inhibited the process of repair
- Enhance the inflammatory process
- Reinitiate the repair process
- Control infection
- Enhance perfusion to the tissues
- Reduce or eliminate edema
- Improve functional ability
- Educate the patient and the caregiver about wound management at home

All of these goals are evidence based and are consistent with expected outcomes from intervention with ES.

In some cases, patients are referred for ES because of an unusually painful wound. Although ES is an effective modality for pain management, the currents and protocols used for pain control differ from the currents used for healing.[9] (See Chapter 7.) In particular, alternating currents are usually used for pain management, whereas **pulsed** or **continuous monophasic currents** are commonly used in wound healing. However, this pattern may change because of recent clinical efficacy studies on alternating current (AC) for wound healing.[10,11,12] More studies on efficacy of wound healing with AC are expected.

## Medical History of Patients

The **medical history** is a critical piece of the diagnostic process for determining candidacy for electrical stimulation. The history provides background information about the course of the wound prior to referral, and factors that could interfere with repair, such as intrinsic factors (eg, cardiopulmonary problems, diabetes mellitus, circulatory impairment, cancer), iatrogenic factors (eg, use of antiseptics, overuse of whirlpool), or extrinsic factors (eg, wound dryness, wound contamination), that could interfere with repair. The **pharmaceutical history** is very relevant to intervention candidacy. There should be a medical diagnosis for each type of medication. Particular medications, such as steroids and calcium channel blockers, will impair the function of fibroblasts. This use of particular medications could interfere with the efficacy of the electrical stimulation treatment. Review of the results of physiologic tests which could impact the treatment outcomes (eg, red blood cell counts, white blood cell counts, pulmonary function, oxygen, growth factors, nutrition, and hydration) is also important.

For example, the medical record may show a history of osteomyelitis. Stimulation of granulation tissue growth with electrical stimulation is considered contraindicated in the presence of osteomyelitis because of a concern that the area of infection will be closed and blinded from observation. This finding should trigger an investigation of the current status of the infection and discussion with the physician before further intervention. If the lesion referred for PT is cancerous, electrical stimulation would be contraindicated because of the risk of stimulating abnormal cell growth.

**Wound location** is another important factor in determining candidacy for ES. Patients with wounds of the anterior chest wall or anterior neck, such as dehisced cardiac bypass, gunshot wounds, or other lesions located over the heart, carotid sinus laryngeal musculature, or the phrenic nerve, would not be candidates for ES because of potential interference with neuronal mechanisms to vital centers.

The history should also determine the presence of electrical implants that regulate body functions, surgical procedures involving metal implants, or presence of metal in the tissue such as shrapnel or bullets. Electrical stimulation may be contraindicated in the presence of electrical implants because the current and electromagnetic fields could disrupt the function of the implant. Metal implants should be considered a precaution because they may conduct excessive electrical current. Also, depending on the type of ES used (eg, continuous direct current), the metal implant could cause tissue trauma.

Concurrent wound treatments should also be determined during the history taking. Treatments with certain topical agents containing petrolatum products (eg, enzymatic debriding agents, antimicrobials) would interfere with the conductivity of the electrical current to the tissues. Other topical agents contain heavy metals, such as povidone–iodine, zinc, mercurochrome, and silver sulfadiazine. These metal ions can be driven into the tissues with ES, can be irritating to tissues, and may be toxic at certain levels.

**Psychosocial information** gathering is also part of the history. This information must be considered by the physical therapist when setting the characteristics for the ES treatment and determining the capabilities of the patient or caregiver to perform the necessary steps of treatment. Both emotional and cognitive status must be considered when planning for the treatment and the instructional component. Depression and hopelessness could interfere with healing even with the correct treatment. In addition, cost of care and reimbursement issues should be discussed.

## SYSTEMS REVIEW

The patient's history will guide the physical therapist to the more specific **review of systems.** For instance, a history of acute trauma will guide the physical therapist to look at the neuromuscular and neuromusculoskeletal problems related to the trauma, such as immobilization for fractures or possible head injuries. Patients with problems of the neuromuscular or musculoskeletal system that impair body mobility may have impaired healing because of reduced muscle autonomic reactions, pumping action, or reduced neurologic responses. These patients could be at risk for trauma. Abnormal sensory feedback could impair important information about excessive skin pressure. Wounds that extend into deep tissue layers have the potential to interfere with voluntary motor control, sensation, range of motion (ROM), and muscle force.

A history of peripheral vascular disease guides the physical therapist to look at the rest of the circulatory system (eg, the cardiac status; the circulatory impairment that may occur at the ankle, the popliteal area, or the cerebral area such as a stroke or transient ischemic attack). A history of medication for pulmonary problems should guide the review of the cardiopulmonary system.

Patients with diabetes mellitus should be reviewed for type of diabetes. For example, type I diabetes is insulin dependent; if of long duration (15 to 20 years), there is increased probability of insensitivity and dysvascularity. Type II diabetes is non–insulin dependent. People with type II diabetes may have dysvascularity; however, their blood sugar levels may be more stable. The sugar levels of a type I diabetic patient may not be readily controlled.

System impairments will affect the prognosis for healing with ES. Time for healing will be longer for patients with comorbidities, and often healing will be less complete. In addition, wounds can affect the life style of the patient and suggest the need for functional examinations to determine levels of activity and independence, which may call for interventions to maximize functional activities during the healing period. Life style can also affect the outcome of treatment. For example, smoking is a risk factor for nonhealing because nicotine causes vasoconstriction.

## EVALUATION AND EXAMINATIONS

After the completion of the history and systems review, the information is evaluated and candidacy for specific examinations is determined. Examinations performed by the physical therapist are divided into two parts. Part 1 is examination of the **comorbidity factors** that will affect the prognosis of the repair efforts. These examinations include musculoskeletal, neurologic, and vascular function; sensation; pain; posture; ventilation; and respiration. It is not within the scope of this book to describe these examinations, but it is well established that these systems contribute to impairment of healing.

Part 2 is the examination of the **wound** and **surrounding tissues.** A key factor in examination of the wound and surrounding tissues is consistency and reliability of the measurement factors. It is important to track the same features of the wound over time to determine the objective outcomes and efficacy of the treatment interventions. Some clinicians focus only on the wound and wound tissues when determining healing, others focus on the wound tissues in conjunction with the surrounding tissues.

**The Sussman Wound Healing Tool (SWHT)** was developed to monitor and track the efficacy of physical therapy technologies for healing.[13] This simple evaluative tool is quickly and easily learned by beginners and experienced wound management clinicians and is to be used as an assessment tool at baseline and for each reassessment. The SWHT offers a methodology that is consistent and reliable. This tool is based on presence or absence of attributes seen in the surrounding skin and the wound. The tool includes five wound attributes **"not good for healing"** and five ranked **"good for healing"** according to severity. Nineteen attributes were identified: ten of tissue type and nine of extent plus location and phase of wound healing. (See Figure 6–1 for the attributes of the SWHT.) The expectation is that as the wound progresses through the biological phases of repair, the wound attributes that characterize "not good for healing" will disappear and the attributes "good for healing" will appear. Scores should change as the wound heals—"not good" scores should be replaced with "good" scores. The expected outcome from intervention with ES can be prognosed from the time of initial assessment and then monitored and tracked by using the SWHT. Wounds that have factors "not good for healing" will require a greater range of visits to heal than those without the risk factors. Coimpairments identified from the medical history will also affect the range of visits.

## Surrounding Skin Examination

Examination of the **adjacent tissues** provides very important information about the impairment of the body tissues, the response to injury, and the predicted response and outcomes of treatment. Characteristics that are observed in the adjacent skin are color, turgor, temperature, and pain, all of which are the characteristics of inflammation. Look for an alteration of color when compared to the normal color of the adjacent skin or comparable area on the opposite side of the body (pink, red, or purplish). Check for skin turgor, which may be hard, firm, or soft. Feel or use instrumentation such as a liquid crystal skin thermometer strip or infrared thermometer to measure skin temperature. Palpate for pain or use a pain scale. A thorough examination of the adjacent skin will determine dryness,

Sussman Wound Healing Tool (SWHT)
WOUND ASSESSMENT FORM

NAME: _____

MEDICAL RECORD NO.: _____     DATE: _____     EXAMINER: _____

CIRCLE WEEK OF CARE:  B  1  2  3  4  5  6  7  8  9  10  11  12

| SWHT Variable | Categorical Tissue Attribute | Attribute Definition | Rating | Relationship to Healing | Score |
|---|---|---|---|---|---|
| 1 | Hemorrhage | Purple, ecchymosis of wound tissue or surrounding skin | Present or absent | Not good | |
| 2 | Maceration | Softening of a tissue by soaking until the connective tissue fibers are soft and friable | Present or absent | Not good | |
| 3 | Undermining | Includes both undermining and tunneling | Present or absent | Not good | |
| 4 | Erythema | Reddening or darkening of the skin compared to surrounding skin; usually accompanied by heat | Present or absent | Not good | |
| 5 | Necrosis | All types of necrotic tissue, including eschar and slough | Present or absent | Not good | |
| 6 | Adherence at wound edge | Continuity of wound edge and the base of the wound | Present or absent | Good | |
| 7 | Granulation (fibroplasia—significant reduction in depth) | Pink/red granulation tissue filling in the wound bed, reducing wound depth | Present or absent | Good | |
| 8 | Appearance of contraction (reduced size) | First measurement of the wound drawing together, resulting in reduction in wound open surface area | Present or absent | Good | |
| 9 | Sustained contraction (more reduced size) | Continued drawing together of wound edges, measured by reduced wound open surface area | Present or absent | Good | |
| 10 | Epithelialization | Appearance and continuation of resurfacing with new skin or scar at the wound edges or surface | Present or absent | Good | |

**MEASURES AND EXTENT (Depth and Undermining: Not Good)**

| MEASURE/TIME | SCORE | Undermining/Location | SCORE | Other | Letter/Number |
|---|---|---|---|---|---|
| 11 General depth > 0. 2 cm | | 16 Undermining @ 12:00 | | Location | |
| 12 General depth @ 12:00 > 0.2 cm | | 17 Undermining @ 3:00 | | Wound Healing Phase | |
| 13 General depth @ 3:00 > 0.2 cm | | 18 Undermining @ 6:00 | | Total "Not Good" | |
| 14 General depth @ 6:00 > 0.2 cm | | 19 Undermining @ 9:00 | | Total "Good" | |
| 15 General depth @ 9:00 > 0.2 cm | | | | | |

Key: Present = 1, Absent = 0. Location choices: upper body (UB), coccyx (C), trochanter (T), ischium (I), heel (H), foot (F); add right or left (R or L).
Wound Healing Phase: inflammation (I), proliferation (P), epithelialization (E), remodeling (R).

FIGURE 6–1.  Sussman Wound Healing Tool.

moisture, flakiness, cracking, hair, pallor, and/or dependent rubor. Changes in these characteristics are used to monitor and track treatment outcomes.[14]

## Wound Examination

The wound examination can be described in two parts: **tissue characteristics** and **wound size.** These characteristics are measured differently in the clinic compared to the research laboratory. In the clinic, instrumentation is usually limited to linear measurements and visual observations. The visual characteristics of the tissues during the progression of wound healing can be observed and recorded with good reliability. These characteristics can be measured as outcomes; however, they do change during the process of healing. The characteristics include **necrosis, exudate, granulation, contraction,** and **epithelialization.** In the research laboratory, there are instruments to measure the quality of healing such as the tensile or breaking strength of the wound, tissue mobility, the cellular response to healing (eg, mast cell degranulation, presence of fibroblasts, and maturity of fibroblasts). Researchers also are more likely to use circumference measurements, planimetry, and stereographic photography, as well as computer-assisted calculations. In the clinic, wound circumference is outlined on a transparency; a handheld calculator and a simple length-by-width measurement is usually used. These have been tested for validity and have high levels of confidence.[15] There are three common methods for measuring wound size: (1) greatest length-by-width surface area, (2) clock method for measuring surface area (eg, by taking the actual measurement and multiplying length from 12 to 6 centimeters and 3 to 9 centimeters); and (3) measurements taken by either method from a wound tracing or a photograph. Reliability of the latter two methods depends on the quality of the tracing or photograph and its consistency from measurement to measurement. Change in wound surface area size is an outcome measure of repair (eg, either epithelialization or wound contraction).

Measurement of wound depth is useful to determine whether the depth is greater than 0.4 cm, which indicates a full-thickness loss of skin. Use of a clock method to measure depth seems to improve the reliability, but this has not been tested. In the research laboratory, depth has been measured using geltrate molds. Change of wound depth is an outcome measure to track fibroplasia during the proliferation phase of healing.

**Wound undermining** or **tunneling** is another wound measurement that has relevance in measurement of healing. Undermining or tunneling is a loss of tissue integrity and a separation of the fascial planes. This loss of integrity allows for tunnels and sinuses to open. These are potential areas for infection and necrosis. As the wound heals, these tissues reestablish their integrity and the tunnels close. Undermining/tunneling is an attribute "not good for healing." Use of the clock method for performing this measurement has been tested and found to have variability, which can be improved with use of a template laid over the wound to mark the four key points of the clock.[16] Addition of the wound undermining at 12 and 6 to the surface area length and addition of undermining at 9 and 3 to the width measurement followed by multiplying length by width gives a conservative estimate of the total wound area involved. This measurement is called the **overall size** estimate.[17] Measurement of the undermined or tunneled areas and the measurement of the wound size at baseline gives an outcome measure indicating reestablishment of tissue continuity and wound healing. Measurements of the undermined or tunneled areas can also be used as an outcome measure for overall reduction of wound size area. Identification of the areas of undermining is particularly important for the ES treatment setup, because it is desirable to pack the tunneled areas and stimulate them as part of the treatment protocol.

# DIAGNOSIS

## Functional Diagnosis

The diagnosis is the bringing together of all the information gathered to outline the problems. Physical therapists use a **functional diagnosis** to describe an impairment, disability, or handicap of an associated body function. For example, the spinal cord–injured patient has a functional diagnosis of "impaired sensation with undue susceptibility to pressure ulceration." The neuropathic patient with an insensate foot would have the same functional diagnosis. The patient with arterial vascular occlusive disease has a functional diagnosis of "impaired circulation with undue susceptibility to ischemia." It could be added that "there is impairment of tissue oxygenation with undue susceptibility to infection." That functional diagnosis would also be applicable for the patient with chronic obstructive pulmonary disease and the patient who is immobile for any reason. "Impairment of the immune system with undue susceptibility to infection and lack of inflammation" could apply to patients with many different disease states, including diabetes, acquired immune deficiency syndrome (AIDS)/human immunodeficiency virus (HIV), or cancer. It could also apply to patients on medications that suppress the immune system. These are examples of patients with impairment of healing at the organ system level.[7]

Patients with chronic wounds fail to progress through the phases of repair, that is, a functional impairment to wound healing at either the cellular or the tissue level. "Absence of inflammation and inability to progress to proliferation" is a functional diagnosis at the cellular or tissue level. This could also be applied equally to a functional impairment of the proliferation phase: absence of proliferation or wound contraction with inability to progress to closure. Chronic wound edges do not produce functional epidermal cells to migrate across the wound to close it. "Absence of epithelialization due to impairment of epidermal cell activity" is another functional diagnosis for lack of wound progression to closure. A poorly or minimally healed wound on an elderly patient would have a functional diagnosis of "absence of remodeling due to integumentary system impairment." A patient who has a functional diagnosis involving an impairment of a body system at the organ level or a combination of impairments related to tissue repair at the cellular or tissue level should be considered candidates for intervention with electrical stimulation.

## Impairments, Disabilities, and Handicaps

Wound healing normally occurs in an organized **biological cascade.** When there is a disruption in the repair process because of related impairments, disabilities, or handicaps, a physical therapist may be engaged to provide an intervention that will mitigate the effects of the problem or reverse them. **Impairment** of an organ system refers to the loss or abnormality of anatomic structure or function at the organ level,[18] for example, a skin ulcer on a patient with an impairment of the cardiopulmonary or the circulatory system, including cardiac or ventilatory pump impairments. Impairments are distinguished from disease. **Disease** includes the intrinsic pathology or disorder such as renal disease, cardiac myopathy, or chronic obstructive pulmonary disease. **Disabilities** are restrictions or lack of ability to perform activities in a normal manner.[19] Persons who have disabling conditions are at risk for developing secondary conditions that lead to deterioration in functional capacity and quality of life,[20] for example, a skin ulcer in a patient with impaired neurologic function who is handicapped in his or her effectiveness and efficacy of self-care. Specifically, they are disabled in mobility, unable to walk or transfer independently. Thus, they are at risk for skin breakdown and bone demineralization because of sensory loss and decreased blood transport. Presence of impairments or disabilities that increase the risk of secondary impairments of organ systems involving healing are indicators that the body could benefit from an intervention to stimulate the biological cascade of healing and educate the patient and family about prevention. This not only impedes the delivery of nutrients and oxygen to the tissues, but also impairs the removal of waste products. Any one or a combination of primary or secondary impairment states are **clinical indicators** that the patient may benefit from ES to enhance perfusion and stimulate healing.

Wound healing impairments can be expected if there is multiple tissue layer involvement or invasion of the wound into the deep tissue structures. For example, a wound of this type cannot be closed by epithelialization but, instead, must go through an extensive repair process of proliferation. Extensive repair takes considerable time before the wound is closed. Surgery may even be needed. The invasion of a wound into deep structures interferes with the normal mobility of associated muscles, nerves, and joints. The consequence is impairment or disablement of the muscle pump function that would normally transport nutrients and oxygen to the tissues for repair.

Patients who have chronic illness and associated handicaps and disabilities are at high risk for impairment at the cellular level, such as inadequate oxygenation to repair tissues in a timely fashion. This leads to prolonged wound healing and increased risk for infection. An open wound is a portal for infection. Patients who are dehydrated and frail and who have multiple comorbidities are likely to have impairment or disablement of the systems required to control infection.

Information about the disability, handicap, or impairment is obtained during the examination and evaluation. This information will guide the physical therapist in terms of determining the expected outcomes of the intervention.

## PROGNOSIS

The functional diagnosis is predictive of the need for the intervention, and the **prognosis** is the predicted maximal improvement and length of time to attain it. There may be different expected prognoses at different intervals during the course of care. Physical therapists must know the expected prognosis specifically related to their services, including how long it will take to reach a predicted result. Intervention with ES must have a predicted outcome that reduces the impairment of the identified systems and increases function. Consider the wound that is diagnosed as "an absence of inflammation phase." This wound would not be able to get to the proliferation phase. It is predictive that the wound needs to have the inflammation phase stimulated, followed by progression through the phases of healing to reach closure. The prognosis for the wound is: initiation of inflammation phase with continued progression through the phases of healing. An expected due date is also required based on the size and depth of the wound and comorbidities. The APTA Guide to PT Practice[21] offers guidelines for expected length of treatment intervention and range for visits based on depth of tissue involvement. The expectation is that 80 percent of patients/clients with wounds of a particular severity will fall in an expected range. Electrical stimulation can be used to achieve the expected outcome by stimulating the cells necessary to synthesize protein and deoxyribonucleic acid (DNA).[22]

Another example of a functional wound diagnosis is "impairment of sensation with undue susceptibility to pressure ulceration." Reflexive neuronal mechanisms are impaired and other methods must be used to stimulate circulatory responses. The prognosis for the wound would be "circulatory perfusion with oxygen and nutrient delivery to tissues."

Use of externally applied ES often needs to be used in conjunction with other interventions necessary for healing. Comorbidities such as diabetes or paralysis that present body system challenges to healing must be managed concurrently. For example, both of these medical diagnoses may have a functional diagnosis such as "undue susceptibility to pressure ulceration" that requires a concurrent intervention of pressure relief or elimination interventions to produce an environment that will allow the enhanced circulatory perfusion to reach the tissues. The physical therapist must apply this methodology to determine the prognosis.

Clinical research studies are very useful to guide the clinician in predicting outcomes, including the date the result will be accomplished. Clinical research studies are usually carried out in ideal settings under optimal conditions. Therefore, the findings serve only as guidelines to be tested in each individual clinical setting. For example, the literature describes wound healing either by closure or by improvement. Improvement is less clearly defined and usually is described by reduction in depth of tissue loss or size of the lesion. Reduction in wound size is an outcome of proliferation. Reduction in wound size is a measure of wound contraction, a component of proliferation and epithelialization. These outcomes are changes at the cellular and tissue systems levels. The time reported in research studies to reach closure or improvement ranges, or both, from 4 to 12 weeks. The prediction of change in the wound phase can be used as a prognosis for wound healing.[7]

# INTERVENTION WITH ELECTRICAL STIMULATION FOR WOUND HEALING

Chapter 5 describes the role of endogenous electrical fields on galvanotaxis of cells and oxygen needed for repair and regeneration. Additional aspects of wound healing are affected by exogenous electrical fields, including blood flow and edema, debridement and thrombosis, infection and pain, and scar formation.

## Blood Flow and Edema

Several studies in the literature reported improved blood flow after treatment with ES. Treatment with high-voltage pulsed current (HVPC) with negative polarity induced greater blood flow in rats than did positive polarity. The blood flow volume was increased nearly instantaneously at the pulse rates tested: 2, 20, 80, and 120 pps. Blood flow was enhanced by increasing the amplitude of the current (eg, stimulating muscle contraction). However, in a small number of cases, blood flow volume increased without visible muscle contraction. Blood flow velocity remained elevated from 4 to 20 minutes after treatment.[23] Necrosis of skin flaps and free full-thickness skin grafts is a major problem following plastic surgery. Several skin flap studies showed greater blood flow increases following ES with a cathode compared to non–electrically stimulated flaps.[24,25,26]

Alon and deDomenico[27] reviewed the literature on the effects of electrical stimulation on venous circulation. As yet, ES is not used extensively for management of venous circulation problems, but merits inclusion in this section for thoughtful application. There is no support for intervention in the acute phase of varicose hemorrhage or deep vein thrombosis, but ES can effectively treat chronic conditions including deep vein thrombosis and venous stasis. When muscle groups in the calf and posterior thigh are stimulated to produce intermittent tetanic muscle contraction, there is very effective enhancement of venous return in cases of venous insufficiency or deep vein thrombosis. The required stimulation characteristics are those needed to provide motor excitation leading to evoked intermittent tetanic muscle contraction. Augmentation of the venous return initiates a response of vasodilation of the arterioles to bring blood flow to the muscles. Enhanced blood flow to tissues supports tissue demands for increased oxygen and nutrients required for healing. In the case of the patient with venous insufficiency, stimulation of enhanced blood flow will need to be evaluated and may require aftercare of compression to avoid pooling of blood at the ankles because of the incompetent valves. If the arterioles are severely occluded, the vasodilation response may not occur, and then electrically evoked muscle contraction may not be desired. In fact, the muscle contraction may cause severe pain by curtailing limited blood flow to the area, leading to ischemia. There is very limited clinical data to support specific protocols for this effect. Therefore, it is up to the physical therapist to evaluate the vascular impairments based on the diagnostic process and select a protocol to support the desired effect. The section on protocols and procedures provides an example for guidance.

Kaada reported a causal relationship between **transcutaneous electrical nerve stimulation (TENS)** and mechanisms involved in widespread microvascular cutaneous vasodilation.[28,29] Results showed that a 15- to 30-minute period of TENS induced vasodilation and produced a prolonged vascular response. Vasodilation lasted several hours, potentially indicating the release of a long-lasting neurohumoral substance or metabolite. Kaada attributed the effects to three possible modes of action: inhibition of the sympathetic fibers supplied to skin vessels; release of an active vasodilator substance, vasoactive intestinal polypeptide (VIP); or a segmental axon reflex responsible for effecting local circulation. The Kaada studies included reports of clinical results wherein patients served as their own controls of stimulation-promoted healing in cases of chronic ulceration of various etiologies.[29]

Edema reduction under the negative pole is attributed to a phenomenon called **cataphoresis.** Cataphoresis is the movement of nondissociated colloid molecules, such as droplets of fat, albumin, particles of starch, blood cells, bacteria, and other single cells (all have an electrical charge because of the absorption of ions) under the influence of a direct current toward the cathode. **Albumin** is a colloidal protein found in blood that is negatively charged. Albumin is repelled by negative polarity, causing a fluid shift and thereby a reduction of edema. Ross and Segal claim benefit in treating postoperative edema, healing, and pain with HVPC[30] and attributed effects of direct current on edema to cataphoresis. They formulated a protocol based on the use of the cathode to reduce edema. Several attempts have been made to learn whether the same effect occurs with HVPC. Reed reported reduction of **posttraumatic edema** in hamsters following HVPC and attributed the effect to reduced microvessel leakage.[31] Posttraumatic edema was curbed in frogs treated with HVPC when the cathode was used. There was no effect if the anode was applied. Treatment effect was significant from the end of the first treatment session until the end of data recording, 17 hours later.[32] A similar study using HVPC on rat hind paws found significant treatment effects after the second 20-minute treatment with the cathode.[33] More investigation is needed to verify this phenomenon in humans.

## Debridement and Thrombosis

A review of the research is a guide for the clinician and provides evidence to support a protocol for wound healing initiated with the negative pole at the wound site. **Debridement** is facilitated if the tissue is solubilized or liquefied, as occurs with enzymatic debriding agents or autolysis. For example, necrotic tissues are made up of coalesced blood elements. Electrical stimulation using negative current can solubilize this clotted blood.[34,35,36]

Reperfusion of tissues is rapidly followed by autolytic debridement. Increased blood flow, stimulated by ES at the negative pole, has been attributed to having this effect. When the clinical studies are compared, the negative pole has clearly been used to initiate treatment in all reported controlled clinical studies. Many of the wounds in the treatment groups included necrotic wounds.

The positive electrode has been found to induce clumping of leukocytes and the forming of thromboses in the small vessels. These effects can be reversed by using the negative electrode.[37] This may explain a clinical observation in which a hematoma, or hemorrhaging at the wound margin or on granulation tissue, is dissolved and reabsorbed following application of HVPC with the negative pole. Hemorrhagic material goes on to necrosis if not dissolved and reabsorbed quickly. Perhaps continuous use of positive polarity produces the clumping of leukocytes and also explains why a protocol of intermittently changing polarity restarts the healing process. These are critical issues that need to be researched.

## Antibacterial Effects

Because infection is an impediment to healing of chronic wounds, methods to control infection are of clinical importance. **Bactericidal effects** have been attributed to ES. Research suggests that there is evidence to support this theory. In vitro and in vivo studies applying direct current have shown inhibition of bacterial growth rates for organisms commonly found in chronic wounds at the cathode.[29,38,39] Passage of positive (anodal) current through silver wire electrodes was found to be bactericidal to gram-negative bacteria in wounds and inhibitive to gram-positive wound bacteria.[40] At low levels of amplitude, 0.4 to 4 $\mu$A, there were negligible bactericidal effects.[12] Kinkaid and Lavoie[41] tested in vitro stimulation using HVPC at the cathode and anode. Szuminsky et al[42] tested HVPC in vitro at the cathode. Both studies found inhibition of *Staphylococcus aureus, Escherichia coli,* and *Pseudomonas aeruginosa* at the site treated with the negative electrode. However, the amplitude of the stimulation reported by Kinkaid and Lavoie was at an amplitude of 250 V, and Szuminsky et al reported 500 V. Patients would likely find this voltage amplitude intolerable. Because there is inconsistency in these findings and there are no chemical changes (acidity or alkalinity) measured under the electrodes of high-voltage pulsed current, it is not clear whether the antibacterial effects are the result of polarity or another mechanism. For example, increased subcutaneous oxygen was found under the anode when a microamperage current (0.3 Hz) was passed through the electrode. Possibly, the oxygen rather than the polarity is the variable that is responsible for the bactericidal effects on pathogens.

### Pain
Noninvasive electrical simulators that stimulate sensory nerves are commonly classified as TENS.[43] A large body of literature supports the use of TENS for both acute and chronic pain management. Techniques for pain modulation can be used along with the wound healing protocols. For example, one electrode may be placed on the painful area, which includes the wound and adjacent tissues, and the other electrode over the related spinal nerve. The electrodes can also be placed bracketed proximally and distally to the areas of pain around the wound, such as with a bipolar technique described later in this chapter.[44] Pain management would be a good reason to use electrodes of equal size so that there would be adequate current density at both electrodes.

### Scar Formation
The goal of wound healing is a **scar** whose characteristics are most like the original skin. Mast cells regulate this process through the healing cycle. A large number of mast cells in the healing wound are associated with diseases of abnormal fibrotic healing such as keloid formation. Following exposure to positive-polarity current, a decrease in mast cells, decreased scar thickness, and better cosmetic results were observed in treated wounds in humans.[45] In animal and human studies, flaps and grafts treated with monophasic pulsed current ES heal without ischemia and result in flatter, thinner scars than in controls.[24,25,26,46]

## Clinical Studies

Since the 1960s, a series of clinical trials have been undertaken to evaluate the effect of ES on wound healing. The early studies are classics in this field.

### Low-voltage Microamperage Direct Current Studies
**Low-voltage continuous microamperage** direct current (DC) was used in three clinical studies. Wolcott et al,[47] Gault and Gatens,[48] and Carley and Wainapel[49] treated ischemic and indolent ulcers. In all

three studies, a positive (anode) polarity was used after a period of 3 or more days using the cathode. The polarity was reversed every day or every 3 days if wound healing did not progress. Rationale for cathode application was the solubilization of necrotic tissue[50] and bactericidal effects.[38,39] The first two studies used an amplitude of 200 to 800 μA and the latter study 300 to 700 μA. Duration of treatment was very long: 2 hours, two or three times per day, or 42 hours per week for the first two studies, and 20 hours per week for the latter study. A combined total of 163 patients were treated, and 29 served as controls. In most cases, the patient served as his or her own control. Mean healing times reported were 9.6, 4.7, and 5.0 weeks, respectively, for these three studies. The difference in healing time among these three studies is not clear. Perhaps in the Wolcott and Wheeler study the wounds were more extensive than in the other studies.

**Microcurrent** stimulation has been studied in animal models in which current was applied only one or two times per day for 30 minutes, for 1 to 2 weeks; no significant clinical effects were demonstrated on wound healing.[51,52] In another study, there were significant increases in subcutaneous oxygen measurements when supplemental oxygen was given by mask during the microcurrent stimulation.[53] There was no acceleration in healing.

### Modified Biphasic Stimulation

Barron et al[54] reported a study of six patients with pressure ulcers who were treated three times a week for 3 weeks for a total of nine treatments with microcurrent stimulation. The waveform reported was a **modified biphasic** square wave, but it was unclear as to the current waveform characteristics and whether positive or negative polarity was used. The treatment characteristics were 600 μA times 50 V (0.3 W), and 0.5 Hz to 5.0 Hz. The electrode probes were placed 2 cm away from the edge of the ulcer and moved circumferentially around the ulcer. Each successive placement of the probes was 2 cm from the prior placement. In this small study, two ulcers healed 100 percent, three healed 99 percent, and one decreased in size by 55 percent.

### High-voltage Pulsed Current Studies

Three controlled clinical studies with **HVPC** have been reported by Kloth and Feedar,[55] Griffin et al,[56] and Unger et al.[57] In the study by Kloth and Feeder,[55] wounds had a mean healing time of 7.3 weeks, and 100 percent of the treatment group healed. Unger et al reported on a controlled study of nine subjects in the treatment group and eight controls. The average wound size in the treatment group was 460 mm², compared with the control group whose average wound size was 118.5 mm². Mean healing time was 7.3 weeks for the treatment group, with 88.9 percent healed.[57] Griffin et al had demonstrated an 80 percent reduction in size in 4 weeks, but the ulcers were not treated until healed.[56] Unger reported an uncontrolled study using HVPC treatment for 223 wounds.[58] The mean healing times for the 223 wounds in the uncontrolled study was 10.9 weeks. In all the above studies, the treatment frequency was five to seven times per week for 45 to 60 minutes. All treatment protocols began with negative polarity. After the wounds were clean of infection, polarity was changed to positive except in the study by Griffin et al[56] where the polarity was kept at negative for the 4-week study period (Table 6–1).

Two additional published uncontrolled studies included 30 patients. Alon et al[59] used positive polarity and stimulated wounds three times a week for 1 hour; 12 of the 15 (80 percent) treated ulcers healed. One patient died, two ulcers did not heal, one did not respond, and the ulcer in one decreased significantly in size, but did not heal in 21.6 weeks. Akers and Gabrielson[60] published a study that compared (1) HVPC direct application to the wound, (2) application of HVPC using the whirlpool as a large electrode, and (3) whirlpool alone. The direct application of the active electrode to the wound site had the best outcome, followed by HVPC using the whirlpool as an electrode. Whirlpool alone was the least effective.

For the best expected outcome, apply HVPC directly to the wound.[60] Conducting current to the tissues during whirlpool is not recommended because it is less effective, and some clinicians report that stimulator leads have become entangled in the agitator. There have even been stories of stimulators falling into the water.

## TABLE 6–1. HVPC CLINICAL STUDIES

| Researchers | Number of Patients | Percentage Healed | Mean Time to Heal |
|---|---|---|---|
| Alon et al[59] | 15 treated, 0 controls (diabetic) | 80% | 2.6 months (10.4 weeks) |
| Griffin et al[56] | 8 treated, 9 controls (pressure ulcers) | 80% reduction in size | 4-week treatment period |
| Kloth and Feeder[55] | 9 treated, 7 control, 3 crossovers (mixed wound etiology) | 100% | 7.3 weeks |
| Unger et al[57] | 9 treated, 8 controls (pressure ulcers) | 88.9% | 7.3 weeks (51.2 days) |
| Unger et al[58] | 223 treated, 0 control (pressure ulcers) | 89.7% | 10.85 weeks (54.25 days) |

## *Low-voltage Pulsed Electrical Current Studies*

Three controlled clinical trials using the Dermapulse® and Vara/Pulse® (Staodyn, Inc, Longmont, Colorado) low-voltage monophasic pulsed electrical stimulation (PES), were located in the literature: Gentzkow et al,[61] Gentzkow and Miller,[62] and Feedar et al.[63] Gentzkow et al[61] reported a study of 40 ulcers in 37 patients. Nineteen pressure ulcers were sham stimulated and 21 were stimulated. The trial lasted for 4 weeks. Treatment characteristics were 128 pps and amplitude of 35 mA for 30-minute sessions twice daily between 4 and 8 hours apart.When the ulcers reached a partial-thickness level, the pulse rate was changed to 64 pps and the electrode polarity was changed daily until healed. Treatment electrode polarity was negative and remained as such until the ulcer debrided and exudate was serosanguineous. Thereafter, the polarity was alternated, from positive to negative, every 3 days. The treated ulcers healed more than twice as much as the sham-stimulated ulcers (49.8 vs 23.4 percent), healing at a rate of 12.5 percent per week compared to 5.8 percent for the sham group. Crossover results for 15 of the 19 sham-treated ulcers showed a fourfold gain in healing during the 4 weeks of stimulation compared to 4 weeks of sham treatment. This difference was statistically significant.

Gentzkow and Miller[62] also published a study on pressure ulcers treated with the Dermapulse. The 61 patients served as their own controls. The treatment phase of the study was preceded by a 4-week control phase of optimal non–electrically stimulated wound care. Only the stage III or IV ulcers with need of surgical debridement, necrotic/purulent drainage, or exudate seropurulent drainage that did not improve during the control phase went on to the treatment phase. After 4 weeks of treatment, 58.8 percent of the wounds had improved in severity. After an average of 8.4 weeks, 23 percent completely healed and 82 percent improved significantly.

Feedar et al[63] treated 47 patients with ulcers of mixed etiology, including pressure ulcers, surgical and traumatic wounds, and vascular ulcers. Forty-seven patients with 50 wounds located at nine facilities were included in this study. To qualify for the wound study, all wounds had to be at least full-thickness loss of the dermis. The treatment characteristics used with the Vara/Pulse were monophasic pulsed current at an amplitude of 35 mA, a duration of 132 µsce, and pulse frequencies of 128 and 64 pps. Treatment was initiated at the negative pole. Two treatments were delivered for 30 minutes each daily, 7 days per week at intervals of 4 to 8 hours. After the wound was clean, the negative polarity was continued for 3 additional days until the wound healed to a partial-thickness depth. Then treatment characteristics were changed so that the polarity was switched daily until closure. Treatment intervention for study participants lasted 4 weeks. After 4 weeks, the wounds in the treatment and control groups were 44 percent and 76 percent of their initial size, respectively. Healing rates per week for the treatment and control groups were 14 percent and 8.25 percent, respectively.

### Biphasic Stimulation Studies

There are reports in the literature by Kaada,[64] Lundberg et al,[65] Stefanovska,[10] and Baker et al[11,12] of clinical trials of wound healing with biphasic waveforms. Benefits were found in patients with spinal cord injury who had pressure ulcers[11] and patients with diabetic ulcers, including those with peripheral neuropathy[12] and venous stasis.[65] Kaada and Lundeberg et al each used biphasic symmetrical waveforms with significant improvement in both ulcer area and healed ulcers. Kaada[29] reported results of TENS on 10 subjects, who served as their own controls, with recalcitriant ulcers of different etiologies. Stimulation was provided indirectly over the web of the thumb daily during three 30-minute sessions with rests of 45 minutes between, for a total of $1^1/_2$ hours of stimulation. Stimulation was below visible muscle contraction. Lundeberg et al[65] performed a controlled study on 64 patients with chronic diabetic ulcers because of venous stasis. All patients received standard treatment with paste bandage in addition to the sham or TENS treatment. Asymmetric biphasic stimulation was determined to produce significant wound healing effects, whereas the other waveforms did not increase the healing rate.

The study by Stefanovska et al[10] compared direct current and asymmetric biphasic current on healing in patients with pressure ulcers who were also spinal cord injured. The control group data were used to represent a normal healing process. For that group, the findings were that the longer the wound duration, the slower the healing. The duration of wound was not an important factor for those treated with DC or AC. Comparing AC group to other groups, AC currents seem to be more effective than DC. However, a very small number of patients were treated with nonoptimized DC treatment. Another interesting finding from this study was that there was a weak positive correlation between the healing rate in the AC-treated group (older patients healed slower) and a weak negative correlation with patient's age in the control group (younger patients healed faster). The older the patient, the greater the likelihood that the AC treatment would be beneficial. Wound size and depth influenced healing rates for all groups, with the larger and deeper wounds healing slowly.

Baker et al[11,12] compared asymmetric biphasic, symmetric biphasic, and microcurrent (DC) in two patient groups that were segregated and evaluated homogeneously by coimpairments of spinal cord injury and diabetes mellitus. Treatment consisted of a minimum of 30 minutes' daily application of the assigned protocol and standard wound treatments. Results are reported in separate studies. For stimulation with the symmetric biphasic protocol, the healing rate did not increase compared with the control subjects. Treatment with the asymmetric biphasic waveform protocol increased the healing rate and enhanced healing by nearly 60 percent over the control rate of healing in the diabetic patient group.[12] The asymmetric biphasic waveform has a potential for some polar effect that should not be discounted. The polar effect may explain why the asymmetric biphasic current was more effective than the symmetric biphasic. However, another likely explanation of the effects are stimulation of neural mechanisms that effect healing.[11]

In all of the studies, except Kaada,[29] stimulation was delivered to the skin at the wound perimeter rather than into the wound bed. An advantage of the stimulation at the perimeter was less disruption of the wound bed, less cross-contamination of the wound, and less interference with the dressing.

### Summary

Electrical stimulation studies have varied from continuous waveform application with direct current to pulsed short-duration monophasic pulses to biphasic pulses. What is known and acknowledged is that electrical stimulation seems to have positive effects on wound healing or on the components necessary for wound healing (eg, blood flow and oxygen uptake, DNA, and protein synthesis). There is still ambiguity about the type of electrical stimulation characteristics that are most important or critical. For instance, polarity has played an important role in protocols used, even though the likelihood of polarity effects of currents with pulses of very short duration is questionable. One possible reason for the wound healing effects of ES with any type of current is the effect of low-level sensory stimulation on the peripheral nerves, which is not wholly dependent on the polar nature of electrical current. Kaada describes effects that include inhibition of sympathetic input to superficial vessels, release of an active vasodilator, and axon–reflex stimulation.[29]

## CHOOSING AN INTERVENTION: CLINICAL REASONING

The previous section evaluated the efficacy of ES on different aspects of healing, as well as clinical trials of wound healing. The studies basically looked at three components:

1. Circulatory effects
2. Effects on pain
3. Effects on repair, regeneration, and completeness of healing

The clinician should consider these variables when selecting ES intervention and choosing a protocol.

## Wound Diagnosis Versus Medical Diagnosis

The specific **medical diagnosis** may not be a significant factor in selecting ES for wound healing. The medical diagnosis of patients in the studies included burns, pressure ulcers, diabetic ulcers (vascular and neuropathic), vascular ulcers, and vasculitic ulcers. The surgical wounds included in the studies were skin flaps, donor sites, and dehiscence. Acute wounds were also included. Electrical stimulation demonstrated efficacy for wound healing across diagnosis and pathogenesis. Reported effects were related to the stimulation of the mechanisms of healing at the cellular, tissue, or systems level. Healing follows a predictable pattern regardless of etiology; what affects the outcome are the intrinsic, extrinsic, and iatrogenic factors that alter healing, described earlier. The physical therapist intervenes in wound management specifically to facilitate the functional mechanisms of healing. Electrical stimulation is just one of the interventions that can be used.

Wound attributes that have positively responded to ES are necrotic tissue, inflammation, wound contraction, infection, and wound resurfacing. Wounds of all depths, from partial-thickness to full-thickness and deeper, have been successfully treated with ES (eg, stage II to stage IV pressure ulcers). Wounds have traditionally been classified by medical diagnosis, by depth of tissue disruption, and/or by phase of wound healing. Depth of tissue disruption is a description of the tissue loss and function that is broader and more generic than that in the medical diagnosis system. This is the wound severity diagnosis. The depth of tissue disruption system can be used for wounds regardless of the wound etiology. Classification by phase of wound healing is also independent of the medical diagnosis. Change in wound phase is an outcome of the process of wound healing. This is the wound healing phase diagnosis.

The typical subjects selected for clinical trials with electrical stimulation had **nonconforming wound healing** with long chronicity. The chronic wounds were the reason for referral for electrical stimulation. There is significant scientific evidence to support that early intervention with externally applied electrical currents will also accelerate healing for the acute healthy wound. **Early intervention** with ES could be a useful method to prevent chronicity and return the individual earlier to a functional status. This early intervention is consistent with other areas of PT practice, such as strokes and low back rehabilitation, in which early intervention can reduce the development of costly chronic health problems.

In summary, selection of ES for wound healing is not dependent on the medical diagnosis. Select ES intervention and treatment characteristics when there are impairments to the systems that interfere with healing at one or more levels: cellular, tissue, or organ. Functional loss at any of these levels suggests that the wound will not or has not healed with the current level of intervention. The reason for referral to the physical therapist is for the development of another strategy to facilitate healing. The use of externally applied currents is one such strategy. The type of stimulation that has been most consistently evaluated clinically and found to be efficacious is high-voltage pulsed current (see Table 6–2).

## Precautions

Signs of adverse effects using ES for wound healing were evaluated in the various clinical trials. The only two adverse signs were some skin irritation or tingling under the electrodes in a few cases and pain in other cases. Patients with severe peripheral vascular occlusive disease, particularly in the lower extremity, may experience some increased pain with ES, usually described as throbbing. An alternative acupuncture protocol has been suggested in these cases: placing the active electrode on the web space of the hand between the thumb and first finger instead of over the ulcer on the leg.[28,29] Transcerebral stimulation and stimulation over the eyes have been suggested as precautions because of conventional approaches possibly producing irritation or other problems. Effects of stimulation to the head in patients with upper motor neuron disorders (eg, stroke, transient ischemic attacks, epilepsy and seizure disorders) are undocumented.[44] Thoughtful application with careful monitoring would be advised. Young children under age 3 years should not be considered candi-

---

### TABLE 6–2.  APPROPRIATE WOUND DESCRIPTORS FOR HIGH-VOLTAGE ELECTRICAL STIMULATION

| Wound Classification | Wound Descriptor |
| --- | --- |
| Wound severity diagnosis | Superficial, partial thickness, full thickness, subcutaneous and deep tissues |
| Etiologies/diagnostic groups | Burns, neuropathic ulcers, pressure ulcers, surgical wounds, vascular ulcers |
| Wound healing phase diagnosis | Inflammation phase: acute, chronic, absent<br>Proliferation phase: acute, chronic, absent<br>Epithelialization phase: acute, chronic, absent<br>Remodeling phase: collagen organization |
| Age | Over 3 years of age |

dates for intervention with ES, because healing mechanisms for this group are not well understood and, although there are no known adverse effects, the benefits are not defined.

## Contraindications

Contraindications for the use of electrical stimulation as described in the literature fall into the following categories: (1) when stimulation of cell proliferation is contraindicated (eg, malignancy); (2) where there is evidence of osteomyelitis; (3) where there are metal ions; (4) where there is placement of electrodes for treatment with ES that could adversely affect a reflex center; or (5) where electrical current could affect the function of an electronic implant.[44,50] Carefully evalute the medical history and review body systems when considering candidates for use of this intervention.

### Presence of Malignancy

When there is a malignancy in the area to be treated, stimulation should not be used (eg, malignant melanoma, basal cell carcinoma). Electrical stimulation stimulates cell proliferation and could lead to uncontrolled cell growth. If the malignancy is distant from the wound (eg, breast cancer in a patient with a presssure ulcer on an ankle), however, local use of ES avoiding current flow through the breast or adjacent lymph nodes would be a precaution but not a contraindication, although this is not consistent with required manufacturer labeling.

### Active Osteomyelitis

Stimulation of tissue growth with ES may cause superficial covering of an area of osteomyelitis. This covering could blind the site from observation. If the medical record documents a history of a bone infection, that should trigger an investigation of the current status of the infection. It is not unusual for the osteomyelitis to be resolved but not to be noted in the medical record.

If a wound penetrates to the bone, as determined by inserting a probe, it must be assumed that osteomyelitis is present and the patient should not be treated with ES. An immediate referral to a surgeon for evaluation[66] must be initiated.

### Topical Substances Containing Metal Ions

Topical substances containing metal ions (eg, povidone–iodine, zinc, mercurochrome, silver sulfadiazine) that may be used as part of the wound treatment regimen should be removed before the application of ES. Direct current ES has the ability to transfer ions into the tissues by ionotophoreseis. Heavy metal ions may have toxic properties when introduced into the body. If removal of the topical substance is not appropriate, ES could be used on other areas of the skin where the topical agent has not been applied.

### Natural Reflexes

There are areas of the body that are particularly sensitive to any stimulation (eg, carotid sinus, heart, parasympathetic nerves, ganglion, laryngeal muscles, phrenic nerve). Sensory levels of ES might create a vasospasm or some type of vasoconstriction that would lead to vasovagal response and other neural responses that could interfere with the function of vital centers and be harmful to the patient. Thus, running current through the upper chest and anterior neck is contraindicated.

### Electronic Implants

Demand-type cardiac pacemakers and other electrical implants raise concerns regarding the use of electrical current. Electrical stimulation is contraindicated *over* electrical implants because the current and electromagnetic fields could disrupt the function of the implant. Safe application of TENS in 10 patients with 20 different cardiac pacemakers at four sites (lumbar area, cervical spine, left leg, and lower arm area ipsilateral to the pacemaker) without ill effects was reported by Rasmussen et al.[67] Therefore, using ES locally in an area away from the implant could be done safely, because it is unlikely to transmit to the electronic implant.

## ELECTRODES

## Electrode Materials

The electrode is the contact point between the electrical circuit and the body. The electrode must be a **good conductor** and provide very little resistance to the current. All metals are good conductors of electricity. Aluminum foil is an excellent conductor to use for electrodes (Figure 6–2). Aluminum foil is nontoxic, inexpensive, disposable, and conformable and can be sized as needed. Carbon-impregnated electrodes are sold to go with most electrotherapeutic devices. They are designed for multiple uses and are relatively inexpensive, but they need to be disinfected between use even if restricted to a single patient. They are nonconformable and will become resistive over time as they lose carbon and accumulate body oils and cleaning products.

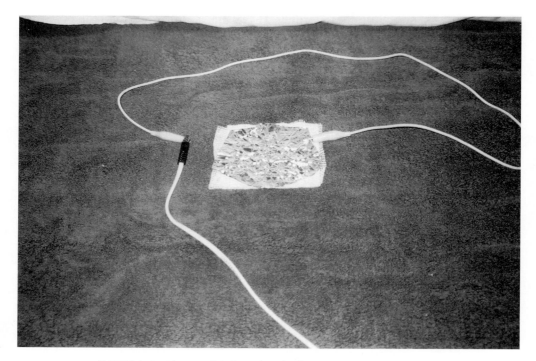

FIGURE 6–2. Aluminum foil electrode with alligator clip and machine leads.

### Size and Shape of Electrodes

Size, shape, and arrangement of electrodes affect the **current density** and **depth.** Current density is the amount of current flow per unit area. Current density is a measure of the quantity of charged ions moving through a specific cross-sectional area of body tissue. The unit of measurement is milliamperes per square centimeter. This measure will affect the reaction of the tissues being stimulated. In general, the greater the current density, the greater the effect on the tissue biology. Two determinants of current density are *size* of the electrode and the *amplitude* of the current applied.[68] Small electrodes concentrate the current for local effects more than larger electrodes, which tend to disperse the charge. Also, the farther apart the electrodes, the deeper the current penetrates.

### Active and Dispersive Electrode

The small electrode is commonly referred to as the active electrode and the large electrode as the dispersive electrode. If the two are nearly equal in size or have equal current, the current will be divided between the two, with the current density at the two treatment sites the same. If the two are not of equal size, the large electrode will have less current density than the smaller electrode. A rule of thumb is that the combined area of the active electrodes should not exceed the overall area of the dispersive electrode. Brown found that the effects of ES extends and affects events 2 to 3 cm beyond the edge of the electrodes.[69] Therefore, avoid placement of the active and dispersive electrodes so that they touch each other. Allow at least 4- to 5-cm spacing between them to avoid the possibility that the wound is receiving stimulation from both poles (Figure 6–3A).

In clinical practice, at times it is necessary to treat multiple wound sites with a single electrical circuit using one or two **bifurcated** lead wires. The advantage of bifurcation is that more sites can be treated simultaneously. A disadvantage is that although the same current passes through all the bifurcated leads, the physiologic responses may vary significantly because the stimulation is perceived under one electrode and the sensory stimulation under the other. Another disadvantage is that if there is a difference in the total surface area of the electrode(s) connected to one lead compared with the other, the stimulation will be stronger under the electrode with the smaller total surface area because there will be greater current density under that electrode. Often, the wound sites are different sizes. The depth and undermining may make the effective electrode size of a small wound larger than the surface area appears. The physical therapist must consider these physical properties when planning treatment and correct them. At this time it is not known what is the optimal current density or the best electrode size to choose.[43] Using a stimulator with two channels or having two treatment sessions if there are multiple wounds with a large discrepancy in wound sizes may be prudent.

### Dispersive Pad Placement

Attempts have been made to apply scientific findings to electrode placement. Most studies use the **active** electrode for direct application (Figure 6–3A) to the site,[55–58] but some use the **bipolar** technique (Figure 6–3B) at the wound edges.[10–12,65] The **dispersive** electrode placement has more variation. For example, in two similar studies, the dispersive electrode was placed differently. In one study,[55] it was placed cephalad on the neural axis, while in the second study it was placed 30.5 cm from the wound.[63] One study on spinal cord injured patients with pressure ulcers in the pelvic region used a protocol where the dispersive electrode was always placed on the thigh.[56] Another method is to place the dispersive electrode proximal to the wound.[57,58] At this time there is not an established proven method that has been shown to change the effect of the treatment. All reported treatment methods had statistically significant treatment re-

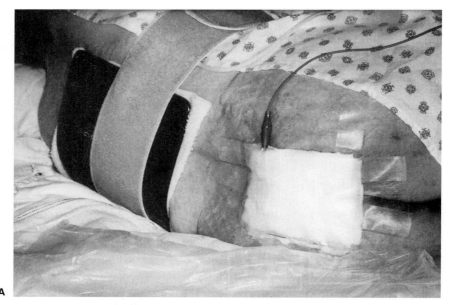

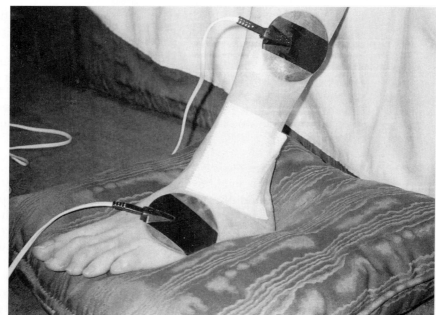

FIGURE 6–3. Positions of electrodes.

sults. Current thinking suggests that the dispersive electrode should be moved around the wound to induce the current to enter the wound from different sides.[70]

## Monopolar Technique

With the **monopolar** technique an electrode is placed to control the polarity at the wound site. Usually, one active electrode is placed on a wet conductive medium in the wound bed and the dispersive electrode is placed in a wet conductive medium at a distance from the wound site, on the intact skin (Figure 6–3A). Polarity for the two electrodes will be opposite. Current will flow through the intervening tissues between the two electrode poles. The current under the active electrode is the polarity selected on the stimulator. The farther apart the two electrode poles, the deeper the current will flow into the intervening tissues. Current will flow through the tissues by following the path with the lowest resistance, which is usually through the muscles and nerves and deeper tissues. Increasing the distance between the electrodes is a good position choice if wounds are deep and extend into underlying tissues (eg, stage III and IV pressure ulcers), having tunneling or undermined spaces or both.

The electrodes can be arranged to target the stimulation to specific tissue sites. Remember to visualize the path of the current flow when locating the dispersive electrode. The poles are usually set up in parallel fashion, enabling current to flow between the positive and negative electrodes no matter how many electrodes are used at either pole. When the surface area of the electrodes is unequal, the current density will not be the same under the two sites. Current density may also vary according to the **impedance** of the intervening tissues and the size of the electrodes. Impedance is the opposition to current flow within the circuit. Different body tissues have different impedances to current flow. Skin, bone, and fat have high impedance and are poor electrical conductors. When there is a break in the skin, however, there is a significant lowering of the skin impedance to current. Techniques to reduce skin impedance include abrasion of the skin surface to remove the hard layers of keratin on the surface, tissue warming, and hydration. High-voltage currents of approximately 100 V have the demonstrated ability to cause sudden, spontaneous breakdown in skin impedance.[68] Because muscles and blood vessels have high fluid content, these tissues are good electrical conductors, and it can be expected that current will flow directly through them with little impedance.

Understanding these principles of tissue impedance and current flow and then appling them correctly to derive the optimal benefits from treatment with electrical stimulation is important. For example, if the dispersive electrode is to be placed on the back, place it *below* the scapula to avoid the resistance to current flow by the bone. Patients with thick layers of callus on the feet will have high impedance to current. Paring the callus should precede ES treatment, or find another placement where the electrode does not lie on callus. A good placement for the dispersive when treating wounds of the lower leg or foot is the muscular tissue of the thigh. One suggestion is to switch the dispersive electrode for each treatment so the current flows into the wound from each side of the wound through different surrounding tissues and through a different wound edge.[70] The active electrodes as well as the dispersive can be bifurcated. This bifurcation allows use of smaller electrodes that can be made to conform to smaller body parts such as an arm or a lower leg. If the dispersive electrode area size must be increased, use a wet washcloth wrapped around a limb or extend a wet washcloth out from the edges of the dispersive electrode to cover a larger skin area. If the wound area size is nearly as large or larger than the skin area under the dispersive electrode, it will be more comfortable for the patient, but the amplitude of the current or the treatment time may need to be increased to deliver the same total amount of current but at a lower current density.

## Bipolar Technique

The definition of **bipolar** technique is the placement of the two leads with their respective electrodes on either side of the target area. This confines the stimulation to the area associated with the clinical problem.[43] For instance, the two electrodes with opposite polarity may both be placed on the intact skin adjacent to the wound site so that the current passes between the electrodes through the wound tissue. The closer together, the more superficial the effect; this is a reasonable choice for superficial or partial-thickness wound disruptions. The bipolar technique is used with either monophasic or biphasic waveforms. An application of the bipolar technique is to place the electrodes on either side of the wound so that current will flow through the wound from all sides at once. Finally, one active electrode could be placed in the middle of the wound and a dispersive electrode fashioned like a donut, made from aluminum foil, slipped over the treatment electrode with an intervening space between so that stimuation would flow into the wound bed from all sides of the wound edges simultaneously. The foil electrode would connect to the dispersive lead with an alligataor clip just like the active leads. (See Figure 6–3B.)

# PROTOCOL CHARACTERISTICS

There are many different ES **protocols** for wound healing. This section first describes some of the aspects of the protocol characteristics including electrode polarity, frequency, and amplitude as described by the researchers.

## Polarity

Polarity must be considered when using galvanic and pulsed monophasic current. Electrode polarity also varies depending on the protocol selected. Most researchers studying ES for wound healing start their protocols with the negative poles as the active electrode and then change the polarity after a period of treatment. However, Griffin et al[56] maintained negative polarity to the wound site throughout the treatment period of 4 weeks. Wounds did not heal but showed improvement. Other researchers[55,61,62,63] recommend using negative polarity for 3 to 7 days and then changing polarity. Another recommendation is to use negative polarity until the wound is clean of necrotic tissue and drainage is serosanguineous, then continue with that polarity for 3 additional days or change to the positive pole.[57,58] Some studies suggest that the polarity should be changed back to negative for 3 days when the wound plateaus. Another method is to change the polarity every 3 days until the wound is healed to a partial-thickness depth.[61,62,63] Once that outcome is achieved, change the polarity by alternating it daily until the wound is closed. Animal studies demonstrate better healing when polarity is initiated at the negative pole and then switched to the positive pole.[71,72,73]

Usually, the negative electrode is used as the active electrode when infection is suspected. The polarity is often alternated during the course of healing. This electrode switching also accommodates the variability in the skin battery potentials that occurs during the course of healing. Thus, electrode polarity may need to be alternated during treatment to achieve an optimal rate of healing. Additional research is needed to ascertain whether wound healing with ES is dependent on matching treatment electrode polarity with fluctuations in wound injury potential polarity.[53] So far, studies have not reported on this important issue. Still, the idea of polarity switching has some demonstrated merit.

## Protocols With Biphasic Current

Protocols demonstrating significant benefit for wound healing with biphasic current are now appearing regularly in the literature. The five studies reported in this chapter (Kaada,[29] Lundeberg et al,[65] Stefanovska et al,[10] Baker et al[11,12]) have similar protocols, except that the two studies by the Baker et al[11,12] research group found that the best outcome was achieved when the biphasic waveform was asymmetric and biased toward the negative pole. Biphasic treatment protocols are shown in Table 6–3.

## Frequency

Frequency or pulse rate is another variable that varies from study to study without much explanation. Several studies used a pulse rate of 100 to 128 pps for treatment with HVPC.[55,56] One investigator starts treatment at 50 pps.[57,58] Sussman uses 30 pps based on evidence that at lower pulse rates HVPC increases blood flow.[23] In some research studies, lower pulse rates produced higher mean blood flow velocity after HVPC than higher pulse rates and had a longer mean recovery time following cessation of HVPC compared to control levels.[23] Frequency switching is also not well understood. For example, in one study the rationale given for reducing the pulse rate from 128 pps to 64 pps was "because we believed the higher pulse frequency might be harmful to the newly healed tissue."[63] This concern is probably because of the higher pulse charge delivered to the tissue at the higher pulse rate.

### TABLE 6–3. BIPHASIC PROTOCOLS

| Characteristics | Kaada[29] | Lundeberg et al[65] | Stefanovaska et al[10] | Baker et al[11,12] |
|---|---|---|---|---|
| Phase duration | Not reported | 1 msec | 0.25 msec | 100 μsec |
| Pulse rate | 100 Hz | 80 Hz | 40 Hz | 50 Hz |
| Waveform | Symmetric | Symmetric | Asymmetric charge balanced | Asymmetric |
| Amplitude | 15–30 mA below contraction | 15–25 mA below contraction | Below contraction | Below contraction |
| Frequency and duration | Daily; three 30-minute sessions (off 45 minutes between sessions) | Twice daily for 20 minutes | Daily for 2 hours | Daily; three 30-minute sessions (off 4 hours between sessions) |
| Location | Web between first and second metacarpal bones | Wound edge | Wound edge | Less than 1 cm from edge, proximal and distal to ulcer |
| Patient sample | Multiple diagnoses | Diabetics with venous stasis ulcers | Spinal cord injury with pressure ulcers | Spinal cord injury with pressure ulcers, diabetic ulcers |

## Amplitude

Wound healing protocols for amplitude are usually constant, reported in either milliamperes or voltage. The HVPC protocols all report amplitudes of 100 to 200 V, the low-voltage direct current protocols call for a 35-mA amplitude, and the low-voltage microamperage stimulation units have an amplitude less than 1 mA.

The ability of the patient to tolerate high-amplitude current will depend on the sensory perception of the individual. For example, in superficial or partial-thickness tissue disruption, if there is intact sensation, an amplitude above 100 V may be very uncomfortable. In deeper wounds or in cases of impaired sensation, these higher amplitudes are well tolerated. Adjust the amplitude to patient comfort. Suggestions have been made to test the amplitude by stimulating until there is a visible muscle contraction under the electrode. This approach is not practical if the active electrode is located in a wound within a muscle because the sensory nerves will not be stimulated. If the dispersive electrode is secure over a large body area, the amplitude of the stimulation required to cause a muscle contraction will be very high and probably uncomfortable, and may not be visible to the physical therapist.

Meters are very useful to the clinican to check on the current flow between two electrodes. Use the device meter if available; if no meter is available on the stimulator, go to other options. Patient sensation is always a good indicator, if the patient can give a report. The use of ES for wound healing is usually done at a sensory level, but many of the patients are insensate, or unable to communicate, or the wounds are deep and below the level of sensation and the patient will not be able to indicate if the current is not felt. Another test method is to position the dispersive/indifferent electrode over a muscle motor point to see whether there is a muscle twitch or tingling under the electrode. The electrode pads can be checked by the physical therapist by placing a wet contact on both positive and negative electrodes and then resting one forearm on the two electrode pads. Ask a colleague to turn up the device until a sensation of prickling is felt.

## Conclusion

Clearly, more investigation is needed to achieve an optimal treatment protocol with electrical stimulation. In the meantime, the protocols presented in this chapter are for use with low- and high-voltage monophasic and biphasic waveforms, which represent these authors' interpretation of the literature and the application to clinical treatment. The authors have used these protocols for several years with good clinical results. Protocols are listed for wound healing for the three phases of repair and for the treatment of an edematous limb where the edema extends beyond the wound area. Protocols change for each phase of repair and have expected outcomes for each. Expected outcomes are based on the literature and clinical experience.

## SELECTING THE DEVICE

The physical therapist is now ready to select the electrical stimulator for treatment. Depending on the stimulator selected, the protocol for treatment will vary. In some cases, the characteristics of electrical stimulation for different current type may not always be based on the wound healing phases. For example, asymmetric biphasic stimulation characteristics are not varied during the progression through the phases of healing.[11,12]

Select a stimulator based on the available waveform, pulse characteristic, and ability to adjust amplitude and polarity. A desirable stimulation should allow for flexibility to set up and deliver a variety of protocols based on changes dictated by clinical trials and current concepts of physiologic rationale. Manufacturers are an important source of helpful information about the characteristics of their devices.

Under what is called **premarket approval** (PMA), manufacturing companies are allowed to make claims of effectiveness and safety about medical devices. PMA requires extensive clinical trials, typically 2000 to 3000 case, for approval. "Off label" means treatment not approved by the Food and Drug Administration (FDA). No electrical stimulators have received PMA by the FDA for wound healing. Externally applied currents for wound healing are considered as off-label use at this time. Off-label use for medical devices is an accepted and common practice in medicine as innovative therapy, as long as the participants are not closely associated with the manufacturer.[74] For example, the "on-label" uses for neuromuscular stimulators, such as HVPC, include application for increased circulation, edema, pain, relaxation of muscle spasms, and muscle reeducation. The on-label use for TENS is pain management.

Expect to find an FDA-mandated instruction manual accompanying each electrical stimulator. Listed in the manual are labeled indications, contraindications, warnings, and precautions (Figure 6–4). The FDA indications and contraindications do not match exactly what is described in this chapter. The physical therapist must be aware of these limitations when selecting a protocol with ES and use thoughtful clinical judgment.

**FDA Indications for Electrical Stimulation**

- Relaxation of muscle spasms
- Prevention or retardation of disuse atrophy
- Increasing local blood circulation
- Muscle reeducation
- Immediate postsurgical stimulation of calf muscles to prevent venous thrombosis
- Maintaining or increasing ROM
- Pain

**FDA Contraindications for Electrical Stimulation**

- Should not be used on patients with demand-type cardiac pacemakers
- Should not be used on persons known to have cancerous lesions
- Should not be used for symptomatic pain relief unless etiology is established or unless a pain syndrome has been diagnosed
- Should not be used over pregnant uterus
- Electrode placements must be avoided that apply current to the carotid sinus region (anterior neck) or transcerebrally (through the head)

FIGURE 6–4. FDA Indications for electrical stimulation. (*Source: Manufacturer Instruction Manuals as required by Food and Drug Administration.*)

Electrical stimulation equipment should have regular calibration checks. In between checks, a multimeter can be used for periodic checking to see that the equipment is functioning properly. Multimeters, which are a combination of volt–ohm–milliammeter, have the ability to determine current flow. They are inexpensive, easy to use, and readily available. A broken lead wire, weak battery, or resistant electrode may not be apparent because the stimulation in the wound bed is below the level of sensation or the patient is insensate or cognitively impaired and cannot report changes in sensation. Checking for good electrical conduction is the responsibility of the clinician.

Many electrical stimulators now use microprocessors with a choice of several waveforms and pulse rates and even include preset protocols for wound treatment. The clinician should not assume that this is the "correct" protocol for the wound. The clinician is responsible for knowing the rationale for protocol characteristics and what the settings are on the chosen stimulator. Most stimulators allow clinicians to override the preset programs.

The most common stimulator used for wound healing today is the high-voltage pulsed current neuromuscular stimulator. This may change in the future. The protocols presented below are based on use of the high-voltage pulsed electrical stimulator. Because the protocol given mimics the studies done with low-voltage pulsed electrical current,[63] the protocol would also be appropriate to use with those stimulators. The protocols are based initially on the wound healing phase diagnosis and require changes in polarity and pulse rate as the wounds progress through the phases of healing.

# SUSSMAN WOUND HEALING PROTOCOL

Sussman uses a wound healing protocol for HVPC based on the completed diagnostic process described earlier. Table 6–4 lists the Sussman Wound Healing Protocols for HVPC for all four phases of wound healing and edema control. In using this method, the clinician initiates an HVPC treatment protocol based on the assessed wound healing phase diagnosis, and predicts an expected outcome for that protocol. Because the polarity of the healing wound changes during the phases of healing, different treatment characteristics are used as wound healing progresses. In the protocol given below, the stimulation selected for treatment is a monophasic current and monopolar technique used with HVPC. For wounds in the acute inflammation phase, with an absence of inflammation phase, or in a

## TABLE 6–4. PROTOCOLS FOR HVPC TREATMENT

| Characteristics | Edema | Inflammation | Proliferation | Epithelialization | Remodeling | Venous Return |
|---|---|---|---|---|---|---|
| Polarity | Negative | Negative | Alternate negative/ positive every 3 days | Alternate daily | Alternate daily | Not critical, adjust for patient comfort |
| Pulse rate (frequency) | 30–50 pps | 30 pps | 100–128 pps | 60–64 pps | 60–64 pps | 40–60 pps |
| Amplitude | 150 V or less depending on patient tolerance | 100–150 V | 100–150 V | 100–150 V | 100–150 V | Surge mode, on time, 3–15 sec, off time, 9–40 sec (1:3 on/off ratio) to motor excitation |
| Duration | 60 min | 60 min | 60 min | 60 min | 60 min | 5–10 min, progress to 20–30 min |
| Treatment frequency | 5–7 times/ week for first week, then 3 times/week for 1 week | 5–7 times/ week, once daily | 5–7 times/ week, once daily | 3–5 times/ week, once daily | 3 times/week, once daily | Daily; modify to biweekly |

Edema and phases of healing protocols from Sussman. Venous Return Protocol adapted from Alon.[27]

chronic inflammation phase, the therapist would start treatment with characteristics to stimulate circulation and cellular responses to healing that are listed under the inflammation phase. The protocol calls for change of characteristics as the wound healing phases progress. Likewise, for a wound healing phase diagnosis of the repair (proliferation) phase and a wound in the remodeling phase, the physical therapist would start treatment using a different set of characteristics as outlined.

## PREDICTABLE OUTCOMES WITH SUSSMAN WOUND HEALING PROTOCOL

Predictable outcomes are expected for each protocol, which are equivalent to a change in the wound phase characteristics. For example, if the wound healing phase diagnosis is **acute inflammation phase,** the expected outcomes are hemorrhage-free, necrosis-free, erythema-free, edema-free, exudate-free red granulation, and progression to the next phase—the **proliferation phase.** If there is absence of inflammation or chronic inflammation, an acute inflammation phase must be initiated, if possible. Expected outcomes would indicate change to an acute inflammation phase, described as increased erythema (change in skin color), edema, and warmth. The phase change outcome predicted is *initiation of acute inflammation phase.* Each wound healing phase has its own diagnosis and expected outcomes that are independent of wound etiology.

When the wound healing phase diagnosis is **acute proliferation phase,** the expected outcomes are reduction in size (eg, open area, depth, undermining/tunneling), red granulation tissue–filled wound bed, minimal serous or serosanguineous wound exudate, no odor, adherence of wound edges, and at the end of the phase a change in wound healing phase to the epithelialization phase. When the wound healing phase diagnosis is absence of or chronic proliferation, the predicted outcome must be acute proliferation: reduction in depth, reduction in open area size, and closing of tunnels or undermining. Chronic proliferation may result from infection of the granulation tissue. There would be clinical signs of infection, including purulent exudate, malodor, and change in appearance of the granulation tissue from a beefy red to dull pink color. The additional expected outcome for a chronic proliferation phase then would enable the wound to become infection free and to restart the proliferation phase.

A wound healing phase diagnosis of **acute epithelialization phase** has the expected outcome of resurfacing and a change in wound healing phase to **remodeling.** A wound in the remodeling phase has an immature scar formation that lacks optimal healing and could benefit from continued stimulation with electrical stimulation to enhance the migration of the epidermal cells and the maturation of the vascular system of the scar tissue. Absence of an epithelialization phase may result from drying out of the wound tissues because of either a poor dressing choice or an absence of dressing. Epidermal cells require a moist environment to migrate across the wound surface. Correction the inadequate wound treatment would be a necessary part of the plan of care. Chronic epithelialization is associated with rolled wound edges that have become fibrotic and stuck without resurfacing the wound. Other adjunctive measures may be required to reinitiate an inflammatory response in the wound edges that will reinitiate the epithelialization process.

Once closure is achieved, the patient is usually discharged from a treatment protocol, including ES. However, the remodeling phase is often overlooked as a point at which treatment with ES can be beneficial in reducing the risk of immature scar breakdown. The remodeling phase is the longest of all the phases of healing, lasting from 6 months to 2 years. A scar that is thicker, better vascularized, softer, and flatter is more resistant to stress from shearing, friction, and pressure, all of which account for a high incidence of recurrence of ulceration on the seating surface or plantar surface of the foot. Electrical stimulation enhances the remodeling of the scar. Of course, other treatment methods also need to be considered to protect the new scar tissue, including pressure-relief devices and dressings. The physical therapist also would include a program of stretching, exercise, and soft tissue mobilization techniques to enhance the elasticity of the mature scar.

## PROCEDURES FOR HIGH-VOLTAGE PULSED CURRENT

The procedure section of this chapter is outlined in a stepwise fashion to help the physical therapist and physical therapist assisant deliver the treatment intervention with electrical stimulation in a systematic and time-efficient way for both the patient and the clinician. Treatment with ES requires a number of supply items and steps. First of all, consider having a PT aide set up the treatment station with the equipment and supplies needed (see list of equipment and supplies needed). The same set of instructions would be useful to give to a patient or caregiver for home treatment. The PT aide can also be responsible to see that the supplies are ordered and available in the department. Always have enough supplies on hand.

## Equipment Needed

- Normal saline (0.9%)
- Clean gloves
- Irrigation syringe, 35-mL with angiocatheter
- Clean gauze pads
- Aluminum foil electrode or carbon electrode
- Alligator clips or electrode lead
- Bandage tape
- Nylon stretch strap
- Wet washcloth
- Dispersive pad
- HVPC machine leads
- Infectious waste bag

## Suggestions for Setup to Maximize Treatment Effectiveness and Efficiency

- Assemble the set-up supplies into kits before the start of the treatment day to make the delivery of service more time efficient.
- Precut and shape the aluminum foil electrodes. Size and shape should be close to the size of the wounds. Round is preferable to rectangular.
- To make an electrode, cut a strip of household aluminum foil the width of the electrode. Fold the strip in half and turn in the edges to make a smooth pad.
- To make a packing strip from gauze, open a gauze pad and pull on the bias or diagonal and twist to make a spaghetti strip, or use stretch gauze strips.
- Warm saline or a package of amorphous hydrogel by placing the bottle between a folded hot pack before use to avoid chilling the wound tissue and slowing mitotic activity. Check the temperature with a digital thermometer. The temperature should not be greater than 100°F to avoid burns. Myer reported keeping the wound care products, including a 16-oz bottle of saline warm for 3 to 4 hours. She observed that warming of the wound care products before electrical stimulation treatment resulted in brighter redness of granulation tissue and contributed to reduction in pain.[75]

  Spray bottles and bulb syringes may not deliver enough pressure (2.0 psi or less) to cleanse wounds adequately. The Water Pik® (Teledyne Water Pik, Fort Collins, Colorado) at middle to high settings may cause trauma to the wound tissue and drive bacteria into wounds; it is not recommended for cleansing soft tissue wounds. Use a cleanser delivery device such as syringe with an angio- catheter to deliver water at 4 to 8 psi. Warm the solution before application.[76]

## Instructions for Patient and Caregiver

1. Explain the procedure, the reason for treatment, and how long it will last. Explain that a mild tingling will be felt and where it will be felt.
2. Advise patient not to handle, replace, or remove electrodes during the treatment. Patients who cannot understand these directions or will not cooperate need to be monitored closely.
3. Give patient a call light to use.

## Setting Up the Patient for HVPC Wound Treatment

1. Have supplies ready before undressing the wound.
2. Position the patient for ease of access by staff and for the comfort of both.
3. Remove the dressing and place in infectious waste bag (usually a red bag).
4. Cleanse wound thoroughly to remove slough, exudate, and any petrolatum products.
5. Complete sharp debridement of necrotic tissue before setting the patient up for HVPC treatment so that the wound packing will act as a pressure dressing to control any bleeding and so that the wound environment will not have to be disturbed again after HVPC treatment.
6. Open gauze pads and fluff, then soak to moisten in warm, normal saline solution; squeeze out excess liquid before applying.
7. Fill the wound cavity with gauze, including any undermined/tunnelled spaces. Gauze pad can be opened to full size and then pulled diagonally to form a thin "spaghetti" strip. Insert into undermined/tunneled spaces like roller gauze. Pack gently.
8. Place electrode over the gauze packing cover with a dry gauze pad and hold in place with bandage tape.
9. Connect an alligator clip to the foil.
10. Connect to the stimulator lead and to the output device.
11. Place the dispersive electrode.
    a. The dispersive electrode is usually placed proximal to the wound (see section on electrode placement for alternative locations).
    b. Place over soft tissues; avoid bony prominences.

    c. Place a moist washcloth over the dispersive electrode.

    d. Place a washcloth against skin and hold it in good contact at all edges with a nylon elasticized strap. (Covering the wet dispersive setup with a plastic sheet to separate it from the bed and the patient's clothing to keep them dry will be appreciated by the patient and the nursing staff.)

    e. If placed on the back, the weight of the body plus the strap can be used to achieve good contact at the edges.

    f. Dispersive pad should be larger than the sum of the areas of the active electrodes and wound packing.

    g. The greater the separation between the active and dispersive electrode the deeper the current path. Use greater separation for deep and undermined wounds.

    h. Dispersive and active electrodes should be 4 to 5 cm apart and *should not touch.* Current flow will be shallow.

## Additional Treatment Methods

Additional treatment methods that have been used to solve clinical problems are described below.

### Simultaneous Treatment of Multiple Wounds

Up to four wounds can be set up with a single-channel HVPC stimulator using double bifurcated leads from the stimulator to the electrodes. However, this will not provide maximal current density at the treatment sites. For a patient with multiple wounds, it may not be practical to run several series of treatments. An alternative is to use two HVPC stimulators, if available. Electrode placement will require careful planning so that the current flows through target tissues. For example, if there is a wound on the right hip, coccyx, left foot, and right heel, the dispersive electrode should be placed on one of the thighs. The thigh has a good blood supply and good conductivity. This setup will send the current flowing through the deep tissues to the feet, the hip, and the coccyx.

### Alternation of Pads

Alternate placement of the dispersive pad for each treatment, if possible, to direct current flow to opposite sides of the wound.[70] This will be more difficult when wounds are located in the feet.

### Increasing the Area of the Dispersive Pad

If a limb is involved, the circumference may be too small to wrap with the large dispersive pad and maintain good contact. An alternative is to use bifurcated leads, which are available to use with the dispersive cable for some stimulators. When using this setup, attach two round carbon-impregnated electrodes to make the surface area of the dispersive electrode larger than the active electrode. Place the electrodes on either side of the limb. Two pads conform easier to a small limb segment than the large rectangular dispersive electrode standard with most stimulators. Use wet gauze under the electrodes; if a greater conductive surface is required, extend the wet gauze out from the edges of the electrode over the surrounding skin. Hold in place with nylon elasticized straps. If the patient complains of excessive tingling under the dispersive setup, check for good contact and see whether the size of the electrode can be increased further.

### Current Conduction to the Wound

Alternative methods of conducting current to the wound using dressing products has been of interest for a number of years. A recent study of conductivity of different wound dressings reported that: (1) **transparent films** are poor conductors; (2) **fully saturated hydrocolloids** will conduct current; and (3) **hydrogel** amorphous gels and sheet forms are good conductors because of their high water content.[77] An animal study using pigs with burn wounds demonstrated that use of a hydrogel dressing with pulsed ES delivered through the dressing increased the levels of collagenase during the critical period of epithelialization initiation. This may be one mechanism by which the electrical stimulation accelerated the wound healing of these burns.[78]

Use an amorphous hydrogel-impregnated gauze to conduct current. Different hydrogel products are constituted differently and have variable conductive capacity. Test a sample of the product to be used before applying it to the patient. Hydrogels can be left on the wound for up to 3 days. This type of dressing is used for partial, full-thickness, and subcutaneous lesions extending into deep tissue wounds. This product class can benefit the wound management by:

- Conducting electrical current when covered with an electrode
- Promoting the "sodium current of injury"
- Absorbing light to moderate wound exudate
- Maintaining a moist wound environment
- Gradually absorbing wound moisture and is also a moisture donor to the wound
- Retaining the cell growth factors in the wound bed
- Reducing trauma and cooling of the wound through less handling
- Reducing product and labor costs by serving a dual purpose

Hydrogel sheets also have high water content and can also be used to conduct current when placed under the electrode.[77] Hydrogel sheets have benefits similar to the amorphous hydrogels except that they should not be left on an infected wound. They are used for lightly exudating wounds and are best used for superficial partial-thickness wounds such as donor sites after skin grafting.

Amorphous hydrogel-impregnated gauze or a hydrogel sheet can be used as the wet contact coupler under an electrode. Although manufacturers say that all that is required is to clip the alligator clips to the dressing to conduct current, Alon explained that this will focus the current at one small area of the dressing and not disperse it throughout the wound areas unless the entire dressing surface is covered with an electrode.[79] Follow the set-up steps described above, but substitute the saline-soaked gauze with the amorphous hydrogel-impregnated gauze or hydrogel sheet. Dressings may be left in place for up to 3 days. The amorphous hydrogel should be warmed before application, but be careful not to overheat the product and cause burns. Check the temperature with a digital thermometer. The temperature should not be greater than 100°F. If wound conditions permit, cover with a moisture/vapor-permeable transparent film or another dressing to retain moisture without maceration and maintain body warmth. For amorphous hydrogel-impregnated gauze, on the second day, lift the secondary dressing and slip an aluminum foil electrode underneath; connect an alligator clip lead to the dressing and the stimulator. Replace secondary dressing. Repeat on the third day. The same approach would apply to the hydrogel sheet.

All petrolateum products, including enzymatic debriding agents such as collagenase (Santyl), and fibrinolysin Elase®, which are petrolatum-based products, must be removed before treatment or current will not be conducted into the wound tissues.

## Aftercare

After the electrical stimulation treatment is complete, slip the electrode out from between the wet and dry gauze. The wound can be left undisturbed. If saline-soaked gauze is the conductive medium, it should be changed before it dries or be covered with an occlusive dressing. If additional topical treatments are required, such as enzymatic debriding agents or antibiotics, the packing will need to be removed. Frequent dressing changes are being discouraged because it disturbs the wound healing environment by removing important substances in wound exudate and cooling the wound. A chilled wound takes 3 hours to rewarm, and during that time leukocytic and mitotic activities slow.[80,81]

## Home Treatment

HVPC stimulation and TENS are very safe and easy-to-apply treatments that a patient or caregiver can be taught for self-treatment at home. HVPC stimulators, as described, are available as portable, battery-pack units. Some units come with compliance meters. TENS are also portable. This is a simple treatment, but it requires several steps and clear instruction. Review the procedures with the person who will deliver the care to ensure that adequate care will be given to achieve the predicted outcomes. If the physical therapist does not believe that the person is able to be taught safe and appropriate procedures, the therapist should document that inability to justify the need for skilled services or another intervention.

To achieve success in a self-care program, psychosocial concerns need to be addressed before establishing the self-care program. Select the patient or caregiver, or both, who is alert, motivated, and able to learn the directions for application. Clinician support and encouragement will be required to convince the patient/caregiver to accept the responsibility for self-care. Patients and caregivers are accustomed to receiving medical care at the clinic or by a home care practitioner rather than doing self-care. The concept of sharing the problem between patient and clinician is new to many people. A step-by-step process is needed to gain patient cooperation. Begin in the clinic with a home visit by encouraging and teaching the patient or the caregiver, or both, to participate in the setup process. Many people are repulsed by the sight of a dirty, smelly, ugly wound. Take it slowly, with patience and understanding of these feelings. Explain in simple language why the wound is dirty, smelly, and ugly and how the treatment will improve the problem. Wound measurements and pictures can be used as motivation to encourage continued participation. Before-and-after pictures of other cases treated this way is a particularly effective way of showing the patient or caregiver how other wounds improved. Move the patient or caregiver increasingly into the role of treatment provider as soon as possible. Observe, instruct, and offer words of support and praise.

### Instructions

Independence in the treatment routine must be established before dismissing the patient with an electrical stimulator for self-care at home. While it may seem overwhelming to give five sets of instructions for a single treatment protocol, understanding the five sets of instructions listed here will ensure that the patient or caregiver is able to achieve the goal of independence in the treatment routine. Keep instructions as simple as possible so the responsible party will not be overwhelmed. Because of the number of steps required, prepared instruction sheets listing the five steps would be helpful. Stick-figure drawings can be helpful in teaching the proper placement of the electrodes. Do not assume that the patient will know where to place the electrodes or how to put on the dressing when he or she arrives home. Two or three visits with the physical therapist may be necessary to complete the instruction. Schedule regular follow-up assessments. The five steps of instructions are as follows:

1. The list of needed supplies. Make sure that the patient can acquire all the necessary items or help make arrangements to acquire those that are needed (eg, a portable HVPC stimulator with dispersive pad and nylon stretch strap).
2. Setup of the patient and the wound for treatment, including all the steps listed: Review what is on paper and then do a demonstration and return demonstration to confirm understanding.
3. The treatment protocol: Review the treatment protocol by dialing in the characteristics for the selected protocols on the stimulator to be used. The dials can be left at the correct setting to help the patient, but they may be moved and should be rechecked at each treatment session. Give *only* the treatment protocol for the current wound healing phase. Tell the patient/caregiver what outcomes to expect and what findings should be reported promptly. Change instructions as the wound heals.
4. The aftercare procedures: Aftercare procedure instructions should include how to apply the prescribed dressing product and disposal of the disposable waste products from the treatment in the home setting. Be sure that the patient or caregiver understands the proper use of the prescribed aftercare dressing products. Damage to the wound and failure to achieve predicted outcomes can be avoided by instruction in use of products. Again, practice and a return demonstration are proven methods of teaching new techniques.
5. A list of expected signs and symptoms: The patient and the caregiver need to be aware of the importance of any expected changes in signs and symptoms related to the treatment and know when to report any undesirable results.

## Protocol for Treatment of Edema

Soft tissue trauma and a closed or minimally open wound would benefit from electrical stimulation to control, eliminate, or reduce edema formation. Edema stimulates pain receptors because of the tension in the tissues, blocks off circulation inflow to the tissues, and impairs mobility. Edema eliminated, controlled, or reduced would be the expected outcome from this intervention. Table 6–4 shows a protocol for treatment for edema reduction using high-voltage pulsed current stimulation. There are limited reports[30] and no clinical trials to support this treatment; however, there are anecdotal evidence and animal studies.[31,32]

### Setting Up the Patient

1. Use the method for setting up the wound for edema control as described under protocol for wound healing.
2. Elevate the limb and support it on a pillow or foam wedge, above the heart if possible.
3. Use three or four electrodes.
4. Place one electrode over the wound and arrange other electrodes over the vascular areas of the limb.
   a. If the wound is on the lower leg, place the second electrode over the medial aspect of the foot and the third over the popliteal area.
   b. If the edema is in the foot distal to the wound, a "foot sandwich" can be made by surrounding the foot with a foil electrode that wraps around the top and bottom of the foot.

*Note:* Apply the same clinical reasoning for the upper extremity.

## Protocol for Infection Control and Disinfection

A clean technique is recommended for treatment of chronic wounds. The use of aluminum foil electrodes is a good method of controlling infection and eliminates the need for disinfection of the electrode pads. If carbon electrodes or electrodes with sponges are used over the wound, they need to be disinfected between each use even if used for a single patient. A cold disinfection solution, such as Cydex+ (Johnson & Johnson Medical, Inc., Arlington, Texas) will disinfect for all organisms within 10 minutes, according to the material data sheet. Cydex+ comes with an activating solution that is added to the main solution when the bottle is opened. The activated solution can be reuseable for up to 28 days. The product is available in quart and gallon sizes. Unless large quantities of electrodes are going to be disinfected at one time, the quart solution has been found to be most cost effective.

Another cold disinfectant, Micro-Quat, (EcoLab Inc, St. Paul, Minnesota) at the dilution of 18.6 g (2/3 oz) in 3.8 L (1 gal) of water has been tested for disinfection of electrodes and electrode sponges after treatment of colonized wounds. The electrodes and sponges were soaked in the disinfecting solution for 20 minutes and then tested for bacterial counts. Both the efficacy of the disinfectant and the protocol for disinfection were evaluated. Samples taken from 92 percent of the posttreatment electrode sponges, after they were disinfected, contained no bacterial growth. The remaining 8 percent contained two or fewer colonies. The results were the same for samples cultured anaerobically.[82] The dispersive pad, which is placed on intact skin, should be cleaned between uses with soap and water or wiped with an alcohol-soaked pad. Alligator clips that come in contact with wound contaminants should be disinfected between uses. One company furnishes alligator clips with packs of hydrogel-impregnated gauze that can be kept for single patient use. Over time, the carbon electrodes will absorb oil and detergent products and become resistant to current flow. A periodic check (eg, every 30 days) of the conductivity of the electrodes is highly recommended.

Aluminum foil electrodes are very cost effective and time efficient for treatment of open wounds. They are easily made, good conductors, can be molded to fit the body part, can be sized for maximum current density to the wound, and are disposable. Saline-soaked gauze packed in the wound and covered with an electrode is also cost efficient and is particularly good on deep lesions.

## Protocol for Treatment of Chronic Venous Insufficiency or Chronic Deep Vein Thrombosis

This protocol from Alon and deDomenico[27] is based on using HVPC to elicit the pumping action of skeletal muscles. (See Table 6–4 showing HVPC protocols.) The best muscle-pumping action is achieved from active exercise, but for some patients this is not an option or is inadequate to facilitate the venous pump mechanisms. Therefore, ES can be used as an intermittent method for stimulation of muscle pump action. Patients with chronic lymphedema may also benefit.

### Setting Up the Patient

1. A bipolar technique is usually used.
2. Place both electrodes over the plantar flexors, one proximal and one over the muscle bellies.
3. Use a surge or interrupted mode with an on time of 3 to 15 seconds and an off time of 9 to 40 seconds. This 1:3 on/off ratio is essential to avoid muscle fatigue.
4. Begin with shorter on/off time and then increase the stimulation time as patient adjusts.
5. Polarity is not critical and can be adjusted for patient comfort.
6. Pulse rate is between 40 and 60 pps and can be adjusted for patient comfort.
7. Amplitude that will produce intermittent, moderate *tetanic* muscle contraction is required. Increase amplitude gradually for patient comfort and compliance.
8. Expect that a few treatment sessions will be required to reach the desired level of muscle contraction.

9. Treatment time is pathology dependent.
   a. Chronic thrombophlebitis: 30 to 60 minutes biweekly
   b. Venous stasis: commence 5 to 10 minutes daily; progress to 20 to 30 minutes biweekly
10. Precaution: Plantar flexors have a tendency to cramp; proceed slowly to avoid cramping. Such cramping must be avoided. To avoid cramping, place the feet against a footboard that limits full range of plantar flexion.
11. Expected outcome: enhanced venous return measured by reduced edema. May facilitate healing of venous ulceration.

## Summary

Patients are usually referred to the physical therapist for ES treatment when a wound has not responded to other treatment interventions and is classified a chronic wound. Patients with "healthy wounds" are usually referred only for purposes of accelerating healing to enable early return to work, sports, and activities of daily living. Both can be helped to accelerate the rate and maximize the quality of the repair. The physical therapy functional diagnosis for the wound and associated impairments will determine the patient candidacy for treatment with ES, type of stimulation needed, protocol, and expected outcomes. Undoubtedly, more investigation is needed to achieve an optimal treatment protocol with ES. However, safe and effective clinical results of wound healing are reported in the literature using the protocols and methods presented in this chapter. The physical therapist should have confidence when using these methods and expect the predicted clinical outcomes. Physical therapists are the most qualified health care practitioners to manage a program of wound healing with ES.

## DOCUMENTATION

Documentation is required at different intervals during the course of care. Below is a case study using a methodology developed by Swanson called a **functional outcomes report (FOR)**.[83] The initial evaluation report and reassessment reports can be written as an FOR. The FOR follows the methodology of the diagnostic process described at the start of this chapter. Items of the FOR fit the boxes of a Medicare HCFA 700 form very well. The FOR serves the function of describing the findings of the diagnostic process and then is used to explain the physical therapist's clinical reasoning for selecting the electrical stimulation intervention. In addition, the FOR lists the prognosis, targeted outcomes, and due dates for each. The FOR example below also includes examinations of related body systems and functional diagnoses of other impairments related to wound healing, along with interventions other than wound care with dressings that require the skills of a physical therapist. The physical therapist should consider the ES as adjunctive treatment to these other interventions. Exercise, for example, will enhance tissue perfusion faster and more effectively than ES. Proper positioning for oxygen transport is an essential part of achieving the optimal outcome with ES. The FOR has been adapted here to present a case study of a patient with a pressure ulcer on the foot and a case study of a patient with a vascular ulcer, both of whom were treated with ES.

## CASE STUDY NO. 1

### PATIENT WITH PRESSURE ULCER TREATED WITH ELECTRICAL STIMULATION

**Patient ID: A.S.**              **Age: 85**              **Onset: May**

■ **Initial Assessment: Brief Medical History and Systems Review**

### Reason for Referral

The patient has developed pressure ulceration along the lateral border of her left foot. She is not a candidate for surgical intervention because of multiple comorbities.

### Medical History

The patient is an 85-year-old woman who is unresponsive, with fetal posture and fixed contractures of all four extremities. She has a history of multiple cerebrovascular accidents. She does not reposition herself in bed and cannot sit up in a wheelchair. She is on nasogastric tube feeding for nutrition; a Foley catheter is in place to control incontinence of urine. The wound onset was 2 weeks prior to referral to physical therapy. The wound has deteriorated and become necrotized. The nurses had been using enzymatic and autolytic debridement methods.

### Systems Review

*Circulatory System*    The patient has systemically impaired circulation because of arteriosclerotic vascular disease. The circulation to the lower extremity is further impaired as a result of contractures of the hips and knees.

*Respiratory System*    The patient has shallow, impaired respiration because of inactivity and her bed-bound status.

*Musculoskeletal System*    The patient has impaired joint mobility because of contractures, resulting in severe disability of the musculoskeletal system.

*Neuromuscular System*    The patient lacks the ability to respond to the need for self-repositioning and is cognitively unaware.

## ▓ Examinations Indicated and Derived Data

### Vascular Examination

Palpation of pulses indicates a weak dorsal pedal pulse. Determination of the ankle–brachial index is not possible because of contractures at the elbow. Pulse oximetry of the great toe shows an oxygen saturation of 96 percent.

### Musculoskeletal Examination

There is limited passive range of motion (less than 90° at either the hips, knees, or elbows). There is no active motor movement.

### Integumentary Examination

The surrounding skin is erythematous, seen as a red glow under darkly pigmented skin. The tissue is edematous. The temperature of the wound is elevated compared with surrounding tissues. There are hemorrhagic areas along the wound margin, and necrotic tissue covers the wound surface.

## ▓ Evaluation of the Examination Findings and Relationship to Function

The specific dysfunction that generated a referral for the services of the physical therapist is loss of wound healing capacity. The patient's loss of function is because of generalized impairments (circulatory, cardiopulmonary, musculoskeletal, and neuromuscular). Limited bed mobility and limited cognitive ability further complicate the ability to heal without physical therapy intervention for integumentary management.

## ▓ Diagnosis

### Musculoskeletal Disability

Impaired flexibility and loss of muscle force leads to increased susceptibility to pressure ulceration of the feet.

## Neuromuscular Disability

The patient has neuromuscular disability associated with insensitivity and inability to reposition and make needs known.

## Wound Healing Impairment

The signs and symptoms identified by the wound assessment, including edema, erythema, heat, and the presence of necrotic tissue, indicate that the wound healing phase diagnosis is a *chronic inflammation phase of healing* and impaired wound healing associated with a chronically inflamed wound.

## Functional Diagnosis

- Undue susceptibility to pressure ulceration on the feet
- Impaired wound healing
- Chronic inflammation phase
- Insensitivity to need for position change

## ■ Need for Skilled Services

The patient has failed to respond to interventions with dressing changes for the last 2 weeks. She now requires the following four interventions:

1. Debridement of the necrotic tissue from the wound bed to determine level of tissue impairment and to initiate the healing process
2. HVPC to enhance circulation to the foot, facilitate debridement, and restart the process of repair
3. Therapeutic positioning to remove pressure trauma on the foot
4. Range-of-motion exercises to all four extremities to maintain tissue extensibility and increase circulation

## ■ Prognosis

Healing is not expected without intervention; however, the prognosis is good for a clean, stable wound. Initiation of the acute inflammation phase with ES is expected in 2 weeks, with progression to a proliferation phase in 4 weeks, and a clean, stable wound in 6 weeks.

## ■ Treatment Plan

- Instruction will be given to nurses' aides in range-of-motion needs of the patient; it will include initial and follow-up for two different shifts (four visits).

- Instruction will be given to the nursing staff in therapeutic positioning; it will include initial instruction and follow-up for two different shifts (three visits).
- HVPC characteristics:
  1. The active electrode will be placed on the wound site.
  2. The dispersive electrode will be placed on the thigh.
  3. Polarity initially will be negative, then alternated between positive and negative, as described under the Sussman Wound Healing Protocol, as the wound changes phases.
  4. The pulse rate will be changed from 30 pps to 120 pps to 64 pps as phases change.
  5. The current amplitude will be set at 150 V throughout.
  6. HVPC will be of a 60-minute duration, seven times a week.
- Debridement will be achieved by HVPC, enzymes, and sharp debridement daily as needed to remove necrotic tissue.

## Interventions

### Passive Range-of-Motion Exercises

Passive range-of-motion exercises will be performed to all four extremities, ranged twice daily by the restorative nurses' aide as instructed by the physical therapist.

*Targeted Outcome*    The nurses' aide will be able to provide the optimal amount of ROM for all four extremities; increase tissue extensibility at elbows, hips, and knees; and increase perfusion to the lower extremities; due date: 2 weeks.

## Healing Pressure Relief

Therapeutic positioning with adaptive equipment will be used to keep the feet off the bed, and a pressure-relief mattress replacement will be provided.

*Targeted Outcomes*    The nursing staff will be able to use therapeutic positions to reduce the risk of pressure ulcer formation on the feet, including elimination of pressure on the lateral border of the foot with the pressure ulcer; due date: 1 week.

### Electrical Stimulation With HVPC 7 Days per Week

*Targeted Outcome*    The intervention will stimulate perfusion and cellular responses of the inflammatory phase, and wound debridement will progress to the acute inflammation phase followed by progression to the proliferation phase; due date: 6 weeks.

## Debridement

Sharp debridement will be used for nonviable tissue; enzymatic debridement will be used to solubilize the necrotic tissue between sharp debridement sessions.

*Targeted Outcome*    The wound will be necrosis free; due date: 4 weeks.

### ■ Discharge Outcome

Within 4 weeks the wound was clean, granulating wound edges were contracting, and epithelialization was starting. Because it was now evident that there was potiential for wound closure, the prognosis was changed to healed wound from clean and stable; HPVC treatment was continued, and at 12 weeks the wound was fully epithelialized and closed.

---

## CASE STUDY NO. 2

PATIENT WITH VASCULAR ULCER TREATED WITH ELECTRICAL STIMULATION

**Patient ID: C.Z.**                    **Age: 80**

### ■ Initial Assessment

### Reason for Referral

The patient came to the physical therapist because a vascular ulcer on posterior right calf would not heal. The patient and his wife reported that they had been caring for the ulcer for more than 6 months, and they wanted it to heal so they could resume their usual activities in the community.

### Medical History

The patient has a history of severe arterial vascular occlusive disease of the lower extremities. Old World War II burn scarring covered the surrounding area of the calf, with hyperkeratotic scarring that kept breaking down. The recurrent skin breakdown on his leg resulted in protracted periods of healing (eg, more than 1 year). One ulcer had healed in 6 months after a course of care using ES (HVPC). The previous ulcer took more than a year and did not heal. The patient was ambulatory and alert, with mild confusion. His wife reported that any moisture left on the surrounding skin caused maceration and skin breakdown. A femoral angioplasty had been done the week before the patient was seen in the outpatient clinic.

## ■ Functional Diagnosis and Targeted Outcomes

### Integumentary Examination

*Surrounding Skin*    Hyperkeratotic scar tissue; flaky, friable, dry skin; and pallor are present.

*Functional Diagnosis*    The patient has loss of functional mobility because of integumentary impairment.

*Targeted Outcome*    The patient will have improved skin texture and integrity; due date: 6 weeks.

### Wound Tissue Examination

The wound edges are poorly defined. There is necrotic tissue along the margins. There is a small island of skin in the middle of the wound bed. The wound has partial-thickness skin loss, with moderate exudate. The wound is about 200 cm$^2$.

*Functional Diagnosis*    There is absence of an inflammation phase.

*Targeted Outcome*    Acute inflammation will be achieved; due date: 2 weeks.

*Associated Impairment*    Necrotic tissue is present.

*Targeted Outcome*    A clean wound bed will be achieved; due date: 4 weeks.

*Functional Diagnosis*    There is absence of a proliferation phase.

*Targeted Outcome*    The wound will have presence of granulation tissue and be ready for grafting; due date: 6 weeks.

### Vascular Examination

*Medical Prognosis*    The patient has severe arterial vascular occlusive disease, status post angioplasty.

*Functional Diagnosis*    The patient has vascular impairment.

*Targeted Outcome*    Perfusion will be enhanced; due date: 2 weeks.

The patient's loss of function in these systems is responsible for the undue susceptibility to skin breakdown on the legs and inability to heal without integumentary intervention. The patient has improvement potential. The wound will heal partially, and the wound bed will be prepared for grafting following intervention.

## ■ Need for Skilled Services

The patient has failed to respond to treatment with wound dressings and conservative managment of his leg ulcer and requires debridement of necrotic tissue to initiate the healing process, and HVPC to initiate healing phases and to enhance perfusion so the wound bed is prepared for grafting.

## ■ Treatment Plan

- The patient and his wife were instructed to perform HVPC as a daily home treatment program with a portable HVPC rental unit.
- Wound debridement will be performed to remove necrotic tissues; methods include autolysis, sharp debridement, and enhanced perfusion with the above-listed HVPC.
- The wife will be instructed in wound dressing changes with an alginate dressing to absorb moderate exudate, including how to cut the dressing to fit the wound to avoid maceration.

## ■ Discharge Outcome

- The patient started care in mid-December.
- The wound was necrosis free.
- The wound phase changed to both proliferation and epithelialization. The wound size was reduced to less than half of the original area.
- The wound was grafted at the end of February.
- The wound graft was successful. A smaller graft was needed than originally expected because of epithelialization.
- Integumentary integrity was improved, skin was softer and smoother, and no new hyperkeratosis developed in the scar tissue area.

## General Comments

The patient and his wife were very compliant with the home treatment regime. The femoral angioplasty apparently opened the vessels enough to permit the enhanced perfusion from the HVPC to reach the tissues. Grafting was a better option for this couple because it provided faster closure and allowed them to live more functional lives without having wound care duties. Grafting also provided a better covering with healthier skin from the oppposite thigh to cover with the open area. New scar tissue was better-quality tissue than surrounding older scars, possibly because of the improved collagen organization and vascularization associated with the HVPC treatments.

## REVIEW QUESTIONS

1. A patient with a history of diabetes mellitus for 15 years has been referred to the physical therapist to determine if use of ES will be beneficial for healing a recalcitrant plantar ulcer. The patient wants to return to work and family activities and is fearful of needing an amputation.
   (A) What information would need to be gathered to determine if the patient is a candidate for treatment with ES for wound healing?
   (B) What type of stimulator and protocols would the patient be given to use for a home program?
   (C) What would be the expected outcomes of an ES intervention for this patient?

2. A patient with a full-thickness ulcer extending into the calf muscle is referred to the physical therapist for ES treatment.
   (A) Describe the electrode arrangement that would be best to treat the ulcer and tell why.
   (B) What type of electrical stimulator would you choose? Why?

3. A patient has multiple full-thickness ulcers with necrotic tissue located over both trochanters, the sacrum, and the left heel secondary to pressure. All have a wound healing phase diagnosis of chronic inflammmation phase.
   (A) What type of electrical stimulator would the physical therapist select? Why?
   (B) Describe the electrode placement for the ulcers and tell why that would be best.
   (C) What wound healing outcomes would be expected? When?

4. The expected outcome of treatment is to convert an infected, necrotic wound from a chronic inflammation phase of healing to an acute inflammation phase.
   (A) What protocol characteristic is associated with this expected outcome?
   (B) When would this protocol characteristic be changed?

5. What might be the response of the circulatory system to application of ES that would effect wound healing? Describe the physiologic basis for the effects.

6. For individuals with chronic wounds, ES has been shown to be effective in reducing wound size, changing wound attributes, and reducing risk of wound complications. Describe the physiologic basis for these effects.

# References

1. Kirschner LB. Electrolyte transport across the body surface of freshwater fish and amphibia. In Ussing HH, Thorn NA (eds), Transport Mechanisms in Epithelia. Copenhagen, Munksgaard, pp 447–460, 1983.
2. VanDriessche W, Zeiske W. Ionic channels in epithelial cell membranes. Physiol Rev, 65:833–903, 1985.
3. Sariban-Sohraaby S, Benos DJ. The amiloride-sensitive sodium channel. Am J Physiol, 250:175, 1986.
4. Barker AT, Kaffe F, Vanable JW. The glabrous epidermis of cavies contains a powerful battery. Am J Physiol, 242:R358–R366, 1982.
5. Illingsworth CM, Barker AT. Measurement of electrical currents emerging during the regeneration of amputated finger tips in children. Clin Phys Physiol Meas, 1:87, 1980.
6. Jaffe LF, Vanable JW. Electric fields and wound healing. Clin Dermatol, 3:34, 1984.
7. Sussman C, Bates-Jensen BM, Tiffany M. The diagnostic process. In Sussman C, Bates-Jensen BM (eds), Wound Care: Collaboration Between Physical Therapists and Nurses. Gaithersberg, MD, Aspen, 1998.
8. Bergstrom N, Bennett MA, Carlson CE et al. Treatment of Pressure Ulcers, Clinical Practice Guideline, Number 15. Rockville, MD, Agency for Health Care Policy and Research (AHCPR), U.S. Department of Health and Human Services Publication No. 95-0652, 1994.
9. Barr JO, Nielsen DH, Soderberg GL. Transcutaneous electrical nerve stimulation characteristics for altering pain perception. Phys Ther, 66:1515, 1986.
10. Stefanovska A, Vodovnik L et al. Treatment of chronic wounds by means of electric and electromagnetic fields, Part 2. Value of FES parameters for pressure sore treatment. Med Biol Eng Comput, 31:213–220, 1993.
11. Baker LL, Rubayi S et al. Effect of electrical stimulation waveform on healing of ulcers in human beings with spinal cord injury. Wound Rep Reg, 4:21–28, 1996.
12. Baker LL, Chambers R et al. Effects of electrical stimulation on wound healing in patients with diabetic ulcers. Diabetes Care, 20(3):1–8, 1997.
13. Sussman C, Swanson GH. The utility of Sussman Wound Healing Tool in predicting wound healing outcomes in physical therapy. Fifth National Pressure Ulcer Advisory Panel Consensus Conference, Washington DC, February 1997.
14. Sussman C. Assessment of the skin and wound. In Sussman C, Bates-Jensen BM (eds). Wound Care: Collaboration Between Physical Therapists and Nurses. Gaithersberg, MD, Aspen, 1998.
15. Gentzkow GD. Methods for measuring size in pressure ulcers. NPUAP Proceedings Advances in Wound Care, 8(4):43–45, 1995.
16. Taylor D. The Sussman Method of Measuring Wounds That Contain Undermining, poster presentation. APTA Scientific Meeting. San Diego, CA, June 1997.
17. Sussman C, Swanson GH. A uniform method to trace and measure chronic wounds. Poster presentation. Symposium for Advanced Wound Care. San Francisco, CA, April 1991.

18. Jette A. Physical disablement concepts for physical therapy research and practice. Phys Ther, 74:380–386, 1994.

19. International Classification of Impairments. Disabilities and Handicaps. Geneva, Switzerland, World Health Organization, 1980.

20. Pope A, Tarlov A, eds. Disability in America: Toward a National Agenda for Prevention. Washington, DC, National Academy Press, 1991.

21. American Physical Therapy Association (APTA). Guide to physical therapist practice. Phys Ther, 77:1163–1650, 1997.

22. Bourguignon J, Bourguignon LY. Electrical stimulation of protein and DNA synthesis in human fibroblasts. FASB J, 1:398–402, 1987.

23. Mohr T, Akers T, Wessman HC. Effect of high voltage stimulation on blood flow in the rat hind limb. Phys Ther, 67:526–533, 1987.

24. Lundeberg T, Kjartansson J, Samuelsson U. Effect of electrical nerve stimulation on healing of ischemic skin flaps. Lancet, 2:712–714, 1988.

25. Politis MJ, Zankis MF, Miller JE. Enhanced survival of full-thickness skin grafts following the application of DC electrical fields. Plast Reconstr Surg, 84(2):67–72, 1989.

26. Pollack S. The effects of pulsed electrical stimulation on failing skin flaps in Yorkshire pigs (abstract). Paper presented at the Meeting of the Bioelectrical Repair and Growth Society, Cleveland, OH, 1989.

27. Alon G, deDomenico G. High Voltage Stimulation: An Integrated Approach to Clinical Electrotherapy. Hixon, TN, The Chattanooga Group, 1987.

28. Kaada B. Vasodilation induced by transcutaneous nerve stimulation in peripheral ischemia (Raynaud's phenomenon and diabetic polyneuropathy). Eur Heart J, 3:303, 1982.

29. Kaada B. Promoted healing of chronic ulceration by transcutaneous nerve stimulation (TNS). VASA, 12:262–269, 1983.

30. Ross C, Segal D. HVPC as an aid to post-operative healing. Curr Podiatry, May 1981.

31. Reed BV. Effect of high voltage pulsed electrical stimulation on microvascular permeability to plasma proteins—A possible mechanism in minimizing edema. Phys Ther, 68:491–495, 1988.

32. Mendel F, Fish D. New Perspectives in edema control via electrical stimulation. J Athlet Train, 28:63–74, 1993.

33. Mohr TM, Akers TK, Landry RG. Effect of high voltage stimulation on edema reduction in the rat hind limb. Phys Ther, 67(11):1703–1707, 1987.

34. Sawyer PN. Bioelectric phenomena and intravascular thrombosis: The first 12 years. Surgery, 56:1020–1026, 1964.

35. Sawyer PN, Deutch B. Use of electrical currents to delay intravascular thrombosis in experimental animals. Am J Physiol, 187:473–478, 1956.

36. Sawyer PN, Deutch B. The experimental use of oriented electrical fields to delay and prevent thrombosis. Surg Forum, 5:163–168, 1955.

37. Williams RD, Carey LC. Studies in the production of "standard" venous thrombosis. Ann Surg, 49:381–387, 1959.

38. Barranco S, Spadaro J et al. In vitro effect of weak direct current on Staphylococcus aureus. Clin Orthop, 100:250–255, 1974.

39. Rowley BA, McKenna J, Chase GR. The influence of electrical current on an infecting microorganism in wounds. Ann NY Acad Sci, 238:543–551, 1974.

40. Kloth LC. Poster presentation. Presented at the Symposium on Advanced Wound Care, Atlanta, GA, April 1996.

41. Szuminsky NJ et al. Effect of narrow, pulsed high voltages on bacterial viability. Phys Ther, 74:600–667, 1994.

42. Kincaid C, Lavoie K. Inhibition of bacterial growth in vitro following stimulation with high voltage, monophasic, pulsed current. Phys Ther, 69:29–33, 1989.

43. Alon G. Principles of electrical stimulation. In Nelson R, Currier D (eds). Clinical Electrotherapy. Norwalk, CT/San Mateo, CA, Appleton & Lange, pp 35–103, 991.

44. Barr JO. Transcutaneous electrical nerve stimulation for pain management. In Nelson R, Currier D (eds). Clinical Electrotherapy. Norwalk, CT/San Mateo, CA, Appleton & Lange, p 280, 1991.

45. Weiss D, Eaglestein W, Falanga V. Exogenous electric current can reduce the formation of hypertropic scars. J Dermatol Surg Oncol, 15: 1272–1275, 1989.

46. Stromberg B. Effects of electrical current on wound contraction. Ann Plast Surg, 21(2):121–123, 1988.

47. Wolcottt L, Wheeler P, Hardwicke H et al. Accelerated healing of skin ulcers by electrotherapy: Preliminary clinical results. South Med J, 62:795–801, 1969.

48. Gault W, Gatens P Jr. Use of low intensity direct current in management of ischemic skin ulcers. Phys Ther, 56(3):265–269, 1976.

49. Carley PJ, Wainapel SF. Electrotherapy of acceleration of wound healing: Low intensity direct current. Arch Phys Med Rehabil, 66:443–446, 1985.

50. Koth LC. Electrical stimulation in tissue repair. In Wound Healing Alternatives in Management, 2nd ed. Philadelphia, PA, FA Davis, p 88, 1995.

51. Byl N, McKenzie A et al. Pulsed microamperage stimulation: A controlled study of healing of surgically induced wounds in Yucatan pigs. Phys Ther, 74:201–218, 1994.

52. Leffmann DJ, Arnall DA, Holmgren PR. Effect of microamperage stimulation on the rate of wound healing in rats: A histological study. Phys Ther, 74:195–200, 1994.

53. Byl N, McKenzie A et al. Microamperage stimulation: Effects on subcutaneous oxygen (II). Presented at the annual conference of the California Chapter of the American Physical Therapy Association, San Diego, CA, 1990.

54. Barron JJ, Jacobson WE, Tidd T. Treatment of decubitus ulcers. Minn Med, 2:103–106, 1985.

55. Kloth LC, Feeder J. Acceleration of wound healing with high voltage, monophasic, pulsed current. Phys Ther, 68(5):503–508, 1988.

56. Griffin J et al. Efficacy of high voltage pulsed current for healing of pressure ulcers in patients with spinal cord injury. Phys Ther, 71(6):433–444, 1991.

57. Unger P, Eddy J, Raimastry S. A controlled study of the effect of high voltage pulsed current (HVPC) on wound healing. Phys Ther, 71:S119, 1991.

58. Unger PC. Randomized clinical trials of the effect of HVPC on wound healing. Phys Ther, 71:S118, 1991.

59. Alon G, Azaria M, Stein H. Diabetic ulcer healing using high voltage TENS. Phys Ther, 66:77(abstract), 1986.

60. Akers T, Gabrielson A. The effect of high voltage galvanic stimulation on the rate of healing of decubitus ulcers. Biomed Sci Instr J, 20:99–100, 1984.

61. Gentzkow GD, Pollack SV et al. Improved healing of pressure ulcers using dermapulse, a new electrical stimulation device. Wounds, 3:158–160, 1991.

62. Gentzkow GD, Miller KH. Electrical stimulation for dermal wound healing. Clin Podiatr Med Surg, 4:827–841, 1991.

63. Feedar JA, Kloth LC, Gentzkow GD. Chronic dermal ulcer healing enhanced with monophasic pulsed electrical stimulation. Phys Ther, 71:639–649, 1991.

64. Kaada B. Vasodilation induced by transcutaneous nerve stimulation in peripheral ischemia (Raynaud's phenomenon and diabetic polyneuropathy). Eur Heart J, 10:651–655, 1985.

65. Lundeberg TCM, Erikson SV. Mats M. Electrical stimulation improves healing of diabetic ulcers. Ann Plast Surg, 71:328–330, 1992.

66. Donayre C. Diagnosis & Management of Vascular Ulcers: Arterial, Venous & Diabetic. Presented at Wound Care Management '96, Torrance, CA, October 1996.

67. Rasmussen MJ, Hayes DL et al. Can transcutaneous electrical nerve stimulation be safely used in patients with permanent cardiac pacemakers? Mayo Clin Proc, 63:443–445, 1988.

68. Cook T, Barr JO. Instrumentation. In Nelson R, Currier D (eds), Clinical Electrotherapy. Norwalk, CT/San Mateo, CA, Appleton & Lange, pp 11–33, 1991.

69. Brown MB. Electrical stimulation for wound managment. In Gogia PP (ed), Clinical Wound Management. Thorofare, NJ, Slack, pp 176–183, 1995.

70. Kloth LC. Electrical stimulation for wound healing. Exhibitor presentation at American Physical Therapy Association Conference, Minneapolis, MN, June 1996.

71. Davis S. The effect of pulsed electrical stimulation on epidermal wound healing. J Invest Dermatol, 90(4):555, 1988.

72. Brown MB, McDonnell M, Menton D. Polarity effects on wound healing using electrical stimulation in rabbits. Arch Phys Med Rehabil, 70:624–627, 1989.

73. Alvarez O. The healing of superficial skin wounds is stimulated by external electrical current. J Invest Dermatol, 81(2):144–148, 1983.

74. Eaglstein W. Off-label uses in wound care. Paper presented at the Symposium on Advanced Wound Care, April 1966.

75. Myer A. Observable Effects on Granulation Tissue Using Warmed Wound Care Products. Presentation, Symposia: Future Directions in Wound Healing, APTA Scientific Meeting, June 1997.

76. Beltran KA, Thacker JG et al. Impact pressures generated by commercial wound irrigation devices. Unpublished research report, Charlottesville, VA, University of Virginia Health Science Center, 1994.

77. Bourguignon GJ et al. Occlusive wound dressings suitable for use with electrical stimulation. Wounds, 3(3):127, 1991.

78. Agren MS, Mertz MA. Collagenase during burn wound healing: Influence of a hydrogel dressing and pulsed electrical stimulation. Plast Reconstr Surg, 94(3):518–524, 1993.
79. Alon G. Panel discussion. Symposia: Future Directions in Wound Healing. American Physical Therapy Association Scientific Meeting, San Diego, CA, June 1997.
80. Lock PM. The effect of temperature on mitotic at the edge of experimental wounds. In Lungren A, Soner AB (eds), Symposia on Wound Healing; Plastic, Surgical and Dermatologic Aspects, Molindal, Sweden, 1980.
81. Myers JA. Wound healing and the use of modern surgical dressing. Pharmaceut J, 229:103–104, 1982.
82. Kalinowski DP, Brogan MS, Sleeper MD. A practical technique for disinfecting electrical stimulation apparatuses used in wound treatment. Phys Ther, 76(12):1340–1347, 1996.
83. Swanson G. Functional outcome report: The next generation in physical therapy reporting. In Stuart D, Ablen S (eds), Documenting Physical Therapy Outcomes. St. Louis, MO, Mosby, pp 101–134, 1993.

# Transcutaneous Electrical Nerve Stimulation for Pain Management

John O. Barr

## Introduction

Pain has been recognized as the symptom which most commonly causes people to seek health care.[1] In the United States, the economic impact of health care and lost productivity associated with chronic pain alone has been estimated to be greater than $80 billion annually.[2] Clinicians who are challenged by a wide range of clinical pain problems have found that transcutaneous electrical nerve stimulation (TENS) can be an important component of many treatment programs for pain management. Although this chapter is introductory in nature, the reader will be encouraged to critically assess factors influencing the efficacy of TENS. The chapter begins with a historical perspective on TENS. Details of commercial equipment are then reviewed, and suggestions are made for improving equipment-related performance. Critical elements of clinical decision making with TENS are reviewed, and key steps in implementing a successful treatment program are presented. Importantly, an algorithm for conducting a trial treatment with TENS is introduced. The theoretical bases for pain management with TENS are next highlighted, and the clinical effectiveness of TENS is subsequently assessed. Finally, a case study is presented in order to illustrate the clinical application of TENS for pain management.

## HISTORICAL PERSPECTIVE

The first recorded use of electricity for pain relief appeared in Compositiones Medicae, written in 46 A.D. by Scribonis Largus, a Roman physician. A live torpedo fish (also called the electric ray) was used for the treatment of gout and headache, its electrical discharge being used to shock the affected body part into numbness.[3] In the 1760s, John Wesley wrote specifically about the use of static electricity for pain relief. With Faraday's discovery of induction in 1831, further interest was directed toward the ability of electricity to relieve a variety of painful conditions by the late 1800s.[4,5] The early 1900s saw a proliferation of questionable therapeutic applications. This proliferation, coupled with an upsurge of promotion by paramedical and occult practitioners, brought about federal and medical society reaction such that most manufacturers of crude stimulators were forced out of business.[6] However, electrical analgesia continued to be described in the literature into the 1950s.[4] In 1967, Wall and Sweet tested a hypothesis central to their gate control theory of pain.[7] They reported temporarily abolishing chronic pain by electrically stimulating peripheral nerves via electrodes on the surface of the skin.[8] This technique soon became known as **transcutaneous electrical nerve stimulation.**

For the 20-year period from 1967 to 1987, Nolan compiled a bibliography of over 300 papers concerning TENS from clinical and basic science literature.[9] In addition, a journal special issue[10] and books[11,12,13] have been devoted to this topic. Although the number of publications concerned with TENS has declined in recent years, TENS continues to be a clinical topic subjected to research and review.[14,15] An array of health professionals, including physical therapists, nurses, physicians, and dentists have employed TENS for a wide range of acute and chronic pain conditions. For example, TENS for acute pain management has been utilized in the emergency room,[16] during minor surgical procedures,[17] postoperatively,[18] during labor and delivery,[19] with acute spinal cord injuries,[20] and for athletic injuries.[21] TENS has commonly been employed for treatment of chronic back pain[14] and headache.[22] TENS has also been used for chronic pain associated with a wide range of diagnoses including angina pectoris,[23] cancer,[24] causalgia,[25] Guillain–Barré syndrome,[26] reflex sympathetic dystrophy,[27] rheumatoid arthritis,[28] multiple sclerosis,[29] and phantom limb.[30] By the late 1980s, Robinson and Snyder-Mackler found that 92 percent of the physical therapists responding to their survey utilized TENS, 67 percent at least once a week.[31]

## COMMERCIAL EQUIPMENT

As has been pointed out by Alon in Chapter 3, all forms of electrical nerve stimulation done through electrodes on the skin's surface represent transcutaneous electrical nerve stimulation. Quite commonly, the terms *TENS (transcutaneous electrical nerve stimulation), TNS (transcutaneous nerve stimulation),* and *TES (transcutaneous electrical stimulation)* are used interchangeably to denote such a technique used for pain management.[32] (In contrast, percutaneous electrical stimulation is done through needle electrodes or surgically implanted wires.) Since 1974, when the Food and Drug Administration (FDA) classified transcutaneous electrical nerve stimulators as class II devices, numerous domestic and foreign-made stimulators have become available. By the late 1980s, there were more than 60 TENS manufacturers registered with the FDA.[33] Some transcutaneous electrical stimulators used for pain management have been classified as class III devices (eg, *cranial electrotherapy stimulators*), and their manufacturers have enjoyed this distinction in the marketplace. Although this discussion of commercial equipment will primarily focus on portable, battery-powered class II stimulators, similar concepts can be applied to the wide range of electrical stimulators used for pain control.

Transcutaneous electrical nerve stimulation systems are usually marketed as a "kit" consisting of the TENS unit, a battery power source, lead wires, electrodes, instruction manual, carrying case, and possibly electrode coupling gel and adhesive patches (Figure 7–1). The TENS unit, a small, portable electrical pulse generator, may be secured by a clip to a patient's belt or clothing, or it can be carried in a pocket.

### TENS Units

Most units produce an electrical output having one characteristic waveform, usually of the symmetric or balanced asymmetric biphasic type with zero net current to minimize skin irritation. The optimal waveform for pain management has not been determined.[34,35] Typically, units can be operated in one or more stimulation modes (eg, conventional, strong low-rate, brief-intense, pulse-burst, modulated, or hyperstimulation). Various arrangements of control dials, switches, or buttons on the unit may allow for regulation of power (on/off), mode, and electrical stimulation characteristics (eg, amplitude, pulse duration, and frequency) for one or two output channels (Figure 7–2). As discussed in Chapter 2, numbers listed on the controls often are nonlinearly related to the actual stimulator output

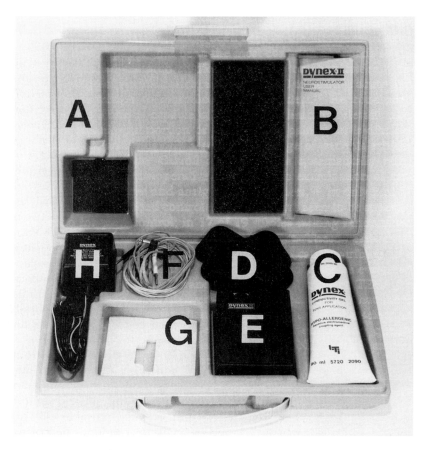

FIGURE 7–1. Typical TENS unit kit components. **(A)** Storage/carrying case. **(B)** Instruction manual. **(C)** Electrode gel. **(D)** Electrodes. **(E)** TENS unit. **(F)** Lead wires. **(G)** Adhesive patches. **(H)** Battery charger. *(Reprinted, with permission, from Clinical Electrotherapy, 2nd ed. Nelson RM, Currier DP [eds]. East Norwalk, CT, Appleton & Lange, 1991.)*

characteristics, which makes it difficult to predict the amount of stimulation a patient will receive. The controls themselves are usually recessed, and they may be internally located to prevent accidental movement or to limit patient access. The unit may have one or more lights to indicate that the unit is turned on, the battery charge is low, or there is a lead wire or electrode malfunction. Although two output channels would seem to provide more versatility and greater likelihood of clinical success than just one,[12] this assumption has been challenged.[36] Some units with independent channels permit asynchronous channel activation, or allow two different TENS modes to be used simultaneously.

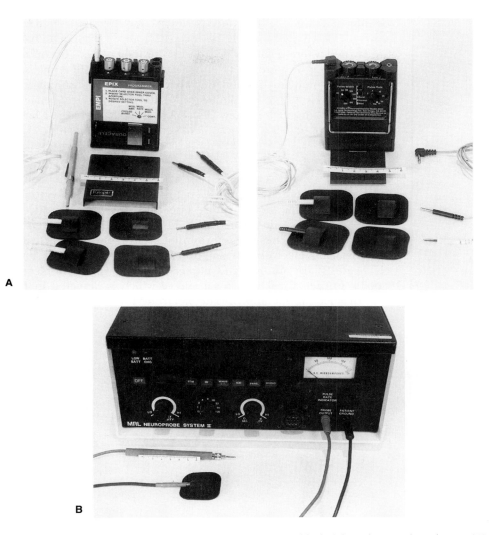

**FIGURE 7–2.** Sample of commercially available TENS units. **(A)** Portable dual-channel units and attachments. **(B)** Stationary single-channel unit (note the small diameter electrode used for hyperstimulation). *(Reprinted, with permission, from* Clinical Electrotherapy, *2nd ed. Nelson RM, Currier DP [eds]. East Norwalk, CT, Appleton & Lange, 1991.)*

The power source is most often a rechargeable battery pack or a long-life disposable battery. Although initially more expensive than the disposable battery, rechargeable batteries are more economical for repeated use if properly maintained. An especially important note is that older-style rechargeable batteries should be fully discharged before attempting to recharge them. If not, a "memory" develops that limits acceptance of a full charge.[36] These batteries have been recommended to be fully discharged at least once per week, and then recharged using a slow "trickle charger," which may take 12 hours.[12] Disposable batteries are favored where reliability is critical or for long periods of continuous stimulation, as in postoperative applications. Battery life is inversely related to the number of stimulating channels employed, stimulator output characteristics (eg, amplitude, pulse duration, and frequency), and duration of stimulation. New disposable or fully recharged batteries should be stored in a cool location to better maintain shelf life.

### TENS Electrodes

The reader should review the important discussion of neuromuscular electrical stimulation (NEMS) unit lead wires, connectors, and electrodes in Chapter 2. Clinical effects of polarity or relative electrode activity on pain treated with TENS have not been well documented.[12] Approaches for determining relative electrode activity and standardizing electrode orientation,[37] and for fabricating low-cost electrodes,[38] are outlined in Chapter 2. A wide variety of electrodes can be utilized for TENS, a sample of which is depicted in Figure 7–3. In selecting the appropriate electrode for a given pain manage-

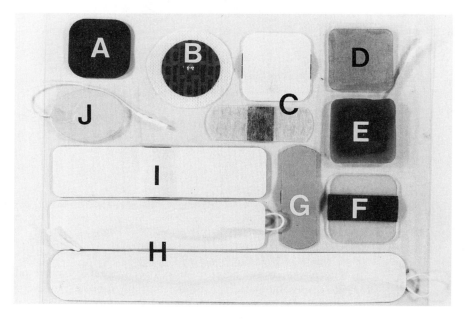

FIGURE 7–3. Sample of TENS electrodes. **(A)** Carbonized silicone rubber. **(B)** Pregelled self-adhering with snap connector. **(C)** Disposable self-adhering. **(D)** Karaya gum pad, to be placed between electrode and skin. **(E)** Karaya gum electrode. **(F)** Reusable synthetic. **(G)** Reusable high heat/humidity. **(H)** Sterile postoperative. **(I)** Non-sterile postoperative. **(J)** Polymer gel. *(Reprinted, with permission, from Clinical Electrotherapy, 2nd ed. Nelson RM, Currier DP [eds]. East Norwalk, CT, Appleton & Lange, 1991.)*

ment problem, a number of factors should be considered, including initial versus long-term cost, durability, ease of preparation and application, and potential for skin irritation. Electrodes come in a variety of sizes, and many can be cut to different sizes and shapes. Electrodes that are reusable or disposable, and nonsterile or presterilized, are available for specific applications. Typically, reusable nonsterile electrodes are employed for long-term repeated use as with chronic pain, whereas disposable presterilized electrodes are used for acute postoperative pain.

Carbonized rubber electrodes are commonly secured to the skin with surgical tape, or with a variety of commercial paper or foam adhesive patches. While such patches are often more convenient than tape, they are considerably more expensive. Electrode placement belts, which hold a pair of electrodes so that they can be secured in difficult-to-reach locations, such as the low back, are also commercially available. At the conclusion of each treatment, siliconized carbon rubber electrodes should be washed with mild soap and warm water, thoroughly rinsed, and patted dry with a soft towel. Alcohol should not be used as a cleansing agent, as this breaks down the electrode. Over a period of months, some electrodes lose their flexibility and demonstrate increased electrical resistance, which renders them ineffective. Thus, some authorities have suggested that this type of electrode be replaced at 6-month intervals.[12] Other types of electrodes, tips for their maintenance, and methods for securing them to patients are described in Chapter 2.

### *Adverse Skin Reactions*

Prevention of adverse skin reactions is especially important with TENS because electrodes may remain in place for hours to days and be utilized over a period of months. The incidence of adverse skin reactions has been widely cited to be quite low, with 4 to 5 percent of the population having reactions to electrolytic gels, for example.[39] Ericksson and colleagues reported a 12 percent occurrence of skin irritation in their long-term study.[40] A nationwide survey of 196 physical therapy departments reported that 79 percent of respondents saw some side effects associated with TENS, of which the most common (68 percent) was skin irritation.[41] Noting that such reactions are the primary reason that otherwise successful TENS programs are discontinued, one electrode manufacturer identified contributing allergic, chemical, electrical, and mechanical factors.[42] Regular inspection of the patient's skin and use of alternate electrode sites may minimize the occurrence of irritation from most of these factors. Although electrodes and related materials (conductive media and adhesives) are usually made from nonirritating or hypoallergenic compounds, instances of localized skin reactions have been noted.[39,43,44]

Electrodes containing mercaptobenzothiazole or having metal components made of nickel, gels containing silicon oxide or propylene glycol, alkaloids in karaya gum, and methacrylate in conductive gel pads have been implicated. The basis for an adverse skin reaction should be identified, with the assistance of a dermatologist to conduct patch testing if necessary. Alternate types or brands of electrodes and related materials may need to be utilized. Skin at electrode sites should be cleaned with mild soap and water before and after treatment. All residues, including those from operative site preparations, soaps, gels, and adhesives, should be removed in order to minimize chemical reactions.

Prior to treatment, electrode sites should be inspected for cuts and abrasions, which can become focal paths of low impedance that produce high-density electrical currents. Undesirably high current density is a primary electrical factor causing skin irritation. This can be minimized by using larger electrodes that are not placed too close together (ie, at least one electrode diameter apart).[12] Griffin reported that direct current densities of less than 1 mA/cm$^2$ will limit the likelihood of skin irritation.[45] Under conditions of extremely intense stimulation (85 mA, 500 μsec, and 185 pps), it has been noted that electrodes larger than 4 cm$^2$ will prevent burns and those larger than 16 cm$^2$ will avoid stimulating nociceptors.[46] Overly dry skin at intended electrode sites can be hydrated by rubbing in a small amount of nonabrasive electrode gel, which overcomes undesirably high skin impedance.

Mechanical reactions are thought to be largely related to poor technique in affixing electrodes to the skin. Electrodes should be positioned to accommodate body movement. Lead wire pins or connectors should be aligned perpendicular to the plane of body segment motion, which allows the electrode to be more flexible in this orientation. A similar alignment should be used for tape, which will stretch and slacken less, thereby minimizing shear forces in the skin. For a similar reason, tape, adhesive patches, and electrodes should not be stretched as they are placed on the skin. Long lead wires can be coiled and taped together at some distance from electrodes in order to provide a relief for tension pulling on the electrodes. Adhesive electrode materials should be removed by slowly lifting them as the underlying skin is held down to prevent skin stripping.

### Critical Evaluation of TENS Units

Unfortunately, only a few publications have critically evaluated specific brands of either domestic or foreign-made TENS units since the mid-1970s.[36,47,48,49] Mason tested TENS unit electrical output characteristics and effectiveness in alleviating pain.[48] Using a simulated body impedance circuit, three of the five units demonstrated changes in current output as resistive loads were varied from 500 to 5000 ohms. Noticeable changes in the sensation produced by TENS were also related to current variations based on different electrode preparations. On one unit, simultaneous adjustment of amplitude and frequency controls from mid to maximum settings resulted in a 37 percent decrease in output pulse duration. All five units were able to produce some degree of pain relief in certain instances. Ultimately, two of the units (Stim-Tech EPC and Avery TNS) were recommended for use in Veterans Administration prosthetic center clinics.

The clinical and engineering staff of *Health Devices* conducted extensive consumer-oriented tests on 18 TENS units.[36] These tests included measurement of various electrical output characteristics, assessment of functional controls, minimization of startle response, safety related to output characteristics, labeling and warning legends, battery life and insertion, construction quality, effects of drops and fluid spills, damage from open- and short-circuit conditions, ease of use, indication of on/off status, quality of operator's manual, and cost of the TENS unit kits. Notably, warranties and service on equipment were not addressed. Most units were judged as being approximately equal and received "acceptable" ratings. Some of the evaluated units had controls that were difficult to see clearly or to adjust. This could present a significant problem to some elderly or disabled individuals. Two units (Bio-Instrumentation TENS-1 and Koken Kogyo Health Point) were not recommended. Although two of the units (Electreat 250 and Koken Kogyo Health Point) exceeded the 75-$\mu$C charge-per-pulse maximum limit proposed in the Association for the Advancement of Medical Instrumentation (AAMI) Standard for Transcutaneous Electrical Nerve Stimulators (1980), they were not seen to pose a risk greater than that associated with most of the other units. (Instead, the *Health Devices* staff challenged the validity of the testing circuit load used with the 1980 AAMI standard.) Given the generally high cost of TENS units, manufacturers were encouraged to review their pricing policies. Although efficacy of the TENS units was not evaluated, it was suggested that clinicians consider having more than one brand of unit available in order to improve the possibility of determining the most effective unit for a given patient.

Stamp briefly summarized the evaluation of 18 TENS units marketed in Britain.[49] Recommended design features were reviewed. Breakage of electrode cables and battery connector wires from mechanical stress were the two most common equipment failures. Although concern for the cost of TENS units was expressed, it was noted that product quality was usually related to unit price.

Campbell assessed the electrical output characteristics of 10 TENS units that were commercially available in the United Kingdom.[47] Some of the measurements were conducted with resistive loads varying between 1000 and 5000 ohms, values that had been derived from actual electrode preparations. None of the units was determined to have either true constant current or constant voltage outputs over this load range. Nonlinear relationships were seen between control settings and output characteristics of amplitude, frequency, and pulse duration for most units. The test load used for establishing the AAMI Standard for Transcutaneous Electrical Nerve Stimulators (revised, 1981) was criticized, but this time in reference to the 25-μC charge-per-pulse threshold for a required label warning against transthoracic use. The more expensive units did not necessarily have the most reliable output characteristics. Several suggestions were given for improvements in TENS unit design.

Equipment-related factors can play a significant role in the success or failure of any clinical treatment with TENS. For example, the lack of independence between unit control settings and other output characteristics is usually not apparent when lower settings are used.[50] Reeve noted that the basic design of modern TENS devices have not undergone any fundamental changes since first being developed.[15] Present standards require that a given control not change by more than 5 percent of its adjusted value when the remaining controls are adjusted over their range in any combination.[51] Practical details discussed above and cited sources of information, including the American National Standard for Transcutaneous Electrical Nerve Stimulators,[51] should prompt those utilizing TENS to be more critical consumers of this equipment. Development and use of equipment rating forms that can be referred to when discussing equipment with colleagues, distributors, manufacturers, and regulatory groups are encouraged.

## CLINICAL DECISION MAKING

The clinician needs to make a number of important decisions prior to, during, and after implementing a TENS program in order to ensure safe and successful pain management. Treatment must be based on a thorough evaluation of the patient's pain and related dysfunction. Indications and contraindications for treatment must be disclosed, taking into account information from the patient's health history and physical examination. The optimal TENS mode, with unique electrical stimulation characteristics and electrode placements, must be determined for each patient. Related decisions should be guided by an understanding of the theoretical basis for pain relief by TENS. In order to carry out successful treatment with

TENS, the treatment protocol may need to be modified in order to provide effective pain relief and improvement in function, or to handle problems that may develop. Ideally, the patient will be actively involved in the treatment after appropriate instruction.

## Overview of Patient Evaluation

Both initial and ongoing evaluations of the patient are important to any treatment program. A wide range of clinical problems present with pain as the major symptom and have associated limitations in physical and psychological functions. An accurate assessment must be made concerning the underlying basis for pain, and aggravating factors should be fully explored. Other sources should be consulted for detailed information about physical and psychological testing, and for functional outcome assessment and documentation.[52] Although the initial evaluation is primarily diagnostic in character and may require more than one session, it provides valuable baseline information. Importantly, the evaluation allows review of indications and contraindications to treatment and guides the clinician in selection of TENS modes and electrode sites. The clinician should also be able to arrive at a prognosis for success in managing pain with a comprehensive program to improve functional outcomes that combines TENS with other relevant treatments (eg, joint mobilization, force-improving exercises, instruction in body mechanics, or education about ergonomic principles). The patient history should include information about medication use or abuse, and about treatments previously used successfully or unsuccessfully for pain management. Ongoing evaluations, conducted during each session, allow the clinician to determine if the patient is progressing adequately or if the treatment program requires modification. In many cases, a multidisciplinary approach to evaluation and treatment of pain may be most beneficial.[53,54] Ultimately, it is important for the clinician to recognize if the patient's response is based upon effective treatment, or if a positive outcome represents a natural resolution of the clinical problem, a placebo effect, or both.[55]

## Pain Assessment

The complexity of the pain experience is well known and has prompted numerous attempts to define pain. In an abstract manner, *pain* has been defined in terms of a multidimensional space comprising several sensory and affective dimensions.[56] More simply, pain has been described as a hurt that we feel.[57] Pain of less than 4 to 6 months in duration is often termed *acute,* whereas pain of longer duration is called *chronic.*[58] **Acute pain,** which occurs with conditions such as trauma and active inflammation, is frequently associated with sympathetic nervous system ("fright/flight") responses. **Chronic pain,** however, may be associated with a decrease in autonomic factors and an increase in psychological factors, particularly depression.[57]

Historically, attempts to measure clinical pain have been confounded by its private and subjective character.[59] The manner in which a person expresses pain has been found to be related to factors of personality, past pain experiences, age, gender, behavioral needs, ethnic membership, and cultural heritage.[56,57] A variety of methods have been developed to permit assessment of clinical pain. Since the late 1970s, clinicians have been increasingly concerned with the validity, reliability, and objectivity of pain assessment techniques.

An assortment of behavioral indicators, which are demonstrable patient pain behaviors, can be documented by the clinician during the patient interview and physical examination.[57] For example, it is possible to qualify facial expression (eg, a grimace). The patient's verbal complaint of pain can provide information concerning the quality, distribution, and duration of pain, and can disclose aggravating or relieving factors. The quality and distribution of pain may be charted by the patient on a body diagram.[60] Other verbal indicators may include crying and changes in mood. Requests for pain medications, including frequency, type, and amount, may be documented. For purposes of comparison, a wide range of pain medications may be converted to a standard morphine equivalent dose.[61] Functional aspects of movement, such as "uptime"[62] and activity patterns,[63] may be quantified using simple automated systems. Various indices and scales have been employed to evaluate functional activities in relation to pain, but lack of sensitivity or limited correlation to changes in pain have been apparent for some measures.[64,65,66]

A number of physical signs may be assessed in relation to pain. In association with acute pain, Sternbach has observed increases in pulse rate, systolic blood pressure, and respiratory rate, as well as dilated pupils, perspiration, nausea, and pallor.[57] Physical characteristics of posture,[67] gait,[68] range of motion (ROM),[69,70,71] muscle force[72,73] and endurance,[73] duration of joint loading time,[28] pressure threshold and tolerance,[74,75] tissue compliance,[74] skin temperature,[76,77] and pulmonary functions[18,78] have also been evaluated in conjunction with pain.

Pain rating scales have been developed in the attempt to more specifically quantify pain that patients are experiencing or have experienced in the past. The **pain estimate** requires the patient to rate his or her pain intensity on a scale of 0 to 100. Zero indicates "no pain," while 100 represents "pain so severe you would commit suicide if you had to endure it more than a minute or two."[79] In less suggestive terms, 100 might be taken to represent "the worst pain that you could ever imagine." With the **verbal rating scale (VRS),** the patient selects one of five or more words that best describes pain (eg, none, mild, moderate, severe, unbearable).[80] The **visual analogue scale (VAS)** utilizes a 100-mm line, with verbal anchors "no pain" next to the line at the left and "pain as bad as it could be" at the right. Pain is rated by the patient placing a mark in one location on the line.[80,81,82,83] A VAS can also be used to assess pain relief by employing anchors of "complete pain relief" and "no pain relief."[84] The **graphic rating scale (GRS)** combines features of the VRS and the VAS, such that word descriptors (eg, mild, moderate, severe) are placed along the analogue line with anchors as previously described.[83] A number of comparative studies have been done with these scales.[80,82,85,86] Although these scales can be quickly administered, patients who have trouble with abstract thinking may have difficulty with some scales (ie, VAS).[82] These scales have also been criticized for focusing primarily on the intensity of pain, for lacking sensitivity in some situations, and for being used with inappropriate mathematical analyses.[87]

Various sensory matching tests have been introduced in the attempt to improve the accuracy of pain assessment. Sternbach and coworkers[79] have advocated use of the **submaximal effort tourniquet** technique originally developed by Smith and colleagues.[88] Essentially, the procedure involves using a blood pressure cuff on the nondominant arm to induce ischemic pain after submaximal isometric exercise. The patient first notes the point at which the induced pain matches the intensity of the clinical pain. Some time later, the patient indicates when the ischemic pain is the maximum that can be tolerated. The time elapsed to the clinical match is divided by the time to reach maximum tolerance; this ratio is multiplied by 100, and result is termed the **tourniquet pain ratio.** Some procedural aspects of this approach were modified by Moore and associates to improve standardization.[89]

**Cross-modality matching** procedures have also been employed, whereby input to another sensory modality is matched to some characteristic of clinical pain. The intensity of an auditory tone,[90,91] grip force,[87] and color matching[92] have been utilized, and comparative studies have been performed.[90] A number of more comprehensive approaches to assessing pain, sometimes in conjunction with function, have been summarized by others.[93,94]

The **McGill Pain Questionnaire (MPQ)**[60] has probably been the most often utilized of these techniques. The questionnaire seeks information relative to the location of pain via a coded body diagram, characterizes the qualities of pain via the Pain Rating Index (PRI), determines how the pain changes with time, and assesses pain intensity through the Present Pain Intensity (PPI) scale. Derived measures have been shown to be sensitive to a number of therapeutic interventions including TENS.[95,96,97,98] Although the original form of the questionnaire required 5 to 10 min to administer, a short-form of the MPQ (SF-MPQ) takes only 2 to 5 min.[99] The author's experience, and that of others,[98] has been that patients sometimes have difficulty understanding pain descriptors used in the original format. Other pain assessment techniques have been compared to this questionnaire.[100] Melzack and Katz have noted that the SF-MPQ and VAS are probably the most frequently used pain self-rating instruments.[101]

## Indications, Contraindications, and Precautions

There are a number of sources of information in both professional literature and commercial publications concerning TENS indications, contraindications, and precautions. The American National Standard for Transcutaneous Electrical Nerve Stimulators[51] will be relied on as a major reference for this section. The primary indications for TENS have been recognized as the symptomatic relief and management of chronic intractable pain, and as an adjunctive treatment in the management of postsurgical and posttraumatic acute pain.[51] The standard notes that TENS is of no known curative value. However, there is evidence that externally applied electrical currents can affect tissue repair, which may be associated with pain relief.[102–105]

Although many types of pain can be effectively treated, some conditions have historically failed to respond well. Long[106] noted that patients with peripheral nerve injuries respond more than 70 percent of the time, and that those with postherpetic neuralgia or acute musculoskeletal syndromes also regularly benefit. In contrast, patients having metabolic peripheral neuropathy with hyperesthesia or serious sensory loss, or those with "central pain states" associated with spinal cord injury and thalamic syndrome generally do not benefit from TENS. Leijon and Boivie determined that 5 of 15 patients with central poststroke pain had temporary increases in pain with conventional or acupuncture-like TENS.[107] Patients who have psychosomatic pain or drug addiction, or who are involved in situations where secondary gain is important, are also rarely helped by TENS.[106] Johansson and colleagues determined that patients with psychogenic or somatogenic pain had significantly poorer results than those with neurogenic pain, and that pain in the extremities was significantly better controlled with TENS than that located on the face, neck, or trunk.[108] However, because exceptional responses can be found despite these general trends, it would seem prudent to permit all pain patients a trial evaluation period with TENS, as will be described later in this chapter.

The use of TENS with some patients having demand-type (synchronous) cardiac pacemakers has been recognized as the sole contraindication for this modality.[51] Eriksson and colleagues assessed the effects of TENS having a pulse duration of 200 μsec, and frequencies of 10 to 100 pps pulsed at 1 to 10 pps.[109] Four ventricular-inhibited synchronous pacemakers were blocked with stimulation at 1 to 3 pps, and in one instance at frequencies up to 6 pps. The current amplitude required for this effect was 5 mA with electrodes on the thoracic wall and 10 mA with electrodes on the lumbar–sciatic region. No blocking was produced with the electrodes distal on the lower extremity, or with modulating frequencies above 6 and not greater than 10 pps. One ventricular-triggered synchronous pacemaker was activated to reach its upper limit (130 beats per minute [bpm]) using TENS at frequencies above 2 pps. An atrial synchronous pacemaker was triggered by unspecified TENS characteristics to operate at its maximal rate of 150 bpm. Electrode position was not noted in these latter two cases. The proper functioning of two asynchronous (fixed-rate) pacemakers, now rarely employed were not interfered with when using any of the frequencies at maximal current amplitude. Chen and associates reported on two cases involving brief inhibition of cardiac pacemaker function, without cardiac symptoms, during extended Holter monitoring. TENS electrodes had been placed paraspinally on the upper back, the lumbar region, or on the right posterior neck and shoulder.[110] Patients had ventricular pacing, ventricular sensing, and inhibition of output in response to sensing pacemakers with unipolar endocardial leads. Interference did not recur after the pacemakers were reprogrammed to lower sensitivity.

Long observed that although TENS should not be used "in the proximity" of demand pacemakers, it could be used on other areas of the body.[106] Shade noted no interference with a temporary demand pacemaker using a dual-channel TENS unit (pulse duration 20 μsec, frequency 35 pps, amplitude not specified), with electrodes simultaneously positioned on the upper thorax in paraspinal and midaxillary locations on one patient monitored in an intensive care unit over a period of days.[111] Rasmussen and associates evaluated TENS effects on 51 patients having 20 models of permanent cardiac pacemakers.[112] Two electrodes from one TENS unit channel alternately stimulated four sites (cervical, lumbar, left leg, and forearm ipsilateral to the pacemaker) for 2-min periods. TENS characteristics included a pulse duration of 40 μsec, frequency of 110 pps, and an amplitude initially producing discomfort that was readjusted to a comfortable level. In no case was there evidence of pacemaker-induced interference, inhibition, or reprogramming. However, the electrodes admittedly had not been placed in what was likely the most hazardous configuration, parallel to the pacemaker electrode vector (eg, for a unipolar pacemaker, one electrode over the right ventricle and the other near the pacemaker).

Although TENS has been safely done on body areas close to fixed-rate (asynchronous) pacemakers and remote from demand-type (synchronous) pacemakers, the range of hazardous stimulation characteristics and electrode positions has yet to be completely determined. In order to ensure safety, and to alleviate both patient and clinician anxiety, all patients with pacemakers should be monitored during an extended initial application of TENS. In the absence of undesirable cardiac-related signs and symptoms, a cardiologist may reprogram the pacemaker to a lower sensitivity in order to prevent interference by TENS.[110] Sliwa and Marinko recently expressed concern about a TENS-produced electrocardiographic (ECG) artifact that was misinterpreted to be a malfunctioning cardiac pacemaker in a patient who did not even have a pacemaker.[113] They suggested that both patients and physicians be made aware of the potential for this artifact. Monitoring devices themselves may require special filters to prevent interference from TENS.[12]

Specific warnings and precautions for TENS use have been identified. It has been recommended to manufacturers that these should be specified in clinician and patient information that is part of the TENS kit.[51] The above-noted use with demand-type cardiac pacemakers should be acknowledged as being hazardous. Some have suggested that electrodes not be placed on the anterior chest wall of patients with histories of any cardiac problems.[12] Stimulation over the carotid sinus, which may reflexly induce slowing of the heart, a fall in blood pressure, or fainting, should also be recognized to be hazardous. Despite a number of studies that have documented safe TENS use during labor and delivery,[19,114,115] it has been thought that the safety of TENS during pregnancy and delivery has not been established. Note that TENS may suppress the sensation of pain in a manner that deprives the patient of this protective mechanism against acute injury, although this could be questioned.[116] The use of TENS in the presence of skin irritation should be warned against, and improper use (eg, prolonged use, contact with metal lead wire tips) should be recognized to be associated with skin burns.

As a precaution, TENS should be used with caution for undiagnosed pain syndromes. TENS may, however, provide a reduction in pain and related muscle spasm, which permits more specific evaluation and diagnosis. TENS appears to be more effective for pain of peripheral than of central origin. Furthermore, treatment outcome can be influenced by the patient's psychological state and by the use of drugs. Specific drugs such as diazepam, codeine, corticosteroids, and other narcotics, as well as drug addiction, have been reported to limit success with TENS.[12] As discussed previously, TENS should be acknowledged to be of no known curative value. Finally, a TENS unit must be kept out of the reach of children. It has been recommended that TENS be used only under supervision of or referral from a physician, which is not consistent with contemporary clinical practice of many other health care professionals.

Aside from the precautions presented in the American National Standard,[51] suggestions from other groups merit consideration.[12,45,106,117] Intense stimulation, especially that associated with muscle contraction, may lead to the disruption of fractures, sutures, and other fragile tissues. Stimulation over the eyes and internally on mucosal membranes has been seen likely to produce irritation or other damage. Stimulation in proximity to the larynx might lead to restriction of the airway. Effects on patients with cerebrovascular accidents, transient ischemic attacks, epilepsy, and seizure disorders, or stimulation on the head or upper cervical regions, are not well established, and thus close monitoring is required. Special precautions will be necessary if attempting to treat the confused or incompetent patient (eg, it may be necessary to cover unit controls to prevent readjustment or to ensheathe the device in protective padding). Manufacturers have traditionally cautioned against the use of TENS units while operating a motor vehicle or other hazardous equipment where unanticipated stimulation might produce a startle response or uncontrolled muscle contraction. Because there is always a probability that a patient will encounter an adverse reaction to treatment, even after some delay, it is important that the clinician provide a follow-up and document the response to treatment.[118]

## Overview of TENS Modes

Six primary types or modes of TENS have been discussed with regularity in the literature.[12] Although descriptive labels have been used in an attempt to classify each mode (ie, conventional, strong low-rate, brief-intense, pulse-burst, modulated, and hyperstimulation), this has led to some confusion. Essentially, each mode is distinguished by unique stimulator output characteristics (Figure 7–4), and sometimes also by electrode placements and other protocol details. In order to improve communication in clinical notes and publications, it is recommended that such detailed information always be specified when describing a TENS mode. To date, some studies have assessed the optimal stimulation characteristics for pain relief within a given TENS mode,[34,98,116,119] whereas others have attempted to determine the most effective TENS mode for given pain management problems.[28,120,121] The following overview will introduce common TENS modes based largely upon stimulation characteristics.

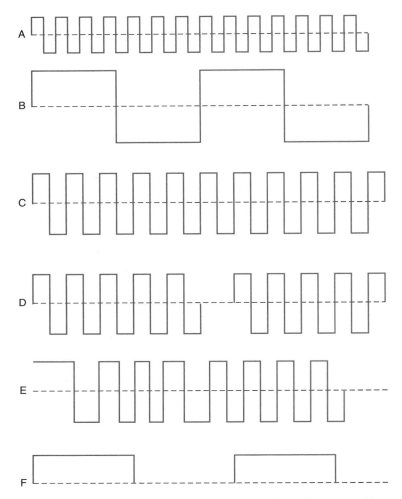

FIGURE 7–4. Schematic representation of common TENS modes. **(A)** Conventional low-amplitude high-frequency. **(B)** Strong low-rate. **(C)** Brief-intense. **(D)** Pulse-burst. **(E)** Modulated (pulse duration). **(F)** Hyperstimulation. *(Reprinted, with permission, from Clinical Electrotherapy, 2nd ed. Nelson RM, Currier DP [eds]. East Norwalk, CT, Appleton & Lange, 1991.)*

The majority of publications dealing with clinical TENS have been concerned with the **conventional mode,** which is generally characterized by a high frequency and a low amplitude (Figure 7–4A).[8,12,18,25,46,116,121] Conventional TENS utilizes frequencies in the range of 10 to 100 pps and an amplitude that produces comfortable cutaneous stimulation without muscle contraction.[40] As a sensation of distinct paresthesia is usually desired, a frequency approaching 30 pps is required before individual electrical impulses will perceptually fuse. Research has indicated that frequencies approximating 60 pps are optimal for producing pain relief with this mode.[34,116,119] Frequencies in the range of 80 to 200 pps have been reported to worsen pain for some patients.[116] Where separate linear unit control adjustments are possible, perception of amplitude is based on a short pulse duration (typically 50 to 100 μsec) and low to mid-range amplitude (eg, a minimum of 24 mA has been seen as necessary for excellent pain relief[119]). A short pulse duration favors preferential stimulation of large-diameter myelinated afferent neurons, the target of conventional TENS.[122] As patients treated with this mode often accommodate to the stimulation, total current must be periodically increased (via increased stimulation amplitude or pulse duration) in order to maintain adequate perception of electrical paresthesia. There have been reports of this mode being done with an amplitude purposefully adjusted to just below that required for sensory perception, a "subthreshold" setting.[116,121,123] Neuronal stimulation has been documented at this low amplitude.[124]

The **strong low-rate mode** (also called *acupuncture-like*) is characterized by a high amplitude and low frequency (Fig. 7–4B).[12,121,125] The stimulating frequency is below 10 pps, most commonly in the range of 1 to 4 pps. Pulse duration typically ranges from 100 to 300 μsec, which can be at mid to maximal control settings. Amplitude is adjusted to produce visibly strong and rhythmic muscle contractions. The beating of these contractions is uncomfortable but within the patient's tolerance to discomfort. This mode and other high-intensity modes are thought to be more resistant to perceptual accommodation.

Some confusion has been associated with the specifications for the **brief-intense mode** of TENS. Commonly denoting stimulation with a high amplitude and high frequency (Figure 7–4C),[28,121,125] considerably lower amplitude is sometimes used.[12] Unfortunately, the term *brief-intense*[95,96] has also been used to define TENS with output characteristics most similar to another contemporary mode (ie, pulse burst). Typical stimulating frequency is from 60 to more than 150 pps, in the range that has been seen to produce significant muscle fatigue with continuous stimulation.[126] Pulse durations of 50 to 250 μsec are commonly employed. Amplitude is adjusted to produce muscle contraction, with high settings yielding uncomfortable tetanic muscle contractions and low settings giving nonrhythmic muscle fasciculations. Either amplitude should also yield a sensation of paresthesia.

The **pulse-burst mode** (also called *burst* or *pulse train*,[12] and even acupuncture-like[40] TENS) is depicted in Figure 7–4D.[28,127] Pulse burst has been utilized in the attempt to improve patient acceptance of high-amplitude stimulation, because some patients have had difficulty tolerating muscle beating associated with the strong low-rate mode.[40,125] This mode is characterized by high carrier frequency (eg, 60 to 100 pps) modulated by a low burst frequency (eg, 0.5 to 4 pps). Pulse durations may range from 50 to 200 μsec. Again, both high- and low-amplitude settings have been utilized.[12] High-amplitude stimulation produces intermittent tetanic muscle contractions and paresthesia, but low amplitude provides just a sensation of pulsating paresthesia.

Although the **modulated mode** has been advocated by some manufacturers and authors to prevent accommodation to stimulation or to improve patient tolerance,[12] few studies have specifically examined this TENS format.[128,129] TENS units with this feature automatically change (modulate) one or more output characteristics (eg, pulse duration, amplitude, or frequency) by a given percentage from an initially set level. Affected characteristics may be modulated in a manner that decreases their values by up to 60 percent one to two times each sec. Figure 7–4E illustrates modulation of pulse duration alone. Output characteristics like the modes discussed above can thus be altered in a manner that may enhance patient acceptance and pain management.

The TENS mode of **hyperstimulation,** also called **noninvasive electroacupuncture**[12] has received limited but promising assessment.[27,71,130,131,132] Undeniably the most noxious form of TENS, it is the only mode that regularly utilizes either direct or monophasic pulsed currents (Figure 7–4F). This mode relies on high current density to produce very noxious cutaneous stimulation that is sharp and burning in character, without resultant muscle contraction. This noxious stimulation is achieved by using a very small probe-type stimulating electrode, with a tip that may be only 1 to 3 mm in diameter, and a very long pulse duration (eg, 500 msec) in some TENS units. Because of these factors, required current amplitude may not need to be higher than 50 μA with some equipment. Although the pulsed frequency can exceed 100 pps, the range of 1 to 4 pps enjoys the greatest empirical use. Progressively higher frequencies become more noxious because the total current per unit time is increased.

## Electrode Placement Options

Effects ascribed to the various TENS modes are not based solely upon electrical stimulation characteristics. A variety of electrode placement options permit specific neuromuscular structures to be targeted and help to ensure the efficacy of stimulation. In Chapter 2, a technique was described for discerning whether one electrode is more "active," and the suggestion was made to standardize placement of the more active electrode distal to its less active paired partner. Discussion will now focus on electrode placement relative to the location or distribution of pain. These placement options may be used as initial or alternative electrode sites. For the sake of simplicity, discussion will begin with placements using just two electrodes from a single TENS unit channel.

Electrodes can be positioned relative to a localized site of painful trauma or inflammation, so that stimulation occurs primarily via cutaneous afferents. There are at least four options that exist for electrode placement when using just two electrodes (Figure 7–5). First, both electrodes may be placed just proximal to the site of pain. This placement is useful if pain arises from a distal extremity location. Second, the electrodes can be positioned just outside the proximal and distal margins of the painful region, in a manner that "brackets" this area. Third, one electrode may be placed on the painful area while the other is situated adjacent to the spine over the related spinal nerve root. The second and third options may not provide sufficient current density to stimulate adequate sensory perception if the electrodes are situated too far apart. Both electrodes may be placed distal to the site of pain. Such distal stimulation, however, has been reported to have more limited effectiveness than the first and second options.[133] Finally, a crisscross or modified interferential placement with two channels might be used.

The site to be stimulated must be sentient, in order to ensure that electrical stimulation is being conveyed to the nervous system. For example, a body region may become denervated from trauma, or a surgeon may purposefully cut an intercostal nerve in the attempt to minimize incisional pain. High-amplitude stimulation, however, may still be capable of producing pain relief in the absence of cutaneous sensation.[120] Generally, it appears important that conventional TENS, and possibly low-amplitude formats of other modes, be done so that stimulation occurs at a site segmentally related to tissues that are giving rise to pain,[12] but conflicting observations have been reported.[116] As illustrated in Figure 7–6, some dermatomes used as sites for stimulation may not spatially overlap painful myotomes or sclerotomes that share the same segmental innervation.[134] If a segmental relationship is indeed important, the proper dermatome must be selected as the site for TENS.

A specific **peripheral nerve** that innervates a painful region can be targeted for stimulation, especially where located superficially. Picaza and colleagues produced more than a 50 percent reduction in pain for 55 of 100 patients in whom peripheral nerves were stimulated.[116] The electrodes from one channel may be placed at varying distances apart along the course of a nerve. Also, the two electrodes can be used to simultaneously stimulate two peripheral nerves (eg, ulnar and median nerves at the wrist). Quite commonly, pain is asso-

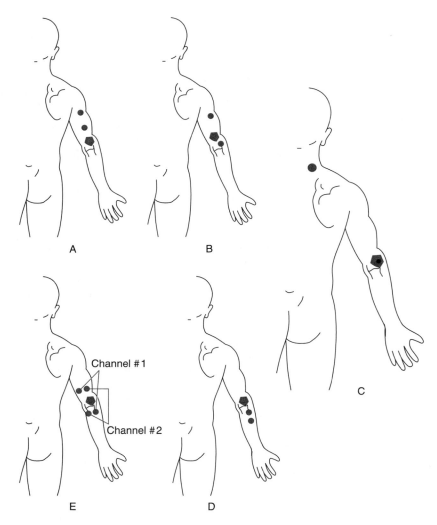

FIGURE 7–5. Electrode site options for localized pain. **(A)** Both electrodes from one channel proximal to area of pain. **(B)** Electrodes bracketing painful area. **(C)** One electrode over site of pain, the other paraspinally over related nerve root. **(D)** Both electrodes distal to area of pain. **(E)** Crisscross placement, two channels. *(Reprinted, with permission, from* Clinical Electrotherapy, *2nd ed. Nelson RM, Currier DP [eds]. East Norwalk, CT, Appleton & Lange, 1991.)*

ciated with injury to the peripheral nerve itself. In such cases, Long has recommended that stimulation be done proximal to the site of nerve injury and that hyperesthetic areas be avoided.[106] Stimulation of peripheral nerves "remote" (ie, not segmentally related) to painful areas has been reported to relieve pain in some instances. In 42 of 280 tests done by stimulating remote nerves, Picaza and associates documented pain suppression, but it was variable and generally

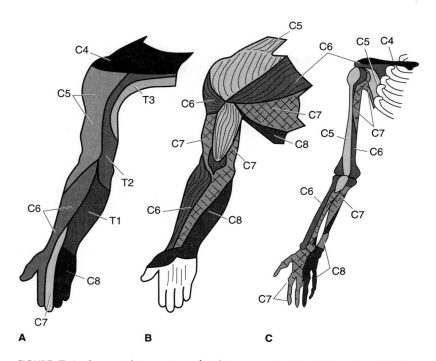

FIGURE 7–6. Segmental innervation of right upper extremity, anterior view. **(A)** Dermatomes. **(B)** Myotomes. **(C)** Sclerotomes. *(From Inman VT, Saunders JB. Referred pain from skeletal structures. J Nerv Ment Dis, 99:660, 1944, with permission.)*

weak. Remote stimulation tended to be positive if stimulation of nerves directly innervating the area was successful.[116]

A **motor point** can be physiologically identified as a specific location on the skin that requires the lowest amplitude of electrical stimulation to produce excitation of an underlying innervated muscle. Anatomically, this area of skin has been found to transversely overlie a muscle's neurovascular hilus, which contains sensory, motor, and autonomic axons, and the zone of innervation, where branches of motor axons terminate on individual muscle fibers.[135,136] Such points would seem well suited to afford input to the central nervous system, permit efficient stimulation of muscle contractions, and influence circulatory control, all of which are desired outcomes for specific TENS modes. Although motor points have been suggested as sites for TENS electrodes,[12] no studies were found that specifically assessed TENS done at these locations.

A **trigger point** exists as a hyperirritable focus in skin, fascia, muscle, tendon, ligament, or periosteum.[137] A trigger point is painful on compression and produces a characteristic pattern of referred pain and related signs. The zone of referred pain often does not follow a segmental pattern. Transcutaneous electrical nerve stimulation electrodes may be positioned relative to a trigger point or relative to its zone of referred pain.[96] Also, one electrode may be placed over the trigger point while the other is located at the reference zone. Travel and Simons have cautioned against using high-amplitude TENS that produces muscle contraction that can aggravate a myofascial trigger point.[137]

An **acupuncture point,** a tender site on the body surface utilized for pain management in traditional Chinese acupuncture,[138] can also be used in TENS. Two approaches have been commonly used for treating these points.[139] One approach involves treating a predefined sequence of acupuncture points for a given pain problem. The other approach involves treating successive points of low pain threshold along the acupuncture meridian that passes through the painful area or points on the auricle, or both, of the ear in locations thought to be related to the pain. Electrodes are placed directly on a single point or on multiple points simultaneously. Fox and Melzack produced greater than a 33 percent reduction in chronic low back pain in 8 of 12 patients using high-amplitude pulse-burst TENS at three predetermined acupuncture points for a total of 30 min.[127] The duration of pain relief averaged 23 hours. Treatment with TENS at appropriate acupuncture points, as opposed to inappropriate points, has resulted in significant pain relief.[96] Lein and associates reviewed a number of studies that used somatic or auricular acupuncture points, or both, for pain control with TENS.[130] The basis for and effectiveness of treatment at auricular points has been controversial.[140,141,142,143]

Mannheimer and Lampe comprehensively summarized the relationships between motor, trigger, and acupuncture points.[12] All of these points can be spontaneously painful or tender to palpation. Palpation can also produce referred pain. These points often present resistance to manual pressure, which may sometimes be associated with fibrositic components. The locations of these points[144,145] and the distributions of their referred pain are very similar.[145] Often, these points are situated over superficial nerves or dense groupings of sensory end organs. Electrically, these points demonstrate locally increased conductivity, and therefore decreased impedance. Taken as a whole, these relationships seem to indicate that motor, trigger, and acupuncture points represent the same entity,[12] although dissent has been voiced.[137]

The preceding discussion has been referenced to single-channel TENS treatment given ipsilateral to a painful body region or related target such as a dermatome, peripheral nerve, motor point, trigger point, or acupuncture point. In some situations, it may be desirable to add a second channel of stimulation or to "piggyback" additional electrodes. Under certain circumstances, it may be appropriate to stimulate contralateral to a painful region, as in the case of limited sensation, skin irritation, herpes zoster, postherpetic neuralgia, or causalgia.[12,146] Bilateral placement of electrodes should provide even greater input to the central nervous system. Although both clinical and experimental pain can be decreased with bilateral electrode placements, results may not be superior to unilateral treatment alone.[147] Electrodes from two separate TENS channels may be crisscrossed so that stimulating current intersects in the painful area (see Figure 7–5E). When such a setup is done without using a true interferential stimulator, this approach has been called the **modified interferential technique.** Additional electrode placement arrangements are discussed in other publications.[12,146]

Except where limited by TENS unit hardware features (eg, limited adjustment of output characteristics, single channel, inability to piggyback electrodes, electrodes that are too large or too small), any of the above electrode site options might be used with any TENS mode. However, as a given TENS mode is characterized by the presence (or absence) of particular perceptual, neural, and muscular responses, certain electrode placements have come to be favored for each mode. Some of this information has already been mentioned earlier in this section. Conventional TENS and low-amplitude formats of pulse-burst and modulated modes can be done using all of the previous electrode sites. Generally, pain relief is better if the sensation of electrical paresthesia is felt throughout the painful area, but exceptions have been noted.[116] Higher-amplitude stimulation (eg, strong low-rate, brief intense, pulse-burst, and modulated TENS) that involves muscle contraction must stimulate the muscle via a peripheral nerve or motor point. Perhaps pain relief is more effective if these sites also represent acupuncture points. Although high-amplitude stimulation that produces muscle contraction at painful trigger points has been warned against,[137] further investigation of this precaution is warranted. Hyperstimulation TENS produces a very noxious sensation through stimulation of cutaneous entities such as nerves, acupuncture points, trigger points, and motor points. The sensation is not nearly as noxious if stimulation is not provided at these low-impedance points. Current density below the skin is not adequate to significantly stimulate muscle at peripheral nerves or motor points with this mode at amplitudes that will be tolerated.

As might be anticipated, various electronic devices have been marketed to assist in the precise location of motor, trigger, and acupuncture points based on their conductive or impedance characteristics. These devices are sometimes incorporated within a TENS unit. However, the validity of relying only on such measurements to locate points is questionable, as Mann has noted many low-impedance sites that do not correspond to acupuncture points.[138] Furthermore, the reliability of such devices has not been adequately documented in the literature. In fact, the small, sharp metal tips on some of the electrodes used to probe the skin can produce minor abrasions that actually lower the measured impedance. Using tips that are smooth and spring loaded to standardize the pressure of application would seem important. The precision with which points can be located becomes a more critical factor when small-diameter electrodes will in turn be used for TENS, as in the hyperstimulation mode.

Berlant has suggested an alternative approach to locating superficial peripheral nerves or related acupuncture points,[148] which warrants further assessment for reliability and safety. Using a single TENS channel, one electrode is placed on the palm of a patient's hand while the other electrode is held by the clinician in the hand used for testing. Transcutaneous electrical nerve stimulation unit pulse duration is set low and frequency is adjusted within the range of 30 to 50 pps. The clinician then probes the patient's skin with the tip of the index finger in the vicinity of a likely peripheral nerve or acupuncture point, while slowly advancing the TENS amplitude. Peripheral nerves and acupuncture points are located at sites where the patient perceives the strongest sensation of radiating paresthesia. Clinicians also feel stronger paresthesia in the tip of their index fingers than elsewhere when these sites are found. Electrode position in this technique has been recommended to be modified to limit unnecessary current flow through susceptible body regions (eg, neck or thorax of the patient being assessed) by placing the patient electrode on the body part being tested.

## THEORETICAL BASES FOR PAIN RELIEF WITH TENS

An understanding of the theoretical basis for pain relief with TENS will guide the clinician in various aspects of decision making (eg, selection of TENS modes and electrode sites). The clinician will also be better prepared to respond to questions from patients and colleagues, and to anticipate patient response to treatment and likely treatment outcomes. Additionally, research is to be encouraged in order to further clarify the bases for the effects of TENS. This section briefly reviews a number of mechanisms by which TENS has been suggested to act.

One action of TENS might be to change the sensitivity of peripheral receptors or free nerve endings responsible for the transduction of nociceptive stimuli. However, evidence for these mechanisms remains limited.[106] Enhanced blood flow in the skin[149] and deeper tissues[150] in response to stimulation producing intermittent muscle contraction[151] (as with strong low-rate, pulse-burst, or modulated TENS) may supply required oxygen and rid the area of stimulating or sensitizing chemical mediators. Similarly, fatigue of muscle spasm produced by sustained muscle contraction[45] (as with brief-intense TENS) may subsequently lead to improved blood flow. Both low-[102,151] and high-amplitude[27] stimulation that does not produce muscle contraction may also be associated with improved blood flow.

Transcutaneous electrical nerve stimulation may block transmission of impulses in afferent nerves (eg, A-delta and C) conveying nociceptive information. Blocking of potassium has been implicated as a possible mechanism.[106] Taub and Campbell assessed averaged compound action potentials from the median nerve during noxious pinprick.[152] High-amplitude TENS (frequency 100 pps, pulse duration 500 μsec) was delivered in two forms. Continuous stimulation (most like brief-intense or high-frequency hyperstimulation), which finally became painless after about 20 minutes, produced analgesia to pinprick and a preferential decrease in the A-delta component of the compound potential. In contrast, bursted stimulation (0.5-sec bursts every 30 sec) was painful throughout, induced no analgesia, and did not produce a change in the compound potential. Using painful electrical stimulation in the range of 0.5 to 10 pps through intradermal needle electrodes, Torebjörk and Hallin observed decreases in induced pain and increased latencies and blocking of averaged C-fiber responses.[153] Similar changes were reported in averaged A-delta fiber responses, but not usually at frequencies below 20 to 30 pps. Ignelzi and Nyquist, however, used stimulation at 15 pps to produce the most dramatic decreases in the A-delta component of compound action potentials from isolated cat peripheral nerves, although changes were also seen in A-alpha and A-beta components.[154] In 30 percent of the experiments there was an enhancement of both the amplitude and conduction velocity of these components after initial poststimulation depression. Devor and Wall determined that ongoing neural activity in experimentally produced neuromas could be stopped by high-amplitude antidromic stimulation (square wave, frequency of 100 pps, pulse duration of 100 μsec).[155] However, an explanation for the effect of stimulation that can be tolerated by subjects or patients, based solely on peripheral mechanisms, has been challenged.[156]

Transcutaneous electrical nerve stimulation may also exert an effect on the autonomic nervous system through peripheral or central mechanisms. Jenkner and Schuhfried employed high-amplitude monophasic pulses to produce an electrical block of the stellate ganglion, which was best associated with increased circulation in the arm or head when using a frequency of approximately 100 pps modulated by an 8-Hz carrier.[157] These stimulation characteristics were also effective for relieving chronic pain. The effect of TENS on angina pectoris was examined by Mannheimer and associates.[23] The chest wall was stimulated using a frequency of 70 pps, pulse duration of 200 μsec, and an amplitude just below that producing pain. In a short-term, 4-day series, 10 patients experienced significantly increased maximal work capacity and decreased ST-segment depression. In a long-term series, 11 TENS-treated subjects had significantly better outcomes than 10 control subjects both during and after a 10-week experimental period with respect to frequency of anginal attacks, nitroglycerin consumption, recovery time, and ST-segment depression. These studies used high-amplitude stimulation similar to pulse-burst and brief-intense TENS modes, respectively.

Since the late 1960s, Melzack and Wall's "gate control" theory of pain[7] has been utilized as the standard explanation for pain relief via TENS, especially that of the low-amplitude conventional mode. This theory has been credited with rekindling interest in electrical control of pain[158] and inspiring research with important scientific and clinical ramifications.[159] An essential tenet of this theory is that large-diameter A-beta afferents excite interneurons in the dorsal horn of the spinal cord, producing inhibition of nociceptive input from smaller-diameter A-delta and C fibers. Both conventional and acupuncture-like (ie, high-amplitude pulse-burst) TENS have been shown to stimulate afferent fibers in the A-alpha–beta range.[160] Descending inhibitory influences from higher centers are also accounted for by this theory. Subjected to critical analyses and experimentation,[159,161,162] the gate control theory has undergone the revisions expected of any theory.[156] However, exact mechanisms of the theory remain to be elucidated.[106,156]

The relationship between TENS and the production of endogenous opiates (eg, endorhpins and enkephalins) has been examined. Mayer and Price critically examined the evidence for endogenous opiate analgesia in man.[163] In only two of ten studies using high-frequency TENS were there indications of endorphin involvement. In contrast, five of eight studies using low-frequency TENS demonstrated endorphin involvement either directly or indirectly. Furthermore, they noted that these studies collectively indicate that it is low-frequency, high-amplitude TENS that is associated with endogenous opiate mechanisms. Langley and coworkers reviewed mechanisms of TENS and placebo therapy.[164] They concluded that intense "acupuncture-like" (ie, pulse-burst) and intense low-frequency TENS (eg, 1 to 4 pps) both act through descending pathways involving endorphins. Intense high-frequency TENS, however, was not seen to be endorphin mediated. In addition, placebo effects were found to be based on both endorphin and nonendorphin mechanisms.

Possible reflex-based effects of TENS have also been examined. Chan and Tsang assessed the lower extremity flexion reflex induced in healthy subjects.[165] Conventional TENS (square waveform, frequency of 100 pps, pulse duration of 1 msec, amplitude two to three times perception threshold) to the L4–S1 region paraspinally for 30 min was associated with significant inhibition of the reflex both during and after stimulation. The time to maximal effect took 20 to 30 min for select muscles, and the effect persisted for as much as 50 min after stimulation. Similar changes were not seen in subjects treated with sham TENS. Of particular interest is the fact that Facchinetti and associates also demonstrated inhibition of the flexion reflex that was correlated with an increase in endogenous opiates (beta-lipotropin and beta-endorphin) after conventional TENS.[166] Effects of TENS on yet other reflexes have also been described.[167,168]

## A STRATEGY FOR SUCCESSFUL TREATMENT WITH TENS

Although TENS is typically but one component in a comprehensive pain management program,[12,169] it alone will be the topic of discussion here. After completing appropriate evaluation procedures, ruling out potential contraindications, and determining that TENS is indeed indicated, the clinician should discuss treatment goals with the patient and proceed with an initial trial treatment of TENS. An algorithm for conducting a trial treatment with TENS, depicted in Figure 7–7, is discussed in detail below.

When introducing the concept of TENS to a patient, steps should be taken to minimize anxiety about electrical stimulation. Emphasize that a small battery-powered unit with well-controlled output is being used. Avoid referring to stimulation as "electrical shocks," no matter how low the amplitude is described to be. Letting the patient experience the sensation of stimulation on a noninvolved body part prior to the actual treatment is often helpful. However, demonstration at the intended site of a surgical procedure is usually used as a part of preoperative patient education. Patients are naturally interested in the likelihood of a successful treatment outcome, although some are skeptical of "high-tech" interventions. A straightforward and nontechnical explanation of both the basis of and plan for treatment is helpful for most patients. The clinician should also be aware that confidence and competence, conveyed by both verbal and nonverbal means, can positively shape patient expectation in a manner that enhances treatment outcome.[55]

With many patients it is possible that significant pain relief can occur as a result of nonspecific factors, including the psychological framework, related to treatment.[170] Fields has noted that "placebo

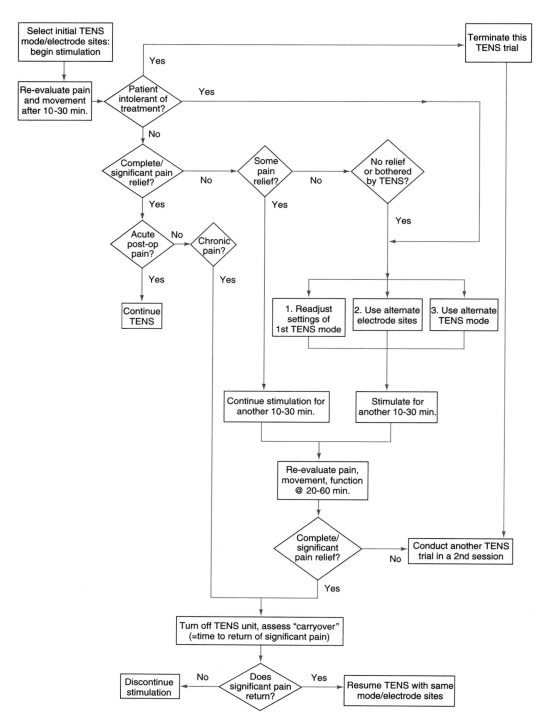

FIGURE 7–7. Algorithm of a trial treatment with TENS.

analgesia occurs when some aspect of the treatment situation causes the patient to expect pain relief and the patient's expectation of relief, rather than any specific action of the treatment, triggers a neurally mediated reduction in pain."[55] Although any patient will respond under the right conditions, the placebo effect is actually enhanced by patient stress and anxiety, and by more severe pain.[55,170,171] Some authorities have suggested that the placebo effect from a given treatment regimen becomes limited after one[6] or two weeks.[58]

While appreciating the concerns of others,[12] it is the author's belief that pain medications should be continued during initial TENS treatments as long as they are not impairing a patient's cognitive function. Continued use of medications is done so that a reduction in pain medications might be documented as a measurable treatment outcome. Similarly, the patient should maintain pretreatment activity levels unless a decrease in mechanical stress is warranted (eg, through the use of a cane in osteoarthritis of the hip, or cessation of jogging for shin splints). However, during the trial treatment with TENS the patient should be positioned for comfort, stability, safety, and good access to intended electrode sites. Most often this involves using a recumbent position for the patient. As pain relief is progressively induced during the trial session, the affected body part should be carefully tested in order to assess if pain relief is due to TENS or to rest from function.

Unfortunately, the clinician must deduce the appropriate TENS mode with which to begin the trial treatment with TENS. Presently, there is not an adequate number of comparative studies to determine the optimal TENS mode for a given pathology or diagnosis associated with pain. Only a few studies have examined patient acceptance or tolerance of TENS modes.[120,128,172] As might be anticipated, patients generally find low-amplitude conventional TENS, and lower amplitude formats of other modes (ie, brief-intense, pulse-burst, and modulated), to be most acceptable. Not considering lower-amplitude formats of established modes, it has been the author's experience that patients are most acceptive of TENS modes in the following rank order: conventional > modulated > pulse-burst > strong low-rate > brief-intense > hyperstimulation. Some studies have suggested that TENS using a low amplitude and high frequency produces a rapid onset of pain relief, whereas stimulation with high amplitude and low frequency gives longer carryover of pain relief.[40,173] Exceptions to these observations, however, have been noted.[25,28,130] Some patients with peripheral nerve injury or radiculopathy require higher stimulation amplitudes to produce satisfactory pain relief.[98] Greater stimulation amplitude, based on a longer pulse duration, higher amplitude, or both, may also be required to stimulate deep peripheral nerves, especially if there is intervening fat or scar tissue. As initial patient acceptance and likelihood of successful outcome are critical to proceeding with treatment, conventional TENS (at a frequency of 60 pps, short pulse duration, and amplitude producing distinct paresthesia in the area of pain) is usually the TENS mode of first choice.[34,119]

Once the initial TENS mode and electrode sites have been selected, the electrodes are prepared and placed on the patient, based on the previously discussed rationale. Regardless of the TENS mode to be used, it is advisable to preset the unit's pulse duration and frequency, then to turn the unit on and advance the amplitude to the desired setting. Although durations of stimulation for clinical pain have ranged from 2 min[8,25] to continuous for up to 5 days,[70] the typical duration of TENS is 20 to 60 min. Thus, a total duration of 20 to 60 min is used during the trial treatment. Stimulation with the high-amplitude modes of strong low-rate, brief-intense, and pulse-burst tend to be on the short end of this range because of limited patient tolerance. Hyperstimulation is often done twice for 15 to 30 sec to multiple acupuncture points.[139]

Continuous monitoring of the patient during treatment for such things as changes in vital signs, adequacy of stimulation, and patient acceptance of treatment is advisable. Minor readjustments of stimulation characteristics within the selected TENS mode may be necessary. After approximately 10 to 30 min of stimulation (see Figure 7–7), the patient's pain should be reevaluated and the effect of body movement (via deep breathing and coughing, active ROM, gait, etc) should be assessed as appropriate. Even by this point, some patients will have attained complete or significant pain relief. In cases of acute or postoperative pain, TENS is typically done continuously to maintain this pain relief while permitting enhanced, but safe, function (eg, effective deep breathing and coughing). Where such relief is obtained in cases of chronic pain, the TENS unit is temporarily turned off until significant levels of pain return, and then stimulation is resumed. If the patient is experiencing some pain relief, the period of stimulation may be continued. If the patient becomes distraught or intolerant of the treatment, it may be necessary to readjust the stimulation parameters, to select alternate electrode sites, to utilize an alternate TENS mode, or to terminate the initial trial session in a dignified manner and to conduct another TENS trial at a second session. If the patient is bothered by the sensation of TENS, or is not getting any pain relief, it is advisable to proceed with one of the following options. First, further readjust the stimulation characteristics within the initially selected TENS mode. Was the stimulation, the resultant of amplitude and pulse duration, too high or too low? Was the frequency optimal? For example, a patient complaining of a sensation of "bugs on my skin" at 60 pps will often have this sensation disappear when a frequency of 10 pps is used instead. Second, relocate the electrodes to an alternative site, with some forethought as to which sites would also be optimal for another TENS mode. Third, select another TENS mode. Stimulation should then be continued for another 10- to 30-min period.

At the end of 20 to 60 min in the TENS trial period (see Figure 7–7), reevaluate pain, ROM, and other functional activities. If complete or significant pain relief has not been achieved, another trial session using an alternate TENS mode should be conducted. If complete or significant pain relief has been attained at this point in the trial, next determine if there is any "carryover" of treatment effect. Assessment of carryover is accomplished by turning off the TENS unit and monitoring the length of time it takes pain to return to a significant level. Patients can either be questioned at the next session, or they can keep a formal log of pain and physical function ratings at regular time intervals (eg, every 2 waking hours). Although very unlikely, it is not impossible that pain will be totally relieved, never to return. Usually, there is a slow return to a level of significant pain over a period of hours, at which point TENS can be resumed. In some instances, pain will immediately return to a significant level as soon as the unit is turned off. This may warrant almost continuous TENS use.

Generally, acute pain responds more rapidly to treatment than chronic pain, although significant relief of chronic pain has been observed with as little as two minutes of conventional low-amplitude TENS.[8,25] In treating acute pain, the primary aim is to decrease pain and related muscle spasm as rapidly as possible. Continuous application of TENS may be required, for example, with postoperative pain.[18,70,78] Although the clinician is concerned with eliminating chronic pain, one should recognize that the patient may become dependent on the TENS unit as an external symbol of pain that evokes a reaction from others. Where chronic pain behaviors are a problem, it may be necessary to administer TENS "by the clock" at fixed time intervals rather than at patient request.[174]

The clinician should be sure that the patient is attaining significant pain relief through two or more treatment/education sessions, either as an inpatient or as an outpatient. Patients seen only for one session of "TENS evaluation and treatment" do not seem to respond as well to TENS. Wolf and colleagues found that only 10 of 114 patients with chronic pain had their best results during the first treatment.[98] Leo and associates determined that 21 of 83 patients achieved additional pain relief when TENS characteristics were changed for a second treatment session.[123] Woolf and Thompson recommended at least a 14-day trial period of TENS.[175] Long noted that up to one month of TENS use may be necessary to determine if treatment will be effective.[106] Some insurance plans have required a trial TENS unit rental period of 1 month before a unit can be purchased. It is important that the patient be taught to operate the TENS unit, and even to trouble-shoot problems with electrodes and batteries. Through such activity, the patient will gain a greater sense of controlling the pain. Similar instruction should also be given to other members of the health care team or family who are vital to the success of postoperative and home pain management programs. Other components of the comprehensive pain management program may also be reviewed at this time.

Both verbal and written home program instructions should include a number of features to ensure patient understanding and compliance. Information should clarify and go beyond that provided in the TENS kit's manual. The schedule for TENS use, be it intermittent or continuous, should be specified. Details of skin and electrode preparation should be outlined. Special electrodes or methods of attachment may be required. Primary and alternate electrode sites can be noted on a body diagram. All unit controls should be reviewed and adaptations utilized as needed. For example, some small control knobs are slotted, which permits the patient to turn them with the edge of a coin. The TENS mode and stimulation characteristics that have proven optimal for the patient should be noted. Battery replacement and recharging, and other unit maintenance procedures, should be reviewed. The TENS unit itself should not be cleaned with solvents that might damage its case (eg, acetone). All warnings and precautions should be summarized and reviewed, and instructions should be provided for care of skin irritation. Finally, an acceptable procedure should be adopted for recording and reporting the patient's response to ongoing and long-term treatment. This may include return-mail pain and function ratings or questionnaires, the use of which the patient should clearly understand. Specific reevaluations have been suggested to be conducted at intervals of 1, 3, 6, and 12 months, and periodically thereafter.[12,175] Decreasing or eliminating the patient's pain medications if adequate relief with TENS permits is desirable. Ultimately, the patient can also be weaned from TENS as intervals of significant pain relief become longer.

Health care professionals should be strongly discouraged from simply sending patients to a medical supply house or pharmacy for instruction in TENS. Aside from risking ineffective treatment and patient injury, legal and ethical questions arise if the practitioner is an owner of such a facility.[176] Additionally, some health care professionals have allegedly been involved in selling TENS units directly to patients, or in benefitting from sales. Such practices have drawn fire from those in the durable medical equipment industry[177,178]; they also have legal and ethical consequences.

## EFFECTIVENESS OF TENS FOR CLINICAL PAIN MANAGEMENT

Numerous reports appearing in the literature since the late 1960s have given credence to the efficacy of TENS in the treatment of both acute and chronic pain. In a series of approximately 300 patients with acute pain, Cohen reported that more than 80 percent of the time patients treated with TENS by Shealy had no need for narcotics.[6] Vander Ark and McGrath determined that 77 percent of patients with acute postoperative pain had a significant reduction in pain.[179] Based on pain control and less use of medications for abdominal surgery, Cooperman and associates found good to excellent results for 77 percent of patients treated with active TENS, but for only 33 percent treated with sham TENS.[180] Outcomes for chronic pain, however, have not appeared to be as successful. Long and Hagfors surveyed five pain treatment centers with a caseload of 3000 patients and found that 25 to 30 percent of patients formerly incapacitated by pain had significant pain relief with TENS alone.[158] Cohen reported that approximately 25 percent of nearly 1000 chronic pain patients treated with TENS by Shealy had their pain relieved to the point at which no other therapy was necessary, whereas this result was seen in 39 percent of a series of 500 patients treated by Long.[6] In 1976, Long noted that of over 900 cases reported in the literature, satisfactory pain relief was noted with TENS alone 35 percent of the time.[181]

Fields has warned that TENS and other nondrug methods of pain control have not truly been established as effective for controlling chronic nonmalignant pain.[55] Furthermore, he cautioned that a specific analgesic effect for TENS has not been proven. Both of his concerns relate to the need to demonstrate that TENS is superior to placebo treatment under a double-blind methodology. Beecher determined that an average of 35 percent of patients obtain satisfactory pain relief from placebo treatment (eg, a sugar pill),[171] although others have noted that up to 100 percent of patients can positively respond to placebos.[182] A double-blind methodology requires that neither the patient nor the clinician know which treatment (active or placebo) is being given. Obviously, it is impossible to disguise some treatments so that the clinician remains unaware of which is the active or placebo treatment. In such instances, it may be sufficient to ensure that whomever performs the patient assessment after treatment is unaware of which treatment has been given.[183] Others have cautioned that the double-blind technique is actually invalid if the perception of stimulation is necessary for pain relief.[184] Additionally, Langley and colleagues have noted that crossover trials may be inappropriate because the patient can easily distinguish active from inactive TENS.[164]

Various approaches to assessing research studies concerned with pain management via TENS have been used in the literature. Historically, the "review paper" has been the most common approach to critiquing published research studies. Recently, Robinson critically reviewed a range of studies concerned with TENS to control acute and chronic pain related to musculoskeletal disorders.[14] He concluded that although TENS is capable of producing clinically relevant pain relief in a meaningful portion of patients, the pain relief is often of short duration, and thus only a small percentage of patients achieve lasting pain reduction. Carroll and associates systematically rated studies about acute postoperative pain through examination of randomization procedures and analgesic effectiveness.[185] In only 2 of 17 studies using randomized control trials, TENS was seen to be superior to placebo for pain control; in 17 of 19 studies lacking randomized controls, TENS had a positive analgesic effect. These researchers noted that the lack of adequate randomization can contribute to a greatly exaggerated treatment effect. Reeve and colleagues evaluated the methodologic quality of randomized control trials of TENS for acute, chronic, and labor/delivery pain. They concluded that there was little evidence for other than limited TENS use.[15] The selection and weighing of the factors used to assess randomization quality could be questioned, however. Assessment of TENS research studies through meta-analysis has yet to become popular.

A chronologic sampling of 18 studies that have been conducted since 1978, and that have examined the effectiveness of TENS by including some type of control procedure in their experimental design, is presented in Table 7–1. Information regarding subjects, study design, TENS mode, electrode site, treatment duration and frequency, and study outcome is presented in order to allow the reader additional insight into the adequacy of these studies. Importantly, comments by the author of this chapter provide information about the type of placebo controls utilized, and about concomitant treatment interventions. These two factors can have a powerful impact on whether active TENS is deemed to be "effective" in controlling clinical pain. Three of these studies provide strong support for the clinical effectiveness of TENS for pain management.[186,187,188] Additionally, eight studies demonstrate moderate support for TENS effectiveness,[16,22,189,190,191,192,193,194] and four studies provide at least fair support.[95,97,195,196] Three studies rated for moderate support[189,191,193] and two rated for fair support[95,195] were seen to be limited by their crossover experimental designs.

Three of 18 studies reviewed initially appear to provide no support for TENS being effective in pain control.[164,197,198] These three studies merit closer scrutiny. Both the study by Langley and colleagues[164] and that by Deyo and coworkers[197] utilized placebo treatments that incorporated "strong suggestion" by the investigators. This strategy could have enhanced the placebo's impact on pain in a manner that was similar to the outcome from active TENS. These investigators also utilized TENS stimulation characteristics not well substantiated for optimal pain control (eg, frequency ≥ 80 Hz). Additionally, both Deyo and coworkers[197] and Herman and colleagues[198] employed a range of concomitant treatment interventions (eg, intensive exercise, thermal agents, and patient education) that likely masked the effect produced by active TENS. Other concerns about Deyo and coworkers' influential study have been presented in the literature.[199,200]

The assessment of long-term pain relief and function with TENS has been difficult. Not only are studies hard to conduct, but researchers have used varying criteria to judge successful pain relief. Stonnington and colleagues noted that of 81 patients who purchased TENS units, 72 percent had partial pain relief and 6 percent had complete pain relief at 3 months.[201] Long determined that of 104 chronic pain patients using TENS for an average of 9 months, 68 percent were able to maintain satisfactory pain relief, 63 percent decreased or eliminated pain medications, and 46 percent significantly increased activity levels.[202] Loeser and associates found that 68 percent of 198 unselected chronic pain patients had significant initial pain relief; yet, approximately one year later, only 13 percent had continued effective pain relief.[203] Ericksson and colleagues reported that of 123 chronic pain patients, 41 percent continued to use TENS after one year.[40] Of this group, 72 percent had significant pain relief, 44 percent significantly decreased their analgesics, and 50 percent had increased social activities. After 2 years, 31 percent of the patients continued to employ TENS, with 79 percent of this group achieving significant pain relief. Keravel and Sindou noted that in following patients with deafferentation pain for a period of 1 to 3 years, 80 percent of those with peripheral nerve lesions most commonly attained partial pain relief.[204] However, only 25 percent of patients with postherpetic pain found stimulation of benefit after 1 year. Johnson and associates assessed 179 patients with chronic pain who had used TENS for an average of 4 years, including the prior 3 months.[205] Via questionnaire, they determined that in 47 percent of patients, TENS reduced pain by more than half, with patients averaging 39.7 hours per week of TENS use. Skin reactions (ie, irritation/rash) had been experienced by 31 percent of patients. Over the 3-month period of time, 58 percent of patients experienced the same degree of analgesia, 32 percent reported a decline in efficacy, and 13 percent had an increase in treatment effect from TENS. Note that 75 percent of patients used TENS along with analgesic drugs. Most recently, Fishbain and colleagues interviewed 376 patients with chronic pain who had used TENS for at least

| Researchers | Subjects | Design | TENS Mode[b] | Electrode Sites[c] | Treatment Duration/ Frequency | Comments[d] | Outcome |
|---|---|---|---|---|---|---|---|
| Thorsteinsson et al (1978)[189] | N = 93, chronic pain[a] | Double-blind, cross-over, random assigned to active and placebo TENS (no current) | Unspecified output | Center of pain, related nerve, and unrelated nerve | Three active/three placebo treatments; follow-up home use of active unit | All told study double-blind. Expectation of positive outcome not given. | (1) During Tx: sig better effect obtained by active vs placebo, stim pain center and unrelated nerve. (2) Subsequent to Tx: sig better by active at pain center. (3) Home treatment: Complete pain relief in 7% at 3 mo, in 2% at 6 mo. |
| Jeans (1979)[95] | N = 16, chronic pain[a] | Double-blind, crossover, 4 Tx conditions (electrode sites) | "BI" (really PB: sine waveform at 60 Hz, in trains 2–3/sec) | 4 Tx conditions: (1) PA; (2) distant TP or AP; (3) sham Tx ("Vanagas"); (4) distant NRP | Two sessions/day for 4 consecutive days | Technician convinced "Vanagas" effective. Pain assessed via McGill pre/post Tx. | Descriptive results: Tx #1, substantially greater decrease in pain than #2–4. |
| Long et al (1979)[195] | N = 150 in first series of unselected patients with chronic pain[a] | Crossover | Unspecified output; treatment for all patients at (1) suprathreshold amplitude; (2) subliminal amplitude; (3) without battery | Unspecified | Duration unspecified; 3 successive days (one type each day); Tx to 1 yr | Results rated as "satisfactory" if patients satisfied with pain relief (possibly not complete) and used no alternate treatment. | (1) "Successful" pain relief at 1 mo: suprathreshold = 35%; subliminal = 8%, no battery = 11% (2) At 1 yr: suprathreshold = 34%, subliminal, no battery = 0%. |

| Study | Sample | Design | TENS parameters | Electrodes | Schedule | Comments | Results |
|---|---|---|---|---|---|---|---|
| Ali et al (1981)[186] | N = 40, elective cholecystectomy | Assignment to 1 of 3 groups: (1) active TENS (2) sham TENS (no stimulation) (3) no TENS | CONV, GR | On either side of incision | Treatment begun in OR; TENS continuous, 48 hr postop; then on demand to 5th day | All had postop PT (deep breathing, coughing, exercise, and ambulation). Pain not directly assessed. | (1) Compared to other 2 groups, active TENS had: (a) sig less medication thru day 3 (b) sig higher vital capacities thru day 5 (c) sig higher functional residual capacity thru day 5 (d) sig higher $PO_2$ thru day 5 (e) no postop complications (2) No differences between sham and control |
| Hansson and Ekblom (1983)[190] | N = 62 acute orofacial pain[a] | Random assigned to either: (1) high-freq TENS; (2) low-freq TENS; (3) placebo TENS | Cefar SIII unit; monopolar square wave; (1) high freq = Conv: 100 Hz, 200 μsec, amplitude at constant tingling; (2) low freq = PB: 71 Hz train, 84 msec long, at 2 Hz, amplitude = nonpainful muscle contraction; (3) placebo TENS = no stim | PA | Schedule unspecified | Avoided suggestion of pain relief. Placebo group advised that stim might not be felt. Verbal pain ratings pre/post Tx. | (1) Nonsig difference in pain relief and induction times of high- vs low-freq TENS. (2) Muscle contractions of low-freq uncomfortable. (3) Active TENS vs placebo: 38% vs 10% with > 50% p. relief; 79% vs 40% some p. relief; 52% vs 20% rated TENS superior to meds. |

**TABLE 7–1.** A CHRONOLOGIC SAMPLE OF STUDIES CONCERNED WITH THE EFFECTIVENESS OF TENS (CONTINUED)

| Researchers | Subjects | Design | TENS Mode[b] | Electrode Sites[c] | Treatment Duration/ Frequency | Comments[d] | Outcome |
|---|---|---|---|---|---|---|---|
| Abelson et al (1983)[187] | N = 32 rheumatoid arthritis (chronic wrist involvement) | Double-blind[f] noncrossover, random assigned to active or placebo TENS (no stim) | Cyrax Mark II: "high intensity" (amplitude) at 70 Hz | Dorsal and ventral wrist | 15 min × 1/wk for 3 wk | Anti-inflammatory analgesics stopped 12 hr prior to Tx. Neutral statement of anticipated effects. Unit light on. Eval pre/post Tx, including VAS. | (1) Active TENS: (a) sig improved resting and grip pain (b) sig improved power and work. (2) Placebo effect = 17%. |
| Lewis et al (1984)[191] | N = 18, osteoarthritis (knee pain) | Double-blind[e] crossover, active vs placebo TENS (no stim) | RDG Tiger Pulse; 70 Hz | 4 APs on knee | Instructed in home program. 30–60 min × 3/day for 3 wk | Unit light on. Standard meds available. Assessed weekly, including VAS. | (1) Median duration p. relief sig dif active (151 min) vs placebo (110 min). (2) Sig improved p. relief after 3 wk active, not placebo. (3) Sig improved "p. index" (knee ROM and wt. bearing) and dec meds—both groups. |

| | | | | | | | |
|---|---|---|---|---|---|---|---|
| Langley et al (1984)[164] | N = 33, rheumatoid arthritis (chronic hand involvement) | Double-blind[f] non-crossover, random assigned to: (1) high-freq TENS; (2) acupuncture-like TENS; (3) placebo TENS | Grass S48; Monophasic waveform; (1) high freq: 100 Hz, 200 μsec; (2) AL: 100 Hz train for 70 msec × 2/sec (#1 and #2 at highest tolerated amplitude on oscilloscope); (3) placebo: no current, but TENS waveform on oscilloscope | Volar and dorsal wrist | 0 min | Initial neutral instructions to all. Strong suggestion provided to placebo group. Meds stopped 24 hr prior to study. Assessed at 15 min intervals post Tx, including VAS. | (1) All groups sig dec resting and grip pain; nonsig between group dif. (2) Nonsig diffs between groups in "overall" pain relief, total joint tenderness or number of tender joints. (3) No sig change in power and work scores. (4) Positive placebo response = 55% for p. relief. |
| Solomon and Guglielmo (1985)[22] | N = 58, migraine or muscle contraction headaches, or both | Random assigned to either: (1) TENS at perception; (2) subliminal TENS; (3) placebo TENS (no stimulation) | Pain Suppressor; GR | Active electrode, PA indifferent electrode opposite active or on hand | 15 min on 1 day | All informed that Tx might be placebo. No meds. In prior 24 hr. Pain estimate pre/post Tx. | (1) "Improvement" in 55% with TENS at perception, 28% with subliminal TENS, 18% with placebo TENS. (2) Perceived TENS sig better than placebo. |
| Smith et al (1986)[88] | N = 18 cesarean section surgery | Single-blind random assigned to either: (1) active TENS; (2) placebo TENS (no current) | Medtronics Comfort burst (#7718); 85 Hz, 80 μsec ≤ tingling sensation | On either side of incision | Continuous from recovery room through 3 days | Unit indicator light on. Equivalent instructions suggestive of pain relief. Meds permitted. Pain assessed up to 3 × day via McGill. | (1) Active TENS sig less cutaneous movement-associated and constant pain. Nonsig dif on day 3. (2) Active TENS, less constant |

| Researchers | Subjects | Design | TENS Mode[b] | Electrode Sites[c] | Treatment Duration/ Frequency | Comments[d] | Outcome |
|---|---|---|---|---|---|---|---|
| | | | | | | | deep incisional pain and uterine pain, but nonsig dif. (3) Nonsig dif in gas pain. (4) Active TENS with nonsig fewer doses of analgesic meds. |
| Ordog (1987)[16] | N = 100 acute trauma outpatients (sprains, lacerations, fractures, hematomas with contusions) | Random assigned to either: (1) functioning unit (2) nonfunctioning unit (sham) (3) functioning unit + med (4) nonfunctioning + med | TENS-PAC; unspecified output | Over or close to injury site | As needed, including continuous | Subjects informed that some would get nonfunctioning units. Both active and placebo units gave slight hum and vibration. Graphic rating scale used to assess pain. Med = Tylenol 3 (acetaminophen + codeine). | (1) Sig dec pain at day 2 for functional vs nonfunctional TENS, nonsig dif at day 30. (2) Nonsig dif in pain for functioning TENS vs Tylenol group at day 2 or 30. (3) 10% using meds, but 0% TENS at day 30. (4) Side effects noted with med, but not TENS. |

| Study | Subjects | Assignment | TENS parameters | Electrode placement | Duration | Comments | Results |
|---|---|---|---|---|---|---|---|
| Finsen et al (1988)[196] | N = 51, amputations (Symes, below and through knee) | Random assigned to either: (1) active TENS; (2) sham TENS (no stim); (3) sham TENS + med | Tenzcare; PB (100 Hz, 90 $\mu$sec in bursts of 7 pulses, × 2/sec, amplitude to discomfort) | 2 at femoral nerve and 2 at sciatic nerve | 30 min × 2/day × 2 wk postop | Unit indicator light on. Analgesic meds on demand. Limited assessment of analgesic effect. Med = chlorpromazine. | (1) At 2 wks: analgesic effect all active TENS and 50% of sham. (2) Nonsig dif in analgesic intake in first 4 wks. (3) Sig more healed BK amputations at 6 and 9 wks, active TENS. (4) Sig fewer incidents of phantom pain, active TENS (10%) vs sham (36%) or sham + med (58%) at 16 wks, but not 1 yr later. |
| Hargeaves and Lander (1989)[192] | N = 75, abdominal surgical wounds | Partial-blind,[g] random assigned to either: (1) active TENS; (2) placebo TENS (no current); (3) no TENS | Grass SD9; 100 Hz 400 $\mu$sec amplitude just below discomfort | Adjacent to incision | 15 min prior to and during wound cleaning and repacking, 2 days after surgery | TENS naive subjects. Each group had pain meds. Pain rated on visual analogue scale. | Active TENS with sig lower pain level than placebo or no TENS groups. Nonsig dif between groups in frequency of meds. |

**TABLE 7–1.** A CHRONOLOGIC SAMPLE OF STUDIES CONCERNED WITH THE EFFECTIVENESS OF TENS (CONTINUED)

| Researchers | Subjects | Design | TENS Mode[b] | Electrode Sites[c] | Treatment Duration/ Frequency | Comments[d] | Outcome |
|---|---|---|---|---|---|---|---|
| Deyo et al (1990)[197] | N = 145 chronic low back pain | Modified double-blind[h]; random assigned to either: (1) TENS alone (2) TENS + ex (3) Sham TENS + ex (4) Sham TENS | EMPI Epix 982 Conv (80–100 Hz); AL (2–4 Hz); (both at modulated pulse rate) | Initially over PA; moved to optimize p. relief. | 4-wk intervention period. Home program: (1) TENS ≥ 3x/day; 45 min each (2) 12 exercises (2–3 reps) (3) Heating pad 2x/day Clinic visits: 2x/wk; included hot pack and evaluation | TENS: 1st 2wks = CONV; patient selected for 2nd 2 wks; all units had "on" lights; strong suggestion provided. Exercise for relaxation and flexibility; groups 2 and 3 had written program for use > 4 wks. Assessed at 2 and 4 wks; 3 mo. | TENS use averaged 25 days/ 4 wks (>120 min/day); 1/3 had minor skin irritation. Home heating pads 23 days/ 4wks (45 min/ day). At 4 wks: Nonsig effect for TENS (TENS vs sham, 52% vs 59% dec p. pain); sig effect for ex. (activity levels, dec p. amplitude and freq). At 3 mo: No effect for ex. |
| Dawood and Ramos (1990)[193] | N = 32 primary dysmenorrhea | Blinded[e] randomized cross-over: (1) TENS (2) placebo TENS (no stim) (3) TENS + ibuprofen (4) Ibuprofen | 3M Tenzcare 6340: CONV (100 Hz; amplitude to comfortable tingling or p. relief) | Adjacent to umbilicus (T10–12 dermatome) | TENS for 1st 8 hrs of assigned cycle; PRN after | Patient adjusted TENS. Ibuprofen also as "rescue med." Menstrual symptoms self-rated at 4 and 8 hrs, and daily after onset. | (1) TENS alone: (a) sig more didn't need rescue med or used less back-up med (b) sig delayed med need (5.9 |

| Study | Population | Assignment | Device | Electrode placement | Treatment | Outcome measures | Results |
|---|---|---|---|---|---|---|---|
| | | | | | | | hrs vs 7 hrs for ibuprofen alone)<br>(c) good to ex. p. relief (42%, vs 3.2% for placebo)<br>(d) sig dec diarrhea, flow, clots and fatigue (vs placebo)<br>(2) TENS and less ibuprofen: p. relief = ibuprofen (in 71% vs 75% of patients). |
| Marchand et al (1993)[194] | N = 42 chronic low back pain | Pseudorandom[f] assigned to:<br>(1) TENS<br>(2) placebo TENS (no current)<br>(3) No Tx control | Medtronic 7720; CONV (100 Hz; 125 µsec) | In dermatome, producing paresthesia in p. area | 30 min, 2x/wk for 10 wks | Pain intensity and unpleasantness rated by VAS: immediately pre/post Tx; at 1 wk, 3 and 6 mo after Tx series. Placebo had visual and sound feedback. | (1) Immediately post Tx:<br>(a) both TENS and placebo dec p. amplitude (43% vs 17%; sig dif) and unpleas. (42% vs 18%)<br>(b) sig cumulative dec p. amplitude, TENS only.<br>(2) Both TENS and placebo sig dec p. and unpleas. to 6 mo.<br>(3) TENS sig dec p. amplitude (vs placebo) only at 1 wk after.<br>(4) No sig changes for control. |

## TABLE 7–1. A CHRONOLOGIC SAMPLE OF STUDIES CONCERNED WITH THE EFFECTIVENESS OF TENS (CONTINUED)

| Researchers | Subjects | Design | TENS Mode[b] | Electrode Sites[c] | Treatment Duration/ Frequency | Comments[d] | Outcome |
|---|---|---|---|---|---|---|---|
| Herman et al (1994)[198] | N = 58 acute low back pain (from work injury) | Modified double-blind[b]; random assigned to either: (1) Active TENS + ex (2) placebo (no output) TENS + ex | Codetron unit | Unit cycled stim among 6 electrode sites every 10 sec (at APs from C7 to popliteal fossa) | TENS for 30 min (15 min at 200 Hz producing strong tingling; 15 min at 4 pps to tolerance) prior to ex. (5 days/ wk for 4 wks) | All patients in intensive rehab (4 hrs/day, 5 days/ wk): hydrotherapy/stretching ex.; force improving ex. for abdominals, trunk extensors and extremities; cycle ergometer for fitness. Pain assessed via VAS. | At end of 4 wks: (1) Both groups had sig dec disability scores (approx. 30%), dec p. ratings (approx. 20%), % predicted work capacity & lumbar flex.; nonsig dif between groups. (2) Immed pre/ post TENS: sig greater dec with active TENS (approx. 12%; deemed "not clinically important"). (3) Nonsig dif in return to work (66% active vs 79% placebo); but 5/29 (17%) active dropped from study due to early return. |

| Benedetti et al (1997)[188] | N = 324 thoracic surgery (postop. pain; 5 surgical procedures) | Random assigned cohorts[e]: (1) Active TENS (2) Placebo TENS (3) Control | Pabisch Tx-3 CONV (100 Hz, 200 μsec, amplitude to strong/comfortable tingling) | 2 unit channels, each with 2 electrodes (at 1 cm from suture line) | Began Tx 1 hr post recovery from anesthesia (1 hr active/sham; 1 hr rest; 1 hr active/sham TENS) | Placebo TENS (no battery) told no sensations produced. Pain meds on request after recovery room. During 12 hr postop. noted: initial p. amplitude by NRS; time to med request; total med intake. | The 5 surgical procedures produced dif amplitudes of postop. p. (mild, mod, severe); cohort initial p. not sig dif. (1) For severe p.: No sig dif between Tx. (2) For mod to severe p. (a) time to 1st med sig dif TENS vs placebo (> 90 min vs < 25 min) (b) total med intake sig less for TENS vs placebo or con. (3) For mild to mod p.: (a) time to 1st med sig dif TENS vs placebo (> 9 hrs vs < 40 min) (b) total meds sig less TENS vs placebo or con |

[a] A variety of diagnoses.

[b] AL = acupuncture-like; BI = brief-intense; CONV = conventional; M = modulated; PB = pulse-burst; GR = only general range of output characteristics given.

[c] AP = acupuncture point; NRP = nonrelated points; PA = painful area; PN = peripheral nerve; TP = trigger point.

[d] Pain rating tool: GRS = graphic rating scale; NRS = numeric rating scale; VAS = visual analogue scale.

[e] Not enough information specified in paper to determine if a true double-blind study.

[f] Patient blinded to treatment; separate therapist and evaluator.

[g] Patient blinded to treatment; therapist rated pain before patient assignment; patient independently rated pain after treatment.

[h] Patient/evaluators blinded to treatment; therapist aware of treatment assignment.

6 months.[206] These patients averaged 12 months of TENS use and reported a significant increase in the amount of pain relief since using TENS; a significant reduction in the use of narcotic/analgesics, tranquilizers, muscle relaxants, nonsteroidal anti-inflammatory drugs (NSAIDs), steroids, and in use of other therapies (eg, physical therapy, occupational therapy, and chiropractic); and a statistically significant reduction in pain interference with work outside of the home, activity inside the home, and social activity.

Long, a pioneer in TENS therapy and research, observed that ". . . it is probable that transcutaneous electrical stimulation represents the single most effective physical entity yet introduced in the management of chronic pain."[106] Noting considerable international uncertainty about TENS since the publication of Deyo and coworkers' study in 1990, Ernst called for more intensive research on clinical TENS.[207] More recently, Reeve and coworkers have suggested that TENS has not been through sufficiently strict and rigorous clinical evaluation.[15] Greater insight should be gained as to which acute and chronic conditions are most amenable to treatment with TENS. Researchers should follow the lead of Benedetti and coworkers[188] in determining the levels of clinical pain severity that realistically respond to TENS. The assessment of the impact of TENS on other dimensions of pain, such as "unpleasantness," warrant further investigation.[194] Additionally, optimal TENS treatment procedures should be more specifically defined. Although most studies have focused on pain management, appropriate functional assessment in relation to pain relief clearly remains a major challenge to those involved in patient care and research with TENS.

# Summary

This chapter has provided a comprehensive introduction to the use of transcutaneous electrical nerve stimulation for pain management. A range of factors important to the safe and effective clinical use of TENS, as supported by the professional literature, have been reviewed. Serious attention to TENS-related factors, including critical review of the algorithm suggested for the initial trial treatment with TENS, requires professional insight and judgment. As illustrated by a case study, successful patient management incorporates TENS in an overall plan of care that includes the control of pain. Well-designed basic and clinical research studies are still needed in order to further clarify mechanisms either supporting or limiting the effects of TENS, and to optimize the effectiveness of TENS in clinical applications.

## CASE STUDY

### ■ Initial Physical Therapy Note, 4/7/98

A 25-year-old male was referred to the physical therapy department 4 days after a motorcycle accident for pain management, gait training, and initiation of knee rehabilitation prior to discharge from the hospital. Related history: a right midshaft femur fracture (repaired by open reduction internal fixation [ORIF]), a partial rupture of the right quadriceps muscle (repaired during ORIF), a fracture of the left wrist (casted), and numerous abrasions and contusions; no head injury (wearing helmet); intolerance of oral pain medications because of gastrointestinal upset; cold, allergy/hypersensitivity; nursing staff not able to ambulate patient because of pain and lack of patient cooperation; patient sleeping poorly because of pain; past history of alcohol abuse; high school graduate, employed as a construction worker; single and currently living alone in a second-story apartment accessible only by stairs with right-sided handrail; parents live in local community.

Examination today revealed:

- Pain (using a 100-point pain estimate): Patient reports that pain is continuous, markedly increased with movement of the right lower extremity (see below); rated as 40/100 during the day at rest, but 60/100 at night; all pain located in the suprapatellar region.
- Girth measurements: (thigh at 5 cm proximal to patella; knee in 20° of flexion): 45 cm on left, 52.6 cm on right; nonpitting edema.
- Joint range of motion: Neck, trunk, and extremities within normal limits except for left wrist (casted); right knee extension (−20° active; −15° passive) and flexion (to 35° active; 45° passive), all limited by pain.
- Muscle force: Neck, trunk, and left extremities grossly 5/5 (except wrist, not tested because of fracture/cast); right upper extremity 5/5; right lower extremity (RLE), hip grossly 4/5, limited by discomfort and recent fixation; quadriceps 2/5, with pain rated 90/100; hamstrings 3/5, with pain rated 80/100; ankle grossly 4+/5.
- Activities of daily living (ADL)/mobility: Able to scoot to edge of bed independently; requires minimum assist of one person, with RLE pain in going from supine to sitting; moderate assist of one in going from sitting to standing; moderate assist of one to ambulate right nonweight bearing (NWB) with crutches 15 ft (lim-

ited by pain, knee ROM, and patient intolerance of activity); patient unwilling to attempt ambulation on stairs with assistance.

*Diagnosis.* Traumatic inflammation of right quadriceps muscle from rupture and related surgical repair. Current disability index is moderate to severe.

*Prognosis.* Recovery potential is good to excellent. Discharge to home/outpatient physical therapy within 3 days based on:

1. Decreased right knee pain (to less than 20/100 at rest and night, permitting more normal rest/sleep cycles; less than 50/100 during ROM/force-improving exercises to permit restoration of ROM/force).
2. Decreased edema formation within right thigh, which has contributed to pain and limited ROM of knee.
3. Increased ROM of right knee (extension to −10° active/full passive; flexion to 60° active and passive) to enhance ADL/mobility and gait on level floor and stairs.
4. Increased force of right knee extensor muscles (to 3/5) and flexors (to 4/5).
5. Increased ADL/mobility: independent in coming from supine to sitting/return; independent in sitting to standing/return.
6. Safe and independent ambulation with crutches right NWB 50 ft on level floor; able to ascend/descend 14 steps with contact safety assistance of one person.

*Physical Therapy Interventions, Beginning This Morning*

1. Trial treatment with TENS for pain management. Following algorithm for a TENS trial (Figure 7–7), began by using conventional mode (100 μsec pulse duration, frequency of 60 pps, amplitude producing distinct sensation of paresthesia over the mid- to distal quadriceps muscle) with a two-channel modified interferential electrode placement from mid-quadriceps to suprapatellar region.
2. Institute program of right knee compression wrapping and elevation to decrease edema, with instruction of nursing staff and family; Ace wrap tension to be monitored/adjusted every 2 hours. Educate patient and nursing staff regarding contraindication to use of cold.
3. Soft tissue mobilization and ROM exercise for right knee twice a day; therapeutic exercise using proprioceptive neuromuscular facilitation to increase knee extensor and flexor muscle force through improved motor unit recruitment.
4. ADL/mobility training, emphasizing preambulatory activities (supine to sit; sit to stand; return) and progressive indepen-

dence in safe crutch gait right NWB (using axillary crutches, forearm platform on left) on both level floor and stairs.

Risks (eg, increased pain, muscle soreness, fall) and benefits (eg, pain reduction, restoration of normal range of motion and muscle force, normal gait, return to full function) of treatment were shared with the patient. He fully understood the ramifications and consented to proceed with treatment.

## ■ Progress Note, 4/7/98, 5:15 P.M.

The initial TENS mode and electrode placements used this morning were revised for a second trial this afternoon. Paresthesia produced by TENS was felt by patient to be only directly under electrodes; patient accommodated to this sensation within 10 min, requiring incremental increases in both stimulation amplitude and pulse duration; this produced painful muscle contractions. No pain relief was obtained and patient became frustrated with the procedure. This afternoon, after additional patient education, a low-amplitude modulated TENS mode (pulse duration automatically decreased from 100 to 50 μsec, × 2/sec; 60 pps frequency) with the two electrodes from a single TENS unit channel placed in the right femoral triangle over the femoral nerve. The patient did not accommodate to the paresthesia, which was felt throughout the anterior thigh without muscle contraction. At the end of the 60-min TENS trial session, pain at rest was rated 20/100, 60/100 with active knee extension, and 50/100 with active knee flexion.

## ■ Inpatient Physical Therapy Discharge Summary, 4/10/98

Now 1 week post-accident, patient is being discharged to home today, to continue outpatient rehabilitation of right knee. Has been using a low-amplitude modulated TENS as the primary method of pain control. After thorough patient education, he understands the TENS unit controls, electrode placement/options, and skin inspection procedure. Skin at right femoral triangle electrode site has not become irritated. Current status is as follows:

- Pain: Rated as being 10/100 at rest for up to 4 hours after 30 min of TENS; pain during ROM/force improving exercises and ambulation with crutches right NWB is 40/100 at worst; TENS use for 30 min prior to bedtime has been associated by patient with sound sleep, with pain less than 20/100 when awakened during night.
- Girth measurement: Thigh at 5 cm proximal to patella; knee in 20° of flexion, 45 cm on left, 48.5 cm on right.

- ROM: Right knee (extension to $-10°$ active/full passive; flexion to $50°$ active and passive).
- Muscle force: RLE hip and ankle primary motions at 4+/5; quadriceps muscle 3/5, with pain rated 40/100; hamstring muscles 4/5, with pain rated 40/100.
- ADL/mobility: Independent in supine to sitting/return and in sitting to standing/return; independent and safe in ambulating up to 50 ft with crutches right NWB on carpeted and tile floors, thus assuring mobility in his apartment; able to ascend/descend 14 steps without handrail using crutches right NWB and stand-by assistance of one person.

*Physical Therapy Evaluation.* This patient has shown good progress in pain management and improved functional mobility during his inpatient subacute stage of treatment. Both ROM and muscle force of the right knee have improved as a result of good pain control with TENS and edema control via compression wrapping and elevation. He has been instructed in and provided with a written home program concerned with TENS, compression wrapping, and ROM/ muscle force improving exercises for the right knee. He will be reassessed for more intensive rehabilitation of the right knee during his first outpatient clinic visit on 4/17/98.

# REVIEW QUESTIONS

1. What equipment-related TENS unit features (eg, electrode type, number/type of controls, durability) are critically important to enhancing patient compliance with, and a successful outcome from, a pain management program that includes treatment with TENS?
2. Given the typical range of patients/clinical problems seen in your practice setting, what clinical tools are most appropiate for assessing pain and related functional limitations?
3. Discuss in detail the primary indications, contraindications and precautions for TENS used in pain management, providing supportive references.
4. Compare and contrast the six primary types/modes of TENS in current use, noting the specific electrical characteristics of each. For a given clinical pain problem, justify beginning the trial TENS treatment with a specific type/mode of TENS.
5. Provide rationales for different electrode placement options that can be used for each of the primary TENS types/modes. What is

the best initial option to use when beginning a trial treatment with TENS?

6. For patients of various ages and levels of cognition/education, provide concise explanations of the theoretical basis for pain relief with TENS.

7. Outline an algorithm for conducting a trial treatment with TENS. What conditions must be met in order for you to recommend ongoing treatment with TENS as part of an overall pain management program?

8. Discuss your views on the clinical effectiveness of TENS for the management of a range of acute and chronic pain disorders, using published references to support your position.

# References

1. Tierney LM, McPhee SJ, Papadakis MA (eds). Current Medical Diagnosis and Treatment, 36th ed. Stamford, CT, Appleton and Lange, p 12, 1997.

2. Bonica JJ. Management of pain. Lecture as visiting professor, Department of Anesthesiology, College of Medicine, The University of Iowa, Iowa City, IA, December 7, 1988.

3. Kellaway P. The William Osler medal essay: The part played by electrical fish in the early history of bioelectricity and electrotherapy. Bull His Med, 20:112–137, 1946.

4. Kane K, Taub A. A history of local electrical analgesia. Pain, 1:125–238, 1975.

5. McNeal DR. 2000 years of electrical stimulation. In: Hambrecht FT, Reswick JB (eds), Functional Electrical Stimulation: Applications in Neural Prostheses. New York, NY, Marcel Dekker, pp 3–35, 1977.

6. Cohen IJ (ed). A new approach to pain. Emerg Med, 6:241–254, 1974.

7. Melzack R, Wall PD. Pain mechanisms: A new theory. Science, 150:971–979, 1965.

8. Wall PD, Sweet WH. Temporary abolition of pain in man. Science, 155:108–109, 1967.

9. Nolan MF. A Chronological Indexing of the Clinical and Basic Science Literature Concerning Transcutaneous Electrical Nerve Stimulation (TENS) 1967–1987. Section on Clinical Electrophysiology, Alexandria, VA, American Physical Therapy Association, 1988.

10. Wolf SL (ed). Transcutaneous electrical nerve stimulation (special issue). Phys Ther, 58:1441–1492, 1978.

11. Ersek RA. Pain Control with Transcutaneous Electrical Neuro Stimulation (TENS). St. Louis, Warren H. Green, 1981.

12. Mannheimer C, Lampe GN. Clinical Transcutaneous Electrical Nerve Stimulation. Philadelphia, PA, FA Davis, 1984.

13. Tapio D, Hymes AC. New Frontiers in Transcutaneous Electrical Nerve Stimulation. Minnetonka, MN, Lec Tec, 1987.

14. Robinson AJ. Transcutaneous electrical stimulation for the control of pain in musculoskeletal disorders. J Orthop Sports Phys Ther, 24:208–226, 1996.

15. Reeve J, Menon D, Corabian P. Transcutaneous electrical nerve stimulation (TENS): A technology assessment. Int J Technol Assess Health Care, 12:299–324, 1996.

16. Ordog GJ. Transcutaneous electrical nerve stimulation versus oral analgesic: A randomized double-blind controlled study in acute traumatic pain. Am J Emerg Med, 5:6–10, 1987.

17. Strassburg HM, Krainick JU, Thoden U. Influences of transcutaneous nerve stimulation (TNS) on acute pain. J Neurol, 217:1–10, 1977.

18. Tyler E, Caldwell C, Ghia JN. Transcutaneous electrical nerve stimulation: An alternative approach to the management of postoperative pain. Anesth Analg, 61:449–456, May 1982.

19. Bundsen P, Peterson LE, Selstam U. Pain relief during delivery, an evaluation of conventional methods. Acta Obstet Gynecol Scand, 61:289–297, 1982.

20. Richardson RR, Meyer PR Jr, Cerullo LJ. Transcutaneous electrical neurostimulation in musculoskeletal pain of acute spinal cord injuries. Spine, 5:42–45, 1980.

21. Roeser WM, Meeks LW, Venis R et al. The use of transcutaneous nerve stimulation for pain control in athletic medicine. A preliminary report. Am J Sports Med, 4:210–213, 1976.

22. Solomon S, Guglielmo KM. Treatment of headache by transcutaneous electrical stimulation. Headache, 25:12–15, 1985.

23. Mannheimer C, Carlsson CA, Vedin A et al. Transcutaneous electrical nerve stimulation (TENS) in angina pectoris. Int J Cardiol, 7:91–95, 1985.

24. Avellanosa AM, West CR. Experience with transcutaneous electrical nerve stimulation for relief of intractable pain in cancer patients. J Med, 13:203–213, 1982.

25. Meyer GA, Fields HL. Causalgia treated by selected large fiber stimulation of peripheral nerve. Brain, 95:163–168, 1972.

26. McCarthy JA, Ziganfus RW. Transcutaneous electrical nerve stimulation: An adjunct in the pain management of Guillain–Barré syndrome. Phys Ther, 58:23–24, 1979.

27. Leo KC. Use of electrical stimulation at acupuncture points for the treatment of reflex sympathetic dystrophy in a child. A case report. Phys Ther, 63:957–959, 1983.

28. Mannheimer C, Carlsson CA. The analgesic effect of transcutaneous electrical nerve stimulation (TENS) in patients with rheumatoid arthritis. A comparative study of different pulse patterns. Pain, 6:329–334, 1979.

29. Winter AW. The use of transcutaneous electrical stimulation (TNS) in the treatment of multiple sclerosis. J Neurosurg Nurs, 8:125–131, 1976.

30. Gessler M, Struppler A. Relief of phantom pain following modification of phantom sensation by TENS. In Bonica JJ, Lindbolm U, Iggo A (eds), Advances in Pain Research and Therapy. New York, NY, Raven Press, pp 591–594, 1983.

31. Robinson AJ, Snyder-Mackler L. Clinical application of electrotherapeutic modalities. Phys Ther, 68:1235–1238, 1988.

32. Standards of Electrotherapeutic Terminology. Electrotherapy Standards Committee of the Section on Clinical Electrophysiology, American Physical Therapy Association, Alexandria, VA, July 1988.

33. Witters D, Hinkley S, Lapp A. Electrical Output Performance Tests on Transcutaneous Electrical Nerve Stimulation Devices. Section on Clinical Electrophysiology Newsletter, American Physical Therapy Association, 4(2):15–16, 18, 1989.

34. Barr JO, Nielsen DH, Soderberg GL. Transcutaneous electrical nerve stimulation characteristics for altering pain perception. Phys Ther, 66:1515–1521, 1986.

35. Lampe GN. Introduction to the use of transcutaneous electrical nerve stimulation devices. Phys Ther, 58:1450–1454, 1978.

36. Mosenkis R (ed). Transcutaneous electrical nerve stimulator (TENS) units. Health Devices, 10:179–195, 1981.

37. Barr JO. The Effect of Transcutaneous Electrical Nerve Stimulation Parameters on Experimentally Induced Acute Pain. Master's Thesis, The University of Iowa, Iowa City, IA, 1980.

38. Lamm KE. Optimal Placement Techniques for TENS: A Soft Tissue Approach. Tucson, AZ, Workshop in TENS, 1986.

39. Fisher AA. Dermatitis associated with transcutaneous electrical nerve stimulation. Cutis, 21:24, 33, 47, 1978.

40. Eriksson MBE, Sjolund BH, Nielzen S. Long term results of peripheral conditioning stimulation as an analgesic measure in chronic pain. Pain, 6:335–347, 1979.

41. Paxton SL. Clinical uses of TENS: A survey of physical therapists. Phys Ther, 60:38–44, 1980.

42. TENS, The Path to Pain Control: Skin Care. Medical Products Division/3M, St. Paul, MN, F-TCBR (421) II.

43. Ronnen M, Suster S, Kahana M et al. Contact dermatitis due to karaya gum and induced by the application of electrodes. Int J Dermatol, 25:189–190, 1986.

44. Marren P, DeBerker D, Powell S. Methacrylate Sensitivity and transcutaneous nerve stimulation. Contact Dermatitis, 25:190–191, 1991.

45. Griffin JE, Karselis TC. Physical Agents for Physical Therapists, 2nd ed. Springfield, IL, Charles C Thomas, 1982.

46. Shealy CN, Maurer D. Transcutaneous nerve stimulation for control of pain—A preliminary note. Surg Neurol, 2:45–47, 1974.

47. Campbell JA. A critical appraisal of the electrical output characteristics of ten transcutaneous nerve stimulators. Clin Phys Physiol Meas, 3:141–150, 1982.

48. Mason CP. Testing of electrical transcutaneous stimulators for suppressing pain. Bull Prosthet Res, Spring, 38–54, 1976.

49. Stamp JM. A review of transcutaneous electrical nerve stimulation (TENS). J Med Eng Technol, 6:99–103, 1982.

50. Barr JO. Evaluation of Transcutaneous Electrical Stimulation Unit Output. Unpublished report, December 9, 1976.

51. American National Standard for Transcutaneous Electrical Nerve Stimulators. ANSI/AAMI NS4-1985. Arlington, VA, Association for the Advancement of Medical Instrumentation, 1986.

52. Stewart DL, Albin SH. Documenting Functional Outcomes in Physical Therapy. St. Louis, MO, Mosby-Year Book, 1993.

53. McCombs D. Current opinions on electrotherapy. Rehab Manage, 2:35–38, 1989.

54. Stieg RL, Williams RC, Gallagher LA. Multidisciplinary pain treatment centers. J Occup Med, 23:94–102, 1981.

55. Fields HL. Pain. New York, NY, McGraw-Hill, 1987.

56. Melzack R. The Puzzle of Pain. New York, NY, Basic Books, 1973.

57. Sternbach RA. Pain—A Psychophysiological Analysis. New York, Academic Press, 1968.

58. Sternbach RA. Evaluation of pain relief. Surg Neurol, 4:199–201, 1975.

59. Chapman CR. Measurement of pain: Problems and issues. In Bonica JJ (ed), Advances in Pain Research and Therapy, vol 1. New York, NY, Raven Press, 345–353, 1976.

60. Melzack R. The McGill pain questionnaire: Major properties and scoring methods. Pain, 1:277–299, 1975.

61. Olin BR, Hunsaker LM, Covington TR et al. Drug Facts and Comparisons. St. Louis, MO, JB Lippincott, 1989:242–244.

62. Sanders SH. Toward a practical system for the automatic measurement of "up-time" in chronic pain patients. Pain, 9:103–109, 1980.

63. Follick MJ, Ahern DK, Laser-Wolston N et al. Chronic pain: Electromechanical recording device for measuring patient's activity patterns. Arch Phys Med Rehabil, 66:75–78, 1985.

64. Barr JO, Forrest SE, Potratz PE, Reed VL. Effectiveness of transcutaneous electrical nerve stimulation (TENS) for the elderly with chronic pain. Phys Ther (abstract), 69:165, 1989.

65. Burton KE, Wright V. Functional assessment. British J Rheumatol, 22(suppl):44–47, 1983.

66. Huskisson EC, Jones J, Scott PJ. Application of visual-analogue scales to the measurement of functional capacity. Rheumatol Rehabil, 15:185–187, 1976.

67. Zacharkow D. Posture: Sitting, Standing, Chair Design and Exercise. Springfield, IL, Charles C Thomas, 1988.

68. Ducroquet R, Ducroquet J, Ducroquet P. Walking and Limping: A Study of Normal and Pathological Walking. Philadelphia, PA, JB Lippincott, 1968.

69. Birkhan J, Carmon A, Meretsky P et al. Modification of TENS by constant-energy stimulation delivered through multiple electrodes: Method and evaluation. In Bonica JJ, Liebeskind JC, Albe-Fessard DG et al (eds), Advances in Pain Research and Therapy. New York, NY, Raven Press, p 3, 1979.

70. Hymes AC, Raab DE, Yonehiro EG et al. Acute pain control in electrostimulation—A preliminary report. In Bonicca JJ (ed), Advances in Neurology, vol 4. New York, NY, Raven Press, 761–767, 1974.

71. Paris DL, Baynes F, Gucker B. Effects of the neuroprobe in the treatment of second-degree ankle inversion sprains. Phys Ther, 63:35–40, 1983.

72. Hoke B, Howell D, Stack M. The relationship between isokinetic testing and dynamic patellofemoral compression. J Orthop Sports Phys Ther, 4:150–153, 1983.

73. Smidt GM, Herring T, Amundsen L et al. Assessment of abdominal and back extensor function. A quantitative approach and results for chronic low-back pain patients. Spine, 8:211–219, 1983.

74. Fischer AA. Advances in documentation of point soft tissue pathology. J Fam Med, Dec: 24–31, 1983.
75. Fischer AA. Pressure algometry over normal muscles. Standard values, validity and reproducibility of pressure threshold. Pain, 30:115–126, 1987.
76. Pochaczevsky R. Assessment of back pain by contact thermography of extremity dermatomes. Ortho Rev, 12:45–58, 1983.
77. Pochaczevsky R, Wexler CE, Meyers PH et al. Liquid crystal thermography of the spine and extremities. J Neurosurg, 56:386–395, 1982.
78. Rooney SM, Jain S, McCornack P et al. A comparison of pulmonary function tests for post-thoracotomy pain using cryoanalgegia and transcutaneous nerve stimulation. Ann Thorac Surg, 41:204–207, 1986.
79. Sternbach RA, Murphy RW, Timmermans G et al. Measuring the severity of clinical pain. In Bonica JJ (ed), Advances in Neurology. New York, NY, Raven Press, 4:281–289, 1974.
80. Ohnhaus EE, Adler R. Methodological problems in the measurement of pain. A comparison between the verbal rating scale and the visual analogue scale. Pain, 1:379–384, 1975.
81. Carlsson AM. Assessment of chronic pain I. Aspects of the reliability and validity of the visual analogue scale. Pain, 16:87–101, 1983.
82. Kremer E, Atkinson JH, Ignelzi RJ. Measurement of pain. Patient preference does not confound pain measurement. Pain, 10:241–248, 1981.
83. Scott J, Huskisson EC. Graphic representation of pain. Pain, 2:75–184, 1976.
84. Huskisson EC. Visual analog scales. In Melzack R (ed), Pain Management and Assessment. New York, NY, Raven Press, pp 33–37, 1983.
85. Downie WW, Leatham PA, Rhind VM et al. Studies with pain rating scales. Ann Rheum Dis, 37:378–381, 1978.
86. Jensen MP, Karoly P, Braver S. The management of clinical pain intensity: A comparison of six methods. Pain, 27:117–126, 1986.
87. Gracely RH. Psychophysical assessment of human pain. In Bonica JJ, Liebeskind JC, Albe-Fessard DG (eds), Advances in Pain Research and Therapy. New York, NY, Raven Press, 3:805–824, 1979.
88. Smith GM, Lowenstein E, Hubbard JH et al. Experimental pain produced by the submaximal effort tourniquet technique: Further evidence of validity. J Pharmacol Exp Ther, 163:468–474, 1986.
89. Moore PH, Duncan GH, Scott DS et al. The submaximal effort tourniquet test: Its use in evaluating experimental and chronic pain. Pain, 6:375–381, 1979.
90. Adams J. The reliability of some techniques utilized in quantifying the intensity of clinical pain. Pharmacol Ther, 4:629–632, 1979.
91. Peck RE. A precise technique for measurement of pain. Headache, 6:189–194, 1967.
92. Eland JM. Minimizing Pain Associated With Pre-Kindergarten Intramuscular Injections. Ph.D. Dissertation, University of Iowa, Iowa City, IA, 1980.
93. Echternach JL. Evaluation of pain in the clinical environment. In Echternach JL (ed). Pain, vol 12. New York, NY, Churchill Livingstone, pp 39–72, 1978.

94. Wall PD, Melzack R (eds). Textbook of Pain. Edinburgh, Churchill Livingstone, 1994.

95. Jeans ME. Relief of chronic pain by brief, intense transcutaneous electrical stimulation: A double blind study. In Bonica JJ, Liebeskind JC, Albe-Fessard DG (eds), Advances in Pain Research and Therapy, vol 3. New York, NY, Raven Press, pp 601–606, 1979.

96. Melzack R. Prolonged relief of pain by brief intense somatic stimulation. Pain, 1:357–373, 1975.

97. Smith CM, Guralnick MS, Gelford MM et al. The effects of transcutaneous electrical nerve stimulation in post-cesarean pain. Pain, 27:181–193, 1986.

98. Wolf SL, Gersh MR, Rao VR. Examination of electrode placements and stimulating parameters in treating chronic pain with conventional transcutaneous electrical nerve stimulation (TENS). Pain, 11:37–47, 1981.

99. Melzack R. The short form McGill pain questionnaire. Pain, 30:191–197, 1987.

100. Walsh TD, Leber B. Measurement of chronic pain: Visual analog scales and McGill–Melzack pain questionnaire compared. In Bonica JJ, Lindblom U, Iggo A (eds). Advances in Pain Research and Therapy, vol 5. New York, NY, Raven Press, pp 897–899, 1983.

101. Melzack R, Katz L. Pain measurement in persons in pain. In Wall PD, Melzack R (eds). Textbook of Pain. Edinburgh, Churchill Livingstone, 1994.

102. Carley PJ, Wainapel SF. Electrotherapy for acceleration of wound healing: Low intensity direct current. Arch Phys Med Rehabil, 66:443–446, 1985.

103. Kaada B. Promoted healing of chronic ulceration by transcutaneous nerve stimulation (TNS). Vasa, 12:262–269, 1983.

104. Kahn J. Transcutaneous electrical nerve stimulation for nonunited fractures. Phys Ther, 62:840–844, 1982.

105. Nordenstrom BEW. Biologically Closed Electric Circuits: Clinical, Experimental and Theoretical Evidence for an Additional Circulatory System. Grev Turegatan 2, S-11435 Stockholm, Sweden, Nordic Medical Publication, 1983.

106. Long DM. Stimulation of the peripheral nervous system for pain control. Clin Neurosurg, 31:323–343, 1984.

107. Leijon G, Boivie J. Central post-stroke pain: the effect of high and low frequency TENS. Pain, 38:187–191, 1989.

108. Johansson F, Almay BG, Von Knorring L et al. Predictors for the outcome of treatment with high frequency transcutaneous electrical nerve stimulation in patients with chronic pain. Pain, 9:55–61, 1980.

109. Eriksson M, Schuller H, Sjolund B. Hazard from transcutaneous nerve stimulation in patients with pacemakers. Lancet, 1:1319, 1978.

110. Chen D, Philip M, Philip PA et al. Cardiac pacemaker inhibition by transcutaneous electrical nerve stimulation. Arch Phys Med Rehabil, 71:27–30, 1990.

111. Shade SK. Use of transcutaneous electrical nerve stimulation for a patient with a cardiac pacemaker: A case report. Phys Ther, 65:206–208, 1985.

112. Rasmussen MJ, Hayes DL, Vlietstra RE et al. Can transcutaneous electrical nerve stimulation be safely used in patients with permanent cardiac pacemakers? Mayo Clin Proc, 63:443–445, 1988.

113. Sliwa JA, Marinko MS. Transcutaneous electrical nerve stimulator-induced electrocardiogram artifact: a brief report. Am J Phys Med Rehabil, 75:307–309, 1996.

114. Augustinsson LE, Bohlin P, Carlsson CA et al. Pain relief during delivery by transcutaneous electrical nerve stimulation. Pain, 4:59–65, 1977.

115. Vincenti E, Cervellin A, Mega M et al. Comparative study between patients treated with transcutaneous electric stimulation and controls during labor. Clin Exp Obstet Gynecol, 9:95–97, 1982.

116. Picaza JA, Cannon BW, Hunter SE et al. Pain suppression by peripheral nerve stimulation, Part I: Observations with transcutaneous stimuli. Surg Neurol, 4:105–114, 1975.

117. Klein J, Pariser D. Transcutaneous electrical nerve stimulation. In Currier DP, Nelson RM (eds), Clinical Electrotherapy. East Norwalk, CT, Appleton-Century-Crofts, pp 209–230, 1987.

118. Griffin JW, McClure M. Adverse responses to transcutaneous electrical nerve stimulation in a patient with rheumatoid arthritis. Phys Ther, 61:354–355, 1981.

119. Linzer M, Long DM. Transcutaneous neural stimulation for relief of pain. IEEE Trans Biomed Eng, 23:341–344, 1976.

120. Andersson SA. Pain control by sensory stimulation. In Bonica JJ, Liebeskind JC, and Albe-Fessard DG (eds), Advances in Pain Research and Therapy, vol 3. New York, NY, Raven Press, pp 569–585, 1979.

121. Leo KC, Dostal WF, Bossen DG et al. Effect of transcutaneous electrical nerve stimulation characteristics on clinical pain. Phys Ther, 66:200–205, 1986.

122. Howson DC. Peripheral neural excitability: Implications for transcutaneous electrical nerve stimulation. Phys Ther, 58:1467–1473, 1978.

123. Leo KC, Dostal WF, Bossen DG et al. Effect of transcutaneous electrical nerve stimulation characteristics on clinical pain. Phys Ther, 66:200–205, 1986.

124. Janko M, Trontelj JV. Transcutaneous electrical nerve stimulation: A microneurographic and perceptual study. Pain, 9:219–230, 1980.

125. Andersson SA, Hansson G, Holmgren E et al. Evaluation of the pain suppressive effect of different frequencies of peripheral electrical stimulation in chronic pain conditions, Acta Orthop Scand, 47:149–157, 1976.

126. Baker LL, McNeal DR, Benton LA et al. Neuromuscular Electrical Stimulation: A Practical Guide. Rancho Los Amigos, CA, Downey, 1993.

127. Fox EJ, Melzack R. Transcutaneous electrical stimulation and acupuncture: Comparison of treatment for low back pain. Pain, 2:141–148, 1976.

128. Leo K. Perceived comfort levels of modulated versus conventional TENS current. Phys Ther (abstract), 64:745, 1984.

129. Miller BA, Smith KB, Real JL et al. A comparison of modulated-rate and conventional TENS. Phys Ther (abstract), 64:744, 1984.

130. Lein DH, Clelland JA, Knowles CJ et al. Comparison of effects of transcutaneous electrical nerve stimulation of auricular, somatic, and the combination of auricular and somatic acupuncture points on experimental pain threshold. Phys Ther, 69:671–678, 1989.

131. McKelvy PL. Clinical report on the use of specific TENS units. Phys Ther, 58:1474–1477, 1978.

132. Santiesteban AJ. Comparison of electroacupuncture and selected physical therapy for acute spine pain. Amer J Acupunct, 12:257–261, 1984.

133. Gammon GD, Starr I. Studies on the relief of pain by counterirritation. J Clin Invest, 20:13–20, 1941.

134. Inman VT, Saunders JB. Referred pain from skeletal structures. J Nerv Ment Dis, 99:660–667, 1944.

135. Gunn CC. Motor points and motor lines. Am J Acupunct, 6:55–58, 1978.

136. Walthard KM, Tchicaloff M. Motor points. In Licht S (ed), Electrodiagnosis & Electromyography, vol 3. Baltimore, MD, Waverly Press, pp 153–170, 1971.

137. Travel JG, Simons DG. Myofascial Pain and Dysfunction. The Trigger Point Manual. Baltimore, MD, Williams & Wilkins, 1983.

138. Mann F. Acupuncture. The Ancient Chinese Art of Healing and How It Works Scientifically. New York, NY, Random House, pp 27–34, 1971.

139. Castel D, Castel JC. Pain Management Desk Reference, 3rd ed. Topeka, KS, Physiotechnology, 1987.

140. Madill PV. Auriculotherapy (letter). JAMA, 252:1856, 1984.

141. Melzack R, Katz J. Auriculotherapy fails to relieve chronic pain. JAMA, 251:1041–1043, 1984.

142. Melzack R, Katz J. Auriculotherapy (letter). JAMA, 252:1856–1857, 1984.

143. Nogier PFM. Auriculotherapy (letter). JAMA, 252:1855–1856, 1984.

144. Liu YK, Varela M, Oswald R. The correspondence between some motor points and acupuncture loci. Am J Clin Med, 3:347–358, 1975.

145. Melzack R, Stillwell DM, Fox EJ. Trigger points and acupuncture points for pain: Correlations and implications. Pain, 3:3–23, 1977.

146. Mannheimer JS. Electrode placements for transcutaneous electrical nerve stimulation. Phys Ther, 58:1455–1462, 1978.

147. Krause AW, Clelland JA, Knowles CJ et al. Effects of unilateral and bilateral auricular transcutaneous electrical nerve stimulation on cutaneous pain threshold. Phys Ther, 67:507–511, 1987.

148. Berlant S. Method of determining optimal stimulation sites for transcutaneous electrical nerve stimulation. Phys Ther, 64:924–928, 1984.

149. Kaada B. Vasodilation induced by transcutaneous nerve stimulation in peripheral ischemia (Raynaud's phenomenon and diabetic polyneuropathy). Eur Heart J, 3(4):303–314, 1982.

150. Currier D. Electrical stimulation for improving muscular strength and blood flow. In Nelson RM, Currier DP (eds), Clinical Electrotherapy. Norwalk, CT, Appleton & Lange, pp 141–164, 1987.

151. Alon G, DeDomenico G. High Voltage Stimulation: An Integrated Approach to Clinical Electrotherapy. Chattanooga, TN, Chattanooga Corporation, 1987.

152. Taub A, Campbell JN. Percutaneous local electrical analgesia: Peripheral mechanisms. In Bonica JJ (ed) Advances in Neurology, vol 4. New York, NY, Raven Press, pp 727–733, 1974.

153. Torebjörk HE, Hallin RG. Excitation failure in thin nerve fiber structures and accompanying hypalgesia during repetitive electric skin stimulation. In Bonica JJ (ed), Advances in Neurology, vol 4. New York, NY, Raven Press, pp 733–735, 1974.

154. Ignelzi RJ, Nyquist JK. Direct effect of electrical stimulation on peripheral nerve evoked activity: Implications in pain relief. J Neurosurg, 45:159–165, 1976.

155. Devor M, Wall PD. The physiology of sensation after peripheral nerve injury, regeneration and neuroma formation. In Waxman SG (ed), The Physiology & Pathobiology of Axons. New York, NY, Raven Press, pp 377–388, 1978.

156. Wall PD. The gate control theory of pain mechanisms. A re-examination and re-statement. Brain, 101:1–18, 1978.

157. Jenkner FL, Schuhfried F. Transdermal transcutaneous electric nerve stimulation for pain: The search for an optimal waveform. Appl Neurophysiol, 44:330–337, 1981.

158. Long DM, Hagfors N. Electrical stimulation in the nervous system: The current status of electrical stimulation of the nervous system for relief of pain. Pain, 1:109–123, 1975.

159. Hoffert M. The gate control theory re-revisited. J Pain Symptom Manage, 1:39–41, 1986.

160. Levin MF, Hui-chan, CWY. Conventional and acupuncture-like transcutaneous electrical nerve stimulation excites similar afferent fibers. Arch Phys Med Rehabil, 74:54–60, 1993.

161. Nathan PW, Rudge P. Testing the gate-control theory of pain in man. J Neurol Neurosurg Psychiatr, 37:1366–1372, 1974.

162. Nathan PW. The gate-control theory of pain: A critical review. Brain, 99:123–158, 1976.

163. Mayer DJ, Price DD. The neurobiology of pain. In Synder-Mackler L, Robinson A (eds), Clinical Electrophysiology. Electrotherapy and Electrophysiologic Testing. Baltimore, MD, Williams & Wilkins, pp 141–201, 1989.

164. Langley GB, Sheppeard H, Johnson M et al. The analgesic effects of transcutaneous electrical nerve stimulation and placebo in chronic pain patients. A double blind non-crossover comparison. Rheumatol Int, 4:119–123, 1984.

165. Chan CWY, Tsang H. Inhibition of the human flexion reflex by low intensity, high frequency transcutaneous electrical nerve stimulation (TENS) has a gradual onset and offset. Pain, 28:239–235, 1987.

166. Facchinetti F, Sandrini G, Petraglia F et al. Concommitant increase in nociceptive flexion reflex threshold and plasma opoids following transcutaneous nerve stimulation. Pain, 19:295–303, 1984.

167. Francini F, Maresca M, Procacci P et al. The effects of non-painful transcutaneous electrical nerve stimulation on cutaneous pain threshold and muscular reflexes in normal subjects with chronic pain. Pain, 11:49–63, 1981.

168. Procacci P, Zoppi M, Maresca M et al. Hypoalgesia induced by transcutaneous electrical stimulation. A physiological and clinical investigation. J Neurosurg Sci, 21:221–228, 1977.

169. Lehmann TR, Russell DW, Spratt KF et al. Efficacy of electroacupuncture and TENS in the rehabilitation of chronic low back pain patients. Pain, 26:277–290, 1986.

170. Beecher HK. Nonspecific forces surrounding disease and the treatment of disease. JAMA, 179:437–440, 1962.

171. Beecher HK. The placebo effect as a nonspecific force surrounding disease and the treatment of disease. In Janzen R (ed), Pain: Basic Principles, Pharmacology, Therapy. Baltimore, MD, Williams & Wilkins, pp 175–180, 1972.

172. Barr JO, Weissenbuehler SA, Bandstra EJ et al. Effectiveness and comfort level of transcutaneous electrical nerve stimulation (TENS) in elderly with chronic pain. Phys Ther (abstract), 67:775, 1987.

173. Andersson SA, Holmgren E. Analgesic effects of peripheral conditioning stimulation III. Effect of high frequency stimulation, setmental mechanisms interacting with pain. Acupunct Electrother Res, 3:22–36, 1978.

174. Fordyce WE. Behavioral Methods for Chronic Pain and Illness. St. Louis, MO, Mosby, 1976.

175. Woolf CJ, Thompson JW. Stimulation-induced analgesia: transcutaneous electrical nerve stimulation (TENS) and vibration. In Wall PD, Melzack R (eds). Textbook of Pain. Edinburgh, Churchill Livingstone, pp 1191–1208, 1994.

176. Relman AS. Dealing with conflicts of interest (editorial). New Engl J Med, 313:749–751, 1985.

177. Morgan S. Examining the ethics of electrotherapy. Rx Home Care, 43–46, June 1986.

178. Paras T. Medical suppliers form alliance to address major TENS changes. APTA Progress Report, p 9, Feb 1986.

179. Vander Ark GD, McGrath KA. Transcutaneous electrical stimulation in treatment of post operative pain. Am J Surg, 130:338–340, 1975.

180. Cooperman AM, Hall B, Sadar ES et al. Use of transcutaneous electrical stimulation in contral of postoperative pain. Surg Forum, 26:77–78, 1975.

181. Long DM. Use of peripheral and spinal cord stimulation in the relief of chronic pain. In Bonica JJ, Albe-Fessard DG (eds), Advances in Pain Research and Therapy, vol 1. New York, NY, Raven Press, pp 395–403, 1976.

182. Wall, PD. The placebo and the placebo response. In Wall PD, Melzack R (eds). Textbook of Pain. Edinburgh, Churchill Livingstone, pp 1297–1308, 1994.

183. Hamilton M. Lectures on the Methdology of Clinical Research, 2nd ed. Edinburgh, Churchill Livingstone, 119–121, 1974.

184. Meyerson BA. Electrostimulation procedures: Effects, presumed rationale, and possible mechanisms. In Bonica JJ, Lindbolm U, Iggo A (eds), Advances in Pain Research and Therapy, vol 5. New York, NY, Raven Press, pp 495–534, 1983.

185. Carroll D, Tramer M, McQuay H et al. Randomization is important in studies with pain outcomes: Systematic review of transcutaneous elec-

trical nerve stimulation in acute postoperative pain. Br J Anaesth, 77:798–803, 1996.

186. Ali J, Yaffe GS, Serrette C. The effect of transcutaneous electric nerve stimulation on postoperative pain and pulmonary function. Surgery, 89:507–512, 1981.

187. Abelson K, Langley GB, Sheppeard H et al. Transcutaneous electrical nerve simulation in rheumatoid arthritis. NZ Med J, 96:156–158, 1983.

188. Benedetti F, Amanzio M, Casadio C et al. Control of postoperative pain by transcutaneous electrical nerve stimulation after thoracic operations. Ann Thorac Surg, 63:773–776, 1997.

189. Thorsteinsson G, Stonnington HH, Stillwell GH et al. The placebo effect of transcutaneous electrical stimulation. Pain, 5:31–41, 1978.

190. Hansson P, Ekblom A. Transcutaneous electrical nerve stimulation (TENS) as compared to placebo TENS for the relief of acute oro-facial pain. Pain, 15:157–165, 1983.

191. Lewis D, Lewis B, Sturrock RD. Transcutaneous electrical nerve stimulation in osteoarthritis: A therapeutic alternative. Am Rheum Dis, 43:47–49, 1984.

192. Hargreaves A, Lander J. Use of transcutaneous electrical nerve stimulation for postoperative pain. Nurs Res, 38:159–161, 1989.

193. Dawood MY, Ramos J. Transcutaneous electrical nerve stimulation (TENS) for the treatment of primary dysmenorrhea: A randomized crossover comparison with placebo TENS and ibuprofen. Obstet Gynecol, 75:656–660, 1990.

194. Marchand S, Charest J, Li J et al. Is TENS purely a placebo effect? A controlled study on chronic low back pain. Pain, 54:99–106, 1993.

195. Long DM, Campbell JN, Gucer G. Transcutaneous electrical stimulation for relief of chronic pain. In Bonica JJ, Liebeskind JC, Albe-Fessard DG (eds), Advances in Pain Research & Therapy, vol 3. New York, NY, Raven Press, 1979.

196. Finsen V, Persen L, Lovlien M et al. Transcutaneous electrical nerve stimulation after major amputation. J Bone Joint Surg, 70B:109–112, 1988.

197. Deyo RA, Walsh NE, Martin DC et al. A controlled trial of transcutaneous electrical nerve stimulation (TENS) and exercise for chronic low back pain. N Engl J Med, 322:1627–1634, 1990.

198. Herman E, Williams R, Stratford P et al. A randomized controlled trial of transcutaneous electrical nerve stimulation (Codetron) to determine its benefits in a rehabilitation program for acute occupational low back pain. Spine, 19:561–568, 1994.

199. TENS for chronic low back pain (letters). N Engl J Med, 323:1423–1425, 1990.

200. TENS for chronic low-back pain (letter). Lancet, 337:462–463, 1991.

201. Stonnington HH, Stillwell GR, Ebersold MJ et al. Transcutaneous electrical stimulation for chronic pain relief. A pilot study. Minn Med, 59:681–683, 1976.

202. Long DM. External electrical stimulation—as a treatment of chronic pain. Minn Med, 57:195–198, 1974.

203. Loeser JD, Black RG, Christman A. Relief of pain by transcutaneous stimulation. J Neurosurg, 42:308–314, 1975.

204. Keravel Y, Sindou M. Anatomical conditions of efficiency of transcutaneous electrical neurostimulation in deafferentation pain. In Bonica JJ, Lindblom U, Iggo A (eds), Advances in Pain Research and Therapy, vol 5. New York, NY, Raven Press, pp 763–767, 1983.

205. Johnson MI, Ashton CH, Thompson JW. An in-depth study of long-term users of transcutaneous electrical nerve stimulation (TENS). Implications for clinical use of TENS. Pain, 44:221–229, 1991.

206. Fishbain DA, Chabal C, Abbott A et al. Transcutaneous electrical nerve stimulation (TENS) treatment outcome in long-term users. Clin J Pain, 12:201–214, 1996.

207. Ernst, E. TENS: Dichtung und wahrheit. Fortschr Med, 110:471–472, 1992.

# Electrical Stimulation to Increase Functional Activity

Lucinda L. Baker

## Introduction

**E**lectrical stimulation has been used to create muscular contractions for more than a century, dating back to the pioneering work of Duchenne.[1,2] Neuromuscular electrical stimulation (NMES) is the actuation of muscular tissue through the intact peripheral nervous system.[3] Throughout this chapter, the necessity of the intact peripheral nervous system will be assumed. Patients who fail to respond with a stimulated muscle contraction when placed on an NMES program with appropriate electrodes and stimulus characteristics require a detailed assessment of the peripheral neuromuscular system. Examples of complicating factors which can interfere with NMES programs are peripheral neuropathies (ie, diabetic neuropathies), partial innervation (ie, from root or peripheral nerve entrapment), and muscle pathology (ie, myopathies or dystrophies). Further discussion of the assessment of peripheral nerves and muscles can be found in Chapter 11.

The perceived usefulness of NMES for management of a variety of patient problems has waxed and waned throughout the years. Since the mid-1970s, major advances in the understanding of stimulation equipment and stimulus characteristics have allowed an expansion of successful therapeutic applications.[2] The purpose of this chapter is to identify the treatment paradigms necessary to ensure success of NMES treatment programs in a wide variety of practice settings. The basic pattern of treatment for each application will be based on clinical research, but the practitioner should use the fundamental pattern of treatment as a springboard from which modifications can be made to ensure the best possible management for his or her own patient. The application of electrical stimulation (ES) to a dynamic treatment process cannot, and should not, be so formalized that the patient or session must follow a stereotypic pattern. On the other hand, each treatment for each individual need not be so individualized that stimulus characteristics must be constantly reset and general guidelines are not usable. Physical therapist creativity and knowledge, of the patient's personal goals as well as his or her pathology, must be the final determinant of when a stimulation program is not only viable but strategically necessary to achieve optimal function. Thus, general guidelines for optimal stimulation outcomes will necessarily be modified as individuals and goals change. Additional information relating the benefits of incorporating an NMES program with traditional therapeutic interventions will be discussed, with an eye to the cost, for both equipment and time, of such expansions.

There are six major categories of treatment programs that use NMES, grouped according to treatment goals. They include the use of NMES to:

1. Improve force or maintain muscle mass both during or following periods of enforced inactivity
2. Maintain or gain range of motion (ROM)
3. Reeducate and facilitate voluntary motor control
4. Temporarily reduce the effects of spasticity
5. Provide an orthotic support
6. Reduce edema formation

Stimulation programs designed to meet the first and sixth goals are discussed elsewhere in this book. This chapter will focus on the middle four treatment goals and address the benefits of integrating stimulation with other treatments for the most effective and efficient patient response.

Sensory intolerance to NMES programs should be anticipated but will vary from patient to patient. Sensory intolerance is generally not indicative of problems in the peripheral nervous system but, rather, a part of the artificial overdrive of intense sensory information that the central nervous system (CNS) interprets as being uncomfortable. Therapeutic applications of NMES are virtually always achieved through surface electrodes. Because the stimulating electrodes are sitting on the skin, sensory nerves in the skin will always receive the highest concentration of electrical current, and some sensory nerves will invariably be activated before motor neuron excitation will be achieved. Thus, NMES programs will universally be accompanied by high levels of sensory nerve excitation, which will result in sensory intolerance in many patients.

The type of sensory nerves activated, especially with low levels of stimulation, tend to be the large discriminative sensory nerves, which generally do not produce pain.[2] The experience, however, is often so unique that patients not properly prepared for the onslaught of sensory information will **interpret** (cortically) the experience as noxious. This interpretation is subject to revision, based on therapist input and repetitive, nonthreatening experience. Thus, a warm-up or training period is often required before the therapeutic level of NMES is achieved. This training period should be anticipated in all NMES programs, even when the desired response is only a 3 or 3+ stimulated contraction. Contractions of greater than 3+ elicited by NMES generally require highly motivated patients or extensive training periods or both. Most programs discussed in this chapter, however, require only the 3+ contraction for success, and some can be effective with NMES used at even lower contraction levels to provide a sensory cue. Only the true force improving program, discussed in Chapter 4, demands that patients accept maximal tolerated stimulation levels to achieve optimal outcomes.

# PRESERVING AND INCREASING ROM

## Problem

**Preserving and increasing range of motion** have similar goals, that is, achieving optimal patient function through complete joint range. Decreased range often leads to impaired use of an extremity, whether the deficit is proximal or distal in the extremity. Preserving ROM can be of major concern in some patients with CNS lesions that result in spasticity. Although passive ROM in the home setting is often successful for the patient with minimal spastic tone, the patient who demonstrates moderate to severe spasticity frequently has difficulty carrying out the home program. This patient is all too often seen in a follow-up visit with markedly decreased range. When this decreased range interferes with function or basic hygiene and positioning of the limb, surgical intervention is often the only plausible treatment. In an attempt to avoid costly and potentially dangerous surgical procedures, NMES can be used as a means of prophylactically maintaining joint ROM for those patients who have a high risk of developing significant ROM limitations.[4,5] The patient recovering from trauma to a joint or the muscles surrounding the joint, or an orthopedic procedure at a joint, may also benefit from the accelerated increase in joint mobility attained through the addition of

ES.[6–10] Many orthopedically involved patients, however, will eventually gain full ROM without the assistance of intensive physical therapy (PT) intervention; efficacy and the value-added benefit of including an NMES program may be more highly questioned in this patient application. The significant exception is the older individual who requires a joint replacement following years of restricted use because of pain.[9] In this situation, the therapist is faced with limited joint mobility, acute pain, and prolonged disuse muscular atrophy. Addition of NMES to a comprehensive treatment program can address each of these problems and, through this multifaceted attack, enhance the total treatment outcome and advance the patient to independence more quickly.

## Evaluation and Prognosis

Increasing joint ROM using any nonsurgical treatment technique is possible only if the restriction is because of intrinsic soft-tissue shortening, and not to bony obstruction of the joint. The shortening usually includes both the connective tissue surrounding the joint and the muscles acting across the joint on the shortened side. Assessment of the source of joint restriction may include physical evaluation of the joint "end-feel," as well as basic radiographic studies. If increased range is not seen over a 2-week treatment period, further objective radiographic evaluation of the joint may be necessary to rule out bony obstruction. Even long-standing soft tissue contractures should demonstrate some increased range after 2 weeks of daily treatment.[2,5,11]

## Intervention

### *Physiologic/Clinical Rationale for NMES and ROM*

Joints most effectively targeted for preserving or increasing ROM through NMES include the elbow, wrist, and fingers in the upper extremity, and the knee in the lower extremity. Although stimulation may assist with ROM at the shoulder, ankle, and hip, the intricacy of the shoulder complex, the biomechanics of the ankle, and the limitations of surface stimulation at the hip restrict the effectiveness of most NMES programs at these joints. That is not to say that stimulation cannot be used at these joints, only that optimal treatment outcomes may be achieved only (1) by combining stimulation with other techniques designed to increase range (eg, casting at the ankle, positioning at the hip), or (2) within limited arcs of range (eg, mobilization of the shoulder though initial ranges, ≤ 30 to 45 degrees). In some specialized applications, even these difficult joints can be adequately managed with an NMES program. Hazlewood et al found that when stimulation was applied to the dorsiflexor muscles in children with hemiplegic cerebral palsy, small but significant increases in ankle dorsiflexion range were attained.[12] While these authors were successful despite the presence of mild spasticity and the biomechanical constraints of the joint, their subjects had no major limitation of ankle range to begin with.[12] When the ankle is plantar flexed by contracture, the anterior tibialis muscle is even further biomechanically compromised and marginally capable of dorsiflexing the joint; thus, stimulation and casting is more appropriate for an optimal outcome.

The inclusion of NMES in an ROM program provides the clinician or patient a means of repetitively moving the joint in question through the available range multiple times. A typical 30-minute NMES program would entail nearly 100 repetitions of the stimulated motion. The physiologic mechanism of action of an NMES ROM program is not very different from manual ROM programs; the automated and repetitive nature of the contractions, however, yields increased compliance, when compared to a similar number of manually repeated gentle stretches.

The technique of NMES to gain ROM is a cross between the traditional high-load, brief-stretch method and the low-load, prolonged-stretch technique.[13] The amplitude of NMES must always be maintained at levels low enough to avoid a "jamming" effect at the end of available range, which is often painful and may lead to swelling and effusion of the joint. Thus, the quality of the stretch placed on the shortened tissues must be relatively low to avoid these complications. Although each electrically stimulated contraction is maintained for a matter of seconds, the number of repetitions inherent in several 30-minute treatment sessions provides a substantial accumulation of time on stretch. In addition to providing stretch, an ROM program incorporating NMES also encourages facilitation and force improvement in the muscles that oppose the contracture. A further potential benefit of a stimulation program is the very real pain management which accompanies tetanic stimulation. When this analgesic effect is coupled with the repetitive nature of the joint motion, the painful patient will often relax and allow enhanced joint motion during a stimulated session, which may be impossible with a one-on-one program. This effect can be readily observed with the patient who has a painfully frozen shoulder. Stimulation of the deltoid muscles, with long ramps for both approach and release, moving the joint through the initial degrees of motion, with or without the addition of a hot pack for patient comfort, will often allow the therapist to move into more active and active-assisted ranges. These latter benefits of facilitation, muscle force improvement, and pain management are not provided by any other singular stretching techniques.

### Clinical Evidence for NMES and ROM

The first report of NMES use to increase ROM came from Munsat et al, who reported that stimulation of the femoral nerve provided activation of the quadriceps femoris muscle group, which provided an increase in knee range, even in the presence of long-standing knee flexion deformities.[11] In this early report, the stimulation program was extremely aggressive (6 hours of cycled stimulation daily) and the deforming force of the spastic hamstring muscles had been reduced by surgical lengthening of the tendons prior to the stimulation program. Under these conditions, two patients demonstrated complete reduction of knee flexion contractures, and two others had a reduction of their contractures to noninterfering levels. The final patient was not treated for an adequate length of time to fully demonstrate the effectiveness of the NMES program, although his contracture did decrease from 60 to 35 degrees over a 3-week treatment program.[11]

More abbreviated reports are found in the literature describing increased knee ROM in children with spina bifida[14] and a child who had scleroderma with hip, knee, and ankle contractures.[8] No prior surgical intervention was reported in the latter two studies. Finally, a recent report of ES for patients with chronic osteoarthritis (OA) reported increased knee range of greater than five degrees in 17 of 38 patients (45%) receiving low levels of stimulation at night.[9] This was compared to 6 of 33 patients (18%) with OA who received placebo stimulation and were found to have similar gains in knee ROM.

In a study reported by Baker et al[4] and expanded by Waters and Bowman,[5] an NMES program was effective in maintaining wrist and finger ROM into extension in nearly 80 patient with spastic hemiparesis without joint limitations. (See Figure 8–1.) The studies also reported an increase in range for an additional 23 patients who presented with contractures of the wrist and fingers in the presence of flexor spasticity. (See Figure 8–2.) Because of the investigative nature of the studies, NMES was used as the only means of maintaining or increasing ROM. Six of six participating clinics were successful in maintaining ROM, and four of five clinics were successful at increasing range in the presence of contracture.[4,5]

The failure to increase range in one participating clinic was attributed to a lack of familiarity with problems associated with stimulation and the inability of the clinical staff to resolve issues relating to the presence of spasticity in the multijoint finger flexors. This inability was based in the clinic's restricted use of stimulation, with only three patients receiving NMES treatment over a 9-month data collection period.[5] The implication of this failure is that clinics and clinicians who use NMES very sparingly may achieve less with each treatment than those who are more comfortable with both the elec-

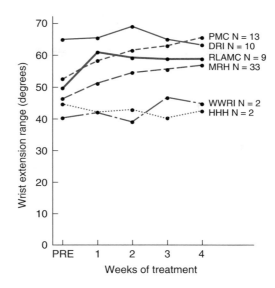

FIGURE 8–1. Effect of an NMES range-of-motion program in hemiparetic patients with finger and wrist flexor spasticity but no signifiant range limitations. Data supplied by six different clinics, including those from a previously reported study (*Phys Ther* 59:1495, 1979). Means and standard error of the means are represented.

trical stimulator and the expected patient response. Experienced and knowledgeable clinicians and clinics can aggressively progress through training periods and problem solve specific situations to achieve optimal patient outcomes. This same pattern of decreased efficacy with less frequent use has been documented in other multicenter studies using ES.[9]

### Application Techniques for NMES and ROM
Treatment programs adequate to accomplish the goal of preserving ROM are relatively less aggressive than those designed to increase range in the presence of a motion restriction. Between 50 and 100 cyclic repetitions of range through full joint excursion will ensure continued mobility of a joint.[2] To gain ROM, especially in the presence of spasticity, the number of repetitions must increase to 200 or more.[2] To be optimal, stimulation programs should be done daily, which is often most effectively managed as a home program.

Short-term stimulation management at home can be successful with most cognitively intact patients, or through the assistance of family members. Electrode placements can be documented through instant pictures, demonstrating both the electrodes and the desired

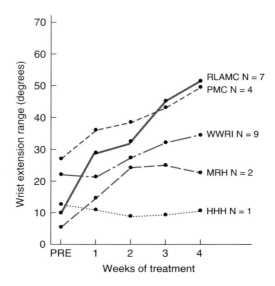

FIGURE 8–2. Effect of an NMES range-of-motion program in hemiparetic patients with finger and wrist flexor spasticity and passive wrist extension range of less than 30 degrees. Data supplied by five different clinics, including those from a previously reported study (*Phys Ther* 59:1495, 1979). Means and standard error of the means are represented.

joint response. The multiuse, self-sticking electrodes greatly simplify home management. Rental of stimulation equipment, if it is not available through the hospital or clinic, can generally be done on a month-by-month basis. This home-based stimulation ensures the outcome of the total treatment plan, without the expense of daily visits to physical therapy. The flip side of the coin is that home treatment assures the therapist the most effective use of a limited number of authorized visits, increasing the probability of achieving the total treatment goal of full ROM to afford optimal return to function for the patient.

NMES may be used as an adjunct to other treatment programs designed to increase ROM. Combining NMES with serial casting or splints has been effective.[15] When casting or splints are used to manage joint limitations, an increase in pressure over bony prominences must be anticipated during the stimulation cycle. Great care in providing snug but compliant stability in a cast or splint is necessary to ensure the integrity of the patient's skin throughout treatment. The combination of stimulation and casting is especially effective in reducing plantar flexion contractures, which are frequently difficult to manage by either technique separately. The combined effectiveness of the two techniques appears to be significantly better than either treatment alone.[15] Stimulation of the hip extensors, coupled with positioning for reduction of hip flexion contractures, is also frequently an efficacious combination.

## Outcome Measures, Benefits, and Efficacy

The goal of all ROM programs is to increase or maintain joint mobility, decreasing the impairment of an extremity and increasing the patient's ability to incorporate that extremity into functional activities. Generally, increases in ROM can be expected within 1 or 2 weeks of daily treatment, even when joint contracture is long standing.[5,11] If increased range cannot be documented within 2 weeks, and radiographic evidence indicates that the restriction is soft tissue, combining stimulation with positional or other ROM techniques is required.

Addition of NMES to ROM programs should greatly decrease the time necessary to achieve functional use of an otherwise unimpaired extremity. This decrease of time to achieve goals is especially true for the patient who is generally debilitated and may have limited reserves available to participate in an active therapy program (eg, a patient with a total joint replacement). An active therapy program also allows the therapist an expedited means of assessing a patient's own voluntary ability to incorporate an extremity into functional activities, determining whether joint restriction or possible poor motor control are the major factors contributing to disabilities. This identification is critical to the development of further treatment programs designed to limit the impact of that disability.

When full range or, in some cases, functional range, is achieved, the continuation of NMES is not warranted, except for the patient with moderate to severe spasticity. In this patient population, an assessment of the probability that the spasticity will cause a second restriction is needed. If the patient is unable to use the extremity functionally to overcome the tone, and the resultant joint restriction is likely to compromise tissue hygiene or positional needs of the patient, continued NMES may be appropriate to preserve the increased range. Part of this assessment must include the ability of the family or caregiver to manage the stimulation, including electrode placement, limb positioning, and determination of appropriate stimulation amplitude. Justification of the home program to third-party payers should be based on the successful gains made under therapeutic supervision and the relative cost benefits between a basic electrical stimulator and its supplies and the possible need for later surgical intervention.

# INADEQUATE VOLUNTARY CONTROL

## Problem

When patients have **inadequate voluntary control** of a muscle, the deficit may be manifest as poor force or a general inability to recruit the muscle(s) at all. This lack may be because of a peripheral inhibition of the central nervous system (eg, pain at the knee may inhibit the quadriceps muscles)[10] or because of decreased descending activation from the cortical and subcortical centers onto the alpha motoneuron pool (eg, immediately following a stroke). In some cases of central nervous system pathology, the descending drive onto a motoneuron pool may be part of a more general movement pattern and result in motion of all joints of the limb, rather than the selective joint motion associated with normal function. Although the presentation of symptoms may be very different, the underlying deficit is an inadequate level of motoneuron drive on voluntary command. This common problem is amenable to amelioration by the application of ES, which necessarily drives sensory input and, in turn, may lead to increased excitation of the motoneuron pool.

Most patients who have experienced an orthopedic trauma or surgery demonstrate a decreased ability to recruit one or more pools of motoneurons, as measured by a marked decrease in voluntary muscle force. Because this problem often resides in the peripheral inhibition of the motoneuron pool,[10] typical interventions include decreasing the patient's pain and increasing the sensory drive, which will excite the motoneurons of the targeted muscle. Even submotor ES over a muscle has been demonstrated to alter the excitability of that muscle's motoneuron pool. This altered excitability was attributed to an enhanced cutaneous,[16] and possible myotatic, sensory drive onto the motoneurons. This altered excitability has been hypothesized to be the source of increased muscle force in patients with orthopedic problems when ES is added to a rehabilitation program.[16] When NMES is used at motor levels in a rehabilitation program, the most common term used to describe the treatment outcome is **strengthening** (improving muscle force); the probable mechanism through which that force gain was attained, however, is the increased recruitment, or reeducation, of the motoneuron pool. This effect, almost immediate in nature but often short lived in duration, would explain the marked gains made in "muscle strength" achieved in the first 2 to 3 weeks of a posttrauma or postsurgical treatment program.[17–21] Because the increased force is largely the result of sensory drive onto the motoneuron pool, high levels of stimulation are not necessary to achieve these early but dramatic gains.[22]

As patients achieve a plateau in strength following the acute rehabilitation, full activation of the available motoneuron pool may be assumed and in some cases tested. At this juncture, a more aggressive muscle force improving program, designed to actually increase the workload of the muscle's contractile elements, becomes necessary to continue the force improving process.[23,24] Chapter 4 covers the force improving programs necessary to enhance the tension output of a muscle in the absence of poor recruitment capabilities.

Patients who demonstrate decreased muscle recruitment because of disruption of the CNS are also candidates for an ES program. In this application, peripheral sensory drive is used to increase the general excitability of one or more motoneuron pools. This increased motoneuron excitability may enhance the effectiveness of compromised descending control, allowing it to exert its influence and be more effective in recruiting motor units. Because CNS-involved patients may have sensory deficits as well as motor recruitment difficulties, stimulation can be graded from high levels, which allow control of the motor activation of a particular muscle group (eg, quadriceps muscle contraction to provide stance stability in gait), to sensory levels, which provide cues for the patient with stimulation simply initiating an appropriate motor sequence (eg, hip extension stimulation to remind a patient to advance the trunk over a stance limb). As found in patients with orthopedic problems, the effects of the stimulation are nearly immediate but are also short in duration.[25–41] The transition to independent voluntary control is typically more prolonged in the CNS-involved patient compared to the orthopedically involved patient; return of voluntary activation generally follows the natural recovery time course associated with the particular CNS pathology. To be considered a truly effective facilitation program, increased voluntary control must be demonstrated independently from the application of ES; that is, patients must be able to demonstrate increased voluntary motor control without the immediately preceding application of the NMES program. Many CNS-involved patients will be unable to assume complete voluntary activation of targeted muscles because of the extent of the central deficit. Stimulation can, however, be used to optimize the voluntary control available to the patient.

## Evaluation and Prognosis

The presence of poor motor recruitment can be demonstrated experimentally through the technique known as an interpolated (superimposed) twitch.[42] First described in the mid-1980s, the technique interposes a supramaximal tetanic burst of stimulation onto the subject's maximal contraction effort. If the subject has contracted all possible motor units voluntarily, the superimposed stimulation will result in no change in torque measurement, or possibly a slight decrease in the tension output of the muscle. If all available motor units are not voluntarily activated, the most common units left unenergized by the patient are those actuated by the largest motoneurons. These large efferents are readily excited by the ES and provide an increased tension output of the muscle, recorded by an external transducer.[42] Thus, in the presence of poor voluntary recruitment, either from peripheral inhibition or lack of adequate central activation, an increased torque during the superimposed twitch would be observed. This technique can be used to monitor a patient's compliance with an aggressive force developing program, as a test to determine the level of inhibition present during a voluntary contraction, or as an approximation of the percentage of the motoneurons which fail to respond to voluntary activation. The technique is experimental, however, most commonly used for study purposes. Clinical assessment of poor motor recruitment is more typically limited to manual or visual assessment of the contraction quality, or objective measurement of tension development across a specific joint through the use of a dynamometer.

When a patient presents with a brief history of limb disuse but marked weakness following trauma or surgery, some degree of compromised recruitment should be anticipated. In addition, the patient who has sustained an insult or lesion to the CNS will often demonstrate poor muscle recruitment on command, although recruitment of the muscle may be evident under a variety of enhanced sensory or movement conditions. These two categories are patients most likely to benefit from a neuromuscular ES program designed to reeducate and facilitate motor recruitment on a voluntary basis. The evaluation and intervention are aimed at the level of the patient's impairment ie, the inability to recruit all or a significant portion of one or more motoneuron pool. The implication of treatment is to decrease the dysfunction (disability) with which the patient is faced and allow him or her to increase independence in all levels of society, thus diminishing the presence of a demonstrable or potential handicap.

In order for a reeducation or facilitation intervention to be optimally effective, one or two key muscle groups should be targeted. When the patient has achieved voluntary control of those key muscle groups and has been able to integrate that control into daily activities, additional muscles may be targeted for similar intervention. Successful outcomes from reeducation programs with patients with orthopedic problems should be anticipated for virtually all individuals, usually within a few days or weeks of treatment.[17–22] Prognosis for the individual with CNS dysfunction is less predictable. Generally, if patients cannot demonstrate some improved voluntary recruitment of a treated muscle/motoneuron system following 2 weeks of therapy, central recovery may not be adequate to allow the control attempted in the treatment. The facilitation program may be withdrawn at that time, but a return to the treatment at a later period of CNS recovery may be appropriate.[2]

## Intervention

### Clinical Evidence for NMES and Reeducation (Peripheral Inhibition in the Presence of Orthopedic Pathology)

Patients who have experienced trauma or surgery to a joint often manifest severe weakness upon voluntary recruitment, even when prolonged disuse is not a problem. This weakness is certainly related to neuromuscular disuse but in many cases is a manifestation of inhibition onto the motoneuron pools through peripheral sensory drive, as well.[10] The addition of an NMES program to the rehabilitation of the relatively healthy individual who has sustained an orthopedic injury has almost universally been beneficial.[17–23] The mechanism of this enhanced force has not been fully established. Early work from authors assessing the components of voluntary force improving programs may shed some light on the means by which NMES increases force in the muscles of the orthopedic patient.

Moritani and DeVries assessed the mechanisms by which normal *voluntary* force improvement occurs.[43] Following a series of studies, they determined that the initial period of increased force, even in healthy subjects, was largely because of increased efficiency in recruiting motor units, with only minor changes in the tension output from the muscle fibers. After 3 or 4 weeks of *voluntary* exercise, the normal young individuals began to demonstrate increased tension from motor units, based on the hypertrophy of the muscle fibers. If the force development programs continued for several weeks more, further changes in force were nearly all attributed to enhanced tension output from the muscle fibers.[43] In patients with orthopedic problems, who have peripheral inhibition from pain and possible disuse, the initial force gains can almost certainly be ascribed to enhanced motoneuron recruitment. Because NMES is very effective at increasing motoneuron excitability, the addition of NMES to the postoperative or posttrauma rehabilitation program *should* allow increased recruitment, with a resultant enhanced voluntary muscle force. Clearly, the clinical literature supports this supposition.[17–23] Virtually every study that has added NMES to a knee rehabilitation program has demonstrated increased force gains in patients receiving stimulation. This increased force has been shown, even when the stimulation program may have been less then optimal because of the constraints of treatment.[23] The enhanced force improvement is not unique to the muscles around the knee, however. In a recent study of chronic back pain patients who demonstrated muscle weakness in a radicular pattern, a reeducation program was successfully used to increase lower extremity (calf and quadriceps) muscle force over a relatively brief period of time.[44] Thus, even in the presence of resolved peripheral nerve lesions, the addition of an NMES reeducation program provided increased muscle force, probably through enhanced recruitment of motoneurons.

### Application Techniques for NMES and Reeducation

NMES reeducation programs always incorporate voluntary effort augmented by stimulation. Because patients who have orthopedic problems are generally able to process sensory and motor information normally, the brief period of excitatory drive following NMES can be used most efficiently. Patients can often demonstrate increased voluntary muscle force for periods of time during and right after stimulation is turned off; the enhanced motor recruitment may be maintained for minutes to hours after the stimulation session. If pain is an ongoing problem, multiple sessions of NMES for reeducation may be necessary, with motoneuron excitability being boosted following each session such that the patient demonstrates enhanced recruitment. As pain becomes less of a factor, the patient will demonstrate maintenance of the increased excitability which follows each NMES session.

Note that patients with orthopedic problems do not require the maximal stimulated contraction typically described in force improving programs, most commonly reported in normal or near normal individuals. While management of the patient with an orthopedic problem is relatively aggressive, and force improving exercises are pushed to the patient's tolerance, the quality of the voluntary/stimulated contraction is often initially 3+ or only slightly better. In some of the older patients, voluntary/stimulated contractions may range downwards to 1+. Despite these very low intensities, reeducation and increased force occur, and the addition of NMES to the total treatment program enhances the outcome. The difference between the levels of stimulation needed to attain "power strengthening" in the healthy individual and the stimulation levels used to enhance the initially very weak muscle of the patient with an orthopedic problem further corroborates the probable mechanism of the initial force enhancing program as being neural enhancement of motoneuron recruitment. Thus, what is needed is a powerful but nonpainful sensory drive to increase motoneuron excitability, allowing more effective volitional recruitment of the muscle. This level of stimulation can be tolerated by virtually all patients. The NMES program may be useful immediately after trauma or surgery, used at the patient's bedside, coupled with isometric contractions. As a patient's muscle force increases, tolerance to the electrical stimulation will usually also increase and more aggressive voluntary/stimulated contractions can be targeted. Stimulation may then move into isokinetic to isotonic contraction levels and be integrated with functional activities, such as increased weight bearing during gait training. Thus, as the patient progresses toward the normal level of strength, he or she may be advanced into the true force improving protocol discussed in Chapter 4.

### Clinical Evidence for NMES and Facilitation (CNS Dysfunction)

Only relatively recently have the potential mechanisms of NMES effects on motor recruitment been examined[16] and those assessments are still in a most incomplete stage. This lack of a physiologic basis for treatment has somewhat limited the clinical applications attempted to date. In a recent review of the efficacy of neuromuscular ES for the rehabilitation of patients with hemiplegia, however, Binder-Macleod and Lee found a good deal of promise for realistic applications of NMES in facilitation programs; many questions were left to be answered as well.[25] Many early studies failed to evaluate the effects of an NMES training program once the stimulation had been discontinued. This evaluation failure precluded the ability to state that patient actually *learned* to use their voluntary control independently, a necessary step before functional integration of that control can be assumed.

An early application of NMES for the patient with CNS dysfunction was reported in 1953, with the addition of **faradism** (ES) to a rehabilitation program for patients with hemiplegia.[40] There was, however, no control program with which to compare the stimulated patients. Even in current literature, reports of intervention without substantial follow-up or without a control treatment for comparison are common. Several studies, however, have undertaken to evaluate the effects of NMES in patients with CNS lesions and to compare that treatment with conventional therapeutic approaches.[26,28,29,32,37,39]

Cozean et al reported the results of a controlled study that compared stimulation with biofeedback, a combination of stimulation and biofeedback and a conventional therapy program.[29] The lower extremity of patients who demonstrated hemiparesis from stroke was the target, and training occurred during gait. Measures of ankle and knee range in swing, step length, stance time, and ground reaction forces were assessed. The authors generated an index that compared each subject's involved side to his or her own uninvolved side. Measurements were taken biweekly during therapy and 4 weeks following the completion of therapy. These authors reported that the group receiving the combined therapy of biofeedback/NMES-facilitated gait training improved the most, while the two groups receiving each of the modalities separately showed significant improvement when compared to the control, standard treatment group.[29]

Similarly, Bogataj et al reported a study that evaluated patients with hemiparesis receiving conventional therapy and gait training, who then crossed into a multichannel NMES gait training program.[26] These data were compared to a group of patients who received the two treatment programs in reverse order, that is, multichannel NMES gait training followed by conventional therapy and gait without stimulation. The authors reported Fugl-Meyer scores, along with stride length, cadence and velocity. Each treatment program lasted for 2 to 3 weeks and assessments were done before any treatment, at the transition between treatments, and at the conclusion of all treatment. No electrical stimulation was used during assessment periods. These authors reported a significant difference in all characteristics measured when the NMES treatment was compared to the conventional therapy. They also reported an order effect. Their interpretation of this interaction was that the NMES treatment was most effective when used early in the rehabilitation program.[26]

Finally, a recent abstract reported not only the presence of improved torque-generating capabilities in patients with hemiparesis using NMES during gait but demonstrated that the increased tension was the result of increased voluntary recruitment of motor units.[37] This change was significantly greater in the stimulated patients, when they were compared with a group of control, nonstimulated subjects.[37] When data from these and other controlled clinical trials are taken in combination with reports that do not include a control treatment group, there is increasing evidence of the enhanced quality of muscle recruitment and subsequently of the directly related functional activity, namely gait, when NMES is added to gait training activities for patients with hemiparesis. A similar finding has been reported in patients who have experienced incomplete spinal cord transection[33]; several case reports of patients with cerebral palsy who have shown improvement in gait after training with NMES have also been recently described.[46–49]

Reports of the effects of NMES in the management of upper extremity dysfunction are somewhat less common but demonstrate similar patterns of effectiveness. An early report by Bowman et al compared wrist and hand function in patients receiving NMES and motion feedback to a second group of patients receiving no stimulation but conventional facilitation and functional training.[28] These authors found a significant increase in voluntary selective wrist extension and wrist extension torque in the patients receiving stimulation, compared to their control counterparts. These gains were maintained in a 6-month to 1-year follow-up, but the patients receiving no stimulation also gradually increased in selective wrist extension and wrist extension torque.[28] Assessment of upper extremity functional use was done with a 17-item scale, ranging from a very simple task (use the involved extremity to stabilize a pillow while putting on a pillow case) to very complex functions (place a dime into a telephone coin slot held at shoulder height, using only the involved upper extremity).[50] Patients receiving the stimulation/feedback program made remarkable gains in functional use of the extremity during the first 3-week treatment period, increasing from a mean score of only three items to the successful completion of a mean of 10 tasks. This improvement was maintained and slightly increased during the follow-up. The control subjects demonstrated less dramatic improvement during treatment, changing from a pretest mean of six items to a total of nine successful completions at discharge. By follow-up testing, the control subjects were able to accomplish as many tasks as the study patients, a mean of 12 items for both groups.[51] These data indicate that the addition of the NMES program provided enhanced **recovery rate,** with patients who received stimulation making marked improvement during the early phases of rehabilitation. The ultimate **level of recovery,** however, was not very different between the two treatment groups, as demonstrated by their performance on all tests at the follow-up assessment. Results appeared, then, that the stimulation accelerated the recovery process but could not alter the ultimate level of recovery, which was more directly related to the CNS pathology than the therapeutic intervention.[51]

Several reports have evaluated the effect of NMES facilitation programs in upper extremity function of patients with **chronic hemiparesis** from stroke. In 1987, Fields reported the effects of electromyographic (EMG)-triggered NMES for 69 patients following CVA.[32] All demonstrated increases in active range of motion, but functional integration of that increased range was not assessed. Smith reported a mean of 68 to 90 percent improvement in upper extremity ROM following an NMES program in 24 patients nearly 2 years following their stroke.[40] Kraft et al reported comparing the effects of sensory-level ES, with EMG-triggered NMES.[35] In addition, a group receiving proprioceptive neuromuscular facilitation training and a control group who received no therapeutic intervention were included in the study. These authors reported that all three treatments were effective in increasing the Fugl-Meyer poststroke motor recovery test scores and grip force, when treatment was compared to the no therapy control group. Small numbers in each of the treatment groups precluded meaningful statistical comparison between treatments. The authors observed that the combination of NMES with voluntary activity appeared to provide the most effective increase, and that increased scores were maintained at a 9-month follow-up assessment.[35] Most recently, Dimitrijevic et al have reported using sensory-level stimulation to enhance wrist control in patients who were more than 6 months following their stroke.[30,31] These authors report a significant increase in wrist extension and total active wrist ROM following daily sessions of sensory stimulation to both flexor and extensor surfaces of the hand and forearm.[30,31]

Although more studies with control treatments and follow-up evaluations should be done, the general body of literature assessing the addition of NMES to the rehabilitation of the poststroke patient generally favors the outcomes. There is evidence for accelerated improvement in the subacute phase of stroke rehabilitation and possible unmasking of latent recovery in more chronic rehabilitation applications. The effect of increased ROM and enhanced muscle tension must also be related to increased functional use of the extremity for complete acceptance of NMES as a primary intervention in stroke rehabilitation.

A specialized program of facilitation, which borders on an orthotic assist, is the use of ES to avoid chronic shoulder subluxation in the patient following a CNS insult. (See Figure 8–3.) Baker and Parker reported an aggressive NMES training program to reduce shoulder subluxation in the subacute hemiparetic population.[52] These authors reported that patients who were nearly 2 months poststroke demonstrated an average acromial–humeral separation of 13 to 15 mm, as measured by bilateral radiograph, before the inception of a stimulation program. Following an aggressive 6-week intervention, those patients receiving NMES had reduced their mean subluxation to 9 mm, whereas the control group maintained a mean of 13 mm. Following the intervention, one third of the sample receiving NMES had subluxation considered to be subclinical (less than 5 mm), while 90 percent of the control group were considered to be significantly subluxed at the shoulder. This subluxation continued despite patients' participation in standard therapy, including sitting support, shoulder slings when upright, and facilitation programs to increase shoulder activation.[52]

More recently a smaller sample of more acute patients with hemiparesis with shoulder subluxation were reported.[53] These patients were an average of 16 days poststroke and presented with 4 to 6 mm of acromial–humeral separation. The 13 patients receiving NMES slightly reduced their shoulder subluxation, decreasing from 6 to 2 mm during the 6-week intervention. The 13 control subjects showed increasing acromial–humeral separation, changing from 4

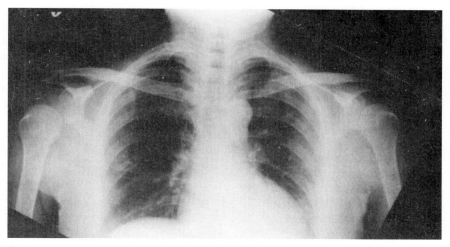

A

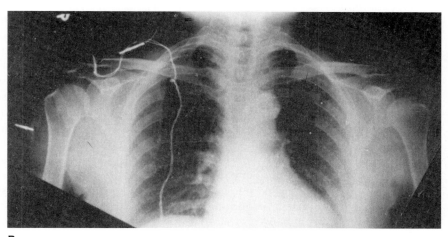

B

FIGURE 8–3.  Example of a hemiparetic patient with a subluxed shoulder **(A)** (right shoulder). Effect of electrical stimulation of the posterior deltoid and supraspinatus muscles is shown in **(B)** (electrode wires can be seen).

mm to 10 mm despite the use of arm support at all times.[53] Both studies report maintained reduction of shoulder subluxation 3 months[52] and 6 weeks[53] after the termination of the electrical stimulation program. These two studies demonstrate the potential to decrease the incidence of shoulder subluxation, and the concomitant problems of pain and further compromise in upper extremity range and function,[54] in the patients following stroke with the addition of an aggressive NMES program. Clearly, slings and supports presently used are inadequate to maintain the integrity of the shoulder capsule in the absence of normal muscle tone (firmness).[55] A daily, all-day stimulation program has been successful in providing that protection when combined with standard supports, and in reducing the incidence of debilitating pain and limiting range of shoulder motion. Management of the problem during the acute phase of stroke recovery is clearly more beneficial than allowing the shoulder capsule to stretch and attempting to reduce the subluxation once it is a clinically recognizable problem. Because most stroke patients do develop at least muscle tone—if not voluntary motor control—around the shoulder, the long-term benefits of the shoulder subluxation program continue, even months after the stimulation has been discontinued.[52,53]

Finally, NMES has most recently been used in a more general manner, with the intent of decreasing the problems of hemi-inattention, most commonly seen with patients experiencing left-sided hemiplegia or hemiparesis.[56] This manner is a controversial application of NMES and has not been fully explored, but one author reported significant improvement in a standard visuomotor exploratory task when stimulation was added either to the left neck extensors or to the dorsum of the left hand. The visuomotor task was a standard letter cancellation test, requiring the patient to cross midline for successful completion. Patients also reproduced several drawings, but analysis of the improvement in copying was not quantified. These authors report the NMES effect to be greatest during the stimulation treatment, with only a minor carry-over following the 15-minute stimulation session, but only single sessions were evaluated.[56] A comprehensive daily treatment to enhance the patient's attention to the hemiparetic side has not been reported to date. Notice should be made that a second author was unable to duplicate the original outcomes, but further study has yet to be reported.[57] The patients were all right handed, with CVA of the right hemisphere, between 2 and 8 months prior to the test.

Applications of NMES facilitation programs are not limited to the patients with strokes, although that population is most often used for study purposes. Patients recovering from traumatic brain injury have also benefitted from NMES facilitation programs,[15] as have children with cerebral palsy.[46–49,58] Some applications of NMES facilitation may be appropriate in the upper extremity of the patient with quadriplegia, but full assessment of innervation status must be considered in this population before NMES is attempted.[59] Awareness of muscles that may be partially innervated because of nerve root damage, along with cognizance of the fully innervated muscles below the level of spinal cord injury and not accessible for voluntary control, are required before aggressive reeducation/facilitation treatment programs can be proposed for the patient with quadriplegia.

### Application Techniques for NMES and Facilitation

NMES facilitation programs are primarily limited by the ease with which a physical therapist can apply the stimulation, the availability of stimulation equipment and the creativeness of the therapist. Stimulation levels will vary depending upon the patient's physical and cognitive capabilities. Patients demonstrating profound hemineglect or with inadequate motor control to contract a muscle on command will probably benefit from stimulation levels high enough to contract specific muscles to achieve a specific goal (eg, quadriceps muscle contraction for a dynamic orthosis during gait training or finger extensor activation in preparation for grasping an object). As motor control becomes more reliable, the patient may still find it difficult to *begin* the muscle contraction, or require assistance with the timing of a contraction during specific activities. Neuromuscular electrical stimulation amplitudes may now be decreased, so that only a sensory cue is provided at the appropriate time, or a small stimulated contraction is used to prime the more powerful voluntary contraction during activities. Thus, ideally the patient can be moved from relying on the stimulated contraction for enhanced function to using it as a cue to achieve smooth transitions in functional activities, to completely assuming the motor control necessary for function. Not all patients with CNS dysfunction will achieve this final goal, but most will demonstrate enhanced motor control with the addition of NMES to their usual muscle force and functional training.

Because the goal in facilitation programs is for the patient's own voluntary control to assume responsibility for function, a great deal of sensory information needs to be sent to the CNS for processing. Thus, facilitation programs are often more effective when stimulation frequencies are set above those needed for tetany. This increased pulse frequency use is done not because the muscle needs to be contracted harder but to increase the amount of total information available to the CNS. This increased information can be used at all levels of the neuraxis, from the spinal-level facilitation of the alpha motoneuron to the cortical processing of the multimodal sensory drive ascending from the thalamus. Since facilitation programs tend to be short, dictated by the patient's ability to cognitively interact with the task at hand, higher stimulation frequencies of 50 to 100 pps are not a major concern and provide a high level of sensory information for central processing. Stimulation cycles also tend to be relatively short when NMES is used in conjunction with functional activities, further reducing concerns about stimulated fatigue during NMES facilitation programs.

In order for NMES to be an effective cue to enhance timing of muscle contractions during functional tasks, it is necessary to control the stimulation ON cycle and the subsequent OFF time. This control is best achieved by the employment of some form of switch that can be used to control the ON and OFF times of the stimulator. Hand switches that can be used to activate a stimulator when contact is made are ideal for controlling stimulation timing during dynamic activities. When a physical therapist requires hands-free activation of the stimulator, a foot switch controlled by the therapist is an additional option. Foot switches can be designed to fit within the therapist's shoe or may be larger and more stationary. These larger switches can often be activated by the patient during activities such as tabletop grasp and release practice. Patient-controlled stimulation must be attempted only when the patient has the cognitive skills to comprehend the task and the physical skills to reliably activate the switch during appropriate periods of the ongoing activity. Use of patient-activated switches during early gait training is not recommended, because the foot-contact pattern is often erratic and unpredictable. Therapist activation of stimulation, either by hand or foot switch, provides reliable muscle contraction and sensory cuing for upright activities, in which patient safety is a paramount concern.

At the beginning of this section, the limitations to NMES use for facilitation in the CNS-involved patient were identified. The first two limitations were ease of therapist use and equipment availability. With today's self-sticking electrodes, which come in a wide variety of shapes and sizes, set-up time for most stimulation programs can be minimized. Some muscles and some patients will require an initial session to probe for an optimal motor point and electrode position, but on large muscles even that inconvenience can be largely overcome with a working knowledge of surface anatomy. Stimulation equipment continues to become ever more sophisticated, and many times manufacturer-set programs can be useful. This equipment potentially reduces the need to modify individual stimulus characteristics such as frequency and cycle times. Still, a therapist who has not used stimulation in more than a week may well feel intimidated and encumbered by the actual application process. General and systematic use of stimulation reduces much of the intimidation factor and provides for a level of problem solving that cannot be attained by only occasional use of NMES. Given the wide range of facilitation programs that can be enhanced by the addition of NMES, there is ample opportunity for most therapists to become both proficient and efficient with stimulation. The question of equipment becomes the next stumbling block, but this too can be overcome with adequate levels of therapist use. When equipment is used, it is not hard to justify additional equipment to further increase use. When equipment sits in the bottom drawer, justification for additional stimulators is difficult to rationalize.

## Outcome Measures, Benefits, and Efficacy

The goal of all reeducation and facilitation treatment programs is to enhance the motor control of the patient. These goals can be demonstrated by increased muscle force and increased voluntary range of motion. These gains generally lead to increased functional use of the extremity or joint. For patients recovering from orthopedic trauma or surgery, the force and functional use is nearly always assured; the addition of NMES to the rehabilitation program may significantly speed this natural process. Many studies have demonstrated increased force improving *rates* with the addition of NMES, and this increased force should be translated into increased ability to meet the functional demands placed on the muscle in question. Generally, the relatively young patient who has sustained an acute orthopedic trauma will demonstrate increased muscle force in as little as one or two NMES treatment sessions, or as much as a month of regular NMES exercise if pain is a persistent problem. The older patient who may be recovering from a total joint replacement, after months or even years of pain and disuse, may require consistent treatment for 1 to 2 weeks, with some patients requiring even longer treatment programs to achieve optimal results. The young athletic patient may progress to an aggressive force improving program, whereas the more sedentary older patient will usually achieve functional results with an appropriate reeducation program alone.

The outcome of an NMES facilitation program is not as assured in the patient with CNS dysfunction. If rehabilitation is occurring shortly after an acute CNS event (physical or vascular), the natural course of recovery must be taken into consideration. A patient who is unable to demonstrate a significant increase in voluntary motor control following a 1- or 2-week trial with NMES, may not yet be ready to display the level of motor control required. In many pathologies, known patterns of return of function are established; the physical therapist should take advantage of those patterns to facilitate volitional control where it is anticipated, as well as where it will enhance functional outcomes. Thus, to begin by attempting to facilitate finger extensors for a patient who has suffered a stroke just 2 weeks before is unwise, if the arm is flail and a dead weight dragging on the glenohumeral joint. A more appropriate treatment approach would be to protect the shoulder from subluxation with both positioning and NMES. As the patient demonstrates increasing control of the shoulder, the subluxation program can be maintained while facilitation of active elbow extension is added. Wrist and finger extension may also be included, so that two channels of NMES can be used to create a pattern of extension in the upper extremity, which will help to counter the flexion synergy that will probably be demonstrated during spontaneous recovery. Similarly, concentrating on a foot drop in the lower extremity when a patient demonstrates poor hip and knee extension control is faulty prioritizing.

Neuromuscular electrical stimulation reeducation and facilitation programs tend to be self-limiting, with patients either achieving the goal of increased motor control, as demonstrated by muscle force and active ROM or clearly not being able to attain that goal because of limitations in the CNS. Neuromuscular electrical stimulation reeducation and facilitation programs are usually successful in weeks, only occasionally extending into 2 or more months. As soon as a patient achieves adequate motor control to voluntarily activate the muscle at the desired level of activity, NMES is no longer needed.

Some types of patients will make very slow progress over rather long periods of time. The most common diagnoses of these individuals include patients who have experienced head trauma or incomplete spinal cord injuries. The child with CNS involvement would also fit into this category. In these instances, the NMES facilitation program should be adapted to home use, with periodic visits to the therapist for updating and modification of programs, so that continued challenges for the patient are provided. Patients who will benefit from long-term facilitation programs must be treated initially in a therapy setting, to establish a pattern of NMES use and the resultant enhanced motor control. Once that pattern has been established, adequate justification for a home unit with appropriate supplies can be generated. In some situations, the patient may have access, through a well-designed NMES program, to quality facilitation in a home setting, using skilled therapy services only periodically for the purpose of incorporating newly acquired motor control into optimal function.

Home facilitation programs typically include one or maybe two key muscles that have been targeted by the therapist for enhanced motor control. These key muscles are identified by their essential performance in providing increased function for a specific task (eg, walking or eating). With the assistance and supervision of family, the patient can engage in daily NMES facilitation, incorporating stimulation with appropriate voluntary activities. When adequate motor control has been attained to allow increased independence, more intensive skilled therapy may be necessary to guide optimal strategies for incorporation of this improved motor control into daily function. The physical therapist may also identify an additional one or two key muscles for facilitation that could further advance the patient's functional capabilities. In this manner, some patients have been able to continue receiving the benefits of neuromuscular facilitation and enhanced activities of daily living for a year or more after discharge from a formal rehabilitation treatment program.

## SPASTICITY

### Problem

**Spasticity** can be elicited with quick stretch in many patients following an insult to the CNS. The appearance of the hyperactive stretch reflex does not always warrant therapeutic intervention, however. Only when spasticity interferes with actual or potential function is it necessary to identify the specific disruptive muscles and attempt to decrease their excessive activity. With this maxim in mind, the elusive nature of measuring the outcome of a spasticity management program becomes significantly more concrete: Has the patient's motor control, muscle force, ROM, or function improved? While problems associated with long-standing spasticity may not resolve in a single intervention session, some improvement should be noted after a short series of trials, or the probability of ultimately increasing function through a stimulation intervention is only slight.

Spasticity is usually associated with motoneuron excitability elicited by some abnormal drive. Considering this, the only way to affect long-term or permanent control of spasticity is to alter the drive onto the motoneuron. Most treatment programs, including those incorporating NMES, provide some means of temporary interruption or balancing of this abnormal drive, either at the source of the drive or at the level of the motoneuron itself. Because the interruption is temporary, the effects of treatment are usually seen as temporary. Long-lasting carryover, as reported in reeducation and facilitation programs, is usually not seen in the area of spasticity management by NMES. Thus, if a treatment is effective, long-term use of NMES would be required to ensure continued increase in function.

Spasticity is a constellation of symptoms that may be caused by any number of sources and different types of pathology. Although the outward signs of the patient with multiple sclerosis and spasticity may resemble the spasticity of a patient with a spinal cord injury, the source of the abnormal muscle firmness may be very different. The effectiveness of NMES treatments will vary according to (1) which structures of the CNS are most sensitive to the particular characteristics of the specific NMES programs, and (2) the source of the spasticity itself. Because the site of action of most NMES programs designed to affect spasticity is speculative at best, and because the source of the spastic drive in any given patient is also largely unknown, the effectiveness of

NMES in the treatment of spasticity is largely unpredictable. Neuromuscular electrical stimulation has been used in a variety of ways to decrease spasticity. Four programs have been described in the literature over the past several years, and all have reported variable success in controlling spastic muscle tone (firmness). These various means of altering CNS processing of information include antagonist muscle stimulation, spastic muscle stimulation, intense point stimulation, and repetitive sensory level stimulation to elicit CNS habituation. These final two treatments have been described in the experimental neurophysiology literature, but have not demonstrated adequate clinical effectiveness and will be discussed only in passing.

## Evaluation and Prognosis

Patients who are most likely to benefit from an NMES spasticity management program demonstrate focal spasticity that either overpowers weak voluntary control or impedes smooth joint motion associated with an ongoing task (eg, gait). When a specific muscle or muscle group can be identified which interferes with function, there is increased probability that an NMES spasticity management program could assist to increase purposeful motion. Patients with generalized muscle tone and spasticity may benefit from intense stimulation of points on the body,[60,61] although specific points do not appear to be critical; intense stimulation almost anywhere on the body has been reported to be effective.[62] Generalized muscle firmness, such as may be seen in individuals following traumatic brain injury or spinal cord injury and in some children with cerebral palsy, is less well managed through the peripheral application of electrical currents. Both the point stimulation[60–62] and the sensory-level habituation stimulation[63–65] have, however, made claims concerning generalized reduction of spasticity that may last for several hours. Clinical assessments of these techniques remain preliminary at this time.

The cornerstone for evaluating the effectiveness of any NMES intervention is not the immediate measure of decreased muscle firmness or change in reflex threshold but rather the patient's ability to demonstrate voluntary recruitment or increased force of a muscle or enhanced ROM at a joint. In order for continued treatment to be justified, the change in control, force, or motion must be translated into purposeful changes in functional ability. For example, a patient experiencing a stiff knee in gait because of quadriceps muscle spasticity following an incomplete spinal cord injury may demonstrate a reduced velocity of walking, increased energy cost of gait and a diminished range for functional ambulation. Neuromuscular stimulation, either of the spastic quadriceps or the antagonist hamstring muscles, can be used to reduce the excessive knee extension in initial and midswing phases of gait. If successful, the patient's velocity will increase, the energy required to functionally ambulate will be reduced, and the range of ambulation will increase. The measurable outcome is not the altered reflex threshold—the probable physiologic response to the treatment—but rather the functional goal of the patient.

Because of the varied nature of the problem, any patient who demonstrates decreased function because of excessive firmness or stretch reflexes, deserves a trial of NMES spasticity management. The trial should consist of a series of NMES treatments given at regular intervals with the program most likely to be effective for that patient's particular problem, as determined by the physical therapist. The NMES effect is often short in duration; therefore, treatments may need to be given several times a day during the trial. Success of the trial would be determined by an increase in function or, more realistically, changes in motor control, muscle force or joint motion, which could eventually lead to an altered functional state.

The appropriate NMES program must be determined by the therapist, based on the proposed physiologic mechanism each program uses and the type (dynamic or static), degree (long standing with joint contractures versus short duration), and extent (focal or generalized) of disruption of function posed by the spasticity. If the patient is recovering from some form of CNS dysfunction, an NMES program may be used for short- to intermediate-term programs, with the patient taking advantage of periods of decreased tone to enhance weak voluntary control/force or to learn functional activities (eg, tabletop activities or transfer training). When the initial spontaneous recovery appears to be completed but spasticity remains as an impediment to function, more long-term treatment programs may be considered, depending on the patient's need and the degree of support available after discharge. Realistic alternatives for long-term management must also include phenol or botulinum toxin (Botox) injections for focal problems, and pharmacologic agents for more generalized spasticity or tone (firmness). In general, NMES is an adjunctive treatment to these more medically managed regimens designed to reduce spasticity.

## Intervention

### *Physiologic/Clinical Rationale for NMES and Spasticity—Antagonist Muscle Stimulation*

One of the earliest reports of decreased spasticity after NMES of the antagonist muscle groups came from Vallejo, California, in 1952.[66] Levine, Knott, and Kabat reported that stimulation of the antagonist to a spastic muscle, followed by vigorous ROM exercises, led to dramatic decreases in muscle tone. The authors emphasized the need to evaluate each patient but found that when spasticity impeded volitional control, the addition of NMES to the treatment program provided significant increases in the management of abnormal muscle tone.[66] These same observations have been made more recently by Seib and coworkers.[67]

Alfieri reported a clinical study of 96 patients with hemiparesis, 90 percent of whom showed evidence of decreased muscle tone (firmness) after multiple treatment sessions of NMES to the antagonists of spastic muscles.[68] Although the immediate effects of the treatment were reportedly decreased within 1 hour after stimulation, Alfieri stated that spasticity tended to decrease and was maintained at a lower level after varying numbers of treatment sessions. The follow-up of those patients who received NMES treatments did demonstrate long-term reduction of muscle tone in this study; however, the author did not report the effects of any other treatment, or the effects of no treatment at all, on the long-term spasticity of similar hemiparetic patients.[68] Whether NMES was more effective than other treatment programs designed to reduce muscle tone or was any different from no treatment in patients with chronic hemiparesis is difficult to determine.

Carnstam and Larsson attributed the long-lasting effects of NMES to an increase in voluntary control, which may potentially overcome the spastic muscle after the initial inhibitory period.[69] Not all authors have reported an effect once stimulation has been discontinued, although a decrease in tone is nearly always seen during the stimulation period.[70–73]

The neurophysiologic rationale for the effectiveness of NMES to the antagonist of the spastic muscle seems to rest on the principle of reciprocal inhibition.[73–75] The time course of reciprocal inhibition, however, is very short, measurable in milliseconds. How is it, then, that clinicians have reported therapeutic decreases in muscle tone (firmness) for up to one hour after a treatment program, and neurophysiologists have measured it for up to 24 hours? The phenomenon known as **posttetanic potentiation (PTP)** may account for some of the therapeutic effects that exceed the length of the treatment program.[75] Although usually described as a prolonged activation of an excitatory reflex pathway, Tan and colleagues have evaluated the effects of tetanization of an antagonist reflex pathway and have reported a decrease in the normal PTP response. The authors refer to this as **posttetanic depression,** and, although they were not evaluating spasticity per se, this may be a significant factor in the effectiveness of NMES in reducing muscle tone in antagonist muscle groups.[75]

The effectiveness of this treatment technique, even in subjects with normal muscle tone, was demonstrated by Liberson and can be evaluated by self-stimulation.[73] Liberson used NMES to establish a contraction of the finger extensors that a healthy subject could not *voluntarily* overcome using the finger flexor muscles. The quality of the stimulated muscle contractions was then graded with a standard manual muscle test. The subject was unable to effectively flex against a grade 3 stimulated finger extension contraction. That the normal finger flexor muscles were unable to counter a grade 3 stimulated extensor contraction can be attributed to the effects of reciprocal inhibition from the Ia myotatic receptors of the extensors onto the flexor motoneuron pool.[74] There has been no documentation of the more prolonged effects of this type of NMES in normal subjects.

### Physiologic/Clinical Rationale for NMES and Spasticity—Spastic Muscle Stimulation

In 1950, Lee and colleagues reported that NMES of spastic muscles with a frequency of 100 to 350 Hz resulted in a "fair" reduction of the spastic tone (firmness) that lasted for several hours.[76] The use of NMES to the spastic muscle for the management of spasticity continued sporadically over the next several years, but no reports of the long-lasting and generalized effects seen by Lee and coworkers were made. When the effectiveness of NMES for improving muscle force, reeducation, and facilitation was documented, some concern about the use of stimulation with spastic muscles was natural.

Several reports were published on the effects of NMES when applied to muscles with spasticity in patients who displayed spasticity following spinal cord injuries.[77,78] These studies reported objective measures of spasticity that, on average, decreased following NMES activation of the spastic muscles. Individual responses varied among measurable decreases in the stretch reflex, no effect from the stimulation, and slight increases in spasticity following stimulation. All of these effects were transient in nature, with no measurable change over the several days of testing and stimulation.[77,78] These studies have largely allayed fears that an NMES program may actually increase spasticity in muscles that demonstrate hypertonia.

The effectiveness of NMES activation of the spastic muscle for the purpose of decreasing abnormal tone appears, however, to be unpredictable, at least in patients with spinal cord injuries. No specific characteristics could be found that distinguished those subjects who demonstrated a decrease in the stretch reflex from those who showed no significant or even increased stretch responses following NMES treatment. Thus, the use of NMES to activate a spastic muscle for some specific therapeutic goal, such as ROM or facilitation of voluntary motor control, would seem merited for most patients. This use of NMES was borne out by the 1995 report of stimulation of the triceps surae muscle in children with cerebral palsy.[47] The goal of treatment was reeducation/force improving of the calf muscles. The results included improved gait, balance, foot alignment, and a plantigrade foot in children who had been toe walkers. No increase in spasticity was noted.[47] The effectiveness of NMES to a spastic muscle *for the purpose of decreasing the spasticity* is somewhat less predictable. Each patient must be evaluated individually before the appropriateness of the NMES treatment can be determined.

A possible neurophysiologic mechanism by which NMES of the spastic muscle could possibly effect a reduction in muscle tone rests in the antidromic activation of the alpha motoneuron axon. With peripherally applied NMES, the electrically elicited action potential is propagated in both directions: orthodromically, toward the motor end plate, and antidromically, toward the spinal cord. Although orthodromic propagation provides the immediately visible muscle contraction, antidromic propagation may provide a spinal-level reflex that could lead to a longer-lasting modulation of the spastic tone.[79] With each voluntary and stimulated action potential, the alpha motoneuron activates the motor unit and excites a pool of Renshaw cells through a recurrent collateral. The Renshaw cells inhibit the alpha motoneurons of the activated pool and the motoneurons of synergist muscles. The function of the Renshaw system seems to be modulation and stabilization of motoneuron firing frequencies. There is some evidence that patients with spasticity may not have normal supraspinal modulation of the Renshaw cells, especially during voluntary contraction.[79] Although the majority of this evidence has been developed with either patients with hemiparesis following stroke or patients with multiple sclerosis, a similar pattern appears to be present in patients with incomplete spinal cord injury as well.[78,79]

In 1953, Eccles and coworker proposed a theory of **synaptic disuse,**[80] and in 1981, Vodovnik invoked this proposal to further theorize that the effects of NMES provide an artificial drive that essentially strengthens synaptic contacts.[81] Thus, the effects of NMES on the spastic muscle group may lead to a reduction of tone (firmness) if a major source of the unbridled alpha motoneuron activity is a lack of control from the Renshaw system. If antidromic activation of the alpha motoneuron acts as a source of posttetanic potentiation onto the Renshaw cells, the therapeutic effect might be expected to follow a time course similar to that seen in NMES programs using activation of the antagonist to the spastic muscle. The time course of both agonist and antagonist stimulation for reduction of spasticity do follow similar time courses.[73,75,77,78] Thus, stimulation of the spastic muscle seems likely to affect hyperactive stretch reflexes through a synaptic mechanism rather than simple fatigue of the myoneural junction. Unfortunately, there is still inadequate information on which types of spasticity may be the result of inappropriate Renshaw cell activity. This inappropriate activity undoubtedly contributes to the variability in the response to NMES programs activating the spastic muscle reported by Bowman and Bajd[77] and by Vodovnik and colleagues.[78]

A variant of the program that activates the spastic muscle has been used for many years clinically, but has not been discussed in recent research or teaching literature. Low-level stimulated contractions for relief of painfully acute muscle spasms has been common clinical practice for over 100 years.[82] In most cases, at least a grade 1 contraction is achieved with the stimulation, taking this program out of the realm of just pain management. The small stimulated muscle contraction can be done by moving an ultrasound head over the muscle, or may be achieved through cyclical stimulus trains. At this time, no literature demonstrating the effectiveness of the technique appears to exist, but the practice persists with excellent anecdotal outcomes. The probable mechanism of the effect is most certainly similar to that achieved by stimulating a spastic muscle.

### Application Techniques for NMES and Spasticity— Antagonist and Spastic Muscle Programs

In order for these NMES programs to be effective, the spasticity that interferes with function must be limited to one or two muscle groups. Stimulation of specific muscles does not appear to effectively decrease hyperactive reflexes in other parts of the body. Because the duration of neurogenic inhibition is relatively short—usually measured in minutes for a single treatment session—NMES should be applied just prior to other forms of therapy. Thus, if the patient is experiencing excessive knee extension during the swing phase of gait, stimulation of the hamstring or quadriceps muscle groups immediately prior to or during a gait training session would be appropriate. Use of a stimulation program to reduce spasticity will also allow the therapist to assess how dependent the patient may be on reflex excitation for stability in upright activities. In some cases, reduction of tone may be detrimental to a patient's function.

The proposed neurophysiologic effect of each type of treatment is mediated through synaptic inhibition onto the motoneuron. Stimulation frequencies can, therefore, be set relatively high, maximizing the amount of information into the CNS. When stimulating the muscle antagonist to the spasticity, sensory stimulation may be adequate, because the Ia afferents have axons that are larger then the alpha motoneurons. If the spastic muscle, or muscle in spasm, is to be stimulated, in order to achieve activation of the Renshaw inhibitory interneuron the alpha motoneuron must be fired. Thus, at least a minimal muscle contraction must be elicited. In either program, the stronger the stimulating current, the more afferents will be driven, potentially increasing the inhibition from the respective interneurons (Ia inhibitory or Renshaw). In both programs, the targeted activation is associated with the nerve to the muscle, so placement of electrodes over the motor point potentially increases the effectiveness of the program.

Stimulation is typically provided either cyclically, with periodic stimulation followed by rest times, or triggered by a switch to coincide with other dynamic activities. If stimulation levels are high enough to cause muscle contraction, some consideration must be given to the hyperactive reflex response. Abrupt onset of even a moderately strong stimulated contraction can cause a stretch reflex, which will probably be counterproductive to the overall treatment goal. Accordingly, spasticity and spasm management programs typically use gradual onset of stimulus amplitude, ranging from 2 sec upward to 10 sec for the patient with high levels of spasticity. This gradual onset of stimulus results in a gradual stretch of the joint when stimulation is used on the antagonist muscle, or a gradual buildup to the stimulated contraction if activation of the spastic muscle, or muscle in spasm, is required. In the presence of a hyperactive stretch reflex, stimulation of an antagonist muscle during dynamic activities, such as gait, may not be possible, because gradual ramps are not an option during short phases of swing or stance. In the presence of severe hyperreflexia, a gradual decrease in stimulus amplitude may also be desirable. Patients who have spasticity on both sides of a joint may benefit from reciprocal stimulation of each set of prime movers, with gradual transitions between activation of the flexors and extensors. In general, optimal regulation of the spasticity can be achieved with 20 to 40 minutes of stimulation, with an anticipated window of decreased reflex activity lasting for 15 to 60 additional minutes.

Spasticity management programs are optimal when immediately followed by other forms of therapy (facilitation, force improving, functional training, etc); therefore, the patient should be positioned in preparation for these additional activities while receiving the NMES program. This position preparation is particularly true in the patient with CNS dysfunction, because repositioning between supine and sitting or upright may cause excessive drive onto the reticular and vestibular motor systems, which in turn can cause abnormally high levels of spinal motoneuron excitability. Thus, in the example of the patient receiving NMES to decrease knee extension during the swing phase of gait, the stimulation program should be carried out with the patient in an upright or semi-upright position. This can be achieved through supported standing in a standing frame or on a tilt table.

### Physiologic/Clinical Rationale for NMES and Generalized Hyperreflexia

Since the early 1970s, neurophysiologists have sought a means of quieting multiple motoneuron pools through the use of sensory-level ES. Dimitrijevic and Nathan reported research that indicated that relatively low-frequency, low-amplitude sensory stimulation could lead to a generalized habituation response, which could be spread to include a large part of the functionally isolated spinal cord in patients with complete cord injury.[63,64] This method for general suppression of interneuron activity, although clearly demonstrated in the laboratory, has been more elusive in the clinical setting.

Sensory habituation is an extremely tenuous clinical treatment program at this time, with insufficient documentation to determine what NMES characteristics are most important to ensure the therapeutic effect. The few areas of agreement seem to rest in the repetitive, consistent nature of the stimulus and in the rather prolonged stimulation programs required to create an observable reduction in muscle tone firmness).[63–65] Sensory-level stimulation done just below motor-evoked responses also appears to be a consistent characteristic of the successful program. Most authors agree that the habituation of a specific reflex (eg, the flexion reflex) occurs in the interneuron network at the spinal cord level; the more generalized interneuron suppression may necessitate potentiation from supraspinal centers. Programs described by Dimitrijevic and Nathan[63,64] and by Walker[65] may also require multiple sites of stimulation.

A newer form of stimulation recently proposed for the management of generalized hyperreflexia includes stimulation of acupuncture points,[60,61] or possibly intense stimulation over any small area of the body.[62] Two recent reports from China have identified high-frequency (100 pps) stimulation over bilateral acupuncture points, which appear to be nonspecific in nature, that resulted in reduction in spasticity.[60,61] The precise measure of spasticity was not clear, however. Similarly, a group using rectal probes for fertility studies initially identified patient reports of decreased frequency of spasms.[62] On more formal assessment, they found objective evidence of decreased stretch reflexes following rectal stimulation, which was generalized to the lower extremities and lasted a mean of 8 hours.[62] Each of these papers found short-term effects after a single treatment and more prolonged effects following daily treatments done for up to 3 months. One paper noted that the stimulation must be done permanently in order to maintain the long-term effects.[61] Another author speculated on the mechanism of reduced spasticity as being linked to the release of metenkephalins associated with the intense stimulation.[60]

Both techniques reported to have generalized effects of reducing spasticity (ie, sensory habituation and intense point stimulation) require additional clinical trials to further define the pertinent stimulus and program characteristics before widespread use in the clinic is advised. However, when all other spasticity management techniques have failed, these techniques may be worth the effort in order to enhance a patient's functional ability or comfort or both.

## Outcome Measures, Benefits, and Efficacy

As has been repeatedly stated, the outcome measure of a successful spasticity management program is enhanced function through improved volitional control or improved joint mobility. When the NMES program is done during the period of recovery from a CNS insult, the stimulation program is used to unmask weak voluntary control or to allow a patient to learn a functional task without the additional encumbrance of a hyperactive reflex. Generally, as a patient increases his or her voluntary control of a limb, spasticity becomes less of a hindrance and can sometimes be used to support specific functional activities (eg, quadriceps muscle tone providing a balance point during a pivot transfer). The patient who demonstrates excessive reflexic activity after central recovery is completed may still use NMES for management of focal spasticity, but will probably be better served by evaluation for a more permanent management technique, such as phenol or Botox injection. The patient with persistent generalized muscle tone will probably be better managed with systemic or localized drug intervention. Neuromuscular electrical stimulation programs for the suppression of spasticity are ideally suited to the dynamic changes being made during recovery from CNS dysfunction but are less than optimal for long-term applications. Stimulation does, however, provide the physical therapist with a tool to evaluate a patient's latent voluntary motor control, dependence on spasticity for functional activities, or actual interaction between helpful and harmful effects of spasticity. Because effects from individual stimulation programs are always short in duration, any changes that occur following an NMES intervention will soon be lost, whether the tone or function was increased or diminished.

# PERMANENT LOSS OF VOLUNTARY MOTOR CONTROL

## Problem

**Permanent loss of voluntary motor control** results when severe damage to the CNS occurs. The use of NMES as a substitute for conventional orthoses provides both the therapist and the patient with a degree of flexibility previously unavailable. This increased flexibility can be critical during functional training sessions, when motor recovery is still ongoing. The addition of dynamic orthoses as permanent means of increasing function—true functional electrical stimulation (FES)—is exciting but has proved difficult to achieve in its practical application. Some of the problems encountered relate to the complexity of seemingly simple tasks, such as standing and walking. Even when the stimulation task is relatively simple, such as the permanent reduction of shoulder subluxation, long-term management with surface stimulation is less then ideal. The very pragmatic problems encountered in the application of any long-term surface stimulation program include variability of electrode placement, skin irritation from repetitive externally applied stimulation and fixation systems, and the mess and bother of electrode preparation. Thus, permanent orthotic substitution would ideally be done through implanted stimulation systems, allowing the patient to easily turn the system on and off with minimal external hardware. This switching of stimulation would make the permanent use of stimulation more like a pacemaker in daily care and set-up time. One such application is now available, designed to enhance manual function in patients with specific levels of quadriplegia. Other potential applications are continuing to make progress toward the fully implanted, user-friendly systems required for long-term home management of an impairment, with the intent of reducing an individual's handicap.

Several applications of dynamic orthoses have been developed but have not yet progressed beyond the use of surface stimulation. In the upper extremities, these include finger extension stimulation to enhance function in the hand of a patient with hemiparesis, and long-term stimulation for shoulder subluxation. Orthotic stimulation of lower extremity muscles to allow standing in patients with complete paraplegia, as well as some primitive stepping activity that can be used for short-distance ambulation, have also been under intense investigation. Finally, the use of electrically stimulated exercise to enhance cardiovascular fitness is an area that may be placed into orthotic substitution. Each of these applications will be discussed separately.

## Patient Evaluation for FES Programs

The patient must demonstrate a functional deficit that contributes to a significant handicap before use of an FES system is appropriate. The status of the impairment that leads to the deficit must be stable, such that neither increasing nor decreasing function is likely without the stimulation intervention. The application of FES is almost exclusively appropriate for the neurologically involved patient, because the electrical stimulation will activate the normal skeletal muscles which fail to respond to voluntary control. In the presence of joint or bony instability, peripheral excitation of muscles, while possible, is ill advised. In the presence of peripheral nerve damage, FES programs are not available, because direct muscle stimulation requires a 10- to 100-fold increase in the stimulus phase duration, which can be very dangerous to skin integrity when used repeatedly. When neurologically involved patients are still demonstrating increasing motor control, dynamic orthoses may be used, with the intent of removing the external excitation once adequate voluntary activation is achieved. This use of NMES falls into the category of neuromuscular facilitation and has already been discussed. Progression from a facilitation program to a permanent orthotic substitute is a possibility for those patients who fail to demonstrate full recovery of voluntary motor control. Only the hand assist for patients with quadriplegia is a fully integrated system designed to be used independently at home, however. Other applications of FES must be evaluated for appropriateness in the home, given the difficulties with long-term surface stimulation.

The specific nature of each FES application, and the persistent problems remaining to be solved for each application, require an altered organization for this section of the chapter. Each area amenable to FES intervention will include a statement of the problem; discussion of the evaluation and patient selection; specific FES application, as now practiced; and, finally, a description of the outcome measures and benefits, as we currently understand them. Because FES is an extremely dynamic aspect of NMES, the reader must look in the current literature for both hardware and clinical advances made following the publication of this text. The references at the end of this chapter may be used as a starting point for the reader's independent investigation, supplying authors' names for searching more up-to-date literature.

## FES Orthosis for Enhanced Hand Function in Quadriplegia

Only one fully implanted stimulation system has been approved for general use in the United States. The goal of the system is to improve hand function in individuals with quadriplegia, and it is designed for those with normal function at the C5 level and a loss of function at level C6.[83] These patients typically have active command of wrist extension but no voluntary control of finger flexion or extension. Full evaluation of the innervation status of all muscles in the forearm is necessary before tendon transfers, joint arthrodesis, and electrode implantation can be considered. Transfer of tendons from muscles controlled by the patient, as well as potentially some controlled by the stimulator, is generally done at the time of electrode and stimulator implantation. At that time, certain joints—notably the metacarpal–phalangeal joint of the thumb—may also be fused to enhance stability of the stimulated grasp. Six to eight muscles, below the spinal injury level but with intact peripheral nerves, are targeted for activation with implanted epymesial electrodes. The implanted receiver is a passive element that allows the stimulation signals to be transmitted through an antenna placed on the skin over the receiver. Stimulation hardware and the power needed for the activation of stimulated muscles is external and maintained in proximity to the patient, usually in a backpack attached to the wheelchair. Daily setup requires the patient to don the stimulation antenna and the external control system, attached to the sternum and the shoulder, which also contains the on–off switch.[83,84]

For increased hand function in the patient with quadriplegia, stimulation must provide both finger extension for hand opening and release of objects, and finger flexion for closure and grasping of articles. The present system provides finger opening and two forms of closure, a key grip (thumb to the side of the index finger) for control of small objects such as a pen or fork, and a palmar or mass grasp (long finger flexor activation) for picking up larger objects like a cup or telephone. The stimulation is proportionally controlled through shoulder movements, typically done by the contralateral extremity.

This system, in development since the mid-1970s, has been shown to significantly increase functional activities for the targeted spinal cord–injured population.[83–85] This increase has been measured under a variety of timed manipulation assessments, as well as personal logs maintained by users detailing their daily routine. Success has been identified as reduced time during manipulation assessments, increased functional use of nonadapted equipment (eg, telephone and fork), and consistent employment of the device throughout the user's routine activities in a typical day. Most, but not all, users have identified the dynamic orthosis as significantly increasing their independence in activities requiring manual dexterity and manipulation. Many of these individuals have used more conventional wrist orthoses, and most prefer the ease of manual tasks with the FES system. Some patients have used the FES as an assist to, and in conjunction with, more conventional orthoses. The success of the FES orthosis largely depends on the innervation status of muscles in the forearm. This assessment must be carefully and thoroughly completed before progressing toward the surgical intervention required for this FES application.[83–85]

### Additional FES Orthoses for Enhanced Hand Function

Conceptually similar orthotic systems designed to improve hand function in other patient populations, such as individuals with hemiparesis from stroke and traumatic brain injury, and use for patients with cerebral palsy, are still being developed and evaluated. Individual patient needs must be kept in mind as FES systems are designed. An orthosis designed to enhance finger extension for the patient with hemiparesis is presently commercially available.[86] Many patients following stroke demonstrate a mass grasp pattern of finger flexion that can be controlled voluntarily, and this pattern is also often seen in traumatic brain injury and cerebral palsy. This grasp is, however, largely useless because these individuals cannot voluntarily extend their fingers adequately to prepare to grasp or to release an object.

A motion-triggered stimulator, mounted on an orthosis worn over the forearm of the patient with hemiparesis, can use slight voluntary wrist extension to trigger a timed cycle of stimulated finger extension.[86,87] Electrodes placed into the orthosis provide a unified system for sensor, stimulator, and delivery systems, while providing additional support for the forearm to minimize excessive ulnar deviation and wrist flexion.[86]

Selection criteria for use of this orthosis include individuals who can initiate voluntary wrist extension to trigger the stimulation cycle, which, in turn, will excite the finger extensor muscles. During the stimulated cycle the patient can position the hand in preparation for grasping an object, which can be accomplished at the completion of the stimulated cycle. In order for the patient to truly benefit from this FES orthosis, some degree of proximal stability and control must be under voluntary regulation. This control includes scapular and shoulder stability, which ideally should be matched with voluntary elbow extension.

When tested under clinical conditions, this type of system has been found to be very effective in increasing guided upper extremity use for persons following stroke and traumatic brain injury (TBI).[86,87] Although encouraging, clinical use does not necessarily equate to independent, spontaneous home use, particularly since many of these patients experience a degree of sensory neglect and hemi-inattention. The functional outcomes with this system are also less rigorous, in the sense that an individual with hemiparesis has one normally functioning upper extremity. Thus, the intent of the orthosis is to provide the patient with (higher-level) functional *assistance* from the involved extremity, not to create a fully functional independent grasp and release. Possibly because of this reduced expectation, and with the assistance of the careful orthosis design, the limitations of surface stimulation in this forearm application have been minimal. Further assessment of orthosis utilization patterns in environments less confined than the clinic is needed in order to fully validate this particular FES application.

## FES Orthosis for Shoulder Subluxation Reduction in the Neurologic Patient

The use of neuromuscular stimulation to reduce and avoid chronic shoulder subluxation was discussed earlier in this chapter. Patients who do not receive adequate protection of the shoulder capsule during the flaccid phase of CNS recovery may demonstrate shoulder subluxation that, although responding to stimulation with reduction, fails to demonstrate maintained reduction when the stimulation is removed. This patient may be a candidate for long-term shoulder stimulation, although a great deal of controversy exists regarding who should be treated for chronic subluxation and which intervention is least intrusive.

Under what conditions should chronic shoulder subluxation be considered for a rehabilitation intervention? Generally, the patient who demonstrates chronic subluxation at the proximal shoulder joint also demonstrates very poor to nonexistent distal motor control. Thus, the upper extremity is relatively incapable of assisting with function for many individuals with chronic shoulder subluxation.[54,88] In these circumstances, the most common reason to attempt a rehabilitation intervention is pain in or around the shoulder. This pain is generally relieved by reducing the subluxation and sustaining that reduction, that is, when the patient lies supine and there is no traction force on the joint capsule. Slings and supports commonly used do not fully reduce the pendulant humeral position and thereby do not significantly diminish the patient's pain.[55] A second patient profile requiring some type of management for chronic shoulder subluxation is the individual who may have some distal function in the upper extremity but no proximal stability and is unable to optimally use that function. This pattern emerges more commonly in patients following traumatic brain injury or sometimes in the child with cerebral palsy.

Management of chronic shoulder subluxation has typically been through orthopedic surgery, with internal reduction of shoulder capsule length through stapling or other stabilizing techniques.[89] Although minimally invasive, this surgical technique may or may not reduce the patient's pain and generally leads to decreased range of shoulder motion, although not to a functionally significant degree. Because voluntary activity is often minimal to begin with, decreased function of the extremity is not typically an issue.

As already stated, long-term management of chronic shoulder subluxation by NMES is not very successful, largely because of difficulties associated with surface stimulation. The potential for implanted stimulation programs, requiring minimal setup and turn-on of the equipment, is a distinct possibility. Several obstacles have impeded the development of such a system, however. The relationship between shoulder pain and the degree of subluxation is not clearly established.[54,88] This may relate to the lack of sensory information from the shoulder complex for some patients with large subluxation, whereas individuals with good sensation may have exquisite pain from much less capsular laxity. Predisposing factors for subluxation, such as joint configuration or prior trauma,[90–92] may further blur the relationship between subluxation and pain. Without a clearly defined relationship between pain and subluxation, there is little reason to attempt restoration of the glenohumeral joint if the upper extremity is marginally functional.

A secondary factor reducing interest in an FES orthosis for shoulder subluxation is the minimally invasive, relatively quick orthopedic techniques presently used, which appear adequate for the low level of function displayed by most patients.[89] Under the present climate of health care, it appears unlikely that an FES orthosis for management of chronic shoulder subluxation will be forthcoming in the near future. This further places the impetus on the *early* management of subluxation, since prevention is the best way to reduce the potential for later complications.

### FES Orthoses for Standing and Walking With Spinal Cord Injury

A great deal of interest in the application of FES to problems related to standing and walking for individuals with complete spinal cord injury was generated in the 1980s.[93] Although walking appears to be a very routine task, the control of multiple muscles in the lower extremities to accomplish that task has proven to be a major stumbling block, both literally and figuratively.[94] There is a U.S. government–approved four-channel stimulation system available for standing and rudimentary stepping,[95] but the expectations generated regarding FES and walking have been next to impossible to meet at this time. Expectations of FES-assisted gait for individuals with some independent walking ability may be more credible in the near future, although a number of problems persist.

Most of the problems associated with FES-generated gait include the following:

- The need to control two to six muscle groups in each extremity, with the concomitant ordeal of surgically placing implanted electrodes
- The presence of spasticity in most walking candidates, with its inherent variability throughout the day and from day to day[96]
- Issues related to control sequences and sensors to ensure that stimulated joint trajectories are being achieved in each step cycle[96–99]

- Adequate levels of training for stimulated muscles, so that fatigue is not a major factor limiting the use of the orthosis[100–102]
- Development of efficient stimulation sequences that would allow users to walk with average velocities at energy levels close to normal[103–105]
- Flexibility in the system to allow ambulation over multiple surfaces, and up and down stairs and ramps, with minimal cognitive input from the user[96]
- Safety of the user in the event of a stimulation system failure

Some of these factors are interrelated, such as the need to control sequences and sensors to ensure the expected joint trajectories, even in the presence of variable spasticity and possible neuromuscular fatigue. Others pose significant individual hurdles to be overcome, such as issues related to implantation in 4 to 12 muscles or muscle groups.

In the United States, the gold standard for mobility of patients with spinal cord injury is the wheelchair. Using this means of ambulation, individuals can go long distances at normal velocities with minimally increased energy expenditure. At this time, FES orthoses, even when mixed with traditional orthoses, cannot approximate these features of wheelchair use, features that are necessary in the daily life of an active individual. Although each area mentioned above as an impediment to FES use is undergoing intense research, it is unlikely that a practical walking system using FES will be achieved in the near future.

Basic standing, with upper extremity support taking a large part of body weight, can be achieved with two to four channels of electrical stimulation.[106–108] Typically, the quadriceps muscles, with or without the addition of the hip extensor muscles, are stimulated to achieve an upright posture. The user must be able to employ his or her upper extremities to both support the trunk and lower body and to control the ascent. Stimulation is generally manually triggered, and if standing is to be sustained for more than a few minutes, some form of a rotating stimulation pattern must be established to avoid neuromuscular fatigue. This level of function is clearly limited to specific applications for only some individuals.

Primitive stepping with stimulation can be achieved through triggered stimulation of one quadriceps muscle paired with the contralateral peroneal nerve.[95,108] Stimulation of the peroneal nerve generally elicits a flexion reflex, with resultant dorsiflexion and hip flexion. In the absence of quadriceps muscles spasticity, the knee will flex passively with the reflex activation of hip flexion. This provides the user with the ability to position the flexed limb forward when the reverse pattern is triggered, stimulating the quadriceps muscles of the formerly flexed limb and the peroneal nerve of the prior stance limb. The commercially available unit ramps the stimulation patterns to reduce the abrupt responses typical of stimulation. An additional safety feature built into the system provides bilateral quadriceps muscles activation any time the stimulation sequence is miscued or there is an apparent fault of an electrode. This form of stepping is usable by select individuals for short-distance gait, but, because of the slow speed, significant upper extremity demands and subsequent high energy cost, this form of gait cannot be considered truly functional except under very limited conditions.[95,108] The added difficulties of placing surface electrodes further reduces the universal application of this orthosis.

### FES Exercise in Paralysis

Exercise regimens have been developed and evaluated, primarily with individuals who have complete spinal cord injury. The beginnings of these exercise programs were necessitated by the increased use of neuromuscular stimulation for standing and walking. Whereas FES-assisted gait has met with major obstacles, the application of NMES to muscles that have experienced prolonged periods of disuse atrophy has become an investigational area of its own. There are two primary physiologic purposes for stimulated exercise, with at least three measurable outcomes. One of the primary purposes of stimulation in the presence of disuse atrophy and complete paralysis is to prepare specific muscles for a planned functional application of stimulation. For example, before the muscles of the forearm can achieve a reliable grip, which can be sustained to allow the user to hold a pen while writing a letter, a systematic exercise program must be instituted.[109] The usual measures of outcome for stimulation used for this purpose are either an increase in strength (force production from supramaximal stimulation) or endurance (the ability to sustain force over a measured time interval of stimulation) or both. When the exercise is applied to the lower extremities, with the larger muscles being activated through stimulation, the potential for a third outcome measure includes an increase in aerobic capacity.

Stimulation exercise programs designed to enhance muscle force and endurance have generally been successful, even with individuals who had experienced prolonged periods of disuse atrophy.[100–102,109,110] Normally, the longer the period of disuse, the longer or more aggressive the exercise program must be to achieve significant force and endurance. Some authors have reported achieving successful force increasing of lower extremity muscles to allow individuals who had experienced disuse for up to 14 years to stand by means of NMES.[108] Training periods may require as much as 6 months or more, but most individuals with complete innervation have been successful in achieving significantly increased muscle force following NMES. These force changes have resulted from increased muscle fiber diameter and are accompanied by increased circulation to the stimulated extremity.[110] Changes in muscular endurance are somewhat less predictable but certainly do occur in most exercise subjects.

The best stimulation and exercise characteristics for achieving increased muscle force and endurance have yet to be defined.[100–102] Most exercise programs begin with isotonic stimulated muscle contractions, usually against the force of gravity. As increased force allows more complete joint ROM against gravity, resistance is typically applied, either in the isotonic mode or with more sophisticated computer-regulated systems. Because of the potential for damage to various aspects of the musculoskeletal system, resistance to a stimulated contraction should be done either with isotonic resistance or with a fail-safe stimulation/limb-resistance shutdown. Individuals participating in an NMES-augmented exercise program will not have voluntary control of the stimulated muscles. Because spinal level reflexes are typically intact, some means of safeguarding the patient in the presence of muscle spasms or structural failure must be provided.

Most programs for improving muscle force are done daily, often with two bouts of exercise each day. Typically, muscles are stimulated to fatigue, as defined by the inability to continue to generate force, even in the presence of increasing stimulus amplitudes. When a 15- to 30-minute stimulation session can be completed without significant fatigue, resistance training is begun, increasing the load slowly and maintaining the specified treatment period. Muscle force and endurance training, because they are associated with specific functional demands, are transitioned to those functional activities when sufficient stimulated contraction will allow. Muscle force training, as a pure exercise to increase tension output from the muscle, has not been explored to determine the limit of stimulated force improvement. This training is largely because of the excessive risk of using high resistances while maintaining the integrity of the musculoskeletal system. Notice should be made, however, that the quality of the stimulated contractions achieved by most patients may be adequate for function but are significantly below torques achieved from those same muscles under voluntary activation by individuals with normal motor control.[100–102,108–110] Typical levels for stimulated muscle contractions required for function range between 3+ and 4 on the standard manual muscle testing scale.

During lower extremity muscle force training exercises it became clear that stimulation provided a potential to increase cardiovascular efficiency, as well as muscular power. Since individuals participating in NMES exercise programs also have the potential for compromised responses to exercise requirements, a full array of general fitness variables have been evaluated during a variety of NMES exercise techniques.[111-120] The general consensus of most studies indicates that stimulation of the large muscles of the lower extremity can produce statistically significant changes in cardiovascular fitness. These changes can usually be augmented with concomitant upper extremity voluntary exercise during the stimulation bout.[115] Many have speculated that the changes in cardiovascular fitness measured during NMES training will, if maintained, lead to a healthier life style and decreased dependence in daily activities.[118-121] The same problem exists with this expected outcome from an NMES training program, as was evidenced in the muscle force improving programs, namely, that the changes measured, while statistically significant, are very small in comparison to the expected changes from a similar level of voluntary training. Evidence for the improved life style and increased independence during continued use of an NMES training program remains anecdotal at this time.

In addition to the general fitness effects of an NMES training program, a number of potential benefits from *sustained* NMES programs have been proposed, including increased bone mineral density,[122,123] decreased incidence of pressure sores; increased healing when an ulcer does develop, and improved urodynamics. At this time, these benefits, although physiologically possible, have not materialized in clinical research trials. Though much has been said of the improved self-esteem reported by some individuals following the increase in muscle bulk from an NMES program, at least one study has found increased depression among users who began stimulation programs with unrealistic expectations.[124] This depression becomes an especially important concern when NMES programs are incorporated into the early rehabilitation of patients with spinal cord injuries. At this time, there is little solid evidence to support the use of NMES general exercise programs for individuals who cannot achieve voluntary control of the stimulated muscles.

The anticipated potential long-term benefits remain speculative, and even if some benefits can be measured in the future, it appears they fall into the category of prophylactic health management. Given the relatively expensive technology involved in NMES fitness programs, the individual's requirement of time and resources for the regular exercise, and the need for health care monitoring of a patient's progress, it appears that this aspect of NMES will remain in restricted use. Unless radical changes are made in how health care is delivered, the high cost and poorly documented outcome benefits are likely to leave NMES fitness programs open to the discretion of the individual. Just as the able-bodied person may choose to purchase a membership in a health club in order to facilitate his or her continued physical fitness, the individual with a disability seeking the potential fitness benefits from NMES is nearly always obliged to pay his own way.

# Summary

Electrical stimulation has been used to enhance a wide variety of treatment goals with a large measure of success. ES is, however, one of a number of tools that the physical therapist brings to resolve problems impeding the function of an individual. While NMES can be used to reduce joint contracture, to facilitate and reeducate voluntary motor control, to reduce the effects of spasticity or to provide a dynamic orthosis, it is generally not the only technique that can meet the patient's need. Treatment goals should be agreed upon by the physical therapist and patient, and NMES can then be judiciously applied to enhance the attainment of specific goals. Electrical stimulation can be used as an extension of therapy hours or as a means of achieving a goal more quickly. The general guidelines provided here must be fit into the context of the individual's total treatment program, always with an eye to achieving optimal function.

NMES has been found to be an effective tool in treatment programs aimed at reducing soft tissue joint contractures. The NMES treatment programs incorporate some aspects of both low-load, prolonged stretching techniques and high-load, brief stretching techniques, while maintaining the efficient use of therapist time. NMES has also been found to effectively maintain joint ROM in the presence of spasticity and, under some circumstances, may be more efficient in doing so than the traditional passive ROM programs.

Stimulation for the enhancement of motor control, whether it is called a facilitation technique or a muscle reeducation program, provides a tremendous amount of sensory information to the CNS through a variety of sensory modalities and afferent pathways, for both automatic and conscious processing. As such, NMES is an extremely powerful tool in programs designed to enhance voluntary control. In addition, NMES can be incorporated into almost any traditional facilitation technique to further enhance a patient's motor control.

The application of NMES to spasticity management programs is the least understood. Because of the lack of clear neurophysiologic rationale, no one set of stimulus characteristics will ensure success with all patients. However, stimulation of either the spastic muscle or its antagonist will result in decreased spasticity, that interferes with function for many patients. Stimulation, however, is an effective tool only when the NMES program is immediately incorporated into other treatments; NMES is not a means of spasticity management for long periods of time. Other, more speculative treatment options, most appropriately used when an individual displays a general increase in muscle tone (firmness), were also discussed.

The final, and most volatile, use of NMES includes orthotic substitution—true functional electrical stimulation. This use of ES continues to be an extremely active research area, but is beginning to impact the daily lives of selected patient populations, and as such will require skilled management by more and more clinicians. The advent of the fully implanted stimulation system makes FES a viable long-term orthosis, and the rehabilitation practioner will be called on for both preimplant muscle strengthening and postimplant functional training. As fully implanted systems expand to include applications beyond the present upper extremity system, more and more clinicians will be involved in both short-term and long-term problem solving, using electrical stimulation to decrease functional impairments and disabilities.

## CASE STUDY

### HEMIPARESIS 2° CVA

Dr. RS experienced a severe right cerebrovascular accident (CVA) 7 weeks before admission to rehabilitation, resulting in a dense hemiparesis in the left upper and lower extremities, with minimal left side neglect. The patient is very self-aware and articulate. Rehabilitation was delayed because of the patient's location at the time of the stroke; Dr. RS was in Africa in the Foreign Service for the U.S. government. He was evacuated to a military hospital in Germany and later air-lifted back to the States.

Dr. RS now presents to inpatient rehabilitation with poor standing balance, and the inability to approximate his left foot to the floor, because of apparent hip flexion and hamstring muscles spasticity. These two problems have led to a need for moderate assistance in all transfer activities and an inability to ambulate. The patient is currently using a wheelchair for all ambulation activities. Upright motor control cannot be accomplished, because of the patient's inability to bear weight on the left lower extremity. Testing of lower extremity motor control in the side-lying position demonstrates patterned movements of the hip and knee, with minimal activity at the ankle. Flexion responses are stronger than extension. Spasticity, as measured on the Ashworth scale, is 2+ to 3 in flexors and extensors throughout the limb, with clonus noted in the plantar flexors. Assessment of ROM reveals a 15° hip flexion contracture, and 20° knee flexion and ankle plantar flexion contractures, all with soft-tissue end-feels.

An attempt was made to reduce the knee and ankle plantar flexion contractures through the application of a splint at night. After use of the splint for two nights, however, the patient experienced pain, swelling and erythema at his knee, precluding its continued use. The splint was cut down to include only the ankle, and the patient was started on an aggressive ROM stimulation program to address the knee flexion contracture. Because of difficulty sleeping, this program was done during the day, while the ankle splint continued to be used at night. The patient also wore a rigid ankle foot orthosis (AFO) during the day. During the first week of the NMES ROM program, the patient participated in one 30-minute session of stimulation to the quadriceps muscles while standing in a supported standing frame, with an additional one or two 30-minute sessions worked into his treatment day. While standing, Dr. RS was engaged in additional upper extremity activities, including general limb placement exercises and developing weight-bearing capabilities. The two additional stimulation sessions were done at lunchtime and at the end of the therapeutic day, while the patient was seated in his wheelchair with the left leg on an elevated leg rest. The quality of the stimulated contraction was sufficient to extend the knee from 60° of flexion through the full available extension range, with the AFO and shoe in place (3+/5). Dr. RS was capable of directing the nursing staff in the removal of the stimulation system after the final treatment session.

Over a 10-day treatment, Dr. RS demonstrated decreased knee flexion contracture, so that neutral extension was achieved. The ankle plantar flexion contracture was also reduced to 5° through the use of the splint and AFO. As a more stable base of support was achieved through contracture reduction, the demand in the upright posture was gradually increased by moving from the standing frame to parallel bars and eventually to the support of a four-point cane. Dynamic weight shifting, side to side and front to back, were instituted early in the upright ROM program, progressing to a facilitation/gait-training activity as the knee and plantar flexion contractures were reduced. A hand switch, controlled by the physical therapist, was used to activate stimulation during more dynamic activities. As Dr. RS progressed from the parallel bars to the cane, a second channel of stimulation was added to the hip extensors, as a reminder to maintain an upright posture. The quality of the stimulated hip extension contraction never achieved a 3/5 level, but the strong sensory cue was sufficient to elicit voluntary activation of the hip and back extensors in order to attain the desired trunk position.

**CASE STUDY** *continued*

As Dr. RS became more functional in the upright position, he was able to decrease the assistance required for transfers to stand-by and eventually to modified independent. Gait activities were limited to therapy sessions, but he was able to walk 50 feet with stand-by assist before his discharge from in-patient at 3 weeks. At discharge, the hip flexion contracture was measured to be 10°, although no specific therapy targeted this joint for ROM, and both the knee and ankle were able to extend to neutral. Upright motor control was moderate to weak in extension, and moderate into flexion. The patient persisted in patterned movements in the upright position, although some selective hip and knee movement were evident in less demanding postures.

This case is presented as an example of a dynamic and multifaceted NMES approach to multiple problems presented by the complex patient. The transition from the ROM program to an aggressive facilitation activity occurred based on the patient's own capabilities. To ensure the continued success of the range program, the two more passive stimulation sessions were maintained until the desired joint range was securely achieved. The active flow from one treatment goal to the next challenge is typical of all good therapy programs, but is too often lacking in the integration of NMES into those programs. As Dr. RS progressed during outpatient rehabilitation, NMES was continued for assistance in achieving an upright posture. During this sequence, however, stimulation levels were gradually decreased, and a diminishing frequency of activation was used as the patient successfully achieved the dynamics of more normal gait. Only one or two muscles were targeted for activation by NMES, recognizing the limitations of most practicing clinicians within the busy treatment environment. Up to eight channels of stimulation have been shown to be effective for the enhancement of hemiparetic gait. Clinical reality, however, dictates choosing one or two key muscle groups to ensure adequate management in order to achieve target goals, and to maintain both patient and therapist tolerance.

# REVIEW QUESTIONS

1. Compare and contrast the NMES management of the following patients:
   a. A 15-year-old with an elbow flexion contracture

   b. A 15-year-old with a plantar flexion contracture
   c. A 55-year-old with a healed Colles' fracture
2. Compare and contrast the NMES management of the following patients:
   a. A 65-year-old with a total knee arthroplasty done yesterday
   b. A 65-year-old individual status post left CVA, with an unstable lower limb
   c. A 24-year-old with a recent anterior cruciate ligament (ACL) repair
3. Discuss the rationale, both physiologic and anatomic, for developing an NMES program to reduce shoulder subluxation in a patient status post CVA. Describe the optimal patient profile for this treatment.

   Would this be an effective intervention for a patient with a high cervical spinal cord injury?

   Would this be an effective treatment for an active volleyball player who periodically experiences recurrent shoulder subluxation? Why or why not?
4. Discuss the key elements in a successful spasticity management NMES program. Include both the stimulus characteristics and patient profile in your answer. Identify the limitations, as well as the strong points, of such a program.
5. Describe the multifaceted use of electrical stimulation interventions for a patient who had a total knee arthroplasty yesterday. Include *all* appropriate stimulation interventions, not just neuromuscular programs. Identify how you would progress this patient through the various applications you identify, including the goal and expected time frame to achieve each goal. (*Hint:* there are at least four different goals that can be augmented through the use of ES.)

## References

1. McNeal DR. 2000 years of electrical stimulation. In Hambrecht FT. Beswick JB eds. Functional Electrical Stimulation: Application in Neural Prosthetics. New York, NY, Marcel Dekker, pp 3–35, 1977.
2. Baker LL, McNeal DR, Benton LA, Bowman BR, Waters RL. Neuro-Muscular Electrical Stimulation—A Practical Guide (3rd ed). Downey, CA, Los Amigos Research & Education Institute, 1993.
3. Section on Clinical Electrophysiology. Electrotherapeutic Terminology in Physical Therapy. American Physical Therapy Association, 1990.
4. Baker LL, Yeh C, Wilson D, Waters RL. Electrical stimulation of wrist and fingers for hemiplegic patients. Phys Ther, 59:1495–1499, 1979.
5. Waters RL, Bowman BR. Multicenter functional electrical stimulation evaluation for contracture prevention and correction. Final report to the Veteran Administration, No V790, p1441, Washington, DC, 1981.

6. Gotlin RS, Hershkowitz S, Juris PM, Gonzalez EG, Scott WN, Insall JN. Electrical stimulaiton effect on extensor lag and length of hospital stay after total knee arthroplasty. Arch Phys Med Rehabil, 75:957–959, 1994.

7. Haug J, Wood LT. Efficacy of neuromuscular stimulation of the quadriceps femoris during continuous passive motion following total knee arthroplasty. Arch Phys Med Rehabil, 69:423–424, 1988.

8. Rizk TE, Park SJ: Transcutaneous electrical nerve stimulation and extensor splint in linear scleroderma knee contracture. Arch Phys Med Rehabil 62:86–88, 1981.

9. Zizic TM, Hoffman KC, Holt PA et al. The treatment of osteoarthritis of the knee with pulsed electrical sitmulation. J Rheum 22:1757–1761, 1995.

10. Young A. Current issues in arthrogenous inhibition. Ann Rheum Dis, 52:829–834, 1993.

11. Munsat TL, McNeal D, Waters R. Effects of nerve stimulation on human muscle. Arch Neurol, 33:608–617, 1976.

12. Hazlewood ME, Brown JK, Rowe PJ, Salter PM. The use of therapeutic electrical stimulation in the treatment of hemiplegic cerebral palsy. Develop Med Child Neuro, 36:661–673, 1994.

13. Light KE, Nuxik S, Personius W, Barstrom A. Low-load prolonged stretch vs. high-load brief stretch in treating knee contractures. Phys Ther, 64:330, 1984.

14. Mizliah J, Naumann S, While C et al. Electrostimulation as a means of decreasing knee flexion contractures in children with spina bifida. Proc Rehabil Eng Soc North Am, 6:63–65, 1983.

15. Baker LL, Parker K, Sanderson D. Neuromuscular electrical stimulation for the head-injured patient. Phys Ther, 63:1967–1974, 1983.

16. Trimble MH, Enoka RM: Mechanisms underlying the training effects associated with neuromuscular electrical stimulation. Phys Ther, 71:273–282, 1991.

17. Delitto A, Rose SJ, McKowen JM et al. Electrical stimulation versus voluntary exercise in strengthening thigh musculature after anterior curcuate ligament surgery. Phys Ther, 68:660–663, 1988.

18. Eriksson E, Haggmark T. Comparison of isometric training and electircal stimulation supplementing isometric muscle training in the recovery after major knee ligament surgery. Am J Sports Med, 7:169–171, 1979.

19. Godfrey CM, Jayawardena H, Quance TA, Welsh P. Comparison of electro-stimulation and isometric exercise in strengthening the quadriceps muscle. Physiotherapy (Canada), 31:265–267, 1979.

20. Jensen JE, Conn RR, Hazelrigg G, Hewett JE. The use of transcutaneous neural stimulation and isokinetic testing in arthroscopic knee surgery. Am J Sports Med, 13:27–33, 1985.

21. Johnson DH, Thurston P, Ashcroft PJ. The Russian technique of faradism in the treatment of chondromalacia patellae. Physiotherapy (Canada), 29:266–268, 1977.

22. Hainaut K, Duchateau J: Neuromuscular electrical stimulation and voluntary exercise. Sports Med, 14:100–113, 1992.

23. Snyder-Mackler L, Delitto A, Bailey SL, Stralka SW. Strength of the quadriceps femoris muscle and functional recovery after reconstruc-

tion of the anterior cruciate ligament. A prospective, randomized clinical trial of electrical stimulation. J Bone Joint Surg, (A) 77:1166–1173, 1995.

24. DeMaio M, Mangine RE, Noyes FR, Barber SD. Advanced muscle training after ACL reconstruction: weeks 6 to 52. Orthoped 15:757–767, 1992.

25. Binder-Macleod SA, Lee SC. Assessment of the efficacy of functional electrical stimulation in patients with hemiplegia. Top Stroke Rehabil, 3:88–98, 1997.

26. Bogataj U, Gros N, Kljajic M et al. The rehabilitation of gait in patients with hemiplegia: a comparison between conventional therapy and multichannel functional electrical stimulation therapy. Phys Ther, 75:490–502, 1995.

27. Bogataj U, Gros N, Malezic M et al. Restoration of gait during two to three weeks of therapy with multichannel electrical stimulation. Phys Ther, 69:319–327, 1989.

28. Bowman BR, Baker LL, Waters RL. Positional feedback and electrical stimulation: An automated treatment for the hemiplegic wrist. Arch Phys Med Rehabil, 60:497–502, 1979.

29. Cozean CD, Pease WS, Hubbell SL. Biofeedback and functional electric stimulation in stroke rehabilitation. Arch Phys Med Rehabil, 69:401–405, 1988.

30. Dimitrijevic MM. Mesh-glove I. A method for whole-hand electrical stimulation in upper motor neuron dysfunction. Scand J Rehab Med, 26:183–186, 1994.

31. Dimitrijevic MM, Stokic DS, Wawro AW, Wun CC. Modification of motor control of wrist extension by mesh-glove electrical afferent stimulation in stroke patients. Arch Phys Med Rehabil, 77:252–258, 1996.

32. Fields RW. Electromyographically triggered electric muscle stimulation for chronic hemiplegia. Arch Phys Med Rehabil, 68:407–414, 1987.

33. Granat HM, Ferguson ACB, Andrews BJ, Delargy M. The role of functional electrical stimulation in the rehabilitation of patients with incomplete spinal cord injury—observed benefits during gait studies. Para 31:207–215, 1993.

34. Hesse S, Malezic M, Schaffrin A, Mauritz K-H. Restoration of gait by combined treadmill training and multichannel electrical stimulation in non-ambulatory hemiparetic patients. Scand J Rehab Med, 27:199–204, 1995.

35. Kraft GH, Fitts SS, Hammond MC. Techniques to improve function of the arm and hand in chronic hemiplegia. Arch Phys Med Rehabil, 73:220–227, 1992.

36. Kralj A, Acimovic R, Stanic U. Enhancement of hemiplegic patient rehabilitation by means of functional electrical stimulation. Prosth Ortho Int, 17:107–114, 1993.

37. Mahdad M, Baker LL. Effect of electrical stimulation on recruitment of motor units in patients with hemiparesis. Phys Ther, 77:S17–S18, 1997.

38. Malezic M, Hesse S, Schewe H, Mauritz K. Restoration of standing, weight-shift and gait by multichannel electrical stimulation in hemiparetic patients. Int J Rehabil Res, 17:169–179, 1994.

39. Merletti R, Zelaschi F, Latella D et al. A controlled study of muscle force recovery in hemiparetic patients during treatment with functional electrical sitmulation. Scand J Rehabil Med, 10:147–154, 1978.

40. Smith LE. Restoration of volitional limb movement of hemiplegics following patterned functional electrical stimulation. Percept Motor Skills, 71:851–861, 1990.

41. Waters RL. The enigma of "carry-over." Int Rehabil Med, 6:9–12, 1984.

42. Rutherford OM, Jones DA, Newton DJ. Clinical and experimental application of the percutaneous twitch superimposition technique for the study of human muscle activation. J Neurol Neurosurg Psych, 49:1288–1291, 1986.

43. Moritani T, DeVries HA. Neural factors versus hypertrophy in the time course of muscle strength gain. Am J Phys Med, 58:115–122, 1979.

44. Adbel-Moty E, Fishbain DA, Goldberg M et al. Functional electrical stimulation treatment of postradiculopathy associated muscle weakness. Arch Phys Med Rehabil, 75:680–686, 1994.

45. Weinstein MV, Gordon A. The use of faradism in the rehabilitation of hemiplegics. Phys Ther Rev, 31:515–521,1951.

46. Carmick J. Clinical use of neuromuscular electrical stimulation for children with cerebral palsy. Part 1: Lower extremity. Phys Ther, 73:505–513, 1993.

47. Carmick J. Managing equinus in children with cerebral palsy: electrical stimulation to strengthen the triceps surae muscle. Develop Med Child Neurol, 37:965–975, 1995.

48. Carmick J. Guidelines for the clinical application of neuromuscular eleectrical stimulation (NMES) for children with cerebral palsy—Clinical Perspective. Pediat Phys Ther, 9:128–136. 1997.

49. Comeaux P, Patterson N, Rubin M, Meiner R. Effect of neuromuscular electrical stimulation during giat in children with cerebral palsy. Pediatr Phys Ther, 9:103–109, 1997.

50. Wilson DJ, Baker LL, Craddock JA. Functional test for the hemiparetic upper extremity. Am J Occup Ther, 38:159–164, 1984.

51. Baker LL. Positional feedback stimulation training—An update. Proceedings of 2nd Post-graduate Course of Restorative Neurology, Department of Neurology, University Malano, Italy, 1990.

52. Baker LL, Parker K. Neuromuscular electrical stimulation of the muscles surrounding the shoulder. Phys Ther, 66:1930–1937, 1986.

53. Faghri PD, Rodgers MM, Glaser RM et al. The effects of functional electrical sitmulation on shoulder subluxation, arm function recovery, and shoulder pain in hemiplegic stroke patients. Arch Phys Med Rehabil, 75:73–79, 1994.

54. Braus DF, Krauss JK, Strobel J. The shoulder–hand syndrome after stroke: a prospective clinical trial. Ann Neurol, 36:728–733, 1994.

55. Zorowitz RD, Idank D, Idai T et al. Shoulder subluxation after stroke: A comparison of four supports. Arch Phys Med Rehabil, 76:763–771, 1995.

56. Vallar G, Rusconi ML, Barozzi S et al. Improvement of left visuo-spatial hemineglect by left-sided transcutaneous electrical stimulation. Neuropsychol, 33:73–82, 1995.

57. Karnath HO. Transcutaneous electrical stimulation and vibration of neck muscles in neglect. Exp Brain Res, 105:321–324, 1995.
58. Carmick J. Clinical use of neuromuscular electrical stimulation for children with cerebral palsy. Part 2: Upper extremity. Phys Ther, 73:514–527, 1993.
59. Carroll SG, Bird SF, Brown DJ. Electrical stimulation of the lumbrical muscles in an incomple quadriplegic patient: Case report. Paraplegia, 30:223–226, 1992.
60. Han JS, Chen XH, Yuan Y, Yan SC. Transcutaneous electrical nerve stimulation for treatment of spinal spasticity. Chinese Med J, 107:6–11, 1994.
61. Yu Y: Transcutaneous electric stimulation at acupoints in the treatment of spinal spasticity: Effects and mechanism. Chinese Med J, 73:593–595, 637, 1993.
62. Halstead LS, Seager SW, Houston JM et al. Relief of spasticity in SCI men and women using rectal probe electrostimulaiton. Paraplegia, 31:715–721, 1993.
63. Dimitrijevic MR, Nathan PW. Studies of spasticity in man. 4. Changes in flexion reflex with repetitive cuntaneous stimulation in spinal man. Brain, 93:743–768, 1970.
64. Dimitrijevic MR, Nathan PW. Studies of spasticity in man. 5. Dishabituation of the flexion reflex in spinal man. Brain, 94:77–90, 1971.
65. Walker JB. Modulation of spasticity: Prolonged suppression of a spinal reflex by electrical stimulation. Science, 216:203–204, 1982.
66. Levine MG, Knott M, Kabat H. Relaxation of spasticity by electrical stimulation of antagonist muscles. Arch Phys Med, 33:668–673, 1952.
67. Seib TP, Price R, Reyes MR, Lehmann JF. The quantitative measurement of spasticity: Effect of cutaneous electrical stimulation. Arch Phys Med Rehabil, 75:746–750, 1994.
68. Alfieri V. Electrical treatment of spasticity—Reflex tonic activity in hemiplegic patients and selected specific electrostimulation. Scand J Rehab Med, 14:177–182, 1982.
69. Carnstam B, Larsson LE. Electrical stimulation in patients with spasticity. Electroencephalogr Clin Neurophysiol Soc Proc, 38:214, 1975.
70. Apkarian JA, Naumann S. Stretch reflex inhibition using electrical stimulaiton in normal subjects and subjects with spasticity. J Biomed Eng, 13:67–73, 1991.
71. Hines AE, Crago PE, Billian C. Functional electrical stimulation for the reduction of spasticity in the hemiplegic hand. Biomed Sci Instrument, 29:259–266, 1993.
72. Katz RT. Management of spasticity. Am J Phys Med Rehabil, 67:108–116, 1988.
73. Robinson CJ, Kett NA, Bolam JM. Spasticity in spinal cord injured patients: 1. Short-term effects of surface electrical stimulation. Arch Phys Med Rehabil, 69:598–604, 1988.
74. Liberson WT. Experiment concerning reciprocal inhibitions of antagonists elicited by electrical stimulation of agonists in a normal individual. Am J Phys Med, 44:306–308, 1965.

75. Tan V, Agar A, Marangoz C. Decreased post-tetanic potentiation of monosynaptic reflexes by simultaneous tetanization of antagonist nerves. Exp Brain Res, 31:499–510, 1978.

76. Lee WJ, McGovern JP, Duvall EN. Cutaneous tetanizing (low voltage) currents for relief of spasm. Arch Phys Med Rehabil, 31:766–771, 1950.

77. Bowman B, Bajd T. Influence of electrical stimulation on skeletal muscle spasticity. Proc Intern Symp External Control Human Extremities. Belgrade, Yugoslavia, Committee for Electronics and Automation, pp 561–576, 1981.

78. Vodovnik L, Bowman BR, Hufford P. Effects of electrical stimulaiton on spinal spasticity. Scand J Rehabil Med, 16:29–34, 1984.

79. Pierrot-Deseilligny E, Morin C, Katz R, Bussell B. Influence of voluntary movement and posture on recurrent inhibition in human subjects. Brain Res, 124:427–436, 1977.

80. Eccles JC, McIntrye AK. The effects of disuse and of activity on mammalian spinal reflexes. J Physiol (Lond) 121:492–499, 1953.

81. Vodovnik L. Indirect spinal cord stimulation—Some engineering viewpoints. Appl Neurophysiol, 44:97–113, 1981.

82. Haynes CM. Elementary Principles of Electro-therapeutics for the Use of Physicians and Students. McIntosh Galvanic & Faradic Battery Co, Chicago, IL, pp 384–395, 402, 1884.

83. Keith MW, Kilgore KL, Peckham PH et al. Tendon transfers and functional electrical stimulation for restoration of hand function in spinal cord injury. J Hand Surg (Am), 21:89–99, 1996.

84. Keith MW, Peckham PH, Thrope GB, et al. Implantable functional neuromusuclar stimulation in the tetraplegic hand: A case report. J Hand Surg, 14A:524–530, 1988.

85. Peckham PH, Marsolais EB, Mortimer JT. Restoration of key grip and release in the tetraplegic patient though functional electrical stimulation. J Hand Surg, 5:462–469, 1980.

86. Alon G, Dar A, Katz-Behiri D et al. Survivors of CVA and head injury can improve selected impairments and functional measures following training with the NESS NMES system. Phys Ther (suppl), 77:S84 1997.

87. Jonkey BW. Upper extremity FES—Evaluation of control signals. Master's Project, Department Physical Therapy, University Southern California, 1979.

88. Zorowitz RD, Hughes MB, Idank D et al. Shoulder pain and subluxation after stroke: Correlation or coincidence? Am J Occup Ther, 50:194–201, 1996.

89. Pinzur MS, Hopkins GE. Biceps tenodesis for painful inferior subluxation of the shoulder in adult acquired hemiplegia. Clin Ortho Related Res, 206:100–103, 1986.

90. Basmajian JV Factors preventing downward dislocation of the adducted shoulder joint. J Bone Joint Surg, 41A:1182–1186, 1959.

91. Chang JJ, Tsau JC, Lin YT. Predictors of shoulder subluxation in stroke patients. Koahsiung J Med Sci, 11:250–256, 1995.

92. Culham EG, Noce RR, Bagg SD. Shoulder complex position and glenohumeral subluxation in hemiplegia. Arch Phys Med Rehabil, 76: 857–864, 1995.

93. Petrofsky JS, Phillips CA, Heaton HH. Feedback control system for walking in man. Comp Biol Med, 14:135–149, 1984.

94. Gardner ER, Baker LL. Functional electrical stimulation of paralytic muscle. In Nelson R, Currier D (eds), Excitable and Connective Tissue: Recent Advances/Clinical Concepts. Philadelphia, PA, FA Davis, pp 182–204, 1992.

95. Gallien P, Brissot R, Eyssette M et al. Restoration of gait by functional electrical stimulation for spinal cord injured patients. Paraplegia, 33:660–664, 1995.

96. Graupe D, Kordylewski H. Artifical neural network control of FES in paraplegics for patient responsive ambulation. IEEE Trans Biomed Eng, 42:699–707, 1995.

97. Durfee WK. Control of standing and gait using electrical stimulation: Influence of muscle model complexity on control strategy. Prog Brain Res, 97:369–381, 1993.

98. Flaherty B, Robinson C, Agarwal G. Determining appropriate models for joint control using surface electrical stimulation of soleus in spinal cord injury. Med Biol Eng Comput, 32:273–282, 1994.

99. Solomonow M, King A, Shoji J, D'Ambrosia R. External control of rate, recruitment, synergy and feedback in paralyzed extremities. Orthopedics, 7:1161–1172, 1984.

100. Gordon T, Mao J. Muscle atrophy and procedures for training after spinal cord injury. Phys Ther, 74:50–60, 1994.

101. Greve JM, Muszkat R, Schmidt B et al. Functional electrical stimulation (FES): Muscle histochemical analysis. Paraplegia, 31:764–770, 1993.

102. Rabischong E, Ohanna F. Effects of functional electrical stimulation (FES) on evoked muscle output in paraplegic quadriceps muscles. Paraplegia, 30:467–473, 1992.

103. Isakov E, Douglas R, Berns P. Ambulation using the reciprocating gait orthosis and functional electrical stimulation. Paraplegia, 30:239–245, 1992.

104. Nene AV. Energy cost of paraplegic locomotion. Arch Phys Med Rehabil, 71:116–120, 1990.

105. Winchester P, Carollo JJ, Habasevich R. Physiologic costs of reciprocal gait in FES assisted walking. Paraplegia, 32:680–686, 1994.

106. Bajd T, Kralj A, Sega J et al. Use of a two-channel functional electrical stimulator to stand paraplegic patients. Phys Ther, 61:526–527, 1981.

107. Kagaya H, Shimada Y, Ebata K et al. Restoration and analysis of standing up in complete paraplegia utilizing functional electrical stimulation. Arch Phys Med Rehabil, 76:876–818, 1995.

108. Kralj AR, Bajd T, Munih M, Turk R. FES gait restoration and balance control in spinal cord-injured patients. Prog Brain Res, 97:387–396, 1993.

109. Peckham PH, Mortimer JT, Marsolais EB. Alteration in the force and fatigability of skeletal muscle in quadriplegic humans following exercise induced by chronic electrical stimulation. Clin Orthop, 114:326–334, 1976.

110. Taylor PN, Ewins DJ, Fox B et al. Limb blood flow, cardiac output and quadriceps muscle bulk following spinal cord injury and the effect of

training for the Odstock functional electrical stimulation standing system. Paraplegia, 31:303–310, 1993.

111. Barstow TJ, Scremin AM, Mutton DL et al. Gas exchange kinetics during functional electrical stimulation in subjects with spinal cord injury. Med Sci Sports Exer, 27:1284–1291, 1995.

112. Bremner LA, Sloan KE, Day RE et al. A clinical exercise system for paraplegics using functional electrical stimulation. Paraplegia, 30: 647–655, 1992.

113. Faghri PD, Glaser RM, Figoni SF. Functional electrical stimulation leg cycling ergometer exercise: Training effects of cardiorespiratory responses of spinal cord injured subjects at rest and during submaximal exercise. Arch Phys Med Rehabil, 73:1085–1093, 1992.

114. Figoni SF, Glaser RM, Rodgers MM et al. Acute hemodynamic responses of spinal cord injured individuals to functional neuromuscular stimulation-induced knee extension exercise. J Rehabil Res Dev, 28:9–18, 1991.

115. Hooker SP, Figoni SF, Rodgers MM et al. Metabolic and hemodynamic responses to concurrent voluntary arm crank and electrical stimulation leg cycle exercise in quadriplegics. J Rehabil Res Dev, 29:1–11, 1992.

116. Krauss JC, Robergs RA, Depaepe JL et al. Effects of electrical stimulation and upper body training after spinal cord injury. Med Sci Sports Exer, 25:1054–1061, 1993.

117. Laskin JJ, Ashley EA, Olenik LM et al. Electrical stimulation–assisted rowing exercise in spinal cord injured people. A pilot study. Paraplegia, 31:534–541, 1993.

118. Ragnarsson KT. Physiologic effects of functional electrical stimulation induced exercises in spinal cord injured individuals. Clin Ortho Rel Res, 233:53–63, 1988.

119. Sipski ML, Alexander CJ, Harris M. Long-term use of computerized bicycle regometry for spinal cord injured subjects. Arch Phys Med Rehabil, 74:238–241, 1993.

120. Sloan KE, Bremner LA, Byrne J et al. Musculoskeletal effects of an electrical stimulation induced cycling programme in the spinal injured. Paraplegia, 32:407–415, 1994.

121. Glaser RM. An evolution of exercise physiology: Effects of exercise on functional independence with aging and physical disabilities—Guest editorial. J Rehabil Res Dev, 34:vi–viii, 1997.

122. BeDell KK, Scremin AME, Perell KL, Kinkel CF. Effects of functional electrical sitmulation–induced lower extremity cycling on bone density of spinal cord–injured patients. Am J Phys Med Rehabil, 75:29–34, 1996.

123. Hangartner TN, Rodgers MM, Glaser RM, Barre PS. Tibial bone density loss in spinal cord injured patients: Effects of FES exercise. J Rehabil Res Dev, 31:50–61, 1994.

124. Bradley MB. The effect of participating in a functional electrical stimulation exercise program on affect in people with spinal cord injuries. Arch Phys Med Rehabil, 75:676–679, 1994.

# 9

# Electrical Stimulation of Denervated Muscle

Neil I. Spielholz

## Introduction

n 1841, Reid reported beneficial effects of electrical stimulation (ES) of denervated muscle.[54] Over the ensuing 150 years, however, so much controversy has developed that even today, there is a question concerning the clinical utility of this procedure. This chapter will review evidence for benefits and for deleterious effects; will discuss how and if the evidence relates to the clinical situations that physical therapists are involved with, namely, human denervated muscle; and will end with some recommendations for future research. To begin, though, a brief synopsis of neuromuscular anatomy and how it relates to the phenomenon of denervation is in order, as is a description of how muscles can become reinnervated if they lose their nerve supply.

## THE MOTOR UNIT

The basic functional component of skeletal muscle is the **motor unit.** This is composed of an alpha anterior horn cell and all the muscle fibers it innervates.[43] A whole muscle is an assemblage of such units.

Different muscles have different numbers of motor units. Depending on the technique(s) used and the assumptions made, numbers reported have ranged from about 100 to over 2000 (although the latter figure may be an overestimation).[15,27,47,48] In addition, the number of muscle fibers in these different units also varies, depending in part on the finesse of the movements the muscle performs. For example, external ocular muscles, the tongue, or muscles innervated by the facial nerve (the muscles of expression) tend to have motor units with relatively few fibers innervated per axon. This low motor unit ratio, in conjunction with other physiologic mechanisms, presumably accounts for how the central nervous system (CNS) can finely gradate the strength of their contractions. Conversely, high motor unit ratios (ie, motor units with hundreds, perhaps thousands, of muscle fibers innervated by a single axon) are found in muscles where exceptionally fine control is not needed. In any one muscle, however, there is a population of motor units of different sizes.

## THE DENERVATED MOTOR UNIT

From the foregoing description of a motor unit, it is apparent that if a single motor axon degenerates, all the muscle fibers innervated by it become denervated. In this hypothetical situation, all other axons, and therefore all their muscle fibers, remain innervated and functioning. In clinical terms, this muscle would be classified as partially denervated. The term **partial denervation** refers to the state of the whole muscle, not the individual muscle fibers. The term means that some muscle fibers—in this case, all the muscle fibers of a single motor unit—have lost their nerve supply, while other muscle fibers remain innervated normally. The denervated muscle fibers are, of course, completely denervated. By itself, the term partial denervation does not indicate how many motor units, or what percentage of motor units in the muscle, have been lost to voluntary control. Furthermore, denervation of a small percentage of motor units in a muscle may not even be noticed clinically.

The term **complete denervation** means that every motor unit in a muscle has lost its motor axon. Clinically, this muscle is paralyzed.

## THE DENERVATED MUSCLE

Let us now turn our attention from the motor unit to the whole muscle and consider the consequences of complete denervation which occurs acutely (such as sectioning of a mixed peripheral nerve).

The first and most obvious consequence is loss of voluntary control of the muscles innervated by the nerve. Paralysis commences immediately. If a sensory examination can also be performed, sensation would be found missing in the appropriate distribution.

Within the ensuing weeks and months, atrophy of the paralyzed muscles becomes apparent, and unless proper steps are taken, joint contractures can occur. Changes in the skin's texture and temperature, usually in the nerve's sensory distribution, may also be noted. If a hand or a foot is affected, swelling of the dependent part is frequent. Some of the changes that occur in denervated muscle are discussed in more detail next.

## Atrophy, Degeneration, and Fibrosis

**Atrophy** is a wasting away, or diminution in size, of a cell, organ, or body part. When we speak of muscle atrophy, the clinical picture that comes to mind is that of a shrunken or wasted muscle. As a result of muscle atrophy, the contour of the affected part flattens (may even appear "scooped out") and adjacent bony structures become more prominent. What are the microscopic changes that produce these macroscopic features?

When denervated muscle atrophies, the individual muscle fibers become progressively thinner. This thinness of the fibers results from each one losing myofibrils (see Chapter 1). As a result of muscle fibers becoming thinner, the weight of the muscle decreases rapidly during the first 3 months and then slows (Figure 9–1). A sort of *steady state* is achieved after about 6 to 9 months.[32] Similarly, the maximal tetanic tension that denervated rat muscle can develop (in terms of percent-of-control side) drops exponentially during the first 3 to 4 months, but then also reaches an *equilibrium* level. After 10 months, this value has been determined as about 0.75 percent for

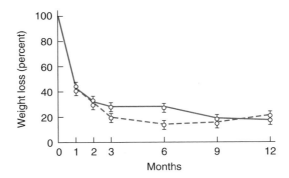

FIGURE 9–1. Percentage loss of weight in the extensor digitorum longus (solid line) and the soleus (interrupted line) muscles in the rat. Abscissa: months after denervation. *(From Gutmann E, Zelena J. Morphological changes in the denervated muscle. In Gutmann E [ed], Denervated Muscle. Prague, Publishing House of the Czechoslovak Academy of Sciences, 1962, with permission.)*

the extensor digitorum longus, and 0.2 to 0.3 percent for the soleus muscles.[3] Therefore, the loss in the ability of the muscle to develop tension far exceeds the loss of weight.

The difference between a denervated muscle's weight loss and its ability to develop tension is not surprising. A muscle's weight reflects not only the size and number of its muscle fibers, but also its connective tissue, blood vessels, and other structural components.[60] Histologically, as muscle fibers atrophy, the proportion of connective tissue (primarily collagen) making up the whole muscle increases. As time goes by, there may also be an actual increase in the amount of collagen as well. Therefore, muscle weight is not as good an index of muscle atrophy as actually measuring fiber diameters[60] or determining the muscle's ability to develop tension.[3]

Furthermore, should the amount of collagen in a denervated muscle increase, the condition known as **fibrosis** ensues. Fibrosis can impede—if not prevent—reinnervation,[31] and might even impair the coordinated activity of groups of muscle fibers.[2] This fibrosis is a condition to be avoided, if possible.

The clinician should also note that during the first few weeks or months following denervation, type II fibers atrophy more than type I fibers (Figure 9–2). The reason(s) for this is not yet known.

Degeneration of muscle fibers is a second major occurrence that must be prevented, or at least retarded. When a muscle fiber degenerates, it is no longer a muscle fiber. The fiber has ceased to be. The muscle fiber is replaced by fibrous tissue, which contributes to the fibrosis described above.[62] If muscle fibers degenerate before a nerve regenerates to them, there is nothing for the nerve to reinnervate. The nerve regeneration now serves no purpose. From the preceding description, muscle degeneration and fibrosis are clearly the real enemies, not simply atrophy. An atrophic muscle fiber, as long as it remains a muscle fiber, is capable of undergoing hypertrophy after it is reinnervated. The race then, so to speak, is between nerve regrowth on one hand and muscle fiber degeneration and fibrosis on the other. Two questions may therefore be legitimate to ask: "How long does it take before degeneration and fibrosis of denervated muscle occurs?," and "Can steps be taken to prevent, or at least retard, degeneration and fibrosis?"

Not surprisingly, there is no unanimity of opinion concerning ultimate degeneration of denervated muscle fibers. Some investigators have reported considerable degeneration within a relatively short time,[1,2,5,17,62] whereas others have reported minimal, if any, at least within the first 1 to 2 years.[10,61] The discrepancy in these findings, however, may relate to the second question mentioned above. If appropriate care is given to the denervated muscles, they remain muscle for longer periods of time. For example, denervated muscle

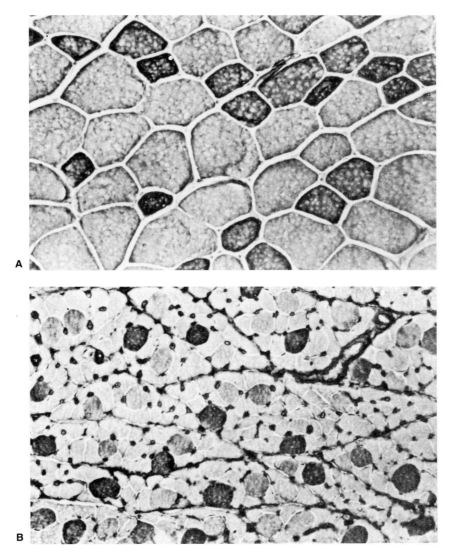

FIGURE 9–2. **(A)** Normal rat extensor digitorum longus (EDL) muscle, ATPase histochemistry, with preincubation at pH 4.6. With this method, type I fibers stain more darkly than type II. Note also that in this muscle, type II fibers are normally bigger than type I. **(B)** Denervated rat EDL (45 days), same stain as in **(A)**. Both fiber types have atrophied considerably, but type I fibers (dark stain) are now bigger than the type II. Both figures taken at same magnification. Calibration bars equal 1 μ. *(Slides for photomicrographs courtesy of Dr. Bruce Pachter.)*

is apparently more sensitive to trauma (including excessive heat or cold) than healthy muscle.[1,22,24,60] In part, this may be because of prolonged intramuscular vascular stasis, which results in impaired nutrition, as speculated by Sunderland.[60] In other words, healthy muscle fibers apparently have all the resources needed to repair even considerable damage to themselves, whereas denervated fibers do not. Because of this deficiency, what might otherwise be minor trauma, or the cumulative effects of it, leads to more and more degeneration as time goes by.

The implication of all this for physical therapy (ignoring for now the question of ES) is that steps must be taken to (1) limit edema and stasis; (2) maintain flexibility of the part, but not overstretch the denervated muscles; and (3) avoid further injury to the muscles as much as possible.[60]

## Contraction and Excitability Characteristics

Since the late 1800s, denervated muscles have been known to lose their ability to respond to short-duration monophasic pulses (those less than 1 msec). To a long-duration pulse, however (greater than 10 msec) denervated muscle will contract sluggishly. A sluggish, or vermicular, contraction is quite different from the brisk twitch of a healthy innervated muscle, but its presence indicates that the muscle is still viable and obviously capable of being stimulated. The fact that denervated muscle requires longer duration stimuli to be activated is related to the well-known changes in chronaxie and strength–duration (amplitude–duration) relationships that help distinguish the innervated from the denervated state. Indeed, it is because denervated muscle retains the ability to respond to long-duration stimuli that we can activate them at all. In addition, because denervated muscle contracts and relaxes slowly, low-frequency stimuli (between 5 and 10 Hz) of appropriate duration can fuse these contractions into a tetany. This ability to tetanize denervated muscle will be of considerable importance to our topic later. Finally, the denervated muscle membrane has poor, if any, accommodation. Accommodation means that, unlike innervated muscle, stimuli which increase in amplitude slowly are still capable of causing the muscle to contract.

## Other Membrane Changes

The resting potential of denervated muscle fibers becomes less negative than healthy fibers,[4,33,64] and the transmembrane resistance increases.[4] Furthermore, the denervated endplate membrane develops pacemaker characteristics, which apparently accounts for the phenomenon of fibrillation,[7,53] which will be described shortly. In addition, denervated muscle fibers become hypersensitive to acetylcholine (ACh),[11] the neuromuscular transmitter that, in the innervated state, causes them to depolarize to begin with. This ACh hypersensitivity is an example of the so-called "Law of Denervation Hypersensitivity," which states that after a period of time, a denervated structure (eg, skeletal muscle, smooth muscle, or gland) becomes even more sensitive to agents that normally activate it.[16] Acetylcholine hypersensitivity of denervated muscle develops because ACh receptors, which are normally present only in the endplate region of the sarcolemma, become incorporated into the entire length of the fiber's membrane.[6] In essence, the denervated muscle fiber becomes one long ACh-sensitive membrane.

## Spontaneous Activity of Denervated Muscle Fibers

Although denervated muscle appears dormant at the macroscopic level, individual fibers are actually twitching spontaneously and randomly. These unsynchronized contractions begin approximately 10 to 14 days after denervation and are too weak to be seen or felt through intact skin. However, if the muscle is exposed to view, small ripplings or undulations of its surface can be seen. These minute movements were originally reported by Schiff in 1851.[57] Such spontaneous and unsynchronized twitchings of individual denervated fibers are known as fibrillation. The electromyographic (EMG) correlate of these fibrillations are the fibrillation potentials, the sarcolemmal activity that precedes the mechanical event. As indicated previously, fibrillation is probably because of the denervated endplate membrane developing pacemaker capabilities as a result of losing its nerve supply.[7,53]

# HOW DO MUSCLE FIBERS BECOME REINNERVATED?

To regain voluntary control of a denervated muscle fiber, a terminal nerve fiber must regrow to the endplate and establish a functional synapse with it. How this reinnervation comes about depends upon whether the muscle is completely or partially denervated.

First, consider what happens when a peripheral nerve lesion disrupts all axons innervating a particular muscle. Although complete loss of voluntary and reflex function starts immediately, wallerian degeneration of axons distal to the lesion proceeds over a period of days to weeks. Along with this progressive distal degeneration, the anterior horn cells that give rise to the axons change their metabolism, gearing to their new priority of replacing what they have lost. If all goes well, regeneration proceeds from the tip of each axon's proximal stump at a rate of about 1 to 2 mm/day, or about an inch per month. Ultimately, the target muscle and its appropriate muscle fibers are reached. Because this regeneration occurs slowly, it may take years before a completely denervated hand or foot muscle is reinnervated following a proximal peripheral nerve lesion.

A totally different scenario exists if a muscle is partially denervated. In this case, denervated fibers can be reinnervated by intact axons, still present within the muscle, which "adopt" them. This reinnervation occurs via the process of **collateral sprouting,**[26,36] of which two types—nodal and terminal—are recognized.[12,13]

In nodal sprouting, an intramuscular axon, lying approximately within 100 μ to 200 μ of a denervated endplate, sprouts an extension originating from a node of Ranvier (ie, where the axon is bared of its myelin sheath).[13] This sprout enters a vacated endoneurial connective tissue tube and follows it to a denervated muscle fiber. In terminal sprouting, a terminal nerve fiber that is already innervating a muscle fiber grows another twig that finds a nearby denervated muscle fiber.[13]

Obviously, reinnervation by sprouting occurs much faster than in the first situation described because sprouts from intact intramuscular nerves need to grow only relatively short distances. Furthermore, reinnervation by either type of sprouting increases the size of the remaining motor units.

On an even more fundamental level is the question of what "guides" a growing axon, from either the tip of a cut nerve or from an intact intramuscular nerve fiber, to the denervated muscle fiber(s)? Apparently, there is something about the denervated state that signals or attracts a growing axon to form a new neuromuscular junction on the fiber, that is, to reinnervate it. What this signal might be, and what aspect(s) of denervation it is related to, is a subject of considerable research. We will return to this later.

## WHY STIMULATE THE DENERVATED MUSCLE?

When the author was a student, denervated muscle was stimulated electrically to prevent atrophy and keep the muscle as healthy as possible until it was reinnervated. This statement has intuitive appeal. The function of muscle is to develop tension, and it is common knowledge that an exercised muscle is bigger, stronger, and usually more efficient than one that is primarily inactive. Because denervated muscle cannot be activated either voluntarily or reflexively, it atrophies and weakens. Cosmetically, the wasting of muscle is not "attractive," and joint contractures, because of imbalance of muscle force, lead to deformities. However, denervated muscle can be made to contract by the application of appropriate electrical stimuli; perhaps this type of artificial activation can substitute for the real thing and prevent the negative changes associated with denervation. Furthermore, if the muscle can be maintained in a healthier condition by stimulating it electrically, perhaps its function would be restored quicker once it was reinnervated. Here is where the discrepancies and controversies have swirled since the aforementioned report of Reid.[54]

## SOME HINTS CONCERNING WHAT TO LOOK FOR

Although a selective review of the relevant literature is included in this chapter, it is more important that readers become independent in their abilities to critically review this literature for themselves. Therefore, as a brief guide, keep in mind the following:

1. Simply knowing whether a study did or did not find a "benefit" is not enough; it is important to know what aspect of the denervated state was studied.

2. If the aspect studied was *atrophy,* it is necessary to know whether this was determined by weighing the muscle or by histology. The latter is the preferred (but more labor-intensive) technique,[60] because it permits the investigator to measure sizes of fibers as well as the connective tissue changes. Weighing is simpler and does indirectly reflect atrophy of fibers, but is also influenced by other factors, such as proliferation of connective tissue and edema. The latter two will tend to make the atrophy appear less than it actually is.

3. If either weighing or histology was used, how much time elapsed between the final "treatment" and removal of the muscle for study? This question is important because an electrically stimulated denervated muscle is swollen and contains more water than usual for some hours after the treatment. Therefore, if removed too soon after ES, these muscles will appear heavier and less atrophic than they really are. In addition, it is important to know what the "control" was to which the treated muscles were compared.

4. Were any functional studies performed? For example, did the investigators determine force or endurance of the treated muscles? (Obviously, this would have to be in response to ES.) Against what controls were they compared?

5. What was the electrical treatment itself? The information needed concerns the waveform, its duration, its strength (in terms of the muscle contraction), its frequency (whether it produced a twitch or a tetanic contraction), whether the contractions produced were isometric, isotonic, or eccentric, the

number of contractions used per treatment session, the number of treatment sessions per day, the length of these treatment sessions, and when these treatments started after denervation.

## REPORTS CLAIMING BENEFITS OF ELECTRICAL STIMULATION

In 1939, 98 years after Reid's original publication, Fischer wondered whether some of the controversy that was already evident concerning possible benefits of stimulating denervated muscle electrically might be because of the different types of stimulation used.[28] He noted that many of the studies since Reid utilized weak stimuli because of the prevailing belief that benefits were because of an influence on the *excitatory* mechanism, not the *contractile* mechanism, of the denervated muscle. Fischer hypothesized that the lack of benefits reported by some investigators was because of inadequate stimulation, which deprived the denervated muscles of a proper training effect.[28]

To investigate this possibility further, Fischer employed daily 12- to 20-minute stimulations of rat denervated gastrocnemius muscles, adjusting the characteristics of amplitude (or strength), pulse duration, and frequency to produce strong tetanic contractions, but without overstimulation (no more stimulation than needed was applied to obtain the strongest possible contraction). Treatments were started the day after surgery. Fischer compared the outcome measures of excitability, weight, water content, $O_2$ consumption, and birefringence (an index of the muscle's ultrastructure) to the contralateral side, which was either not denervated or denervated but not stimulated. As a historical aside, Fischer used birefringence as the index of the muscle's ultrastructure because at that time the electron microscope had not yet been developed for this purpose.

Fischer noted that for the first few days, faradic current was able to fulfill the requirement for producing a strong tetanic contraction. However, as time went by and the denervated muscles' chronaxies increased, the faradic current (whose negative phase is only 1 msec in duration) became ineffective, so galvanic (monophasic) pulses of longer duration had to be employed. In addition, as the chronaxies increased, stimulation frequency could be reduced and still obtain the tetanic contractions that were wanted. In this study, then, Fischer tailored stimulation to the excitability needs of each muscle (determined by each muscle's chronaxie), a refinement of treatment not usually done. Unfortunately, the paper does not specify whether the contractions were isometric or isotonic, nor how long each one was sustained. The report is also unclear as to the exact number of contractions employed during the "12–20 minutes of treatment"; however, it does state, "Thus 60 short but strong contractions were produced per minute. After 2 to 3 minutes of stimulation a rest period of 1 to 2 minutes was interpolated and then the direction of the current changed."

Fischer's results can be summarized as follows:

1. Although chronaxies increased in the denervated muscles, the increase was not as great in the ones stimulated. Absolute values, however, are not given, and it is also unclear as to exactly how many days after denervation these were followed. The report states, "The maximal differences observed were not more than 18 per cent during the first two weeks, while later on with marked lengthening of the chronaxies the differences occasionally reached almost 25 per cent."

2. The loss of both wet and dry weights was retarded (but not prevented) by the electrical treatment for the time period investigated (up to 40 days).

3. There were few beneficial effects on birefringence changes; that is, both stimulated and nonstimulated muscles lost birefringence equally compared to healthy muscles.

4. Toward the paper's end, Fischer talks about the "power" of the contractions, but does not define what this means. Power probably refers to a qualitative assessment of the visible contractions that occurred. He states, however, that compared to innervated muscle, the denervated–treated muscles had little power, although these appeared stronger than the denervated–nontreated ones. In the absence of quantitative measures, and the nonblinded nature of these subjective evaluations, this comment must be regarded with caution. Fischer also comments that the little power of the treated muscles, coupled with the lack of a beneficial effect on birefringence, indicate that the treatment appeared to have little effect on the contractile machinery of the muscles.

Fischer concluded that "the best results are obtained with a treatment starting immediately after denervation, and that the amplitude and the duration of the electrical currents must be adapted to the changing excitability of the atrophying muscle."[28] He also speculated that "it seems reasonable that a treated muscle with its higher excitability, its greater weight, its lower water content, and its larger metabolism, may more easily be restored to normal function than an untreated muscle."[28] This, however, was speculation.

Fischer's paper was followed by two by Gutmann and Guttmann,[30,31] the second of which has become one of the most frequently referenced when discussing the benefits of ES. These investigators studied a number of characteristics that might be affected by strongly stimulating denervated rabbit muscle, including muscle weight, circumference of limbs, fiber diameters, connective tissue changes, quality of contractions (in response to the electrical stimulation), and the presence of fibrillation. They also systematically varied treatment protocols in terms of treatment duration, number of treatments per day, and when treatment was begun after denervation. Their treatments used monophasic pulses (called *interrupted galvanic* in those days) strong enough to produce "vigorous" contractions. A typical 20-min treatment would produce 500 to 600 single twitches. Treated and nontreated muscles were removed at various times after denervation (ranging from 30 to 150 days) and examined. They reported the following:

1. There was delayed or diminished atrophy of treated muscles.
2. Best results were obtained with daily treatments of 20 to 30 minutes' duration.
3. The earlier the treatments were started after denervation, the better. The earliest their treatments started was 7 days after surgery (to permit healing to begin), and the latest was 90 days after surgery.
4. Treated muscles had larger muscle fibers and less connective tissue than untreated muscles. (See Figure 9–3.)
5. Treated muscles were preserved better in superficial areas than in deeper areas.
6. Muscle fatigue caused by the treatment did not seem to matter.
7. Treated muscles appeared to have brisker and stronger twitches than nontreated.
8. The rate of reinnervation, as evidenced by return of reflex or voluntary function, was neither hastened nor retarded by the treatment.
9. In animals in which reinnervation occurred within a few months (crush denervation, or **axonotmesis**, as opposed to cutting the nerve, or **neuronotmesis**), there was little if any difference between treated and nontreated muscles after both had been reinnervated for a while.

In 1945, Wehrmacher, Thomson, and Hines also used the denervated gastrocnemius muscle of the rat. Their outcome measures were weight, creatine content, and force (in grams). They reported that strong contractions were needed to get an effect, but that this effect was also dependent on the muscle contracting isometrically (ie, against an immovable resistance) and in the stretched position. When these two conditions were satisfied, the authors argued that the stimulated muscles were able to generate the most tension possible, and this was required for the optimal benefits. They also reported that tetanic contractions should be maintained for at least 2 sec, but longer than that did not add much.[65]

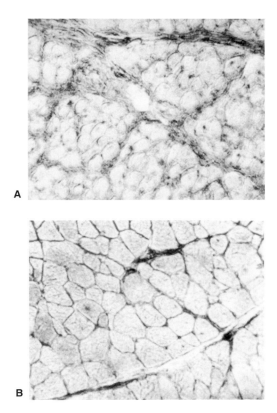

**FIGURE 9–3.** Cross-sections of untreated **(A)** and treated **(B)** muscles of a rabbit 67 days after denervation. Treatment sessions were for 20 minutes daily, commencing 7 days after neurectomy. Fibers are more atrophic and connective tissue more plentiful in the untreated muscle. *(From Gutmann E, and Guttmann L. The effect of galvanic exercise on denervated and reinnervated muscles in the rabbit. J Neurol Neurosurg Psychiat, 7:7–17, 1944, with permission.)*

Similar to Fischer, they found that atrophy and loss of creatine were retarded, but not the loss of force that follows denervation. In a side study, they reported that ES was unable to retard the atrophy that follows tenotomy, presumably because the tenotomized muscle cannot generate sufficient tension to get the benefit. However, the clinical significance of this study is questionable because it was not extended beyond 14 days of denervation.[65]

Kosman, Osborne, and Ivy presented back-to-back papers,[40,41] which looked at a number of factors that might influence the effectiveness of stimulation. They also utilized the denervated gastrocnemius muscle of the rat, with treatments starting the day after surgery. Again, the outcome measures were atrophy (in terms of weight) and tension developed (although how this was done is not described beyond the statement, "The amount of tension developed was determined . . .").

Their best results were obtained under the following conditions:

1. The current was a 25-Hz alternating current (AC), at an amplitude that produced a strong contraction. Although the authors did not comment further on this, the reader should note that the negative phase of a 25-Hz AC waveform has a duration of 40 msec, which is long enough to satisfy a denervated muscle's chronaxie. Also, this frequency would be fast enough to produce a tetanic contraction.

2. The muscle was made to contract isometrically while maintained in a stretched position.

3. The muscle was treated two to three times daily, but the duration of stimulation did not have to be longer than 30 sec. Increasing this treatment time did not improve the results (described below).

4. The rest between treatments (ie, these single 30-sec contractions) was vitally important; at least 10 min was required.

5. The reason for items 3 and 4 was the easy fatigability of denervated muscle. By the end of the 30-sec stimulation interval, the denervated muscles were no longer developing tension, and they required at least 10 min of rest before they fully recovered. The authors therefore explained their findings on the basis that if the retardation of both atrophy and force loss requires strong tension development, stimulating fatigued muscle is wasted time and effort. Also, resuming stimulation before the muscle has recovered its ability to contract maximally again is also wasted effort.

6. Even with these best-case scenarios, the maximal retardation of atrophy was about 90 percent of normal, but force was maintained only at about 56 percent of normal.

7. A shortcoming of this study, however, is that most animals were stimulated only up to 14 days after denervation, with only 10 animals stimulated up to 28 days. Thus, this investigation, like others described earlier, gives no information concerning whether the benefits noted are maintained over longer time intervals.

8. In an aside, the authors mention, "For man, we have found that alternating current with a carrier frequency of 5 to 25 cycles per second can produce strong contractions of paralyzed muscles with little discomfort to the patient. A first requisite, then, is the proper stimulation of paralyzed muscles with a

stimulator that furnishes such currents." (This comment will be discussed later in the chapter.)

In 1955, taking a more functional approach to the question, Wakim and Krusen investigated how ES in rats affects denervated muscle functionally instead of histologically.[63] In eight groups of animals, lower extremities were denervated by removing segments of both the sciatic and femoral nerves. Treatment consisted of square wave pulses, 1 msec in duration, 16 pulses per sec, and strong enough to produce maximal contractions of the entire extremity. The independent variables were the durations of treatments and the number of treatments given per day. The dependent variables were the mechanical work and endurance of the treated muscles tested 25 to 30 days after denervation.

They found that 30 min of stimulation once daily was of some benefit (compared to no stimulation); 30 min twice a day was considerably better; 5 min every half hour over an 8-hour day (with one hour off for lunch) was as beneficial as longer periods of stimulation also performed every half hour. Unfortunately, though, while the stimulated muscles were stronger and more endurant than nonstimulated controls, treated muscles at best achieved only 50 percent of the power and endurance found for innervated muscles.[63]

That these percentages of innervated muscles continue to drop with longer durations of denervation was shown by a more recent study, which treated denervated rat extensor digitorum longus (EDL) and soleus muscles for up to 10 months. Though stimulated EDL muscles had about seven times the force-generating capacity of nonstimulated EDLs, and stimulated soleus muscles were 20 to 55 times stronger than nonstimulated, these stronger muscles were still only 4 to 5 percent of normal innervated values.[3] In a companion study, the denervated–stimulated muscles were histologically better than nonstimulated, but still well below "normal."[59]

How should these data be interpreted? On one hand, stimulation clearly resulted in muscles that were stronger than nonstimulated (evidence that stimulation is beneficial), but on the other hand, the actual retention of force-generating capability was very low (which questions whether the results are worth the time, effort, and expense). It should be noted, though, that no evidence of accelerated degeneration of muscle was noted in these articles.

So far, we have reviewed a number of animal studies of relatively brief durations, which have shown that if any benefits are to be obtained with ES, certain guidelines must be met. The problem with these studies, however, is whether they are applicable to humans where months or years may be required for nerves to regenerate. Some studies have attempted to address this issue.

In 1943, Doupe, Barnes, and Kerr reported their experiences with 12 patients who had suffered radial nerve injuries with subsequent suturing.[24] The level of injuries was noted, as well as the time for return of volition of the extensor carpi radialis muscle. Six of these patients received electrical treatments for 5 months or longer, while the other six received little or none. All (except for two) received massage three to five times a week for a period of 6 to 8 months, and all had cock-up splints applied. The electrical treatment consisted of "15–30 moderate contractions of each muscle 5–6 times a week, induced by interrupted galvanism applied longitudinally to the muscle." (Note the lack of details concerning the contractions themselves, how long they were sustained, or the rest between them.)

The authors reported no significant differences between the patients who received treatment for periods of 5 to 18 months and those who did not with respect to the "time of the first return of voluntary contraction or in the rate of subsequent recovery." They concluded that "electrical treatment in its customary method of application has no beneficial effects on the return of motor power"; and later they state, "Electrical therapy does not aid the recovery of denervated muscles except insofar as it assists in reeducation and in maintaining the mobility of the tissues." Note, however, that the electrical treatment described in this paper was not of the type thought to be optimal by other investigators.[24]

In 1951, Osborne used a different approach to determining efficacy of ES in humans.[52] Obviously, removing a muscle to weigh it or examine it microscopically is not a viable option. Instead, Osborne developed a volumetric technique that gave very similar side-to-side findings in a group of 20 healthy subjects. He reasoned, therefore, that the method could be used "to estimate the probable volume of one limb from the actual volume of the other." Once the probable volume was determined, the difference between the affected limb's actual volume and its estimated probable volume became the probable degree of atrophy.

Of 15 patients who began the study, only 7 "were able or willing to continue treatment over a minimal period of five to a maximal of 18 ½ months." Treatment was described as follows: "The denervated muscles of each patient were stimulated once daily and five times a week. The current used was selected in accordance with an experimental intensity–frequency curve and was either a sinusoidal or a modulated sinusoidal current with a low carrier frequency. For the maximal effectiveness of the therapy, it was deemed essential to secure a vigorous muscular contraction and the degree of contraction was limited only by the patient's tolerance to the current. . . . Muscle reeducation exercises were given in addition to stimulation with the electrical current."[52]

A total of 106 muscles were treated in the seven patients. Manual muscle testing at the beginning and end of the study showed the following grades:

|       | At Beginning | At End |
|-------|--------------|--------|
| Zero  | 93           | 8      |
| Trace | 5            | 32     |
| Poor  | 6            | 13     |
| Fair  | 2            | 21     |
| Good  | 0            | 32     |

Therefore, there appeared to be considerable overall clinical improvement.

With respect to atrophy, however, Osborne reported mixed results. He concluded that although stimulation seemed to stop further atrophy once the stimulation was started, it did not reverse the atrophy that had already occurred prior to starting the treatment. While on this point, Osborne discussed a number of logistic problems that are encountered when humans are being treated but that are absent in animal experimentation. In the "real" world, human nerve injuries are usually associated with other medical and surgical problems that preclude immediate institution of ES. Thus, patients actually start their first treatment after atrophy has already had a chance to move forward. Also, as shown by the high drop-out rate in his study, many patients found it impossible to continue treatments on a daily basis. What happens to treatment efficacy if patients miss treatments at various times is likewise unknown.

More importantly, and especially in light of what will be said later, it should be noted that improvements in muscle force (ie, reinnervation) were found for most muscles. Claims cannot be made that these improvements resulted from the ES (there was no "control group" in this study), but at least the stimulation did not appear to prevent reinnervation in these patients. This last point—that the stimulation did not appear to prevent reinnervation—is especially important considering what will be discussed.

The lack of a "control" group was not a factor in a study by Boonstra et al.[9] These authors reported results on 73 patients with 81 nerve injuries involving the median, ulnar, brachial plexus, and peroneal nerves. Surgical interventions were required in 52, which included 39 primary repairs, 11 secondary repairs, and 2 neurolyses. None of the brachial plexus or peroneal nerve injuries underwent surgery. Of these 81 injuries, 35 did not receive "treatment," which consisted of supramaximal stimuli (1/sec), using the shortest pulse duration with the same amplitude as the rheobase (called the *utilization time* or *Hauptnutzzeit* in the older literature) determined by each patient's strength–duration curve. The denervated muscles that were treated received one of four regimens:

1. Thirty stimulations 5 days a week until reinnervation was determined by EMG investigation
2. The same treatment until voluntary effort was a clinical grade 2 (ie, beyond the time that reinnervation was noted)
3. Thirty stimulations twice a day (60 contractions per muscle), 7 days a week, until reinnervation was visible on the EMG
4. The same as 3 (above) until a clinical grade 2 was reached

Like Osborne, these authors also describe the delay they encountered in humans before this treatment began. In this series, the delay averaged 6.9 weeks (standard deviation [SD], 4.7 weeks), while the mean duration of therapy was 35 weeks (SD, 22.1 weeks). Outcome measures included EMG, dynamometry of handgrip, clinical muscle force, computerized tomography (CT) scans determining cross-sectional area and x-ray density of the hypothenar muscles (in patients with ulnar nerve lesions), and ultrasonography to measure cross-sectional area of the thenar muscles in patients with median nerve injuries, or of peroneal muscles in those with peroneal lesions.

In summarizing their findings, the authors state, "From this study it can be concluded that electrical stimulation as performed in our study has no delaying effect on denervation atrophy and no beneficial effect on muscle recovery."[9] They also properly point out, however, that a different stimulation paradigm (such as tetanic contractions instead of twitches) might produce different findings. Just as important, they also emphasized the fact that neither did their study show a detrimental effect. Why they specifically addressed this issue is described next.

## STUDIES REPORTING ADVERSE EFFECTS OF ELECTRICAL STIMULATION

In keeping with the adage, "Above all, do no harm!," it is more important to know whether a treatment may adversely affect a condition than simply be of no benefit. This situation has existed with ES of denervated muscle. As previously shown, by the early 1950s the controversy concerning this treatment was whether it was effective. Studies which had shown no effectiveness (mostly based on animal experimentation) were considered "flawed" because they did not employ the proper stimulation characteristics. With stronger stimulation, and with the introduction of histologic techniques that could distinguish between muscle fiber types, other problems started to be reported.

In 1939, Chor et al had already reported a possible problem in a study using rhesus monkeys with sciatic nerve sections and repair (suturing) at the level of the greater trochanter of the femur.[17] In a series of experiments (ranging from 6 weeks to 6 months), these investigators compared atrophy of the gastrocnemius muscle and time to return of voluntary movement in three groups of animals: Group 1 was treated with ES (described only as galvanic current giving 10 good contractions daily); group 2 received passive range of motion (ROM) and massage, and group 3 only immobilization in a plaster cast. They reported that the best results, including the fastest return of voluntary motion, was in group 2 (the group that received passive ROM and massage), with the poorest results in group 3 (the group with prolonged immobilization). With respect to return of voluntary motion, four animals in group 2 showed this return in 76, 92, 95, and 96 days, while five animals in group 1 showed this return in 103, 118, 122, 158, and 158 days. In addition, Chor et al stated that in one series, the electrically stimulated muscles "showed slightly more wasting than the untreated."[17]

In 1977, Schimrigk, McLaughlin and Gruninger studied two groups of rats (n = 20 in each) with denervated quadriceps muscles, but whose surgery was such as to permit reinnervation.[58] Starting 4 days after surgery, the treated group received galvanic stimulation "three times 2 minutes a day . . . using supramaximal intensities . . . and a frequency of 5 per second." (*Note:* By today's standards, this is inadequate information for a Methods section. Furthermore, the authors state that their supramaximal amplitudes were 5 to 8 volts and a current of "4 to 6 Amps," which the author assumes should be mAmps, not Amps.) Muscles were removed for histologic examination at various intervals, ranging from 3 to 7 weeks after surgery. These authors reported that as reinnervation occurred, the diameters of the stimulated fibers were less than the nonstimulated. They concluded, "We can say that we observed delayed regeneration of denervated rat muscles under electrical stimulation therapy. This causes us once more to doubt the efficiency of this therapy in human medicine."[58]

In 1982, Girlanda et al crushed the sciatic nerves of 12 rabbits just above the bifurcation into the tibial and peroneal nerves (a crush injury permits nerves to regenerate in most mammals).[29] Six animals received "square waves, 400 ms in duration at a frequency of 40 stimuli/min delivered through surface electrodes. This treatment was carried out twice daily after the nerve crush, each muscle group being stimulated for 5 minutes in every session. A current amplitude sufficient to produce strong contractions of the denervated muscles was chosen. During the sessions, the limbs were held manually in a rest position so as to obtain isometric contractions" (clearly a more informative Methods section than the previous paper, but why the investigators chose 400 msec pulse durations is not explained). Electromyograms were performed starting 2 weeks after nerve crush to determine the reinnervation time in the two groups.

Fifty days after surgery, soleus and EDL muscles were removed for weighing as well as histologic and histochemical examination. Prior to removal, it was determined that the average reinnervation to the anterior tibialis muscles of the treated group was 40.8 ± 1.7 days (± SD), whereas in the untreated group it was 41.3 ± 1.8 days. These groups were not significantly different. With respect to the soleus and EDL muscles, the treated EDLs lost significantly less weight than did the nontreated EDLs, but no difference was noted between treated and nontreated soleus muscles. Treatment, however, affected fiber types differently in the two muscles. In treated EDLs, type 2b fibers atrophied less than in the nontreated, but type 1 fibers atrophied more. A similar greater atrophy of type 1 fibers was found in treated soleus muscles compared to the nontreated controls.

This study indicates, as others before it had done, that (1) weight measures by themselves do not tell the whole story, (2) fiber types may be affected differently by the treatment, and (3) that different muscles may be affected differently. The latter finding warns that generalizing the results from one muscle may not be valid for other muscles, even in the same animal. However, the generalizability of this study could be questioned because it used 400 msec pulse durations, which are considerably longer than needed to stimulate denervated muscle. Note also that because pulse durations were so long, the stimulation frequency was given in terms of stimuli per minute, not the usual stimuli per second.

In 1987, Nix and Dahm revisited the question of strong stimulation and its effect on denervated muscle architecture.[51] Using the rabbit EDL muscle, animals were divided into three groups. Group 1 received no treatment; group 2, daily 20-minute treatments with 7-msec square wave pulses delivered 1 per sec, adjusted to produce vigorous isometric twitches, Group 3 received 1-msec pulses at a frequency of 40 per sec, for 100 msec each sec, also producing vigorous isometric tetanies. Treatments were started 2 days after denervation and conducted daily for the next 4 weeks. Muscles were then removed for further mechanical testing and histology.

In the group that received the strong tetanic stimulation, contractures developed about the end of the second week (even though these animals were permitted unrestricted use of their limbs when not being treated). In addition, these muscles became unresponsive to the stimulation as time went by. Morphologically, these muscles "demonstrated atrophic muscle fibers surrounded by large masses of connective tissue." Nix and Dahm speculated, "The tissue proliferation was presumably caused by microtrauma. The high tetanic tensions in denervated muscle may have caused ruptures within single muscle fibers or lacerations of connective tissue."[51]

This finding, of course, is noted to be contrary to the one of Gutmann and Guttmann,[31] who reported *less* fibrosis in denervated muscles stimulated similarly. Why the differences? Both groups used the lower extremities of rabbits; both used 20 min of galvanic stimulation producing strong isometric contractions. Two differences, however, concerned (1) when treatments started after denervation, and (2) the electrodes used to administer the treatments.

With respect to the start of treatments, Gutmann and Guttmann began stimulating 7 days after surgery, whereas Nix and Dahm started theirs after 2 days. Could this have been a factor? Might the institution of vigorous treatment so soon after denervation be deleterious to the outcome? Possibly, but this factor is perhaps not as important as the one described next.

Gutmann and Guttmann administered their stimulation through moistened surface electrodes (similar to how our patients are treated) and moved these electrodes periodically over the muscles. Conversely, Nix and Dahm used implanted wire electrodes—one on the proximal and the other near the distal end of the EDL. Although they state, "The polarity of the stimulus was reversed after each stimulus to minimize damage to the tissue caused by possible polarization at the electrodes," the current may have been so concentrated by the thin wires that damage was indeed done that would not have occurred had surface electrodes been employed. Therefore, though it is important to know that this paper reports an adverse reaction, this must be viewed with caution because it does not reflect the clinical manner in which the treatment would be done to humans. Alternately, unlike previous suggestions extolling the need for strong contractions to obtain the proper "training" effect, denervated muscle cannot tolerate such contractions, and they should be avoided. These results represent another example of contradictory findings that have been plaguing this field for almost a century and a half. Other types of possible adverse effects, however, have also been reported. These include delaying the reinnervation process and possible "overworking" of recently reinnervated muscle fibers.

# POSSIBLE DELAY OF REINNERVATION

As previously described, how denervated muscle fibers can be reinnervated depends in part on how they were denervated to begin with. A completely denervated muscle, such as resulting from its nerve being cut, must await regeneration of its axons growing down from the proximal stump. Conversely, denervated fibers in a partially denervated muscle can become reinnervated by sprouting from remaining intramuscular axons.

Some studies have reported that terminal sprouting is inhibited by ES of partially denervated muscles.[14,37] This condition is interesting physiology, but does it have clinical significance? The answer here, in the author's opinion, is "no," because there is no reason to stimulate a partially denervated muscle to begin with. This reason is so because in partial denervation, reinnervation by collateral sprouting (whether nodal or terminal) occurs relatively quickly, so what would be gained with ES?

There is still the issue of how ES might retard or prevent reinnervation. Recall that earlier the question was raised as to how a denervated muscle fiber signals a growing nerve fiber to reinnervate it. Without going into the details of this very fascinating area of neuromuscular physiology, the strong possibility exists that by stimulating the denervated muscle, that is, by keeping it more active than it would be if left alone, the muscle is kept so "healthy" that it fails to express its denervated state, thus "fooling" the nervous system into not reinnervating it! But is there evidence to support this possibility?

Earlier in this chapter, denervation was shown to be accompanied by a number of structural, physiologic, and biochemical changes in the affected muscles. The presumption is that one or a combination of these alterations is the signal that says, "Come and reinnervate me." What might it, or they, be?

Without going into details (because this could easily be a review in itself), just two will be mentioned:

1. The proliferation of Ach receptors of denervated sarcolemmas, which, as indicated earlier, accounts for the increased Ach sensitivity of these muscle fibers, has been suggested as a possible "guide." Electrical stimulation of denervated muscle has also been shown to reduce considerably this hypersensitivity.[25,44]

2. A second possible guidance factor is the neural cell adhesion molecule (N-CAM),[18,55] a glycoprotein that is present in embryonic muscle prior to innervation, or in muscle that is inactive because of denervation or long-standing neuromuscular blockade. N-CAM is not present in muscle that is innervated and nor-

mally active. Considerable evidence suggests that profound inactivity (secondary to denervation or long-standing neuromuscular block) causes the reexpression of this substance, and it, either alone or in combination with others, guides growing axons to the denervated or inactive muscle fibers.[18,55] The point is that inactivity is required for this substance to be synthesized. The possiblity exists, therefore, that the activity of denervated muscle produced by ES might inhibit the expression of this substance, so that reinnervation is retarded or prevented.

The question may then boil down to determining whether a "happy medium" may be found between enough stimulation to keep denervated muscles as healthy as possible, but at the same time below the level that might keep them "too healthy." This would not be an easy task.

## OVERWORK OF MUSCLE

As far back as 1915, Lovett reported that unaccustomed use or overuse of paretic muscles was frequently associated with loss of force in patients recovering from poliomyelitis.[45] Lundervold and Seyffarth confirmed this, not only in patients with poliomyelitis but in healthy subjects who underwent compression of their peroneal nerves for 20 to 30 min.[46] In this latter situation, subjects who did not walk until some hours had passed after the compression was released showed full return of function by day's end, but those who walked immediately after release of the compression took 3 to 4 days before their normal force and endurance returned.[46]

Similarly, Bennett and Knowlton described four patients with poliomyelitis and one with C5–6 quadriplegia in whom excessive exercise of weak muscles was followed by considerable clinical deterioration.[8] Overuse was also the reason given by Johnson and Braddom to explain why all except one member of a family with facioscapulohumeral muscular dystrophy had more weakness and atrophy on the dominant side compared to the nondominant side.[38] In other words, regardless of whether a muscle is weakened because of neuropathy or myopathy, overuse must be avoided.

Keep in mind, however, that all of the studies mentioned, and the data now available concerning late-onset weakness in patients who had poliomyelitis decades ago, may not be directly applicable to the situation we are discussing. In all of the studies, overuse was occurring because of *voluntary activity,* not artificial stimulation. Therefore, it is not clear (at this time) whether the site of lesion for the weakness following voluntary activity is at the level of the anterior horn cell (ie, the anterior horn cell is metabolically unable to meet the demands put upon it), or distally at the neuromuscular junction, or the muscle itself. If the cause of weakness in these situations is overuse of anterior horn cells, ES applied to the muscle might not be contraindicated. The problem is that, at present, the site of the lesion in all these situations is yet to be determined.

## MIGHT THERE BE A BETTER WAY TO STIMULATE DENERVATED MUSCLE?

In 1952, Kowarschik described using "exponential" or slowly rising currents, which presumably stimulated denervated muscle selectively, but not innervated muscle.[42] Kowarschik presented clinical evidence that this selectivity reflected the fact that the excitable membrane of the denervated muscle, the sarcolemma, has poor accommodation, whereas the innervated muscle accommodates as expected. In this way, the innervated muscle fibers of a partially denervated muscle, or the innervated muscles in the vicinity of a denervated one, are not stimulated.

In this same paper, Kowarschik describes how he was able to stimulate muscles paralyzed by poliomyelitis 20 to 30 years later, and remarks from this how long it may take before denervated muscles are transformed into fat and connective tissue. He goes on to note that to get the most stimulation of denervated muscles using slowly rising currents, the target muscle should be stimulated with the **bipolar technique**—that is, one electrode near the muscle's origin and the other near its insertion. He then mentions that he also used these currents to treat patients who had suffered nerve injuries during World War II, but says nothing about the number of patients or their results.[42]

So is this technique worth using? From a theoretical standpoint, there are a number of reasons not to. First, the fibers that are being stimulated selectively (ie, the denervated ones) are exactly those that some data show should not be stimulated. If these fibers are more susceptible to mechanical (and possibly electrical) trauma than innervated fibers, they are the ones we should be trying to protect, not stimulate. Second, if a muscle is partially denervated, why stimulate it at all? As has been described earlier in this chapter, the denervated fibers in a partially denervated muscle stand a fairly good chance of being reinnervated by collateral sprouting in a relatively short period of time anyway. Finally, evidence has been mentioned that one form of collateral sprouting (ie, terminal sprouting) may be inhibited by ES. Existing data indicate, then, that exponential current stimulation may be precisely what we want to avoid, but this is certainly not written in stone. The field is still awaiting a controlled study that will either show or refute that exponential current stimulation is a safe and effective method to treat denervated muscle.

## OTHER ISSUES TO BE CONSIDERED

Let us return for a moment and reconsider why ES has not been shown to prevent denervation atrophy completely. The most obvious possibility is that the quality and quantity of stimulation that has been employed in the different studies still did not approach the exercise that a healthy innervated muscle receives.

There is another possibility for which some evidence exists, namely, that certain aspects of muscle metabolism, including those relating to a muscle fiber's size, are controlled in part by trophic substances released by nerves. These trophic factors are presumed to exert their effects independent of activity. For example, extracts of peripheral nerves have been reported to:

- Delay atrophy (measured as loss of weight and loss of muscle proteins) in denervated muscles, especially type IIb fibers,[19,20]
- Prevent more than half the slowing of twitch times that occur in denervated muscles[21]
- Lessen the reduction in sizes of individual mitochondria, mitochondrial volume per fiber, sarcoplasmic reticulum, and t-tubules that occur in denervated fibers[35]
- Reduce the increase in carbonic anhydrase III activity that occurs with denervation of type II fibers[49]
- Decrease the Ach-receptor content of denervated muscle[56] (which has also been shown to be affected by activity)

Therefore, if some of the consequences of denervation result from the absence of trophic factors, then one cannot expect electrical stimulation, regardless of its quality and quantity, to fully substitute for the innervated state.

Not surprisingly, and fulfilling a prediction made in previous versions of this chapter, a 1997 article now reports what appears to be quite beneficial effects of electrically stimulating denervated muscle in humans.[50] Although this paper can be criticized for omitting considerable detail (see below), its findings are such that I believe it deserves a more in-depth review.

This paper reports biopsy, computed tomography (CT) scans, and stimulated-force changes following an 8-month training period of ES of the quadriceps muscles of 14 patients with paraplegia. Four of these individuals had conus-cauda lesions (ie, a lower motor neuron or denervated group), while the other 10 had higher thoracic lesions (ie, an upper motor neuron or spasticity group). The subjects "averaged 3–4 years after the spinal cord injury" before entering the study. This last point is important because it confirms what was said earlier in this chapter about the ability of denervated human muscle to remain viable for many years.

This study compared the long-term effects of ES tailored to whether the muscles were denervated or not. What follows is a description of the methods used, some comments on these descriptions, and what was found.

## STIMULATION PROTOCOL

- **Electrodes and their location:** two conductive rubber electrodes, 250 cm$^2$ in area, fixed to both upper legs.
  *COMMENT:* Inadequate description. For example, is the area the size of one electrode or both together? Were these electrodes circular, elliptical, or rectangular? What does "upper legs" mean?
- **Stimulus characteristics:** (1) For the persons with spasticity: biphasic pulses, 1.3 msec in duration, at a frequency of 27 Hz, and a peak-to-peak voltage of up to 70 V. (2) For the individuals with denervation: treatment started with 200-msec pulse durations, at a frequency of 1.25 Hz, and peak-to-peak voltage of 60 to 100 V. As the strength of contractions increased over time, stimulus characteristics were changed to 25- to 30-msec pulse durations and frequencies of 15 to 20 Hz.
  *COMMENT:* Adequate description of waveform, pulse durations, and pulse frequencies. Note the much longer duration pulses employed in the denervation group.
- **Treatment durations and frequencies:** twice a day, starting with 15 min, but then increased throughout the 2 months to 30 min.
  *COMMENT:* Inadequate description of the "treatments" themselves. All we are told is, "The legs were stimulated until complete extension of the knee joint was achieved." This does not tell us, for example, how many total contractions were elicited per treatment session, nor how long each contraction was held, nor how long the rest periods were between successive contractions. The omission of these points prohibits readers from replicating the methods.
  *NOTE:* None of the above criticisms negate the findings, just the ability of others to replicate the methods used.

## OUTCOME MEASURES

- **CT scans** before and after the 8-month program to determine the cross-sectional areas of the quadriceps and adductor/flexor muscles groups at three different levels of the thigh.
- **Muscle biopsies** before and after the 8-month program to determine percentage of type I and type II fibers, as well as fiber diameters.
- Although not specifically measured, the **force** of the electrically stimulated contractions was noted. Here is what they reported:

### Fiber Sizes (median diameter in μm)

|  | Spasticity | | Denervated | |
|---|---|---|---|---|
|  | *Before* | *After* | *Before* | *After* |
| Type I fibers | 34 | 56 | 24 | 37 |
| Type II fibers | 52 | 70 | 24 | 42 |

$P < 0.05$ for changes in both fiber types

Note, however, that by the end of the study the denervated type I fibers were only slightly larger than the innervated type I fibers had been *before* stimulation, and that the denervated type II fibers were still considerably smaller than the innervated type II fibers had been *before* stimulation.

### Fiber Type Proportions

|  | Spasticity | | Denervated | |
|---|---|---|---|---|
|  | *Before* | *After* | *Before* | *After* |
| Type I fibers | 16.2% | No change | 27% | 19% |
| Type II fibers | 83.8% | No change | 73% | 81% |

Increased percentage of type II fibers in denervated muscles after stimulation

### CT Scans (to determine change in cross-sectional areas of muscles)

| Cross-sectional area of: | Spasticity | Denervated |
|---|---|---|
| Quadriceps | Increased by 27.5% | Increased by 10% |
| Adductor/flexors | Increased by 22% | Increased by 7% |

# FORCE OF ELECTRICALLY STIMULATED CONTRACTIONS

No specifics were given except that in both groups, ES was ultimately able to achieve full knee extension. In the patients with spasticity, 4- to 5-kg weights were added to the knee extension exercises after 2 months, but no similar comment is made concerning the patients with denervation. Whether the weights against which the spastic group exercised were increased beyond 4 to 5 kg as time went on was also not stated.

There are a number of "take-home" lessons from this study:

1. As already mentioned, this study confirms that denervated human muscle can remain viable (though atrophied) for many years following denervation.
2. Because the authors did not comment on any apparent increase in connective tissue or fibrosis of the stimulated muscles, the stimulation paradigm used (which is unfortunately inadequately described) was not deleterious to the muscles.
3. The ability of denervated muscle to increase its stimulated force is again shown, although it apparently falls far short of what can be achieved by innervated (spastic) muscle.
4. The ability of ES to partially reverse denervation atrophy is again shown. However, the increase in size still leaves them quite atrophied.
5. Note also the discrepancy between the percentage increases noted by CT scan and the measurements made on biopsy. According to the CT scans, the cross-sectional area of the denervated quadriceps muscle increased just 10 percent, while the adductor/flexor group (which must have received some stimulation as well), increased 7 percent. However, the biopsy measurements, which determined individual fiber diameters, showed that the median diameter of type I fibers increased 54 percent, whereas the median diameter of type II fibers increased 75 percent. However, because these are not mean values, it cannot be claimed that the average diameters increased. The reason for not determining mean values is unclear, especially since the authors state that for each biopsy, "about 600–1,100 muscle fibers were evaluated."
6. The authors conclude, but prematurely because they present no supporting data, that, "This allows for better rehabilitation with an increased blood flow and prevention of decubital ulcers and osteoporosis. Finally, this stimulation technique will enable active walking even in patients with denervated muscles after improvements of the technology." Perhaps.[50]

# Summary

Despite the almost 150 years since the original report suggesting that electrical stimulation might be beneficial to denervated muscle, controversy still exists. Although some experimental studies on animals have reported benefits, their major shortcoming is that they did not mimic the realities encountered in human injuries. The major differences between these animal experiments and human peripheral nerve lesions relate to how soon after injury treatment can begin (usually delayed considerably in humans because of many practical issues), but more importantly, to the length of time required for human nerves to regenerate compared to the short durations of the animal studies. Therefore, these experimental conditions did not reflect the realities of clinical practice. The situation is further complicated by other investigations which showed that ES is either of questionable benefit, of no benefit, or actually harmful to the denervated muscle. Reports of supposed benefits in humans are few, and in most cases of questionable validity. In some of these, the "benefits" ascribed to the treatment may simply have been because of lack of understanding of the natural history of the condition itself. This chapter reviews many of the above reports, both pro and con, and alerts readers to the types of details they should look for to determine a study's clinical relevance.

Therapists involved with the care and treatment of persons with peripheral nerve injuries are encouraged to design and perform the quality of clinical studies needed to either confirm or deny the benefits of stimulating denervated muscle.

## CASE STUDY

On September 23, a college football player (strong safety) was struck forcefully on his right shoulder pad. He described feeling instantaneous "electric shock" down the entire right upper extremity, and then the weight of many other players falling on top of him. He was unable to arise from the pile-up. He described to the trainers and team physician who ran to him that the entire upper extremity was now numb and he could not move any of its joints, from shoulder to fingers. All other extremities were healthy. After about 10 minutes at the sidelines, feeling began to return to his hand, as did the ability to move his fingers. This return of function then slowly continued in a distal-to-proximal direction, so that after 12 hours he was able to voluntarily contract all muscles except the right deltoid. He was also left

**CASE STUDY** *continued*

with a sensory deficit over the belly of the middle deltoid. X-rays of the neck and shoulder were negative.

Forty-eight hours later, the only neurologic deficit was the complete absence of deltoid muscle function and sensory loss in the axillary nerve distribution. The patient was treated symptomatically for pain in his right shoulder with hot packs and gentle ROM exercises. After one week, atrophy of the deltoid was discernable. Electromyographic examination on October 26 revealed profuse fibrillation potentials and positive sharp waves in all three heads of the right deltoid, and no motor unit potentials on attempted volition. Electromyography of the right biceps, brachioradialis, infraspinatus, triceps, and paracervical muscles was "normal." The findings were consistent with the clinical diagnosis of right axillary nerve lesion.

As pain subsided, the patient progressed to active exercises of his remaining musculature (see below for more details). Repeat EMG shortly before Christmas showed no changes; however, on February 20, a few long-duration polyphasic motor units were present on attempted volition in both the posterior and middle deltoid muscles (with more in the posterior than in the middle). Abnormal spontaneous activity was still present in these heads, but less than previously. The anterior deltoid remained devoid muscle of voluntary activity. On April 26, more of these polyphasic units were found in the posterior and middle deltoid muscle, along with some normal motor units. In addition, long-duration polyphasics were present in the anterior deltoid muscle. More important than these electrical improvements, clinical examination showed clearly visible and palpable contractions of all three heads.

By mid-July, he began practicing again with the team. His right deltoid muscle was still not quite as bulky as his left (although quite well developed), there was mild weakness on manual muscle testing of the anterior head, and he still described sensation over the middle deltoid as "funny." However, ROM was full, and he was able to perform all drills and exercises with the team.

On September 28, he competed in his first intercollegiate game since the injury. Although this sounds like a Hollywood ending, he made the game's first tackle as a member of the the specialty kick-off squad. A local newspaper described this tackle as "jarring." He also "led the defense with nine tackles."

The lessons of this case are many:

1. Because the method of injury was a severe blow to the shoulder, followed by rapid return of function, the lesion was first considered "neurapraxic."

2. When deltoid muscle function did not return, it was apparent that the axillary nerve had suffered a more severe type of injury, probably axonotmetic. Axonal degeneration was confirmed by the EMG findings 1 month later of fibrillation potentials and positive sharp waves in all heads of the deltoid, although these, by themselves, did not distinguish axonotmesis from neuronotmesis. The latter, though, was considered unlikely given how the injury occurred.

3. In the presence of an axonotmesis, the prognosis for regeneration was considered good. In addition, experience with these axillary nerve lesions also favored recovery, usually within a year.[39]

4. Based on this, treatment was directed at maintaining ROM of all joints, as well as maintaining and increasing the force of all other muscles. As voluntary control returned to the different heads of the deltoid muscle, highly directed muscle reeducation (including EMG biofeedback using a Verimed Myoexorcisor III) was added. This approach was necessitated by the substitution patterns he was using. Electrical stimulation, however, was avoided.

5. The athlete was also counseled to maintain good nutrition, as well as to avoid alcohol and drugs. (Although there was no history of using them, this advice is given routinely as a precaution.)

6. As described above, recovery was quite gratifying. Would it have been "better" if ES had been employed? We do not know. Would regeneration have been "retarded" had electrical stimulation been employed? We do not know. What we do know is that this type of injury in a young, highly motivated individual who receives good, comprehensive treatment carries a very good prognosis.

This case demonstrates how we must guard against claiming a beneficial effect of a treatment when the natural history of a particular condition is that it carries a good prognosis anyway. Nerve injuries that are either neurapraxic or axonotmetic, such as Bell's palsy or Saturday night palsy, are other examples. In the former, the lesion is neurapraxic in a high percentage of patients (shown by preserved facial nerve excitability and conduction 7 to 10 days after the onset of paralysis or paresis), and only partially denervating (axonotmetic) in others.[23] Indeed, even in the absence of any treatment, approximately 80 percent of them regain full function within a year,[66] while those with neurapraxia recover in weeks to months. Therefore, these are ideal patients to "treat" electrically, because most of them are destined to go on to recover. If a patient whose lesion is primarily neurapraxic is given ES when the condition becomes manifest, and then

**CASE STUDY**  *continued*

function returns in a short time, it is human nature to say, "See, my therapy worked. Don't tell me electrical stimulation is useless!" But this is classical *post hoc, ergo propter hoc* reasoning; it demonstrates more enthusiasm than basic understanding of the condition being treated.

For those who believe that ES should be used in these situations, their task is to show that return of muscle force and function is either faster or attains a higher final level than when ES is not employed. That will not be an easy study to perform, but it is certainly needed. The use of ES for denervated muscle cannot be based on arguments that fall back on "tradition" (although the tradition may indeed be valid), or on studies that only superficially represent the clinical situations that physical therapists encounter.

The area where we really need clinical data relates to neuronotmesis, that is, situations in which an entire nerve trunk is severed and repaired, possibly microsurgically or with nerve grafts. Physical therapists who have the opportunity to work with patients who have undergone limb salvage procedures, such as reattachment of an amputated part, have the ideal opportunity to document the type of treatments given and the extent of neurologic return that occurs over the months or years. The comparative experiences of these clinicians can contribute the most to determining whether ES is needed or necessary. Because any one therapist probably does not see a large number of these patients, perhaps some sort of "central registry" can be established to which individual clinicians can contribute their experiences.

In conclusion, the final chapter obviously has not been written concerning the possible benefits of ES for human denervated muscle. Will that goal ever be reached? Not until long-term human studies are properly conducted, reported, and subjected to critical, unbiased scrutiny.[34] Until then, the question is unresolved.

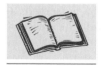

## REVIEW QUESTIONS

1. When reviewing a paper which reports that "electrical stimulation is beneficial to denervated muscle," what is the overriding issue that you should be concerned about? What specific issues should you look for to determine whether or not the study satisfies your main concern?

2. A patient is sent to you 4 weeks after anterior dislocation of his right shoulder. You note marked atrophy of the right deltoid and decide to use ES to help "strengthen" this muscle. The only stimulator you have is a battery-operated neuromuscular electrical stimulator, which you have used in the past on patients with conditions such as patellar tracking problems. You set the unit up as you usually do with your orthopedic patients, and find that even with maximal amplitude, there are no responses from any head of the involved deltoid. Why?

3. You have a clinical stimulator that permits you to choose between three sinusoidal frequencies: 1000 Hz, 100 Hz, and 10 Hz. Which of these would probably be capable of stimulating a denervated muscle? Why?

## References

1. Adams RD, Denny-Brown D, Pearson CM. Diseases of Muscle: A Study in Pathology. New York, NY, Paul B. Hoeber, 1954.
2. Aird RB, Nafziger HC. The pathology of human striated muscle following denervation. J Neurosurg, 10:216–227, 1953.
3. Al-Amood WS, Lewis DM, Schmalbruch H. Effects of chronic electrical stimulation on contractile properties of long-term denervated rat skeletal muscle. J Physiol, 441:243–256, 1991.
4. Albuquerque EX, McIsaac RJ. Fast and slow mammalian muscles after denervation. Exp Neurol, 26:183–202, 1970.
5. Altschul R. Atrophy, degeneration and metaplasia in denervated skeletal muscle. Arch Path, 34:982–988, 1942.
6. Axelsson J, Thesleff S. A study of supersensitivity in denervated mammalian skeletal muscle. J Physiol, 149:178–193, 1959.
7. Belmar J, Eyzaguirre C. Pacemaker site of fibrillation potentials in denervated mammalian muscle. J Neurophysiol, 29:425–441, 1966.
8. Bennett RL, Knowlton GC. Overwork weakness in partially denervated skeletal muscle. Clin Orthop, 12:22–29, 1958.
9. Boonstra AM, van Weerden TW, Eisma WH et al. The effect of low-frequency electrical stimulation on denervation atrophy in man. Scand J Rehab Med, 19:127–134, 1987.
10. Bowden REM, Gutmann E. Denervation and re-innervation of human voluntary muscle. Brain, 67:273–313, 1944.
11. Brown GL. The actions of acetylcholine on denervated mammalian and frog's muscle. J Physiol, 89:438–461, 1937.
12. Brown MC, Holland RL, Ironton R. Nodal and terminal sprouting from motor nerves in fast and slow muscles of the mouse. J Physiol, 306:493–510, 1980.
13. Brown MC, Holland RL, Hopkins WG. Motor nerve sprouting. Ann Rev Neurosci, 4:17–42, 1981.
14. Brown MC, Ironton R. Suppression of motor nerve terminal sprouting in partially denervated mouse muscles. J Physiol, 272:70P–71P, 1977.

15. Brown WF. A method for estimating the number of motor units in thenar muscles and the changes in motor unit count with ageing. J Neurol Neurosurg Psychiatry, 35:845–852, 1976.

16. Cannon WB, Rosenblueth A. The Supersensitivity of Denervated Structures. New York, NY, Macmillan, 1949.

17. Chor H, Cleveland D, Davenport HA et al. Atrophy and regeneration of the gastrocnemius-soleus muscles: Effects of physical therapy in the monkey following section and suture of sciatic nerve. JAMA, 113:1029–1033, 1939.

18. Covault J, Sanes JR. Neural cell adhesion molecule (N-CAM) accumulates in denervated and paralyzed skeletal muscles. Proc Natl Acad Sci, 82:4544–4548, 1985.

19. Davis HL, Kiernan JA. Neurotrophic effects of sciatic nerve extract on denervated extensor digitorum longus muscle in the rat. Exp Neurol, 69:124–134, 1980.

20. Davis HL, Heinicke EA, Cook RA, Kiernan JA. Partial purification from mammalian peripheral nerve of a trophic factor that ameliorates atrophy of denervated muscle. Exp Neurol, 89:159–171, 1985.

21. Davis HL, Bressler BH, Jasch LG. Myotrophic effects on denervated fast-twitch muscles of mice: Correlation of physiologic, biochemical, and morphologic findings. Exp Neurol, 99:474–489, 1988.

22. Denny-Brown D. The influence of tension and innervation on the regeneration of skeletal muscle. J Neuropath Exp Neurol, 10:94–96, 1951.

23. Dumitru D. Cranial neuropathies. In Dumitru D, (ed) Electrodiagnostic Medicine, Philadelphia, PA, Hanley & Belfus, pp 689–740, 1995.

24. Doupe J, Barnes R, Kerr AS. The effect of electrical stimulation on the circulation and recovery of denervated muscle. J Neurol Psychiat, 6:136–140, 1943.

25. Drachman DB, Witzke F. Trophic regulation of acetylcholine sensitivity of muscle: Effect of electrical stimulation. Science, 176:514–516, 1972.

26. Edds MV. Collateral regeneration of residual motor axons in partially denervated muscles. J Exp Zool, 113:517–552, 1950.

27. Feinstein B, Lindegard B, Nyman E, Wohlfart G. Morphologic studies of motor units in normal human muscles. Acta Anatomica, 23:127–142, 1955.

28. Fischer E. The effect of faradic and galvanic stimulation upon the course of atrophy in denervated skeletal muscles. Am J Physiol, 127:605–619, 1939.

29. Girlanda P, Dattola R, Vita G et al. Effect of electrotherapy on denervated muscles in rabbits: An electrophysiological and morphological study. Exp Neurol, 77:483–491, 1982.

30. Gutmann E, Guttmann L. The effect of electrotherapy on denervated muscles in rabbits. Lancet, 1:169–170, 1942.

31. Gutmann E, Guttmann L. The effect of galvanic exercise on denervated and re-innervated muscles in the rabbit. J Neurol Neurosurg Psychiat, 7:7–17, 1944.

32. Gutmann E, Zelena J. Morphological changes in the denervated muscle. In Gutmann E (ed). Denervated Muscle. Publishing House of the Czechoslovak Academy of Sciences, Prague, 1962.

33. Guth L, Kemerer VF, Samaras TA et al. The roles of disuse and loss of neurotrophic function in denervation atrophy of skeletal muscle. Exp Neurol, 73:20–36, 1981.

34. Harris SR. How should treatments be critiqued for scientific merit? Phys Ther, 76:175–181, 1996.
35. Heck CS, Davis HL. Effect of denervation and nerve extract on ultra-structure of muscle. Exp Neurol, 100:139–153, 1988.
36. Hoffman H. Local reinnervation in partially denervated muscle: A histo-physiological study. Aust J Exp Biol Med Sci, 28:383–397, 1950.
37. Ironton R, Brown MC, Holland RL. Stimuli to intramuscular nerve growth. Brain Res, 156:351–354, 1978.
38. Johnson EW, Braddom R. Over-work weakness in facioscapulohumeral muscular dystrophy. Arch Phys Med Rehabil, 52:333–336, 1971.
39. Kessler KJ, Uribe JW. Complete isolated axillary nerve palsy in college and professional football players: A report of 6 cases. Clin J Sports Med, 4:272–274, 1994.
40. Kosman AJ, Osborne SL, Ivy AC. The comparative effectiveness of various electrical currents in preventing muscle atrophy in the rat. Arch Phys Med Rehabil, 28:7–12, 1947.
41. Kosman AJ, Osborne SL, Ivy AC. The influence of duration and frequency of treatment in electrical stimulation of paralyzed muscle. Arch Phys Med Rehabil, 28:12–17, 1947.
42. Kowarschik J. Exponential currents. Br J Phys Med, 15:249–252, 1952.
43. Liddell EGT, Sherrington CS. Recruitment and some other features of reflex inhibition. Proc R Soc Lond (Biol), 97:488–518, 1925.
44. Lomo T, Slater CR. Control of acetylcholine sensitivity and synapse formation by muscle activity. J Physiol, 275:391–402, 1978.
45. Lovett RW. The treatment of infantile paralysis: Preliminary report, based on a study of the Vermont epidemic of 1914. JAMA, 64: 2118–2123, 1915.
46. Lundervold A, Seyffarth H. Electromyographic investigations of poliomyelitic paresis during the training up of the affected muscles, and some remarks regarding the treatment of paretic muscles. Acta Psychiatr Neurol, 17:69–87, 1942.
47. McComas AJ, Fawcett PRW, Campbell MJ, Sica REP. Electrophysiological estimation of the number of motor units within a human muscle. J Neurol Neurosurg Psychiat, 34:121–131, 1971.
48. McComas AJ, Galea V, de Bruin H. Motor unit populations in healthy and diseased muscles. Phys Ther, 73:868–877, 1993.
49. Milot J, Cote CH, Tremblay RR. Putative effects of nerve extract on carbonic anhydrase III expression in rat muscles. Muscle Nerve, 17: 1431–1438, 1994.
50. Neumayer C, Happak W, Kern H, Gruber H. Hypertrophy and transformation of muscle fibers in paraplegic patients. Artific Org, 21:188–190, 1997.
51. Nix WA, Dahm M. The effect of isometric short-term electrical stimulation on denervated muscle. Muscle Nerve, 10:136–143, 1987.
52. Osborne SL. The retardation of atrophy in man by electrical stimulation of muscles. Arch Phys Med Rehabil, 32:523–528, 1951.
53. Purves D, Sakmann B. Membrane properties underlying spontaneous activity of denervated muscle fibers. J Physiol, 239:125–153, 1974.
54. Reid J. On relation between muscular contractility and the nervous system. Lond Edinb Month J Med Sci, 1:320, 1841.

55. Sanes J, Covault J. Axon guidance during reinnervation of skeletal muscle. Trends Neurosci, 18:523–528, 1985.

56. Sayers ST, Yeoh HC, McLane JA, Held IR. Decreased acetylcholine receptor content in denervated skeletal muscles infused with nerve extract. J Neurosci Res, 16:517–525, 1986.

57. Schiff M. Ueber motorische Lahmung der Zunge. Arch Physiol Heilkunde, 10:579–593, 1851.

58. Schimrigk K, McLaughlin J, Gruninger W. The effect of electrical stimulation on the experimentally denervated rat muscle. Scand J Rehab Med, 9:55–60, 1977.

59. Schmalbruch H, Al-Amood WS, Lewis DM. Morphology of long-term denervated rat soleus muscle and the effect of chronic electrical stimulation. J Physiol, 441:233–241, 1991.

60. Sunderland S. Nerves and Nerve Injuries (2nd ed). Churchill Livingstone, Edinburgh, 1978.

61. Sunderland S, Ray LJ. Denervation changes in mammalian striated muscle. J Neurol Neurosurg Psychiat, 13:159–177, 1950.

62. Tower SS. Atrophy and degeneration in skeletal muscle. Am J Anat, 56:1–43, 1935.

63. Wakim KG, Krusen FH. The influence of electrical stimulation on the work output and endurance of denervated muscle. Arch Phys Med Rehabil, 36:370–376, 1955.

64. Ware F, Bennett AL, McIntyre AR. Membrane resting potential of denervated mammalian skeletal muscle measured in vivo. Am J Physiol, 177:115–118, 1954.

65. Wehrmacher WH, Thomson JD, Hines HM. Effects of electrical stimulation on denervated skeletal muscle. Arch Phys Med Rehabil, 26:261–266, 1945.

66. Wolf SM, Wagner JH, Davidson S, Forsythe A. Treatment of Bell's palsy with prednisone: A prospective, randomized study. Neurology, 28:158–161, 1978.

# Contemporary Application of Electrotherapeutic Examination and Intervention

# 10

# Evaluating New Treatments in Electrotherapy

Jane E. Sullivan

## Introduction

A s health care providers, physical therapists continually strive to improve the quality of life of the clients we serve. We talk with each other, read articles and textbooks, and attend courses. We ponder difficult cases and we look for newer and better methods to make a difference for our patients. We scrutinize established methods to determine whether they really produce the positive outcomes that we once thought they did. At times, we choose to abandon interventions when positive clinical outcomes are not borne out by studies or in practice. There are examples of abandoning unsuccessful treatments in the field of electrotherapy. In 1950, Lee and coworkers described a "fair" reduction in abnormal firmness (defined as tone) achieved by stimulating a spastic muscle.[1] Unsuccessful attempts to reproduce these beneficial effects led clinicians to look for more successful methods for spasticity management. Techniques that produce a contraction of the antagonist to the spastic muscle through electrical stimulation[2,3] and submotor levels of stimulation[4,5] both appear to yield more positive results.

Just as we analyze established interventions, we need to critically examine developing techniques and equipment. We should continually question whether the new methods we try are better than the old. We need to become experts at analyzing the evidence regarding our clinical methods. Evidence to support efficacy is critical on three levels: ethics, economics, and the continued growth and development of our profession. Ethical practice demands that we choose treatments that have a high probability of achieving successful outcomes for our clients. Economically, our services are unlikely to be reimbursed unless we can demonstrate efficacy based on outcome studies. Finally, our profession will continue to survive and grow only if we can offer evidence that the skills and services we provide constitute a critical and integral component of health care.

## EVIDENCE-BASED PRACTICE

Reading professional literature is a common method of keeping up-to-date. However, what we read and how we interpret what we read will affect our clinical choices. We need to use our reading not only to get new ideas but also to provide us with evidence to support our clinical decisions. **Evidence-based medicine (EBM)** is a term that has been used to describe an approach to practicing medicine in which clinicians are aware of the evidence and the strength of that evidence in support of clinical practice.[6] Evidence-based medicine recognizes the importance of three types of information:

1. **Systematic overviews**—reviews that use explicit and rigorous methods to identify, critically appraise, and synthesize relevant studies from medical research
2. **Meta-analysis**—reviews that use quantitative methods to summarize the results of research, preferably randomized controlled trials
3. **Practice guidelines**—recommendations that provide bottom-line messages that are clinically applicable and scientifically valid[6]

The Agency for Health Care and Policy Research (AHCPR), an arm of the U.S. Public Health Service, was established in 1989 to "enhance the quality, appropriateness, and effectiveness of health care services and to improve access to that care."[7] The AHCPR conducts research in general health care and medical effectiveness, and develops and disseminates clinical practice guidelines. These guidelines are "systematically developed statements and recommendations to assist practitioner and patient decisions about appropriate health care for specific clinical conditions."[7] Because clients with the diagnoses addressed in these guidelines are seen frequently by physical therapists, the guidelines themselves and the studies cited in each guideline may aid clinicians in making choices based on the strength of available evidence.

In addition to reading professional literature, physical therapists attend continuing education courses in an attempt to learn about new techniques and equipment. We are anxious to return to our clinics and try out our new techniques and equipment. Harris expresses concern that when physical therapists learn a new treatment approach at a continuing education course given by an acknowledged "expert" in the field, they are often satisfied that their roles as responsible consumers of this new knowledge have been achieved. She comments that even seasoned clinicians may have vested interests in believing that their newly acquired intervention techniques are effecting positive changes in their clients.[8]

As we try new techniques and equipment, we continually hope that these newer methods will prove more effective and efficient. However, in trying new skills or tools, we often tend to overestimate their effectiveness. Sackett discusses three reasons why experienced clinicians tend to overestimate the efficacy of nonexperimental evidence.

1. Clinicians are more likely to recognize and remember when clients are compliant and keep their appointments. Increased compliance with treatment generally leads to better outcomes. Therefore, we remember those clients and may conclude that the interventions we used with them are more successful than interventions used with less compliant patients.
2. Unusual patterns or symptoms tend to return to a more normal result, a regression toward the mean. Treatments that are initiated in the interim may appear efficacious.
3. Routine clinical practice is never blinded. The placebo effect and the client's and clinician's desire for success can cause both to overestimate efficacy.[9]

Harris[8] has provided us with a blueprint for analyzing new treatment approaches. She describes six criteria to use in evaluating the scientific merit of developing treatments. This systematic analysis of information could also be useful in evaluating both new equipment and continuing education courses. As our resources are not limitless, we need to make informed choices about the techniques we use, the courses we attend, and the equipment we purchase and recommend.

## CRITERIA FOR EVALUATING NEW TREATMENTS

In this chapter, Harris' criteria will be used as a framework for assessing new techniques, equipment, and continuing education offerings in electrotherapy. Discussions about three electrotherapy techniques will be used to illustrate this analysis. The therapies analyzed will include: a technique of nighttime submotor electrical stimulation (ES) that has been called **therapeutic electrical stimulation (TES),**

**pelvic floor electrical stimulation (PFES)** used to treat urinary incontinence (UI), and a technique using subsensory levels of electrical stimulation commonly referred to as **microcurrent electrical neuro stimulation (MENS).**

Harris' first criterion analyzes the theory supporting the use of the technique. She states, "Theories underlying the treatment approach are supported by valid anatomical and physiological evidence."[8] I propose expanding this criterion to include not only the scientific evidence but also the logical design of the characteristics of the intervention. Therefore, I propose that the first criterion related to the theory behind the approach, equipment design, or course be: **The theory supporting the approach is logically sound and supported by valid anatomic and physiologic evidence.**

Harris' second criterion[8] is that the treatment is designed for a specific type of patient population. Because multiple diagnostic groups may share impairments based on similar etiology, a focus on the etiology of the impairment or functional limitation versus the diagnosis seems more appropriate. This leads me to reword Harris' criterion as follows: **The treatment approach is designed for specific impairments or functional limitations based on etiology.**

Harris' third criterion[8] deals with the potential risks of the intervention. I agree that this information must be presented and discussed openly. Therefore, the third criterion is: **Potential side effects of the treatment are presented.**

Harris' fourth and fifth criteria[8] address the evidence supporting the treatment intervention. She recommends analyzing three characteristics: where the studies are published, the support offered by these studies, and the design of the studies themselves. The first recommendation is that the studies are published in peer-reviewed journals. Reports appearing in these publications have been subjected to review by acknowledged experts. This review represents additional scrutiny that clinicians should welcome. Increasingly, medical information is disseminated in the lay press. Use of the lay press can be both educational and misleading. We have become accustomed to hearing about studies published in reputable medical journals on local news broadcasts. When this information is presented accurately and coupled with a commentary by an unbiased expert, the public is well served. Often, the information is in the form of clinical anecdotes and patient testimonials, which can lead clients to develop unrealistic expectations from treatment or to seek treatments that are not appropriate for them. The situation is more serious when clients abandon clinically proven treatments to pursue interventions that have not been validated.

When information from medical studies or developing medical therapies is presented in the lay press, it may be difficult to control the content. The proponents of the interventions have a responsibility to the public to attempt to present the information as factual and unbiased. The public should understand whether the approach has been tested, how it compares in terms of costs and benefits to conventional treatments, and for what population the intervention is recommended.

An example of this phenomenon in electrotherapy is in the area of functional electrical stimulation (FES). Techniques to achieve standing and limited ambulation in clients with spinal cord injuries had already been documented in the professional literature for almost a decade[10] when these techniques were profiled on several television news magazine shows and made-for-television movies. There was an immediate flurry of attention. Patients and their families were excited by the possibility that they might be able to walk. The small percentage of clients for whom this technique was appropriate, the time and money involved in the training, and the limited number of subjects that achieved any measure of functional ambulation were not apparent in the initial reports. Subsequent research in this area has delineated candidates, costs,[11] outcomes[12] and equipment.[13] Later studies looked at stimulated cycling, which was initially utilized for improving muscle force for ambulation. These techniques have been shown to provide benefits in the prevention of cardiovascular disease.[14,15] Although the stimulated cycling programs were developed in the hopes of providing functional locomotion, the impact of demonstrating that this tool can improve cardiovascular function in the patient population with spinal cord injuries is very significant.

In short, initial public attention was drawn by the limited information presented in dramatic fashion in the lay press (both TV and magazines). Eventually, more balanced accounts of the techniques were disseminated in professional literature. Although these scientifically based, peer-reviewed reports may not have the emotional impact of those presented in the popular media, they must form the basis of both our clinical decision making and the education of our clients.

Harris also recommends that the data and conclusions from the studies actually support the efficacy of the intervention.[8] One must consider the study design. Ideally, the trial should be randomized, controlled, and blinded. Outcome measures should be valid and reliable. Single-subject studies should be designed with multiple repeated measures and withdrawal phases. Comparisons with conventional treatments should be included wherever appropriate and possible. My fourth criterion therefore summarizes Harris' considerations of the relevant literature: **Studies from peer-reviewed journals are provided that support the treatment's efficacy. These studies include well-designed, randomized, controlled clinical trials or well designed single subject experimental studies.**

## TABLE 10-1 SUMMARY OF TREATMENT CHARACTERISTICS

| CHARACTERISTIC | MENS | PFES | TES |
|---|---|---|---|
| Waveform | Variable, slow rise to square wave[16]<br>Alternating polarity[88] | Interferential[38,69,94]<br>Symmetric biphasic[39–42,68, 70,75,95,97,99] | Alternating coupled current pulses[44,96]<br>Balanced biphasic[66] |
| Current amplitude | 10–600 μA[16]<br>30 μA[88]<br>100 μA[79,80,89] | Sufficient for subjects to perceive stimulation[37,76]<br>Sufficient for visible or palpable pelvic floor contraction[41]<br>Highest tolerable[42,69,94] | Less than 10 mA[44,64]<br>Sensory level[116] |
| Phase duration | 0.5 sec[37] | 20–700 μsec[40,41,68,70,95,97]<br>1.0–50 msec[39,42,72,91] | 300 μsec[65,66] |
| Frequency | 0.1–990 Hz[16]<br>0.3 Hz[79–80,88–89]<br>1 Hz[22] | General recommendations:<br>0–100 Hz[94]<br>0–20 Hz[7,79,99]<br>20–50 Hz[40,68,95,96]<br>For SUI:<br>10–50 Hz/2 kHz<br>50 Hz/2 kHz[69]<br>10–50 Hz[39,42,76]<br>For UUI:<br>20 Hz or less[39,42]<br>5–10 Hz/2 kHz[69]<br>12.5 Hz[40,41]<br>For mixed UI:<br>50 Hz in A.M., 12.5 Hz in P.M.[40]<br>Adjusted for the dominant condition[42] | 35 Hz[65,66,116] |
| Duty cycle | 50 %[22,79,80] | General recommendations:<br>1:3 ON:OFF cycle[40–42,97]<br>1:3.5 ON:OFF cycle[92]<br>Continuous[94] | 1:! ON:OFF cycle[65,66,116] |
| Ramp/fall | Gentle wave slope[16]<br>0.5 sec[88] | Not addressed | 2 second ramp[65,66,116] |
| Treatment time | Few seconds—several minutes, averages 15–20 min[16,22]<br>10 min[89]<br>1 hr[80]<br>2 hr[79] | 15–30 min[38,40–41,68–70, 94,95,97]<br>up to 24 hr[37,99] | 8–10 hr/night[116]<br>8–12 hr/night[65] |
| Treatment frequency | Daily[16,79,80]<br>Three times weekly[89] | 2–3 times/week[68,94,95]<br>Daily[38]<br>2–3 times/day[40–42,96,97]<br>Continuously[98] | Nightly[44,65] |
| Treatment duration | Varies with diagnosis[16]<br>5 days[80]<br>14 days[79]<br>3 weeks[89] | 6 sessions[38]<br>4–8 weeks[42,68,94–97]<br>12–20 weeks[41,67,70] | Several months to several years[71] |

| TABLE 10–1   SUMMARY OF TREATMENT CHARACTERISTICS (CONTINUED) | | | |
| --- | --- | --- | --- |
| CHARACTERISTIC | MENS | PFES | TES |
| Electrode placement | Varies with diagnosis[16] Anode at wound site[79] Cathode at wound site for 3 days, then reverse polarity[78] | Surface[38,68,93,98] Internal[38,40–42,67,70,94–96] Surgically implantable[70] | Tibialis anterior, quadriceps muscles[64] Overantagonist to spastic muscle[65] |

Harris' final criterion[8] considers the collegial atmosphere of information sharing that has enabled the development and refining of many important clinical interventions. As students, we are taught to self-assess and invite peer assessment to further our ideas. Authors who are willing to share their information seek feedback and recognize the limitations of their studies can make greater contributions to clinical practice. The final criterion expands Harris' criterion in considering the proponents' willingness to discuss all aspects of the interventions: **The proponents of the treatment are open and willing to discuss the approach's methods, benefits, and limitations.**

Microcurrent electrical neuro stimulation, PFES for incontinence, and TES are popular topics in physical therapy clinics but have been noticeably absent in electrotherapy textbooks and in the curricula of entry-level electrotherapy courses. Students frequently return from clinical experiences with questions about techniques that they have observed but not discussed in the classroom. The analysis that follows is based on the modified Harris criteria, the available literature, and input from the numerous faculty and students who have participated in many lively discussions about this analysis. Each criterion will be identified and the corresponding evidence regarding MENS, PFES, and TES will be presented followed by a commentary. Table 10–1 has been provided to illustrate the general characteristics utilized in these approaches.

## ASSESSMENT CRITERIA

### Criterion 1

**The theory supporting the approach is logically sound and supported by valid anatomic and physiologic evidence.** MENS treatment has been proposed for two primary goals, tissue healing and pain reduction. Microcurrent electrical neuro stimulation proponents[16,17] have suggested a mechanism for the role of electrical stimulation in healing based on the theory of a "current of injury." Becker and Murray[18] have described a current that can be measured on the surface of wounds after injury. Others have theorized that there is a flow of charged particles from healthy to injured dermis.[19,20] that triggers the tissue repair process by enhancing the migration of macrophages and fibroblasts. Burr and coworkers[21] observed that chronic wounds demonstrate a reduced injury current relative to noninjured tissue and theorized that this reduced current is responsible for the lack of healing. Microcurrent electrical neuro stimulation proponents have advocated the application of electrical currents to damaged tissue to augment the existing injury current and accelerate healing.[16,17]

Wallace[16] and Picker[22] cite the Arndt–Schultz Law ("weak stimuli increase physiologic activity and very strong stimuli inhibit or abolish activity") as a rationale for MENS strategies. They utilize this law to support their position that higher amplitudes of ES may inhibit the desired response, whereas lower amplitudes of ES may facilitate this response.

How does MENS theory measure up on the basis of the first criterion? The theory of electrical enhancement of an injury current, while unproven, does have a basis in anatomic and physiologic observations. If this error recognition system does exist in the body, it may be possibly augmented via externally induced electrical fields. Baker suggests that some effect may be achieved by enhancing peripheral circulation via ES[23]; however, the amplitude of stimulation necessary to achieve this effect is not known.

Application of the Arndt–Schultz Law to ES in the clinic is not clear. Dose–response relationships have yet to be determined for wound healing and pain reduction. Electrical stimulation at very high amplitudes is known to be painful and cause tissue irritation. Electrical stimulation delivered at levels that cause strong muscular contraction can improve muscle force (strength), increase range of motion, decrease spasticity, and enhance motor control. We need to determine whether there is an amplitude below which no benefit is observed. Finding the point at which the dose–response curve flattens out—the point at which there is too little input to achieve a therapeutic effect—is critical.

We also need to consider the logic of the relationship between input dosage and time needed to achieve a beneficial effect. For example, if a comparable beneficial outcome can be achieved by both low-dosage, low-duration inputs and treatment with a higher (although tolerable) dosage given over a shorter time duration, the latter treatment is more cost effective. An example of this relationship between dosage and treatment duration can be seen with the application of ES in wound healing. Studies with continuous or pulsed direct current[24–28] demonstrated a beneficial effect in wound healing, but shorter duration; higher, yet tolerable, current amplitudes have also produced positive outcomes.[29–31] This later intervention is very efficient in terms of resource utilization. Finally, from the client's perspective, there is often additional value in the treatment that yields results in a shorter period of time.

Pelvic floor electrical stimulation has been recommended for urinary incontinence resulting from striated muscle malfunction. In cases of stress urinary incontinence (SUI), there is often inability to generate sufficient force (strength) or sustain contractions over time (endurance) in the pelvic floor musculature.[32] Difficulty achieving urethral closure may result from this muscle weakness. If a client is unable to contract the pelvic floor muscles voluntarily, PFES may help them to identify the location of these muscles and experience the feeling of appropriate muscle contraction. Pelvic floor electrical stimulation may also be utilized to help train sufficient force production and endurance capabilities.

Hahn suggests that a sufficient number of fast-twitch pelvic floor muscle fibers is necessary to prevent a drop in urethral closing pressure during stressful activities (eg, coughing, jumping).[32] Conversely, slow-twitch fibers are necessary to maintain adequate resting tone of the urethra. The transformation of fast-twitch fibers to fibers that have slow-twitch characteristics in response to low-frequency ES has been suggested.[33,34] Conversely, stimulation delivered at higher frequencies can cause slow-twitch muscle fibers to behave like fast-twitch ones.[35] Depending on a patient's presenting problems, stimulation can be delivered at frequencies consistent with the desired muscle fiber characteristics.

In contrast to SUI, urge urinary incontinence (UUI) results from uninhibited detrusor activity or an unstable bladder. Pelvic floor electrical stimulation is hypothesized to elicit a pudendal-to-pelvic reflex that depresses or eliminates these uninhibited detrusor contractions.[36] Fall has theorized that improving the performance of the pelvic floor muscles also results in better reflex inhibition of the detrusor.[37]

Because the mechanisms of SUI and UUI are different, different PFES treatment characteristics are recommended. For SUI, stimulation is designed to elicit contraction of the striated muscle of the pelvic floor and delivered at an amplitude and pulse frequency sufficient to achieve strong tetanic muscle contraction.[37,38,39] For UUI, stimulation is aimed at activation of the pudendal-to-pelvic reflex and delivered at a pulsed frequency of 20 Hz or less.[38,39,40,41] For mixed incontinence (with characteristics of both UUI and SUI), a combination of frequencies may be employed,[40] or stimulation pulse frequency may be directed toward improving the dominant condition.[42]

The theory behind PFES to treat SUI is grounded in the goal of achieving either better force production or fatigue resistance in the pelvic floor muscles. This application is similar to the force (strength) and endurance applications that have long been advocated and documented in patients with orthopedic problems. The anatomic and physiologic basis of this intervention is sound. The theory of UUI treatment by PFES is based on reflex inhibition of the detrusor muscle. Treatment characteristics for PFES derive logically from the intended physiologic action.

Therapeutic electrical stimulation techniques were developed by Dr. Karen Pape, a Canadian physician, and her coworkers. Pape discusses the development of the theory of TES in the description of the first child on whom the technique was performed. She describes a "child born in 1982 with C1, C3 spinal cord injury."[43] At 2 weeks of age, the child had "some movement in her right index finger" and was given "full support." At 3 years of age, the child was tried on a "standard neuromuscular paradigm" using ES; however, this protocol was reportedly "not well tolerated" secondary to "breath holding." Pape says that the research team was "frustrated" and reasoned that if "high intensity, short duration therapy would have an effect, it would be valid to see if low intensity over a long duration would have a similar effect."[43] Assuming that motor control is the goal of this treatment, what is confusing is the fact that conventional techniques utilizing ES for improving motor control and muscle force (strengthening) employ an electrical current amplitude sufficiently high enough to activate motor nerves and cause muscle contraction. How muscles can achieve greater force production or improved motor control without contracting is unexplained by Pape.

Much of the rationale for the development of TES techniques appears to be a reaction to more conventional ES treatments. Pape and colleagues say that TES was developed to address the problems associated with daytime, high-amplitude stimulation protocols. They state that "traditional electrical stimulation techniques cannot be easily used by young children."[44] Carmick, however, has demonstrated that ES is well tolerated with children as young as 18 months of age.[45] Numerous other authors have reported that ES can be utilized effectively in children to improve motor control and muscle force (strength).[46-57] Pape expresses concern over the "time and cost of supervised daily treatment programs."[58] However, most authors advocating conventional ES paradigms for treatment of motor control problems in children recommend stimulation sessions one[51,52] to three times weekly.[47-49,55]

Following the publication of two case studies on motor level ES utilized with children,[51,52] Pape expressed concern about risks to children using motor-level stimulation. She discussed numerous "ill effects" observed in her clinic including "overwork syndromes, stress fractures, tendon and epiphyseal plate disruptions and small joint dislocations."[59] In her response to Pape's concerns, Carmick elaborated on how safety can be ensured by close monitoring of the child's response and of the equipment characteristics. She recommended that Pape "document both the programs and injuries and present them through some appropriate forum."[60] To date, no reports of these ES-related injuries have been offered by Pape or other TES proponents.

Pape has hypothesized that the effect of TES is mediated by changes in regional blood flow in response to the current.[43] She speculates that this increased blood flow occurs during the nighttime treatment, at the same time that there is an increase in the production of growth hormone. She states that "by applying the current during sleep, we believe that we have tricked the body into growing muscle." There is, however, evidence that in order to increase blood flow via ES, a muscle contraction must occur.[61,62] Therapeutic electrical stimulation authors have not presented evidence to support their contention that nighttime submotor ES results in an increase in regional blood flow, nor have they shown evidence for an increase in the levels of growth hormone regionally or systemically.

Pape offers another explanation for the use of TES: "Neural pathways short-circuited by, say CP or spina bifida, or damaged by spinal injuries can be reactivated so long as they are artificially given muscles to operate by means of TES."[63] This explanation appears to presuppose that the intervention has some effect on spinal pathways. The mechanism of such an effect or the evidence of its existence is not discussed.

Because spasticity is reported to be a problem for many of the clients who have used TES, Pape theorizes that the intervention might be useful to reduce this abnormally high reflex sensitivity. In a pilot study utilizing TES on children with cerebral palsy, Pape and coworkers stated, "Our investigations were aimed at determining whether the beneficial effects of ES could reduce spasticity for the long term."[64] The theory of reciprocal inhibition is offered to support spasticity reduction via TES. One rationale for the delivery of stimulation during sleep has been that spasticity is lower during this time. Aside from anecdotal information from clinicians and parents, the literature about TES does not present quantitative information detailing spasticity measurement. That the researchers chose not to measure spasticity when they state that their aim was the reduction of this abnormal tone is puzzling. Other researchers have published reports that describe the objective reduction of spasticity achieved by ES delivered at cutaneous levels in subjects with spinal cord and traumatic brain injuries[4] and in subjects with hemiplegia following stroke.[5]

Pape acknowledges that there is weakness in spastic muscle but argues that the nonspastic antagonist muscle is even weaker.[44] This logic appears to drive the decision of where to place the stimulating electrodes. However, because the stimulation amplitude is below the threshold of the motor fibers and muscle activation is not desired, the logic of electrode placement over a muscle belly of the antagonist to the spastic muscle is unexplained.

Pape comments that the intervention "requires ongoing therapy be conducted to improve the muscle's force and to channel the added force into function."[63] If this additional therapy is a necessary component of the intervention, how can one determine if any beneficial effects are as a result of the ES or the "functional retraining"[63] or both? The answer of course is to compare subjects using stimulation only, functional retraining only, a combination of the two interventions, and controls. Data on these comparisons have not been published. Pape and coworkers do not appear to advocate a particular form of exercise therapy. "All but one child [in their study] continued to have standard rehabilitation procedures administered by community rehabilitation centers."[64] Whether the outcomes for the child who did not receive conventional therapy were different from those who did is not reported. In a TES study by Steinbok and colleagues, it was similarly reported that "parents were instructed to continue with any other therapy that the child was receiving and not to modify any ongoing therapy program."[65] The authors further report that the treating therapist was "contacted and given similar instructions." This raises some concern about the effect of the treating therapist knowing that the child was participating in a TES study.

In addition to the question of which intervention—the TES or the functional retraining—produces the outcome, the issue of utilization of resources is raised. Other authors have demonstrated that motor control can be improved by utilizing ES during task specific therapy.[45,51–55] If TES protocols require "functional retraining"[63] in addition to nighttime stimulation, and if ES during functional activities alone has proved beneficial, the latter approach appears to be more cost effective than the former. The best interests of our clients would be served by comparing the two approaches to determine if one proves to be not only more efficient but equally or more effective.

How does TES rate on the first criterion? The literature on TES is unclear about what the proponents see as the primary goal of the intervention. Spasticity reduction, muscle growth, and treatment of disuse atrophy have all been identified as goals. The logic of how stimulation at the recommended characteristics would achieve the desired physiologic effects on the target tissues is not clearly elucidated by the proponents of the approach. Much of the design of the approach appears to be a reaction to conventional and tested paradigms of ES without explanation or evidence of why changes of the characteristics are recommended. Hopefully, as TES is examined more critically, we will be able to determine whether this labor-intensive, lengthy treatment produces significantly better functional outcomes than motor level ES delivered during functional tasks.

## Criterion 2

**The treatment approach is designed for specific impairments or functional limitations based on etiology.** MENS proponents advocate the intervention for a variety of diagnoses and impairments of multiple body systems. Table 10–2 illustrates the indications that have been identified by MENS writers. Wallace[16] and Picker[22] list contraindications common to other electrotherapeutic interventions.

In addition to identifying specific diagnoses and impairments for which MENS is indicated, Wallace recommends MENS as a treatment

## TABLE 10–2.  IMPAIRMENTS AND DIAGNOSES FOR WHICH THE APPROACHES HAVE BEEN RECOMMENDED

| MENS | PFES | TES |
|------|------|-----|
| Temporomandibular joint problems[88] | Urinary stress incontinence[38,68,69,94] | Brachial plexus injuries[116] |
| Osteoarthritis of the knee[73,89] | Urinary urge incontinence[38,40,67,75,93,88] | Spina bifida[116] |
| Stroke[16] | Mixed stress/urge urinary incontinence[40,67,75,93,95,97,98] | Acquired brain injury[116] |
| Multiple sclerosis[16] | Mixed urinary incontinence with low pressure urethra[96] | Spinal cord injuries[116] |
| Peripheral nerve injury[16] | | Cerebral palsy[116] |
| Spinal cord injury[16] | | Multiple sclerosis[72] |
| Obstetric–gynecologic diagnoses[16] | | Geriatric fitness[72] |
| Dental diagnoses[16] | | Chronic sports injuries[72] |
| Rheumatologic conditions[16] | | Post polio syndrome[103,104] |
| Ear–nose–throat diagnoses[16] | | Bowel and bladder incontinence[71,72] |
| Pain[22] | | Weakness[63,105] |
| Swelling[22] | | Atrophy[63,117] |
| Wounds[22] | | Spasticity[64,117] |
| Inflammation[22] | | Dependence on bracing[72,116] |
| Atrophy secondary to pain and muscle guarding[22] | | |
| Immobility and reduced function after injury[66] | | |

for "bizarre symptoms," saying "unresolvable cases will sometimes respond to MENS."[16] Stanish et al[67] recommend MENS for greater mobility and the earlier return to function. Wallace advocates MENS as a diagnostic aid, which is "less expensive than an EMG (or) CAT scan."[16] He says that in some cases "EMG testing (was) avoided." Wallace asserts, "if pain increases (with MENS), confront the patient (MENS does not increase pain), and if MENS does not provide relief quickly—find out what has been missed in the diagnosis."[16]

In conclusion, to rate MENS on the second criterion, one needs to look for the common denominator in the diagnoses for which MENS is recommended. For example, many of the diagnoses and impairments have their physiologic basis in the inflammatory process. If MENS is found to have a positive circulatory effect or decrease the release of inflammatory substances, it might be of benefit in these conditions. Weakness, atrophy, and spasticity have a basis in disruption of the neuromuscular system. If MENS could be demonstrated to have a positive effect on this system, an application in these conditions could be explained. The recommendation of any intervention for bizarre and unresolvable cases is unacceptable.

The recommendation to use an unproven treatment modality that is intended for pain and tissue healing as a substitute for diagnostic testing does not appear to be responsible. Electromyography and CT scans are designed to identify specific anatomic and physiologic abnormalities. Microcurrent electrical neuro stimulation does not have these capabilities. This application could result in undiagnosed and inappropriately treated clients and gross misuse of health care funds.

Pelvic floor electrical stimulation has been recommended for SUI, UUI, and mixed incontinence in women, men, and children (Table 10–2). One study has offered recommendations about which clients are good candidates for PFES. Susset et al[67] studied 64 women with SUI, UUI, and mixed incontinence using electromyography biofeedback (EMGBF) alternated with PFES. They reported an overall success rate of 64 percent. This study identified five factors as being most predictive of successful outcomes: age, presence of estrogen (present in women before menopause or in women taking estrogen regularly), the absence of detrusor muscle instability and intrinsic sphincter deficiency, low urethral hypermobility, and, most significantly, compliance. Factors that did not appear to influence outcomes were also identified by these authors as being obesity, type of incontinence, initial digital testing, parity, and previous surgery. Because this study combined PFES with biofeedback, the results may only be suggestive of results in clients receiving PFES alone.[67]

Pelvic floor electrical stimulation is not recommended for clients with abnormal neurologic status.[40,68,69] Merrill et al note treatment failures in several subjects with traumatic lower motor neuron lesions and myelomeningocele.[70] Siegel and coworkers found that nonresponse correlated with the number of previous therapies and the number of vaginal deliveries.[41]

Numerous authors have identified contraindications common to other electrotherapeutic interventions (eg, pacemaker, malignancy, and pregnancy).[67,68,69,70] Other contraindications are identified that would interfere with function of the pelvic floor structures or use of the intravaginal ES device (eg, pelvic implanted device, menstrual abnormalities, atrophic vaginitis, vaginal infections, genital prolapse into the introitus, intrinsic sphincteric deficiency, pelvic irradiation).[40,67,69]

In summary, on criterion two, PFES proponents are specific about the limited number of indications for the intervention. Several authors have gone a step further to identify those clients who are and are not good candidates for the treatment.

Therapeutic electrical stimulation has been recommended for multiple diagnoses and impairments. Table 10–2 summarizes these recommendations. Functional changes in clients receiving TES are also discussed. Pape claims, "One of the expected benefits is a decrease in the use or level of bracing or assistive aids required (ankle–foot orthoses, knee–ankle–foot orthoses, crutches, walkers, and wheelchairs). If there is no functional gain, a partial refund is available for used equipment."[71] "In cases of children with mild diplegia, we can usually have them out of ankle–foot orthoses and walking quite normally within 2 years."[72]

Therapeutic electrical stimulation proponents list the following contraindications to treatment: major sensory disabilities,[63] fixed contractures,[63] medication for seizures,[44] clients with uncontrolled seizure activity,[44] severe retardation,[44] and children younger than two years of age.[44] In discussing the population with cerebral palsy, Pape notes that there are "strict entry requirements" including "proven ability to comply, high motivation to work towards change and type and severity of cerebral palsy."[63]

As in the case of MENS, the underlying cause of the impairment or dysfunction is at issue. For example, the weakness noted in clients with cerebral palsy is of a different etiology than that seen in cases of spina bifida. Because the effect of TES is unclear on tissues and systems it is similarly unclear about its appropriateness in these very different pathological conditions. As discussed with MENS, various diagnoses for which TES has been recommended have their etiology in dysfunction in the neuromuscular system. If TES is shown to have an effect here, it might prove appropriate for treatment of disuse atrophy, spasticity reduction, or even effecting functional changes in clients with neuromuscular impairments. As to the claims of improving fitness, the necessary stimulus to bring about changes in an individual's fitness level is to stress the cardiovascular system. There is no physiologic explanation to support TES having this cardiovascular effect.

Claims or apparent guarantees of results are uncommon in medical literature. The proponents of TES make numerous claims of functional expectations. These claims raise concern, since studies of the intervention do not support these claims. Clients considering the treatment may not look beyond these claims to consider the results of available data. We owe our clients accurate information upon which to base decisions about the allocation of their health care resources.

## Criterion 3

**Potential side effects of the treatment are presented.** Using a treatment intervention much like traditional MENS, Zizic and colleagues reported that almost a quarter of their subjects with osteoarthritis of the knee developed a skin rash from the electrode gel. This reaction was seen in both the active and sham device groups. The rash resolved once the treatment was discontinued. These subjects received ES for hours at a time, which is considerably longer than treatment duration with traditional MENS applications.[73] Picker noted that lightheadedness can occur in clients receiving MENS treatment, but that this symptom dissipates after treatment.[22]

Wallace stated that, "essentially no risk is involved, MENS is very safe—patients don't get worse."[16] He goes on to comment that "if a patient complains of an increase in symptomology and are adamant that the unit increased the symptoms, be suspicious (almost all of these patients are workman's compensation, legal or individuals who have some secondary pain [sic] incentive)."[16]

Of concern here is the notion that if the patient does not get better, the fault is with the patient, not the treatment. If this logic is implemented clinically, ineffectual treatment would be continued and, more seriously, the client might not receive an accurate diagnosis and effective treatment. In summary, on criterion three, minimal side effects have been reported with MENS treatment, but these appear to resolve once the intervention is discontinued.

In the AHCPR summary of findings on the treatment of urinary incontinence (UI) by PFES, the conclusion is drawn that this technique can be administered with minimal side effects.[74] While numerous studies identify side effects with the treatment, the number of subjects experiencing them is low. Merrill et al reported that most patients treated with transrectal stimulation experienced abdominal cramps and often mild diarrhea during stimulation, but noted that the symptoms usually subsided after several days.[70] In 1984, Fall reported some degree of constipation in 2 of 40 subjects.[37] Of 40 subjects in a later study, Fall found 4 patients who said that the device (an inflatable intravaginal electrode) was uncomfortable, 2 had slight bleeding, and 5 found the treatment mode unaesthetic.[75] Bent and colleagues reported that 4 of 45 subjects reported pain.[42] In a study by Sand and coworkers,[69] 35 subjects used an active device and 17 used a sham stimulator. These authors reported vaginal irritation in 5 of 35 subjects using the active device and 2 sham subjects, occasional episodes of pain in 1 sham and 3 active subjects, a vaginal infection in 4 active and 2 sham subjects, and urinary tract infections in 1 active and 2 sham subjects. Siegel reported on three subjects who withdrew from treatment; one with of right lower quadrant pain and bladder spasms during treatment, one subject with a history of uterine fibroids who experienced cramping during treatment, and one subject with a history of diarrhea who experienced increasing symptoms. All side effects resolved with discontinuation of device.[41] In summary, while side effects from PFES for treatment of UI are documented, they appear to be relatively minor in severity and low in number, and resolve when the treatment is discontinued.

Writers on TES note minimal side effects from the treatment. Of 86 clients Pape and Kirsch described, one child had seizures after six months of treatment and another child developed a problem sleeping.[44] In the pilot study by Pape and coworkers on TES, one child is reported to have developed slight recurrent skin irritation.[64] Steinbok and colleagues note minor technical problems such as dislodged lead wires and electrodes detaching. They also report one child who had an exacerbation of a previous problem with extrusion of subcutaneous sutures.[65] In conclusion, few side effects from TES are reported and they appear to be relatively minor and infrequent.

Side effects are usually considered to be physiologic, but if a client continues to spend time and money on a treatment without demonstrated efficacy, could a side effect also be functional, psychological, or economic in nature?

## Criterion 4

**Studies from peer-reviewed journals are provided that support the treatment's efficacy. These studies include well-designed, randomized, controlled clinical trials or well-designed single subject experimental studies.** There are two primary problems for which MENS has been advocated: wound healing and pain reduction. In 1969, Wolcott et al described the preliminary results of wound healing in patients with ischemic ulcers that had not responded to conventional therapy. Direct electrical current was administered for a total of 6 hours per day, with a current amplitude of .200 to .800 mA.[76] Other authors reported positive results with similar current characteristics.[25,26,27] Gault and Gatens called this intervention **low-intensity direct current (LIDC).**[25] These early studies used a current amplitude similar to MENS as described by Picker[22] and Wallace[16]; however; the treatment time was significantly longer.

In 1965, Barron and colleagues treated chronic decubitus ulcers in six geriatric patients with an electrical technique they termed **micro-electro medical stimulation (MEMS).** A "modified" biphasic square waveform, with a frequency of 0.5 to 5.0 Hz, and amplitude of .200 to .600 mA was used. Treatments were delivered three times per week for an unspecified duration. The authors reported that five of the six ulcers were healed or "essentially healed" in one month.[77] The similarity between this treatment and MENS is in current amplitude, but treatment duration cannot be compared.

In 1995, Leffman et al and Byl et al presented controlled studies of MENS usage in wound healing.[78,79] These studies were published in a respected, peer-reviewed journal. In each study, MENS was used to treat surgically induced wounds in animals. Both studies utilized random subject assignment into stimulation or control (sham stimulation) groups. Neither study found a significant difference in wound healing between the experimental and control group wounds. Robinson points out that, although the two studies appear similar, they differed in the duration of treatment and current density.[80] Despite these differences, neither study demonstrated evidence of wound healing. In the authors' response to the invited commentaries on their article, Leffman and colleagues state, "It is time for health care practitioners in general and physical therapists specifically to abandon the use of 'microamperage stimulation' for wound healing."[81]

Baker and colleagues studied the effect of healing rates for decubitus ulcers in clients with spinal cord injuries. They used one of four treatment protocols: asymmetric biphasic waveform, symmetrical biphasic waveform, microcurrent stimulation, or a sham stimulation protocol. Analysis showed significantly better healing rates for those receiving stimulation with the asymmetrical biphasic waveform, compared with the control and microcurrent groups. However, while the authors label the stimulation one treatment group received as microcurrent stimulation, the amplitude utilized (4 mA) was higher than that described by Picker (< 1 mA).[22] The authors theorized that low-amplitude stimulation might enhance healing by activation of cutaneous nerves to create a centrally mediated circulatory response.[23] This increased circulation may increase the delivery of nutrients to damaged tissue thereby increasing healing. However, the authors caution that the threshold for activation of these sensory fibers must be reached. This stimulation would therefore not be subsensory stimulation.

The AHCPR Clinical Practice Guideline No. 15 addresses the treatment of pressure ulcers.[82] The guideline recommends that ES be utilized in the treatment of pressure ulcers that do not respond to conventional treatment. The guideline cites studies that utilize either a high voltage current[29,30,31] or a low-amplitude direct current applied for 6 hours/day.[27] None of the studies cited in the guideline utilize MENS characteristics.

In summary, several well-designed studies of MENS have not supported the efficacy of this intervention for wound healing. However, ES delivered at higher amplitude or longer duration than conventional MENS characteristics has been shown to be effective for this problem.

The second general topic of MENS studies is for pain reduction. Lerner and Kirsch reported on the effect of microstimulation compared with a placebo in the treatment of patients with chronic back pain.[83] Forty subjects were randomly assigned to a stimulation or sham stimulation group. A biphasic current with a frequency of 0.5 Hz and an amplitude of less than 1 μA was delivered. Two 6-sec treatments were given three times per week for 2 weeks. Because the current was subsensory, subjects were unaware whether they were receiving MENS or sham stimulation. While the authors reported that the MENS group had significantly better pain reduction, details of how their data were analyzed were not included in the report.

Wallace presented data on 1531 patients with pain who were treated with MENS in his clinic.[16] While these clients are noted to have generally positive results, the outcome measures are vague. These results were not based on controlled studies and the data have not been subjected to peer review.

Three posters were presented at the American Physical Therapy Association's 1991 conference dealing with MENS treatment for pain. Two of the studies[84,85] noted some preliminary positive effects with MENS used to treat delayed-onset muscle soreness (DOMS). Wolcott et al compared the effects of HVPC and MENS in the treatment of DOMS. The authors concluded that HVPC delivered at the submotor level was more effective in reducing DOMS than MENS.[86] To date, none of these studies has appeared in article form in a peer-reviewed journal.

Weber and coworkers examined subjects' experience of DOMS following a bout of high-amplitude eccentric exercise. Subjects were randomly assigned to one of four groups: massage, upper body ergometry, MENS, or a control group. These investigators found no significant differences in pain reduction among the groups for any of the measures of DOMS. They concluded that none of the interventions tested was effective at reducing DOMS.[87]

Bertolucci and Grey studied clients who had degenerative joint disease of the temporomandibular joint. In their study, 48 patients were randomly assigned to microcurrent electrical stimulation, mid-laser, and placebo treatment groups. Patients were noted to have significant mobility and pain improvements with both mid-laser and MENS compared with the placebo treatment; however, mid-laser was found to be superior to MENS in pain relief.[88]

Zizic and colleagues conducted a multicenter, randomized, placebo-controlled study of pulsed ES used on patients with osteoarthritis of the knee. A stimulator or sham device was used 6 to 10 hours per day for 4 weeks. Stimulation was delivered in a monophasic spiked waveform at 100 Hz. Amplitude was adjusted to a subsensory level. The authors reported that the stimulation group demonstrated significant improvements in the patient's evaluation of pain and function and in the physician's global evaluation.[73] In a related report, with a similar population, Zizic et al stated that 85 of 137 subjects treated with stimulation were able to defer total knee replacement surgery a mean of .95 years. These authors concluded that ES delivered at these characteristics is a cost effective alternative to earlier surgical intervention.[89] While the amplitude of the stimulus delivered in these studies is comparable to MENS, the treatment duration proposed is significantly longer.

Based on demonstrated efficacy in the studies reviewed, the AHCPR Guidelines do not recommend any form of electrotherapy for the treatment of acute pain,[90] acute back pain,[91] or cancer pain.[92]

In summary, of the studies reviewed, while Lerner and Kirsch[83] reported better pain relief in subjects receiving MENS than sham stimulation, how their data were analyzed is unclear. These results were not published in a peer-reviewed journal. Bertolucci and Grey demonstrated a beneficial effect on pain with traditional MENS characteristics, but their study also showed that mid-laser treatment was more effective than MENS.[88] While Zizic and colleagues recommended subsensory electrical stimulation for patients with osteoarthritis of the knee, their study utilized a stimulation duration that was considerable longer than traditionally recommended in MENS protocols.[73,89]

Studies of UI treated by PFES have been reported in literature for almost 30 years. Much of the earlier work was performed in Europe, with a more recent volume of studies originating in North America. The bulk of what has been written is presented in urology- and gynecology-related journals; however, nursing and allied health publications have included limited reports.

The available studies on PFES can be classified several ways. A variety of current characteristics have been used. Current waveform has either been interferential[68,93] or low-frequency (10–50 Hz) biphasic.[37,42,75,94,95] Treatment time has varied from several times daily[40–42,69,95,96] to several times weekly.[93,94] Two studies have compared the outcome of treatment given daily or every other day and found no significant difference.[40,41] Treatment duration has lasted from four weeks[95] to several months.[40,95] The majority of studies have utilized an internally worn electrode (vaginal probe for women[40–42,69,75,94–97] or anal probe for men[95]). However, surface electrodes[68,93,98] and implanted electrodes[70] have also been employed. Table 10–1 contains specific details on the current characteristics used in the studies cited.

Subjects in the PFES studies have primarily been adult women, although reports of PFES use in men[70,95,98] and children[4,98] are available. The type of incontinence has varied in published studies. Several studies have enrolled subjects with SUI only.[40,68,69,94] Other studies have included subjects with UUI and SUI or mixed incontinence or both.[37,41,42,67,75,93,96–98] Reports of treatment compliance have been quite high, ranging from 77 percent[40] to 93 percent.[41] Richardson and coworkers found that subjects that were treated every other day had significantly higher compliance than subjects treated daily.[40]

Two studies have examined the effects of PFES and EMGBF.[67,94] Meyer and colleagues treated 36 subjects having SUI with six sessions of PFES followed by six sessions of EMGBF. They concluded that when either PFES or EMGBF alone is compared to combined treatment, the therapeutic effect is unchanged.[94] Susset and coworkers alternated PFES and EMGBF during each of 12 sessions delivered over the course of 6 weeks. They concluded that there was no evidence that the combination of techniques produced superior results to those achieved with each treatment when given alone.[67]

Several prospective, double or single-blind, randomized clinical trials have been published. Laycock and Jerwood reported on two trials in a 1993 paper. The first trial randomly assigned 46 women with SUI to receive either pelvic floor exercise (PFE) with weighted vaginal cones or PFES with interferential current. Women in the PFES group were instructed not to practice PFE so that PFES could be assessed independently. Both groups demonstrated a significant decrease in the frequency and severity of urine loss. However, there was not a significant difference between the groups. There was however, a significant difference between the groups in muscle force (strength), assessed digitally. The PFES group was reported to have a significant increase in muscle force while no significant change was seen in the PFE group. In the second trial reported in the same paper, 30 women with SUI were randomly assigned to a PFES or a sham stimulation group. The authors reported significant improvements only in the PFES group on pad wetness tests, muscle force (as measured by perineometer), subjective reporting of frequency and severity of voiding and on a visual analog scale (VAS) of perceived severity of incontinence.[68]

Hahn and colleagues randomly assigned 21 women with SUI to 6 months of either PFE or PFES. They reported significant improvements in both pad wetness tests and in the subject's rating of success in both groups. There was no significant difference in the outcomes of the two groups.[32]

Sand and colleagues conducted a multicenter, prospective, randomized, double-blinded study comparing PFES with a sham device. Fifty-two women with SUI were randomly assigned to an active transvaginal stimulation or sham stimulation group. Treatment was carried out twice daily for 12 weeks. The PFES group demonstrated significant improvements over baseline on several outcome characteristics: weekly and daily leakage episodes, pad wetness testing, muscle force (on perineometer), VAS scores of urinary and stress incontinence, and urine loss with sneezing, coughing, or laughing. Results of pad wetness testing demonstrated that 62 percent of subjects in the active device group and 19 percent in the sham group were improved by 50 percent or better. This latter result indicates the potential of a placebo cure or improvement rate.[69] Laycock and Jerwood have commented that the results of a placebo effect in the treatment of this population may not be surprising, but may be the result of the clinician listening and responding to the concerns of incontinent clients.[68]

Yamanishi and colleagues conducted a randomized, double-blind, placebo-control trial to study the effectiveness of PFES. Thirty-eight women and six men with SUI or SUI with mild UUI were randomly assigned to a stimulation or sham stimulation group. Treatment was given two to three times daily for 4 weeks. The active device group demonstrated a significant reduction in the number of leaks, the frequency of daily pad changes, and the amount of leakage on the one-hour pad test. There was a significant improvement in the scores of disturbance in daily activities in the active device group.[95]

Brubaker et al reported on a multicenter trial of 121 women with SUI, UUI, and mixed incontinence. Subjects were treated for 8 weeks with either an active or sham device. This study demonstrated a significant improvement in UUI in the active device group but no significant difference between groups in the subjects with SUI.[97] Fall and colleagues reported similarly better results with subjects having UUI versus SUI.[75]

Numerous authors have reported better subjective than objective results in PFES incontinence studies.[37,42,68,94] Hahn and coworkers explain this discrepancy by noting that subjects who have experienced incontinence frequently adapt their life styles to avoid activities that would provoke their symptoms. Subjective ratings of improvement based on daily experiences may therefore be higher that those obtained during a short-term provocative test performed in the clinic.[32] Laycock and Jerwood discuss the effect that various psychological factors have on the client's perception of satisfaction with treatment. They conclude by agreeing with the International Continence Society in recommending the "more scientific, quantifiable pad test as an objective measure of treatment outcome."[68] The revised AHCPR Guidelines on the treatment of adult urinary incontinence acknowledged that there are "limits and issues surrounding current outcome measures while evaluating the available data on assessment and treatment methods for UI. The current outcome measure of UI treatment is to stop urine leakage or reduce its amount, frequency, or both. Monitoring urine leakage or wetting is difficult, however. The panel agreed that UI outcome can be measured in many domains (eg, patients' opinions, diaries, pad tests, quality-of-life scales, urodynamic tests) and that each of these domains is continuous and not discrete. There is variability in outcome measures across different PFES studies which makes it difficult to assess treatment efficacy. Because the subjective outcome of 'cure,' improvement, or both was cited in studies much more often than objective measures, this was the outcome the panel generally relied on."[74]

Several studies have examined follow-up after the active treatment period. Dogall was able to contact 20 of 40 subjects one year after treatment. Fourteen of these reported that they had maintained a successful improvement and six reported regression of symptoms.[93] Fall reported that of the 45 percent of subjects who remained free of symptoms after withdrawal of treatment, two thirds of these subjects had carryover at follow-up at 6 years.[37] Hahn and coworkers surveyed 19 of 20 subjects after 4 years. One of these subjects reported further improvement, 8 were unchanged, and 5 had deteriorated.[32] Laycock and Jerwood sent questionnaires to 15 subjects in the active treatment group a mean of 16.2 months after treatment. Of those contacted, 20 percent reported that they had sustained their improvement.[68] Yamanishi and colleagues reported that "satisfactory improvements" continued in 7 of 12 subjects for 3 to 11 months. In the sham device group, 3 subjects were improved, but 2 of these had recurrence of symptoms on follow-up.[95]

Richardson and colleagues reported that carryover at 1 year was 70 percent. These subjects continued to use their active devices to maintain their status. These authors recommend that "a long-term maintenance program of approximately 3 days/week is necessary to maintain treatment outcomes."[40]

The AHCPR Revised Guidelines for the treatment of urinary incontinence conclude that PFES can significantly reduce incontinence in men and women having SUI and may be useful in cases of UUI and mixed incontinence. The Guidelines recommend that PFES be combined with pelvic muscle rehabilitation.[74] Further studies to determine the optimal characteristic choices for PFES and the effectiveness of PFES alone or in combination with other interventions is recommended.

Several abstracts describing TES appeared in the literature during the late 1980s and early 1990s.[99–102] Numerous descriptions of the intervention followed in textbooks,[44] client-oriented[103–105] and nonrefereed medical publications.[106] Lechky's article in a 1993 issue of the Journal of the Canadian Medical Association on Pape and the Magee Clinic generated considerable controversy among the medical community.[72] Concern was expressed about the lack of published evidence in peer-reviewed journals,[107] the lack of well-designed clinical trials,[108] and the "one size fits all" claims of the intervention.[109] Rosenbaum and colleagues cautioned about attributing changes to TES when the treated children were both growing and maturing and receiving physical therapy.[109] Several authors[109,110] were critical of the comment that TES' focus on self-care was "quite revolutionary in chronic neurological conditions."[72] Pape responded to these concerns, stating that she felt that the controversy was one of how to test new therapies. She commented that the delay from study design to publication can often be as long as 10 years.[111] Pape expressed concern over denying clients access to new treatments during this interval. Pape argued that "most of what we now accept as rehabilitation therapy has never been subjected to a controlled trial." She posed the question, "Do we demand a different standard of proof for new ideas?"[111]

In 1993, a long-awaited study on TES was published in a peer-reviewed journal. Pape and coworkers reported on a study of six children with mild cerebral palsy who used nighttime sensory-level ES to their lower extremities.[64] Improvement was measured by the Peabody Developmental Motor Scale scores of gross motor, locomotor, and receipt/propulsion skills. The authors reported a statistically significant improvement on these scales during the six months of treatment and a reduction in scores when the stimulation was withdrawn. Harris has expressed concern over the design of this study, stating, "This 'pilot study' failed to satisfy some of the most basic criteria required of a (replicated) single-subject research design such as using repeated measures throughout each phase of the study, including visual analysis of graphed data, and establishing interrater reliability of the outcome measures during the course of the study."[8] If instead of being viewed as a replicated single-subject design, this study is considered a small group pre/post design, there are also flaws. The study lacks a control group and therefore cannot control for subject maturation or the effects of other concurrent therapies.

Steinbok et al reported on a randomized, controlled, singly blinded trial of utilizing TES in subjects having cerebral palsy. All subjects were children who had undergone selective posterior rhizotomy

(SPR) at least one year earlier. The children were randomly assigned to receive TES for one year or not receive TES. The primary outcome was the score on the Gross Motor Function Measure (GMFM). The authors reported significantly higher GMFM scores in the TES group. No significant difference between the two groups was noted in the secondary outcome measures of physiologic cost index, sitting scale score, lower extremity muscle force (strength) or spasticity. This led the authors to conclude that their "study does not lend support to the hypothesis that TES works by increasing muscle bulk and contractility."[65]

Mayatek, Inc. operates an Internet Website that disseminates information about TES. This site lists several clinical trials that are either in process or have been completed. Trials are reported that would: (1) compare TES and therapy with therapy alone, (2) examine the effect of TES on motor function and speech in quadriplegia and (3) compare TES with "sham" stimulation.[112] Well-designed studies that compare TES to "sham" stimulation and TES to therapy alone have the potential of providing valuable information. Hopefully, these investigators will submit their data and conclusions for peer review and make their findings available to the medical community in refereed publications.

In summary, a considerable amount of information has been published about TES since 1987. The technique's primary proponent, Pape, has written much of this information. Pape has provided this information largely through the lay press, the Internet, and nonrefereed journals. Two studies utilizing TES have appeared in peer-reviewed journals. The first of these studies has been criticized for methodological flaws.[64] The second report offers some support of the technique's effect on functional abilities in children with cerebral palsy who have undergone selective posterior rhizotomy, but does not offer evidence to support TES use for improving muscle force or reducing muscle spasticity.[65] No study to date has compared TES effectiveness to motor level ES delivered during functional activities. Since positive outcomes have been reported with motor ES, we need to look at whether one of these techniques produces better outcomes. Since there are differences in time and additional therapy required for each of these interventions, our recommendations must consider both efficacy and costs. Clearly, clinicians need more objective information from controlled studies before we can recommend TES to our clients based on the strength of available evidence.

## Criterion 5

**The proponents of the treatment are open and willing to discuss the methods, benefits, and limitations of the approach.** The majority of authors discussed in this chapter have evidenced this willingness.

Those who have submitted their reports for publication in peer-reviewed journals have already received feedback from their peers. They have demonstrated their willingness to receive constructive criticism and to make modifications so that their work can be widely disseminated. Studies that are presented in peer-reviewed publications must address not only the outcomes and conclusions of the authors, but the limitations of the study and the intervention as well. Clinicians need this information to determine how to interpret and use the study.

Reading the discussions at the end of published studies can shed light on the authors' openness. As we read these comments, we need to ask: Is the discussion balanced? Do the authors attempt only to explain why their results were not as positive as they might have been? Where appropriate, are comparisons made to other interventions? Are recommendations for future studies offered?

Several MENS authors have offered recommendations on future MENS studies including studies to clarify; critical characteristics, polarity issues, electrode size and placement,[79] and the effects of different frequencies.[83] Based on the outcomes of their studies, other authors have concluded that MENS is not indicated for wound healing[78] and the treatment of delayed onset muscle soreness.[87] Consistent with these conclusions, these authors have not recommended future MENS studies for the impairments they studied.

Comparisons of MENS with conventional treatments are found in two studies. Weber and coworkers compared MENS with massage and upper body ergometry in the treatment of delayed onset muscle soreness. None of the interventions resulted in significant improvements in symptoms.[87] Bertolucci and Grey found that both MENS and mid-laser were effective in reducing TMJ pain, but mid-laser treatment produced superior outcomes.[88]

Reading the comment and discussion section of PFES studies, one frequently finds examples of openness and self-assessment. Numerous PFES authors have demonstrated a willingness to critically analyze their studies, discuss limitations, compare PFES to conventional treatment approaches and make recommendations about the direction of future research.

Laycock and Jerwood acknowledge that early literature was somewhat "promotional," because it was supplied by manufacturers and the physical therapy profession could be criticized for adopting the intervention before sufficient numbers of controlled studies were published. These authors are to be commended, however, for moving the body of knowledge on PFES beyond promotional literature with their clinical trials.[68]

Numerous authors have acknowledged issues with the design of their studies that may have affected the results. Dogall and coworkers[93] and Laycock and Jerwood[68] have discussed the limitation of their small sample size. The potential effect of a study with a duration of several weeks has been acknowledged.[37,42,68] One study noted that despite randomization, subjects in the control group were a mean of 6.8 years older.[69] The possible effect on outcomes is discussed. Two studies discuss the problems encountered in attempting to objectively assess the force (strength) of the pelvic floor muscles.[32,68]

Recommendations have been offered regarding PFES characteristic selection. Fall and colleagues acknowledged the need to standardize characteristics in study design, but recommended the individualization of treatment characteristics based on a client's primary presenting problems in the clinical application of the technique. These authors also concluded that sufficient stimulus amplitude may be the most important characteristic when treating SUI.[75] Two studies have recommended that, in many subjects, continued or intermittent treatment may be necessary to ensure sustained continence.[37,40]

Traditional treatment for UI has included medication, pelvic floor exercise, bladder training, and surgery. Several authors have made comparisons between PFES and these more conventional treatments. PFES has been acknowledged to have a lower cure rate than surgery[37,68,75,96] but with significantly lower risks and costs.[37,41,69] PFES studies have reported similar outcomes to bladder training[32] and PFE.[32,42,66,67] Susset and coworkers, however, comments that although PFE has proved useful in cases of SUI, this intervention has not been shown to be effective in clients with UUI.[67] In clients with UUI, therefore, PFES may produce better results. Two studies[42,95] report that PFES produces similar outcomes to drug therapy. The risks and potential side effects of pharmacologic interventions coupled with a comparable response with PFES may make PFES a more desirable choice for some patients.

Study results may be affected by other factors. Laycock and Jerwood comment that some effects may be enhanced by increased patient information about the etiology of his or her condition (regarding diet and voiding schedule). These authors also acknowledge the placebo effect and feel this may be related to psychological impact of clinicians listening to the concerns of incontinent clients.[68] Sand and colleagues have reported a 19 percent placebo effect in a recent controlled study.[69]

Numerous recommendations have been made for future research. These have included studies with longer duration treatment,[42,68] larger samples,[42,68,96] and more sensitive, objective outcome measures.[32,42] Because of the positive correlation between compliance and successful outcome, studies to evaluate the psychological factors that contribute to patient compliance have been recommended.[67] Because clinical intervention is often multimodal, studies comparing PFES, EMGBF,[67] and PFE[68] alone and in combination are advocated.

Merrill and coworkers cite an example of how the information gleaned from one study can help contribute to the understanding of the theoretical underpinnings of the approach and shape future studies. These authors state that their initial beliefs were that PFES activates "electrical vesical stimulation to empty the bladder."[70] This contrasted with their results and led them to the interpretation that PFES activates the pudendal nerve. From this, they concluded that PFES is inappropriate in patients with denervation.

TES proponents have acknowledged limitations to their studies. The authors of a pilot study on TES-treated children with cerebral palsy and acknowledged that their subjects were drawn from a small select group. The question is posed, "Would the CP in these children be likely to improve as a result of natural growth and development?[64] Steinbok and colleagues cited a lack of sham stimulation as a drawback of their study. They note that they dismissed the idea of a sham stimulation group as impractical because sham stimulation would need to be without a "tickling sensation" and therefore would affect blinding of subjects.[65]

Limited comparisons of TES with conventional treatment are offered. Since motor-level ES is a similar and acceptable treatment intervention, this inclusion would be logical and helpful. Pape and colleagues comment that TES does not increase the "burden of care." With what intervention TES is being compared in terms of care requirements is unclear. Nightly application of equipment and morning removal would involve some additional care. TES is reported to be at least as beneficial as selective posterior rhizotomy in mildly affected children.[64]

TES proponents make other recommendations about the future research needed in this area. These include studies to define optimal duration,[64] identify selection criteria,[64] differentiate the effects on ambulatory versus nonambulatory subjects,[65] and determine the underlying mechanism of effect.[64,65] Steinbok and coworkers identify limitations to the generalizability of their results, stressing that "results are not generalizable to the larger population of children with spastic CP who have not undergone SPR." These authors also concluded that their study did not lend support to the hypothesis that TES increases muscle bulk and contractility.[65]

Table 10–3 summarizes how the recommended criteria have been used to analyze MENS, PFES, and TES. Hopefully, physical therapists will find this approach useful to analyze both new treatment interventions as well as conventional ones.

Everyone has the responsibility to look critically at all the interventions we use. Criticism of conventional interventions without sup-

TABLE 10–3. APPLICATION OF CRITERIA TO MENS, PFES, AND TES

| CRITERIA | MENS | PFES | TES |
|---|---|---|---|
| 1. The theory supporting the approach is logically sound and supported by valid anatomic and physiologic evidence. | • Theory based on injury current has anatomic and physiologic support.<br>• Theory based on Arndt–Schultz Law not supported by evidence.<br>• Logic behind choice of stimulation characteristics is unclear. | • Theory for SUI treatment is to achieve either better force production or fatigue resistance in the pelvic floor muscles via ES. This is physiologically sound and has been demonstrated with other applications.<br>• Theory for treatment of UUI is based on reflex inhibition of the detrusor muscle. This is physiologically sound.<br>• Some PFES parameters derive logically from the intended physiologic action (amplitude, frequency, phase duration). Specific recommendations on other characteristics need to be tested. | • Supporting theory unclear.<br>• Anatomic and physiologic evidence in support of theory not presented.<br>• Primary goal is unclear—spasticity reduction, muscle growth or treatment of disuse atrophy or both?<br>• Logic behind choice of stimulation characteristics is not clear. |
| 2. The treatment approach is designed for specific impairments or functional limitations based on etiology. | • Recommended for numerous impairments and diagnoses of multiple body systems. Appropriateness of intervention based on etiology unclear.<br>• Contraindications common to other electrotherapeutic interventions discussed. | • Specific indications identified (SUI, UUI, and mixed UI) based on etiology and PFES mechanism of action.<br>• Predictors of successful outcomes have been suggested.<br>• Contraindications common to other electrotherapeutic interventions discussed.<br>• Specific contraindications relative to PFES identified. | • Recommended for numerous diagnoses of neuromuscular origin. Also advocated for genitourinary and cardiopulmonary conditions.<br>• Appropriateness of intervention based on etiology not discussed.<br>• Contraindications identified. |
| 3. Potential side effects of the treatment are presented. | • Minimal side effects reported. These appear to resolve following treatment.<br>• Statements suggesting that if clients do not improve, the problem is with the patient, not the intervention.<br>• Evidence of cost effectiveness compared with conventional treatment not presented. | • Side effects appear to be relatively minor in severity, low in number, and resolve with when the treatment is discontinued.<br>• General statements made comparing costs favorably to surgery. | • Side effects from TES appear to be relatively minor and infrequent.<br>• Proponents state that trained practitioners individually evaluate clients for appropriateness.<br>• Cost comparisons made to bracing, wheelchairs, and traditional therapy; however, data to support clients not needing these devices/care not presented. |

| | | | |
|---|---|---|---|
| **TABLE 10–3.** | **APPLICATION OF CRITERIA TO MENS, PFES, AND TES (CONTINUED)** | | |
| **CRITERIA** | **MENS** | **PFES** | **TES** |
| 4. Studies from peer-reviewed journals are provided that support the treatment's efficacy. These studies include well-designed, randomized, controlled clinical trials or well-designed, single-subject, experimental studies. | • Early information available largely through the lay press and nonrefereed journals.<br>• Two well-designed studies of MENS have not supported its efficacy for wound healing.[78,79]<br>• One study demonstrated a beneficial effect on pain with MENS, but found mid-laser treatment to be more effective.[88]<br>• One study recommended subsensory ES for patients with osteoarthritis of the knee; stimulation duration was longer than conventional MENS.[73] | • Large volume of literature, spanning three decades.<br>• Earlier reports supported the intervention, but were largely anecdotal.<br>• Literature in the last decade has contained several large, randomized, control trials, which support efficacy. | • Early information available largely through the lay press, the Internet, and nonrefereed journals.<br>• Two studies in peer-reviewed journals. One article has been criticized for methodological flaws.[64] The second report offers some support of a positive effect on functional abilities in children with cerebral palsy but does not support TES use for improving muscle force or spasticity reduction.[65] |
| 5. The proponents of the treatment are open and willing in discussing the approach's methods, benefits, and limitations. | • Information on methods available.<br>• Variability among authors as to willingness to discuss limitations. | • Details of treatment are clearly identified, however inconsistently rationalized and referenced.<br>• Limitations of studies are discussed openly.<br>• Comparisons have been made between PFES and conventional treatment. | • Treatment protocols available only from trained practitioners.<br>• Limitations of studies are identified.<br>• Proponents have expressed concern over the safety of motor-level ES. |

portive data and failing to look critically at new treatments does little to identify the potential risks to clients or to advance effective care.

There are other characteristics that may be associated with new treatments that should signal caution. We need to be wary of financial interests on the part of treatment proponents in the promotion of a treatment regimen or sale of equipment. The risk here is that the financial interests will supercede scientific integrity. We should be cautious when "new" language is utilized to describe established concepts. The Section on Clinical Electrophysiology of the American Physical Therapy Association has provided us with an excellent source for the standardization of terminology in electrotherapy.[113] The use of nonstandard terminology conveys the impression that new concepts are being discussed. We should be cautious if we are asked to agree not to disclose information about a treatment intervention. Nondisclosure results in clients' being denied potentially beneficial services and physical therapy professionals' being denied the opportunity to examine the method scientifically.

Proponents of some new treatment interventions offer certification in their methods. Certification is not a new concept in medicine. To identify an individual as certified in an approach connotes an additional level of study and hopefully skill. To offer continuing education courses in an attempt to aid the participants' understanding and clinical expertise is acceptable. To utilize certification courses as the sole means of information dissemination denies responsible clinicians the opportunity to investigate and evaluate new ideas. Competencies necessary for physical therapists to perform electrodiagnostic and electrotherapeutic procedures have been established.[114] The suggestion that physical therapists require postgraduate education in order to incorporate ES into a treatment program demonstrates a lack of awareness of the educational and clinical preparation all therapists undergo.

The above list is certainly not exhaustive. In short, statements or behaviors that betray biased perspectives or personal agendas do a disservice to good clinical practice. They are often symptoms of an approach that is not well thought out or studied.

# Summary

Health care providers are likely to continue to be faced with new equipment and developing treatment interventions. Assessing the merit of both current and developing techniques and equipment can ensure optimal care. The following criteria may be useful in making these important assessments:

1. The theory supporting the approach is logically sound and supported by valid anatomic and physiologic evidence.
2. The treatment approach is designed for specific impairments or functional limitations based on etiology.
3. Potential side effects of the treatment are presented.
4. Studies from peer-review journals are provided to support the efficacy of the treatment approach. These studies include well-designed, randomized, controlled clinical trials or well-designed, single-subject experimental studies, or all.
5. The treatment proponents are open and willing to discuss the methods, benefits, and limitations of the approach.

There are additional characteristics or behaviors associated with a new intervention or piece or equipment that should make us wary. These include:

- Financial interests on the part of the proponents
- Use of new terminology to describe established concepts
- Restrictions on the disclosure of information about the intervention
- Postgraduate education requirements to access information on the intervention or to teach skills already covered in an entry-level curriculum

The profession of physical therapy is committed to providing the highest quality care for all clients who require our services. Critical analysis will enable us to choose interventions that have a high probability of achieving successful outcomes. The evidence for efficacy should be weighed against the required inputs of time, labor, and funds. Ultimately, consideration of this balance of evidence and costs will allow us to provide and recommend high-quality, cost-effective health care.

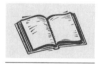

## REVIEW QUESTION

1. Consider the last continuing education course you attended or the last presentation you heard on a treatment intervention or piece of equipment. Use the following questions to help you to rate the merits and limitations of the approach/equipment:

- Was logically sound theory presented?
- Was the theory supported by anatomic and physiologic evidence?
- Was the treatment approach or equipment designed for specific impairments or functional limitations based on etiology?
- Were potential side effects of the treatment presented?
- Were studies from peer-review journals provided to support the efficacy of the treatment approach?
- Were these studies well-designed, randomized, controlled clinical trails or well-designed, single-subject experimental studies, or both?
- Were the treatment proponents open and willing to discuss the approach's methods, benefits, and limitations?

If information provided by the presenter(s) is insufficient to answer these questions, what additional sources could you utilize to supplement the information provided by the presenter(s)?

# References

1. Lee WJ, McGovern JP, Duvall EN. Continuous tetanizing (low voltage) currents for relief of spasm. Arch Phys Med, 31:766, 1950.

2. Levine MG, Knott M, Kabat H. Relaxation of spasticity by electrical stimulation of antagonist muscles. Arch Phys Med, 33:668–673, 1952.

3. Alfieri V. Electrical treatment of spasticity—reflex tonic activity in hemiplegic patients and selected specific electrostimulation. Scand J Rehab Med, 14:177–182, 1982.

4. Seib TP, Price R, Reyes MR et al. The quantitative measurement of spasticity: Effect of cutaneous electrical stimulation. Arch Phys Med Rehabil, 75(7):746–750, 1994.

5. Dewald JPA, Given JD, Rymer WZ. Long-lasting reductions of spasticity induced by skin electrical stimulation. IEEE Trans Rehabil Eng, 4(4):231–242, 1996.

6. Evidence Based Medicine: Finding the Best Clinical Literature. Library of Health Sciences: University of Illinois at Chicago. http://www.uic.edu/depts/lib/health/ebm.html#evidence.

7. Clinical Practice Guidelines. Agency for Health Care Policy and Research. http://text.nlm.nih.gov/ftrs/display?ftrsK=64916&t=886711691&collect=ahcpr&sc=ftrs%2fpick&dt=1&du=/ahcpr/copyright.html.

8. Harris SR. How should treatments be critiqued for scientific merit? Phys Ther, 76:175–181, 1996.

9. Sackett DL. Rules of evidence and clinical recommendations on the use of antithrombotic agents. Chest, 95(2)(suppl):25–45.

10. Kralj A, Grobelnic S. Functional electrical stimulation–A new hope for paraplegic patients? Bull Prosth Res, Fall:75–102, 1993.

11. Marsolais EB, Edwards EG. Energy costs of walking and standing with functional neuromuscular stimulation and long leg braces. Arch Phys Med Rehabil, 69:243–249, 1988.

12. Ragnarsson KT, Pollack S, O'Daniel W et al. Clinical evaluation of computerized functional electrical stimulation after spinal cord injury: A multicenter pilot study. Arch Phys Med Rehabil, 69(9):672–677, 1988.

13. Jaegar RJ. Design and simulation of closed-loop electrical stimulation orthoses for restoration of quiet standing in paraplegia. J Biomech, 19f:825–835, 1986.

14. Twist DJ. Acyanosis in a spinal cord injured patient: effects of computer-controlled neuromuscular electrical: A case report. Phys Ther, 70:45–49, 1990.

15. Faghri PD, Glaser RM, Figoni SF. Functional electrical stimulation leg cycle ergometer exercise: Training effects on cardiorespiratory responses of spinal cord injured subjects at rest and during submaximal exercise. Arch Phys Med Rehabil, 73:1085–1093, 1992.

16. Wallace LA. MENS Therapy Clinical Perspectives: Volume 1. Cleveland, OH: privately published, pp 7–82, 1990.

17. Picker RI. Current trends: Low-volt pulsed microamp stimulation. Part 1. Clin Manag Phys Ther, 9:10–14, 1989.

18. Becker RO, Murray DG. Method for producing cellular dedifferentiation by means of very small electrical currents. Trans NY Acad Sci, 29:606, 1967.

19. Illingsworth CM, Barker AT. Measurement of electrical currents during the regeneration of amputated fingertips in children. Clin Phys Physiol Meas. 1:87–89, 1980.

20. Becker RO, Selden G. The Body Electric: Electromagnetism and the Foundation of Life. New York: William Morrow, 1985.

21. Burr HS, Harrey SC, Taffell M. Bio-electric correlates of wound healing. Yale J Biol Med, 11:103–107, 1938.

22. Picker RI. Current trends: Low-volt pulsed microamp stimulation. Part 2. Clin Manag Phys Ther, 9:28–33, 1989.

23. Baker LL, Rubayi S, Villar F et al. Effect of electrical stimulation waveform on healing of ulcers in human beings with spinal cord injury. Wound Rep Reg, 4:21–28, 1996.

24. Wolcott LE, Wheeler PC, Hardwicke HM et al. Accelerated healing of skin ulcers by electrotherapy: Preliminary clinical results. South Med J, 62(7):795–801, 1969.

25. Gault WR, Gatens PF. Use of low intensity direct current in management of ischemic skin ulcers. Phys Ther, 56(3):265–268, 1976.

26. Alvarez OM, Merits PM, Smerbeck BS et al. The healing of superficial skin wounds is stimulated by external electrical current. J Invest Dermatol, 81:144–148, 1983.

27. Carley PJ, Wainapel SF. Electrotherapy for acceleration of wound healing: Low intensity direct current. Arch Phys Med Rehabil, 66:443–446, 1985.

28. Brown M, McDonnell MK, Menton DN. Polarity effects on wound healing. Using electric stimulation in rabbits. Arch Phys Med Rehabil, 70(8):624–627, 1989.

29. Feedar JA, Kloth LC, Gentzkow GD. Chronic dermal ulcer healing enhanced with monophasic pulsed electrical stimulation. Phys Ther, 71(9):639–649, 1991.

30. Gentzkow GD, Pollack SV, Kloth LC et al. Improved healing of pressure ulcers. Using Dermapulse, a new electrical stimulation device. Wounds, 3(5):158–170, 1991.

31. Griffin JW, Tooms RE, Mendius RA et al. Efficacy of high voltage pulsed current for healing of pressure ulcers in patients with spinal cord injury. Phys Ther, 1(6):433–442, 1991.

32. Hahn I, Sommar S, Fall M. A comparative study of pelvic floor training and electrical stimulation for the treatment of genuine female stress urinary incontinence. Neuro Urodynam, 10:545–554, 1991.

33. Bazeed MA, Thuroff JW, Schmidt RA et al. Effect of chronic electrostimulation of the sacral roots on the striated urethral sphincter. J Urol, 128(6):1357–1362, 1982.

34. Pette D, Vrbova G. Neural control of phenotypic expression in mammalian muscle fibers. Muscle Nerve, 8(8):676–689, 1985.

35. Hennig R, Lomo T. Effects of chronic stimulation on the size and speed of long-term denervated and innervated rat fast and slow skeletal muscles. Acta Physiol Scand, 130(1):115–131, 1987.

36. Teague CT, Merrill DC. Electric pelvic floor stimulation. Invest Urol, 15:65–69, 1977.
37. Fall M. Does electrostimulation cure urinary incontinence? J Urology, 131(4):664–667, 1984.
38. Laycock J, Green RJ. Interferential therapy in the treatment of incontinence. Physiotherapy, 74(4):161–168, 1988.
39. Ohlsson B, Lindstrom S, Erlandson BE et al. Effects of some different pulse parameters on bladder inhibition and urethral closure during intravaginal electrical stimulation: An experimental study in the cat. Med Biol Eng Comput, 24(1):27–33, 1986.
40. Richardson DA, Miller KL, Siegel SW et al. Pelvic floor electrical stimulation: A comparison of daily and every-other day therapy for genuine stress incontinence. Urology, 48:110–118, 1996.
41. Siegel SW, Richardson DA, Miller KL et al. Pelvic floor electrical stimulation for the treatment of urge and mixed urinary incontinence in women. Urology, 50(6):934–940, 1977.
42. Bent AE, Sand PK, Ostergard DR et al. Transvaginal electrical stimulation in the treatment of genuine stress incontinence and detrusor instability. Int Urogynecol, 4:9–13, 1993.
43. Pape KE. Therapeutic electrical stimulation: the past, the present, and the future. NDTA Network. July/August, pp 1996, 1–2. http://www.mayatek.com/ndta.n&m:1-4.
44. Pape KE, Kirsch SE. Technology-assisted self-care in the treatment of spastic diplegia. In Sussman MD (ed), The Diplegic Child: Evaluation and Management. Rosemont, IL, American Academy of Orthopedic Surgeons, p 244, 1991.
45. Carmick J. Guidelines for the clinical application of neuromuscular electrical stimulation (NMES) for children with cerebral palsy. Pediatr Phys Ther, 9(3):128–136, 1997.
46. Carnstam B, Larsson I, Prevec TS. Improvement in gait following functional electrical stimulation. Scand J Rehab Med, 9:7–13, 1977.
47. Dubrowitz L, Finnie N, Hyde SA et al. Improvement of muscle performance by chronic electrical stimulation in children with cerebral palsy (letter). Lancet, 12:587–588, 1988.
48. Laborde JM, Solomonow M, Soboloff H. The effectiveness of surface electrical stimulation in improving quadriceps strength in young CP patients (abstract). Dev Med Child Neurol, 53(28)(suppl):26–27, 1986.
49. Atwater SW, Tatarka ME, Kathrein JE et al. Electromyography-triggered electrical muscle stimulation for children with cerebral palsy: A pilot study. Pediatr Phys Ther, 3:190–199, 1991.
50. Hazelwood ME, Brown JK, Rowe PJ et al. The use of therapeutic electrical stimulation in the treatment of hemiplegic cerebral palsy. Dev Med Child Neurol, 36:661–673, 1994.
51. Carmick J. Clinical use of neuromuscular electrical stimulation for children with cerebral palsy, Part 1: lower extremity. Phys Ther, 73: 505–513, 1993.
52. Carmick J. Clinical use of neuromuscular electrical stimulation for children with cerebral palsy, Part 2: upper extremity. Phys Ther, 73:514–527, 1993.

53. Carmick J. Managing equinus in children with cerebral palsy: electrical stimulation to strengthen the triceps surae muscle. Dev Med Child Neurol, 37:965–975, 1995.

54. Carmick J. Use of neuromuscular electrical stimulation and a dorsal wrist splint to improve the hand function of a child with spastic hemiparesis. Phys Ther, 77:661–671, 1997.

55. Comeaux P, Patterson N, Rubin M et al. Effect of neuromuscular electrical stimulation during gait in children with cerebral palsy. Pediatr Phys Ther, 9(3):103–109, 1997.

56. Mulcahey MJ, Betz RR. Upper and lower extremity application of electrical stimulation: a decade of research with children and adolescents with spinal injuries. Pediatr Phys Ther, 9(3):113–122, 1997.

57. Bertoti D, Stranger M, Betz RR et al. Percutaneous intermuscular functional electrical stimulation as an intervention choice for children with cerebral palsy. Pediatr Phys Ther, 9(3):123–127, 1997.

58. Pape KE. Electrical stimulation for the treatment of disuse muscle atrophy in cerebral palsy. http://www.mayatek.com/muscles.htm.

59. Pape KE. Caution urged for NMES use (letter). Phys Ther, 74(3):265, 1994.

60. Carmick J. Caution urged for NMES use (author's response). Phys Ther, 74(3):266, 1994.

61. Mohr T, Aker TK, Wessman HC. Effects of high voltage stimulation on blood flow in the rat hand limb. Phys Ther, 67:526–533, 1987.

62. McMeeken J. Tissue temperature and blood flow: a research based overview of electrophysiological modalities. Aust J Physiol, 40:49–57, 1994.

63. Pape KE. Therapeutic electrical stimulation (TES) for the treatment of disuse muscle atrophy in cerebral palsy. Pediatr Phys Ther, 9(3): 110–111, 1997.

64. Pape KE, Kirsch SE, Galil A et al. Neuromuscular approach to the motor deficits of cerebral palsy: A pilot study. J Pediatr Orthop, 13: 628–633, 1993.

65. Steinbok P, Reiner AM, Beauchamp R et al. A randomized clinical trial to compare selective posterior rhizotomy plus physiotherapy with physiotherapy alone in children with spastic diplegic cerebral palsy. Dev Med Child Neurol, 39(3):178–184, 1997.

66. Stanish WD, Rubinovich M, Kozey J et al. The use of electricity in ligament and tendon repair. Phys Sports Med, 13(8):109–116, 1985.

67. Susset J, Galea G, Manbeck K et al. A predictive score index for the outcome of associated biofeedback and vaginal electrical stimulation in the treatment of female incontinence. J Urol, 153(5):1467–1468, 1995.

68. Laycock J, Jerwood D. Does pre-modulated interferential therapy cure genuine stress incontinence? Physiotherapy, 79(8):553–560, 1993.

69. Sand PK, Richardson DA, Staskin DR et al. Pelvic floor electrical stimulation in the treatment of genuine stress incontinence: a multicenter placebo-controlled trial. Am J Obstet Gynecol, 173:72–79, 1995.

70. Merrill DC, Conway C, DeWolf W. Urinary incontinence. Treatment with electrical stimulation of the pelvic floor. Urology, 5(1):67–72, 1975.

71. Pape KE. Electrical stimulation for the treatment of disuse muscle atrophy in cerebral palsy. http://www.mayatek.com/muscles.htm.

72. Lechky O. Toronto clinic takes new approach to neurologic injury, damage. Can Med Assoc J, 148(1):72–74, 1993.

73. Zizic TM, Hoffman KC, Holt PA et al. The treatment of osteoarthritis of the knee with pulsed electrical stimulation. J Rheumatol, 22(9): 1757–1761, 1995.

74. Urinary Incontinence in Adults: Acute and Chronic Management. Clinical Practice Guideline No. 2, 1996 update. Rockville, MD: U.S. Department of Health and Human Services, Public Health Service, Agency for Health Care Policy and Research. AHCPR Publication No. 06-0682, March 1996.

75. Fall M, Ahlstrom K, Carlsson C. Contelle pelvic floor stimulator for female stress-urge incontinence. Urology, 3:282–287, 1986.

76. Wolcott LE, Wheeler PC, Hardwicke HM et al. Accelerated healing of skin ulcers by electrotherapy: Preliminary clinical results. South Med J, 62(7):795–801, 1969.

77. Barron JJ, Jacobson WE, Tidd G. Treatment of decubitus ulcers: a new approach. Minn Med, 68(2):103–106, 1985.

78. Leffman DJ, Arnall DA, Holmgren PR et al. Effect of microamperage stimulation on the rate of wound healing in rats: A histological study. Phys Ther, 74:201–219, 1994.

79. Byl NN, McKenzie AL, West JM et al. Pulsed microamperage stimulation: A controlled study of healing of surgically induced wound in Yucatan pigs. Phys Ther, 74:201–219, 1994.

80. Robinson AJ. Invited commentary. Phys Ther, 74:213–215, 1994.

81. Leffman DJ, Arnall DA, Holmgren PR et al. Author's response. Phys Ther, 74:216, 1994.

82. Treatment of Pressure Ulcers, Clinical Guideline Number 15. AHCPR Publication No. 95-0652. December 1994.

83. Lerner FN, Kirsch DL. A double-blind comparative study of micro-stimulation and placebo effect in short term treatment of the chronic back patient. ACA J of Chiropract, 15:S101–S106, 1981.

84. Kulig K, Jarski R, Drewek E et al. The effects of microcurrent stimulation on CPK and delayed onset muscle soreness (abstract). Phys Ther, 71(6)(suppl):S115–S116, 1991.

85. Rapaski D, Isles S, Kulig K et al. Microcurrent electrical stimulation: Comparison of two protocols in reducing delayed onset muscle soreness (abstract). Phys Ther, 71(6)(suppl):S116, 1991.

86. Wolcott C, Dudek D, Kulig K et al. A comparison of the effects of high volt and microcurrent stimulation on delayed onset muscle soreness (abstract). Phys Ther, 71(6)(suppl):S116, 1991.

87. Weber MD, Servedio FJ, Woodall WR. The effect of three modalities on delayed onset muscle soreness. J Orthop Sports Phys Ther, 20:236–242, 1994.

88. Bertolucci LE, Grey T. Clinical comparative study of microcurrent electrical stimulation to mid-laser and placebo treatment in degenerative joint disease of the temporomandibular joint. Cranio, 13(2):116–120, 1995.

89. Zizic TM, Hoffman KC, He YD et al. Clinical and cost effectiveness of pulsed electrical stimulation treated knee osteoarthritis in total knee

replacement candidates. San Francisco, CA, American College of Rheumatology, 1995.

90. Acute Pain Management: Operative or Medical Procedures and Trauma. Clinical Practice Guideline No. 1. Rockville, MD: U.S. Department of Health and Human Services, Public Health Service, Agency for Health Care Policy and Research. AHCPR Publication No. 92-0032, 1994.

91. Acute Low Back Problems in Adults: Assessment and Treatment. Quick Reference Guide for Clinicians. No. 14. Rockville, MD: U.S. Department of Health and Human Services, Public Health Service, Agency for Health Care Policy and Research. AHCPR Publication No. 95-0643, 1994.

92. Management of Cancer Pain. Clinical Guideline Number 9. Quick Reference Guide for Clinicians. No. 9. Rockville, MD: U.S. Department of Health and Human Services, Public Health Service, AGency for Health Care Policy and Research. AHCPR Publication No. 94-0592, 1994.

93. Dogall DS. The effects of interferential therapy on incontinence and frequency of micturition. Physiotherapy, 71(3):135–136, 1985.

94. Meyer S, Dhenin T, Schmidt N et al. Subjective and objective effects of intravaginal electrical myostimulation and biofeedback in the treatment of patients with genuine stress urinary incontinence. Brit J Urol, 69:584–588, 1992.

95. Yamanishi T, Yasuda K, Sakakibara R et al. Pelvic floor electrical stimulation in the treatment of stress incontinence—An investigational study and placebo controlled double-blind trial. J Urol, 158(6):2127–2131, 1977.

96. Sand PK. Pelvic floor electrical stimulation in the treatment of mixed incontinence complicated by a low-pressure urethra. Obstet Gynecol, 88(5):757–760, 1996.

97. Brubaker L, Benson JT, Bent A et al. Transvaginal electrical stimulation for female urinary incontinence. Am J Obstet Gynecol, 177(3):536–540, 1997.

98. Nakamura M, Sakuria T. Bladder inhibition by penile electrical stimulation. Br J Urol, 56:413–415, 1984.

99. Pape KE, Herbert AM, Galil A et al. Electrical stimulation as an adjunct to rehabilitation in childhood spinal cord injury: A pilot project (abstract). Pediatr Res, 21:495A, 1987.

100. Pape KE, Galil A, Boulton J et al. Therapeutic electrical stimulation (TES) in the rehabilitation of children with cerebral palsy (abstract). Pediatr Res, 23:656A, 1988.

101. Pape KE, Kirsch SE, White MA, et al. Therapeutic electrical stimulation (TES) in the rehabilitation of spastic hemiplegia, (abstract). Clin Invest Med, 13:B100, 1990.

102. Pape KE, Kirsch SE, Boulton JE et al. Therapeutic electrical stimulation measured by the peabody developmental motor scales (PDMS) and the progressive ambulation scale (PAS) (abstract). Clin Invest Med, 14(suppl):A91, 1991.

103. Pape KE, Kirsch SE, Castagna LA. New hope for people with post-polio syndrome. Abilities, 11, 1992.

104. Bell C. TES therapy. Polio Network News. 7(4): 1991.

105. Head T. Stimulating therapy. Insights into Spina Bifida. November/December: 4–5, 1991.

106. Lechky O. New technique helps reverse effects of brain injuries. Canadian Living, September:153, 1992.

107. Armstrong R. Toronto clinic's new approach (letter). Can Med Assoc J, 148(8):1270, 1993.

108. Smith KM, Bayley M. Toronto clinic's new approach (letter). Can Med Assoc J, 148(8):1272, 1993.

109. Rosenbaum P, Gowland C, King G et al. Toronto clinic's new approach, (letter). Can Med Assoc J, 148(8):1271–1272, 1993.

110. Teasell RW. Toronto clinic's new approach (letter). Can Med Assoc J, 148(8):1272, 1993.

111. Pape KE. Toronto clinic's new approach (letter). Can Med Assoc J, 148(8):1270, 1993.

112. Mayatek-http://www.mayatek.com/

113. Electrotherapeutic Terminology in Physical Therapy. Alexandria, VA, Section on Clinical Electrophysiology, American Physical Therapy Association, 1990.

114. Guidelines on Competencies Necessary to Perform Physical Agent Modalities/Electrotherapy. Alexandria, VA, American Physical Therapy Association. BOD 03-93-23-61, 1996.

115. Beck S. Use of sensory level electrical stimulation in the physical therapy management of a child with cerebral palsy. Pediatr Phys Ther, 9(3):137–138, 1997.

116. TES course offerings. http://www.mayatek.com/. Mayatek Incorporated.

117. Pape KE, Kirsch SE. Bugaresti JM. New therapies in spastic cerebral palsy. Contemp Pediatr, May/June:6–13, 1990.

# 11

# Therapeutic Uses
# of Biofeedback

Timothy A. Hanke

## Introduction

Physical therapists routinely provide feedback to their patients. This feedback is typically presented in the form of verbal information regarding the outcome (result) or some aspect of the performance of the movement task. As it relates to movement function, the result of the task is often obvious to the physical therapist and the patient. For example, in the case of a sit-to-stand transfer, the patient and therapist would typically know that the patient successfully moved from a sitting to a standing position. So instead of providing information on the outcome generally, physical therapists often provide information about specific characteristics of the movement such as the amplitude, direction, or speed of movement as this information relates to the intended goal of the task. Continuing with the example above, the sit-to-stand movement may have lacked sufficient excursion anteriorly in order to transfer the patient's mass to the new base-of-support configuration.

Feedback, in general, can be intrinsic or extrinsic.[1] **Intrinsic (inherent) feedback** is information provided as a natural consequence of making an action. Examples of intrinsic feedback include vision, proprioception, audition, somatosensation (touch), and smell. A patient may have difficulty using intrinsic feedback when a disease, trauma, or birth injury affects the peripheral or central nervous system (CNS). **Extrinsic feedback** consists of information from the measured performance outcome that is fed back to the patient by some artificial means.[1] Extrinsic feedback is considered augmented feedback and is supplied beyond intrinsic feedback.[1] Examples of extrinsic feedback include knowledge of performance and knowledge of results (described in the previous paragraph), videotape replays, and biofeedback.

**Biofeedback (BF)** is a type of extrinsic, augmented feedback. The *Guide to Physical Therapist Practice*[2] defines biofeedback as "a training technique that enables an individual to gain some element of voluntary control over muscular or autonomic nervous system functions using a device that produces auditory or visual stimuli." BF is categorized as an electrotherapeutic modality.[2] There are a number of differences between BF and the other electrotherapeutic modalities described in this text. First, when **electrical stimulation (ES)** is used to improve muscle performance, tissue repair, or pain management, an electrical stimulus is applied to the client. No electrical stimulus is applied to the patient with BF; rather, a physiologic process (eg, blood pressure, skin temperature, electromyographic [EMG] activity) is recorded from the patient. Instead of putting some entity into the patient, BF takes some entity out—information that the patient and therapist may use in order to improve voluntary movement control or decrease pain. Second, the patient typically remains relatively passive during ES. Exceptions exist, of course, such as using functional ES to augment the force-generating capacity of certain muscles during gait. With BF, the patient is frequently active throughout the session and must access and interact with the technology used to measure and display the physiologic process in order to benefit from it. Even when BF is being used to decrease or inhibit an excessive physiologic process, the patient is very involved in using the information to modify that physiologic behavior. Therefore, the active involvement of the patient in transforming some entity previously unconscious to the conscious level[3] is what makes BF unique from other electrotherapeutic modalities.

A very common form of BF used in physical therapy and physical medicine and rehabilitation is **electromyographic biofeedback (EMGBF).** EMGBF is simply an application of BF in which an individual receives visual or auditory information about his or her muscle activity. The purpose of EMGBF is to change electrical activity of the muscle into auditory or visual cues so that the patient may learn to increase or decrease the physiologic activation of a skeletal muscle or muscles.[3–5] EMGBF has been used to improve muscle activation control in patients with diagnoses of orthopedic problems such as arthritis,[6] low back pain,[7] and following surgery,[8,9] as well as in patients with neurologic dysfunction.[10–13]

There are several key issues to consider when reviewing the definition and purpose of BF. First, Binder-Macleod has rightly pointed out that EMGBF is a tool and not a treatment. The treatment a physical therapist provides is the activity or exercise that the patient is performing.[5] EMGBF produces a signal (or information) that the clinician[14] and patient use to modify the treatment or activity. In summary, EMGBF is a component of a treatment plan used to augment other active or functionally oriented procedures. Second, EMGBF affords the patient some element of voluntary control over a physiologic response (in this case, the EMG signal) that is not usually perceived at a conscious level. That is, a patient does not usually know how much muscle activity he or she is using while producing a movement. EMGBF allows the patient to gain insight into the level of muscle activity he or she is using. Finally, the information fed back to the patient is usually in the form of an auditory or visual cue. A major advantage to the incorporation of EMGBF into a treatment plan is that even the smallest increases (or decreases) in muscle activity can be identified during a therapeutic exercise procedure. If the detection of small changes of muscle activity is indicated, EMGBF will more accurately accomplish this than the clinician's observation or palpation skills. This cue of BF provides an opportunity for the clinician to objectively observe which techniques or activities are having the desired effect.[14]

Other forms of BF used in physical therapy (PT) settings include **force feedback** using a weight scale, limb load monitor,[15] force platform,[16] position or kinematic feedback[17,18] (some using electrogoniometric devices[19]), and to a lesser extent skin temperature. Additionally, with the growth and use of technology in PT, **virtual reality BF** may be used. Biofeedback in a virtual (simulated) environment is presently being studied in the research setting.[20] The key to all of these types of feedback and their success is in how accurately and quickly information is provided to the patient (ie, is the information provided to the patient through the instrumentation proportional to the physiologic process being recorded?[3]) These forms of BF will not be the focus of this chapter.

## GENERATION OF A MUSCLE ACTION POTENTIAL

The EMG signal provides a window to the nervous system. An understanding of how the neural signal is transformed into a muscle action potential is important in understanding what information EMGBF is providing to the patient. A thorough description of the electrical and mechanical events underlying a muscle contraction are not within the scope of this chapter and can be found elsewhere.[21,22] There are, however, several key steps in the process worth reviewing. First, the neural action potential leaves the spinal cord and travels to the neuromuscular junction in order to produce

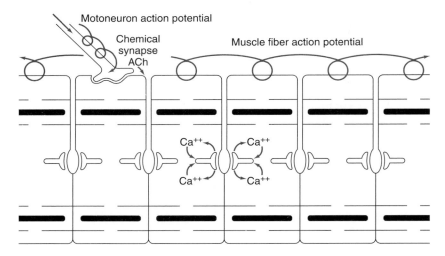

Motoneuron action potential

Chemical synapse ACh

Muscle fiber action potential

Ca++     Ca++

Ca++     Ca++

FIGURE 11–1. Electric and chemical events of the transmission of a neural action potential to the neuromuscular junction. See text for details. EMGBF records the resultant muscle action potential and not the subsequent muscle contraction (binding of actin and myosin filaments). *(From Loeb G, Gans C. Electromyography for Experimentalists. Chicago, University of Chicago Press, 1986. Used with permission.)*

a muscle action potential. Acetylcholine (Ach) travels across the synaptic cleft and interacts with receptors on the sarcolemma. Acetylcholine increases the permeability of the postsynaptic membrane to sodium and potassium which, causes an **endplate potential.**[21] The endplate potential is conducted away from the neuromuscular junction and can result in the generation of a muscle action potential in the adjacent sarcolemma.[21,22] The depolarization of the sarcolemma (muscle action potential) is what the EMGBF instrumentation is detecting. (See Figure 11–1.)

## THE PATIENT'S PROBLEM AND EXPECTATIONS

Why would a patient seen by a physical therapist require BF as a direct therapeutic intervention? As with other electrotherapeutic modalities, BF may be indicated when a patient presents with impaired motor function, impaired muscle performance, muscle spasm, pain, or a combination of these.[2] In this connection, too much or too little muscle activity contributes to the movement dysfunction or pain syndrome. That is, the patient's functional ability is hindered by a muscle or muscle group that has either too much or too little muscle activity necessary to perform the particular functional task. Biofeedback is used to decrease unwanted muscle activity (through inhibition or relaxation training) or promote muscle contraction (through recruitment training) during a functional posture or activity.

Because of the significant active involvement of the patient in each BF training session, open communication between the clinician and the patient as well as an understanding of the patient's expectations are important for success. Patient expectations are obtained during the examination. Subsequently, as the therapist reviews the identified problems with the patient, goals can be established. The therapist must document these patient goals in conjunction with his or her goals and review the patient's expectations. The therapist is responsible for explaining each treatment's purpose and expected outcome to the patient. In situations in which communication may be hampered by the primary diagnosis (eg, aphasia following cerebrovascular accident), including the patient's family or designated caregiver may be useful.

## Examination and Evaluation

To address the patient's problem, the physical therapist conducts an examination, which begins by taking a history and reviewing all pertinent information. Complaints of pain, weakness, joint stiffness, muscle spasm, and decreased movement function in general are identified during the patient interview. After analyzing all relevant information, the physical therapist decides what groups of tests and measures should be included in the examination of the patient.[2]

Specific tests and measures outlined within the *Guide to Physical Therapist Practice*[2] such as gait, locomotion, and balance; joint integrity and mobility; motor function; muscle performance; neuromotor development and sensory integration; pain; and posture may assist in identifying movement dysfunction that may be amenable to BF. Assessment of motivation, orientation, and cognition (arousal, attention) will help the therapist evaluate whether the patient has the perceptual–cognitive capacity to participate in BF training. Assessment of joint pain, range of motion (ROM), muscular force (strength), coordination, selectivity,[23] and the use of functional performance scales such as the **Patient Evaluation and Conference System (PECS)**[24] will assist the therapist in identifying the presence of a movement dysfunction and will provide baseline information as to the integrity of the essential components of movement. Surface EMG may also be used during the examination process as an indicator of muscle performance during movement tasks.[14,25] Subsequently, the technology may also provide the clinician with evaluative information related to the success of the treatment interventions and help with prognosis and discharge planning.

## Impairments, Disabilities, and Handicaps

In 1980, the World Health Organization (WHO) drafted a document entitled "International Classification of Impairments, Disabilities, and Handicaps."[26] One purpose in its development was to provide uniformity of terminology in health care and to improve information on the consequences of disease. EMGBF directly addresses a patient's problem at the level of impairment. Impairment is defined as "any loss or abnormality of psychological, physiological, or anatomical structure or function."[26] Although eight impairment categories were described in the document, three specific impairment categories—visceral impairments, skeletal impairments, and generalized, sensory, and other impairments—include the major impairments that may be discovered in an examination and be associated with the application of BF within the context of PT. Table 11–1 lists the impairments within these three major impairment categories.

### TABLE 11–1. COMMON IMPAIRMENTS ASSOCIATED WITH THE APPLICATION OF BIOFEEDBACK AND PHYSICAL THERAPY

| | EMGBF Goal |
|---|---|
| Visceral impairments (impairments of internal organs and of other special functions) | |
| Urge incontinence | Recruitment |
| Stress incontinence | Recruitment |
| Skeletal impairments (mechanical and motor disturbances of the face, head, neck, trunk and limbs) | |
| Impairment of head and trunk regions | |
| Facial paralyis | Recruitment |
| Torticollis | Relaxation |
| Impairment of posture | Recruitment or relaxation |
| Impairment of the limbs (spastic paralysis of more than one limb: hemi-, para-, or tetra-paresis/plegia) | |
| Muscle weakness | Recruitment |
| Spasticity | Relaxation |
| Other paralysis of limb | |
| Flaccid paralysis | Recruitment |
| Weakness of limb | Recruitment |
| Other generalized impairment | |
| Generalized pain | Relaxation |
| Sensory impairment of head, trunk, limb | |
| Headache | Relaxation |
| Back pain | Relaxation |

The classification system lists nine disabilities. **Disability** refers to the tasks, skills, or behaviors of the person.[26] Major disabilities resulting from **impairments** in motor function, pain syndromes, or both may include disabilities of personal care, locomotion, body disposition, and dexterity. Applying BF to specific impairments hypothesized to be primarily contributing to the patient's disability may subsequently minimize that disability (eg, improved control over voiding; walking with less dependence). Finally, as part of the WHO's classification system, specific **handicaps** may be associated with the disabilities and impairments listed above. These handicaps, as defined by the WHO, include handicaps of physical independence, and mobility.

The *Guide to Physical Therapist Practice*[2] has described preferred practice patterns for selected patient–client diagnostic groups. Consistent with the examination and evaluation, patients may exhibit impaired posture, impaired muscle performance, or impaired motor function and sensory integrity associated with neuromuscular diagnostic categories such as the following:

1. Congenital or acquired disorders of the CNS in infancy, childhood, and adolescence
2. Acquired nonprogressive disorders of the CNS in adulthood
3. Progressive disorders of the CNS in adulthood
4. Peripheral nerve injury
5. Acute and chronic polyneuropathies
6. Nonprogressive disorders of the spinal cord.

Impaired posture, joint mobility, ROM, muscle performance, motor function, or combinations of these may be evident subsequent to musculoskeletal diagnoses associated with spinal disorders (eg, disk disease), ligament or other connective tissue disorders (eg, sprains, strains), joint arthroplasty, and following soft tissue surgical procedures (eg, muscle, tendon, or ligament repair). The use of BF may be applicable to conditions in these diagnostic groups.[2]

In summary, patients who exhibit muscular weakness because of either immobilization, deconditioning, or some musculoskeletal or neurologic trauma, disease, or surgery are potential candidates for BF (recruitment training). Likewise, those patients with excessive muscle activity secondary to pain or changes in resting muscle tone may also be candidates for EMGBF (relaxation training). The assumption is and the examination findings should support, however, that these impairments have resulted in some disability.

## DIAGNOSIS/PROGNOSIS

The *Guide to Physical Therapist Practice*[2] lists 12 anticipated goals related to the use of electrotherapeutic modalities. Several of these goals are pertinent to EMGBF intervention. (See Table 11–2.) The

---

### TABLE 11–2.  ANTICIPATED GOALS OF EMGBF

Through increasing insufficient EMG activity or through decreasing unwanted EMG activity and in conjunction with an integrated treatment plan, any or all of the following anticipated goals may apply:

- Ability to perform physical tasks is increased.
- Complications are reduced.
- Joint integrity and mobility are improved.
- Muscle performance is increased.
- Neuromuscular function is increased.
- Pain is decreased.
- Risk of secondary impairments is reduced.

---

physical therapist should be aware of the literature regarding the application of EMGBF to the specific condition within a category of interest. This awareness is necessary in order to identify appropriate patients, develop a realistic plan, and determine anticipated outcomes.

As an example of the diagnosis/prognosis process, the provision of EMGBF in patients with movement dysfunction following a cerebrovascular accident is common and well described in the literature, but not all stroke patients are appropriate for EMGBF. As it pertains to recovery of motor function of the upper extremity, Wolf, Baker, and Kelly[27] and Wolf and Binder-Macleod[28] have concluded that chronic stroke patients with at least some general element of voluntary control of the upper extremity (shoulder, elbow, wrist) and finger extension control specifically,[28] and presence of proprioception[27] may benefit more from EMGBF than those patients without such control or sensory capacity. These findings, however, do not preclude the use of EMGBF during treatment sessions for those stroke patients unable to minimally control the wrist or fingers. At a minimum, EMGBF may be useful for the physical therapist in identifying if the therapeutic exercises instituted to target movement deficiencies are, in fact, eliciting the appropriate muscle responses.[14]

Other patients' conditions may benefit from EMGBF, and information from federal clinical practice guidelines and the research literature can help the clinician determine potential length of treatment and outcomes. For example, BF has been used alone and in conjunction with **neuromuscular electrical stimulation (NMES)** to address the problem of stress and urge urinary incontinence. However, the use of BF for incontinence is not a new idea. Kegel[29] first developed a perineometer, which was a type of force measurement BF used during the process of improving (strengthening) pelvic floor muscle force.

Although the WHO classifies urge and stress incontinence under the category of visceral impairments,[26] the *Guide to Physical Therapist Practice* likely includes the problem of incontinence under the musculoskeletal diagnostic category of impaired muscle performance, which includes dysfunction of the pelvic floor musculature.[2] In this connection, anorectal or vaginal BF is used to assist the practice of pelvic floor muscle exercises in order to learn isolated sphincter control. A goal in this application of BF is to learn to contract and relax the pelvic floor muscles while keeping abdominal muscles relaxed.[30] For women, this is done by using surface electrodes on a vaginal probe and anorectal manometry to measure intra-abdominal pressure and external sphincter pressure. Patients are trained to contract pelvic floor muscles and sustain a contraction from 5 to 10 sec before relaxing. When patients with incontinence are identified as being able to learn new skills and actively participate in treatment (patient selection criteria), BF therapy appears to readily assist in identifying the appropriate muscles to control and also serves to promote a sense of accomplishment as therapy progresses.[31] Outcomes in the treatment of incontinence with BF can be measured at the impairment and disability levels via the amount of EMG activity of pelvic floor muscles, the ability to develop quick contractions,[31] and the frequency of accidents.[30] In light of the psychosocial impact of this type of problem in elderly people, quality-of-life measures are appropriate measures of success as well.

With a minimum number of treatment sessions,[30,32] improvement in incontinence has been demonstrated. The Clinical Practice Guidelines for the management of urinary incontinence have identified that 54 to 87 percent improvement in incontinence has been demonstrated when BF is combined with behavioral treatment.[33] When BF using multimeasurement techniques (abdominal and sphincter pressure) are used, studies show a further (75 to 82 percent) reduction in urinary incontinence, leading the Agency for Health Care Policy and Research (AHCPR) to conclude that the treatment for urinary incontinence (including behavioral therapies and BF) can improve or "cure" most patients.[33]

## INTERVENTION

## EMGBF Components and Instrumentation

EMGBF components consist of the **electrodes, lead wires** (some computerized systems use infrared technology), and the BF **unit** itself. The unit, which could be a small handheld device, desktop device, or a computerized system, has two purposes: to process the

EMG signal and to produce auditory or visual feedback proportional to the input signal. A graphic summary of the process by which the raw muscle EMG signal is transformed into an auditory or visual cue for the patient is provided in Figure 11–2.

Although electrodes come in subdermal (needle) and surface types, physical therapists most frequently use the surface electrode (Fig. 11–3). Electrodes record the summated muscle EMG activity. To convey this concept to the patient, electrodes are often described as sensors. *Sensor* is a preferable term to use when describing the EMGBF intervention to the patient because it is potentially less threatening than the term *electrode.*

Surface electrodes usually come in pairs and are usually made of some type of metal. Silver–silver chloride or gold-based electrodes are popular because of their good electrical conductivity.[3] A third electrode, the **ground** (or reference) **electrode** is also part of the patient–BF unit interface. The ground electrode helps the BF unit discern the muscle activity recorded from the surface (recording) electrodes from extraneous electrical activity or "noise" such as wide-band noise (amplifier filters, electrode impedance), narrowband noise (fluorescent lights, television and radio signals), and biological noise (muscle cross-talk, respiratory artifact).[34] Lead wires

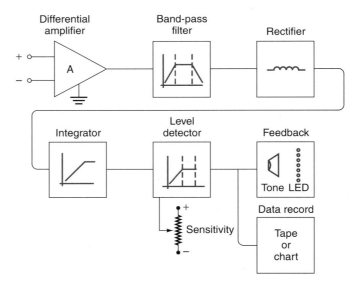

FIGURE 11–2. Major components of the BF unit and steps in transforming the raw muscle EMG signal into auditory or visual feedback to the patient. See text for details. *(From Basmajian JV [ed]. Biofeedback: Principles and Practice for Clinicians, 3rd ed. Baltimore, MD, Williams & Wilkins, 1989. Used with permission.)*

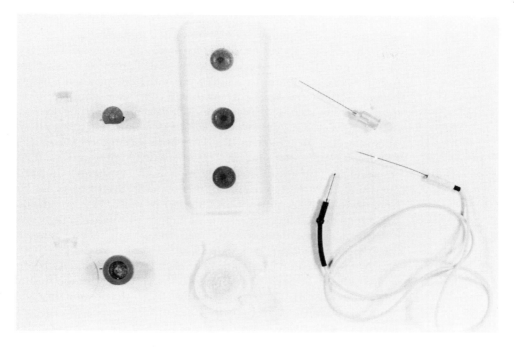

FIGURE 11–3. Examples of electrodes used during biofeedback. **Left,** large and small permanent surface electrodes with associated adhesive patches. **Center,** disposable surface electrodes. **Right,** monopolar and fine-wire percutaneous electrodes. *(From Wolf SL. Electromyographic biofeedback: An overview. In Nelson RM, Currier DP [eds], Clinical Electrotherapy, 2nd ed. Norwalk, CT, Appleton & Lange, 1991. Used with permission.)*

connect the electrodes to the BF unit. Sometimes these wires, when moved, produce unwanted signals in the EMG tracing. Shielded wires help to reduce electrical noise. Lead wires can be secured to the patient to minimize movement once the electrodes have been applied.

In order to adequately display the signal to the patient, the signal must first be processed. This processing is a major function of the BF unit. An amplifier will increase the amplitude of the signal. The signal amplitude is controlled through adjusting the gain (or sensitivity) of the device. The term *sensitivity* is often used in operator's manuals of BF devices. The greater the amplification, the more sensitive the device.[5] The **gain** describes the relationship between the input signal and the output amplitude of the amplifier. Gain is the factor by which the input signal is multiplied to obtain the output. BF units generally have a range of sensitivity scales (eg, 0–1, 0–10, 0–100, 0–1000 μV). In EMG, differential amplifier is needed, and not a simple amplifier, because a differential amplifier will reject signals common to both electrodes and enhance signals that are different.[35] Differentiation is an important concept in the elimination of unwanted signals.

There is no specific formula for defining the sensitivity setting of the BF unit during a treatment session. Rather, one must assess the patient's capability to control the targeted muscle in order to properly adjust the sensitivity of the BF unit. For example, if a patient with significant weakness or paresis is just learning to recruit motor units of a particular muscle and that muscle is presently producing only 5 μV of activity, then the appropriate range would be 0 to 10 μV. That is, the unit must significantly amplify the small EMG signal. This amplification results in a high sensitivity. Conversely, choosing a 0 to 100 μV range in this scenario would be of little use because the low sensitivity (large range) of the device would not allow adequate monitoring of small changes in muscle activity. Without this adequate detection, the patient will not receive important information about small changes in muscle EMG activity.

A filter in the BF unit will further aid in the elimination of unwanted electrical signals and enhance the recording of the desirable muscle activity signal. Depending on the sophistication of the BF unit, the clinician may have the opportunity to set the frequency range in which to allow specific signals to pass into and through the amplifier. Because most EMG signals generally fall within a 100- to 1000-Hz range,[5] the filter could be set to eliminate those frequencies above and below these values. This screening of frequencies may be done through high-pass and low-pass filters, which allow higher- and lower-frequency signals, respectively, to pass through the amplifier.

**Rectification** is needed in order to integrate the EMG signal. Rectification is simply taking the positive and negative values of a signal and making them all positive. **Integration** is a calculation that obtains the area under the signal (since the signal is positive because of rectification).[36] The EMG integral can be thought of as the amount of EMG activity acting over a period of time. Therefore, the measurement value resulting from integration is V·s (volt-seconds). Integration is important because clinicians usually have the opportunity to adjust the time constant in the BF unit. The **time constant** determines the rate at which the integrated EMG signal will increase or decrease.[5] This constant may be considered as the smoothing option of the BF unit.[25] However, this should not be confused with the filtering components of the BF unit described earlier. (See Figure 11–4.)

As with setting the sensitivity, there is no specific formula for setting the time constant. However, most BF units tend to have fewer choices for setting the time constant than the sensitivity. The determination of the time constant is based on the goal of the treatment session and how proficient the patient is at understanding and using the EMG activity to change the response. For example, if general relax-

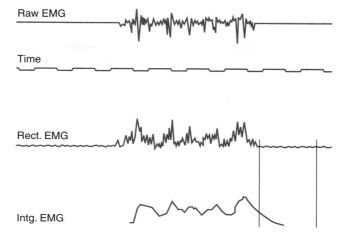

Raw EMG

Time

Rect. EMG

Intg. EMG

FIGURE 11–4. Processing of the EMG signal generated by a brief contraction of the right forearm flexor mass. Upper trace, raw amplified (×1000) EMG; second trace, time markers every 100 msec; third trace, rectified raw amplified signal; fourth trace, integrated EMG (time constant of integrator = 100 msec). *(From Wolf SL. Electromyographic biofeedback: An overview. In Nelson RM, Currier DP [eds], Clinical Electrotherapy, 2nd ed. Norwalk, CT, Appleton & Lange, 1991. Used with permission.)*

ation was the goal and the patient was relatively new at using this technique, then a longer time constant might be appropriate. However, if a patient was just learning to identify and activate a very weak muscle, then a shorter time constant would be appropriate because it would more quickly reflect the changes at the muscle. In this way, the shorter time constant more closely mimics the rectified EMG signal so that the patient can identify whether he or she is actually recruiting or inhibiting that muscle. However, a time constant that is too short could result in a rapidly changing signal (approaching the characteristics of a raw signal) that could be difficult to follow, thus making it difficult for the clinician and patient to interpret the effect of the movement action or exercise. Binder-Macleod[5] recommends a time constant of approximately one third of a second (300 ms) for most muscle training applications; however, some BF units allow adjustment only at fixed intervals such as one tenth, one half, and 1 sec.

When the EMG signal reaches a desired or set voltage level, a threshold detector will provide either an "on" signal or an "off" signal (feedback) depending on the desired effect during the intervention. For example, if the goal is to minimize excessive EMG activity in a trapezius muscle of a patient with chronic neck pain, the clinician may choose to have the auditory or visual cue turned on when the EMG activity exceeds the set threshold and have the auditory or visual cue turned off when the patient relaxes the trapezius muscle (decreasing the EMG activity) to a point below the set threshold. Additionally, the intensity of the feedback cue may also be adjusted as the input EMG signal increases or decreases. For example, the tone of the auditory cue may become proportionally higher with increased EMG activity, or the visual feedback may become a more vivid color with increased EMG activity. Continuing with this example, as the patient is able to relax the upper trapezius muscle, the physical therapist adjusts the threshold level detector down so that further relaxation can be achieved through training. Conversely, when training a patient with weakness to recruit a particular muscle, the threshold would be set just above the amount of activity the patient could generate through motor unit recruitment. As the patient is able to increase activity, the threshold could then be adjusted to a higher level. The modification of the threshold level up (higher $\mu V$ EMG activity) or down (lower $\mu V$ EMG activity) as the patient changes his or her control over the targeted muscle during BF treatment is called **shaping.**[3]

The choice to use auditory or visual feedback depends on the specific patient and therapeutic situation. There are several factors to consider: patient age and preference (an EMG signal tracing on a visual display may have little value to a child, whereas music that turns on and off in accordance with changing behavior may be more valuable to that child), the type of movements that will occur (eg, gait training may be more amenable to the use of auditory feedback because the patient has to use vision to scan his or her environment during walking,[37] while targeting muscles necessary for successful reaching in sitting may afford visual or auditory feedback to be equally effective), and training approach. For example, if the goal is general relaxation and the patient is in a reclined posture, visual cues may be difficult to track in that position; auditory cues would allow the patient to close his or her eyes, further aiding in a relaxation response.

The choice of electrode size is determined largely by the size of the muscle or muscles being monitored during a treatment session. The best choice of size of electrodes is one that provides an appropriate sample of muscle activity while avoiding undesired activity (muscle cross-talk) from neighboring or antagonistic muscles.[38] Therefore, larger electrodes tend to be used for limb muscles because a larger recording area monitors more muscle volume and potentially will record greater EMG activity.[5] Using a large electrode over a small muscle, however, increases the chance that the electrode will record EMG activity from surrounding or antagonistic muscles. The same holds true for interelectrode distance. A wider spacing results in an increased volume of muscle monitored,[39] therefore potentially recording more EMG activity. A narrow spacing may provide more specific recording from a single muscle or local group. In cases of recording from hand and face muscles, interelectrode distance should be minimal in order to accurately capture the specific activity of these smaller muscles. Treatment goal and the patient's ability to access the muscle also affect the choice of interelectrode distance. This situation will be addressed in upcoming sections on recruitment and relaxation. The physical therapist should select the identical electrode size used previously when repeating EMGBF training on subsequent occasions. This approach enables a comparison of recorded data.

A major area of resistance (impedance) for the EMG signal is the skin–electrode interface. A conductive medium, usually in the form of a gel or paste, is added to the recording surface of the electrode when electrodes are applied to the skin. This use of a gel is done in order to remove air in the space and improve contact between the electrode recording surface and the patient's skin. Preparing the skin by clipping or shaving any excess hair in the area, wiping or cleansing the area with rubbing alcohol, and lightly sanding the skin with a coarse substance (usually fine sandpaper or scrub pad) is usually necessary to decrease skin resistance. This procedure, however, will have no impact on scars or excessively thickened skin over the recording area, or adipose tissue and fascia beneath the skin. These barriers, along with trying to record from deeper muscle tissue, may hinder adequate recording of the EMG signal when using surface electrodes.

Most surface electrodes used in the clinic setting are disposable and come pregelled and pretaped so that they are easily applied to the skin. Placing the electrodes on the skin directly over the area of the muscle fibers targeted for treatment is desirable. The placement of the ground electrode is less important and need not be between the recording electrodes as commonly recommended. Application of the ground electrode to a nearby bony prominence is sufficient. To maintain the highest level of accuracy during a treatment session, the recording electrodes should be applied in such a way as to be on the skin over the area of the targeted muscle fibers when the segment is in the desired training position or posture.[40] For example, electrode placement and interelectrode distance will be different if a physical therapist is training the elbow flexor biceps brachii muscle with the elbow in full extension versus full flexion. In this case, the electrode placement would need to be more proximal if the biceps muscles were being targeted when the elbow was in greater flexion. Finally, the electrodes should generally be placed parallel to the direction of the muscle fibers of interest as most texts that describe electrode placement for surface EMG and BF demonstrate.[25,39]

The physical therapist is obligated to record the locations and sizes of electrodes for use in subsequent training sessions. This approach enables a more accurate assessment of the EMG results for comparison with EMG data recorded during different sessions.

## EMGBF: Therapeutic Application

### Patient Preparation and Instructions
EMGBF requires active and attentive participation by the patient (as well as the clinician). The following is a fundamental list of considerations to determine whether EMGBF is appropriate for a particular patient:

- Patient receptiveness to the concept
- Patient motivation
- Motor planning skills
- Presence and degree of neglect or aphasia in cases of neurologic disorders
- Adequate vision and hearing
- Rehabilitation potential
- Presence of initial voluntary control[38]

The amount of instruction or orientation given to a patient depends on whether the patient and the clinician or the clinician alone will be using the feedback information. Initial instructions should include purpose and expected outcome, overview of the equipment, description of the type of feedback information that will be provided, and any exercise- or movement-related information. If a patient has difficulty understanding how BF works, a simple demonstration using an uninvolved muscle may be helpful.

### Recruitment Training
The goal here is to assist the patient in increasing EMG activity through shaping the muscle EMG activity responses upward, activating a muscle or muscles in isolation and during a functional movement task, and to make the patient aware of any neural connections that remain during the acute (or chronic) stage of an injury or disease state. There is at least one prerequisite when EMGBF training for recruitment is initiated. The patient must have some minimal (detectable by the BF unit) ability to voluntarily activate the muscle or muscles of interest. For example, targeting wrist flexor muscles for recruitment in a patient with a complete spinal cord injury at the C4 level would not be appropriate.

Training recruitment in cases of impaired muscle performance following a musculoskeletal injury or orthopedic surgical procedure can be fairly simple.[3] These patients usually have adequate cognitive ability to understand BF and a normal CNS, that is, sufficient central motor coordination and sensory feedback from the muscles, joints, and skin. Additionally, the goal of treatment is usually targeted to a single muscle or muscle group, such as is the case following anterior cruciate ligament (ACL) repair,[9] meniscus repair[8] or in the management of chronic arthritic knee pain, which can result in decreased muscle performance of the quadriceps muscles.[6]

In all of these examples, BF is used to augment the present muscle function through increasing awareness of actual muscle EMG activity and through shaping procedures to progressively increase the desired response during isometric quadriceps muscle setting and terminal knee extension exercises. A wider interelectrode distance may be required early in training if the muscle is very weak and minimal muscle activation is present. However, spacing should not be so wide as to contaminate the EMG signal with extraneous muscle activity. Choosing the best interelectrode distance in cases of electrode spacing is a delicate balance in which close inspection and evaluation of the muscle EMG signal by the clinician is required. This balance is true for the quadriceps muscle and the vastus medialis muscle component in particular. In this case, specific electrode placement is important. Cram, Kasman, and Holtz recommend electrode placement for the vastus medialis to be an oblique positioning in line with the muscle fiber orientation, 2 cm medial from the superior rim of the patella, and the inter electrode distance at 2 cm.[25] Generally, the gain or sensitivity of the system may be set higher in the early stages of rehabilitation in order to convey small changes in EMG activity to the patient, particularly when the initial EMG signal is very small. As treatment progresses the sensitivity can be decreased along with the interelectrode distance.[3]

Providing an attainable goal for any patient early in the training is important. The threshold level should therefore be set just above resting baseline EMG level. Specific approaches for determining the threshold within operant conditioning paradigms exist but are infrequently reported. Brucker and Bulaeva argue that the inclusion of operant conditioning procedures (essentially the procedure for shaping the desired response) is essential for successful outcomes when using BF. Specifically, these researchers have used the standard deviation of the patient's integrated EMG from a baseline examination as the criterion for the initial threshold level.[13] The patient then has the opportunity to attempt the desired movement. As the magnitude of the volitional response increases, the threshold is readjusted, based on the new EMG activity levels. This readjustment of threshold is an example of a systematic approach to shaping the EMG responses during recruitment training. Despite the abundance of research published on BF in PT and physical medicine and rehabilitation, few studies actually detail the shaping procedures.

The use of BF in patients with neurologic conditions can be complex, in part because of potential cognitive–perceptual issues, alterations in central neural drive onto motor neurons, and changes in sensory feedback processes that may accompany lesions of the CNS. Review chapters on recruitment training using BF have traditionally described the use of EMGBF in light of procedures related to traditional neurotherapeutic approaches.[41–44] Specifically, through an emphasis on neurophysiologic data from the first half of the 1900s, these approaches advocated recruitment of proximal muscles, emphasizing stability before targeting distal muscles and training mobility, and inhibiting abnormally hyperactive muscles before recruiting weak muscles. Advances in motor control and motor learning research since the 1960s have resulted in some physical therapists' questioning the assumptions underlying the treatment approaches advocated by these traditional neurotherapies.[45,46] As such, EMGBF should be used in conjunction with neurotherapeutic approaches based on the foundation science of **motor control,** which emphasizes biomechanical and behavioral factors of movement as well as neurophysiologic factors.[23] The use of motor control science includes the application of motor learning principles[1] related to part/whole task transfer, practice schedule, and the nature and frequency of feedback within a therapy session in which EMGBF is used.

Patients with diagnoses of neurologic conditions such as stroke, spinal cord injury, and brain injury initially receiving recruitment training with EMGBF may be unable to initiate or complete the necessary movement. EMGBF traditionally progresses from training isolated muscle control to training muscles during the desired functional movement or activity. Therefore, component movements are usually targeted first over training the whole movement action, and EMGBF is usually targeted to one muscle or an agonist–antagonist muscle pair. For example, Tries has emphasized the recruitment of necessary biomechanical elements of upper extremity elevation during a treatment session. She argues that it is insufficient to target only the typically hyperactive upper trapezius muscle for inhibition and the typically weak anterior deltoid muscle for recruitment. The essential synergists of upper extremity elevation such as serratus anterior (scapular protraction) and infraspinatus (external rotation) muscles are frequently weak and should be targeted for recruitment as well. This way, often neglected elements of the movement are trained and incorporated into a treatment session.[47]

This example, however, raises an important issue related to the concept of part/whole task transfer. Part practice implies that meaningful units (or parts) of a whole movement task are isolated and practiced separately.[1] The implication of part/whole task transfer for the provision of EMGBF is in how the BF session is designed and integrated in order to achieve some functional goal. An example of part practice during the relearning of a movement such as reaching for a cup and bringing it back to the mouth would be isolating the scapular protraction component (serratus anterior muscle recruitment) before practicing the whole reaching movement. This part practice technique may be performed very early in training when the patient has little control and is just learning about BF and the role of the serratus anterior muscle in forward reaching. However, there is little evidence to suggest practicing a part of a relatively short-duration, discrete task such as forward reaching will transfer to the whole task.[1] This technique is probably even more important when a component part such as scapular protraction is practiced in the supine position while the task or goal may be reaching in the sitting position at a kitchen table. Not only is part of the task being practiced, but the practice position significantly changes biomechanical factors associated with performance such as the effect of gravity generally, the influence of the upper limb as an additional load specifically, postural support of the trunk provided by the plinth or treatment table, and length–tension relationships of scapulohumeral and scapuloaxial muscles. In this example, the physical therapist should progress to practicing serratus anterior muscle recruitment within the context of forward reaching in the sitting position as soon as possible.

This concept must also be applied to the lower extremity. Clinical observation frequently identifies that knee flexion is diminished in the gait pattern of patients with cortical lesions.[48] Traditionally, hamstring muscle activation for knee flexion may be trained with EMGBF in a position such as sidelying. However, training knee flexor muscles to improve knee flexion during gait is inconsistent with gait studies that demonstrate that the hamstring muscles are not active during early swing phase and that the examination of biomechanical variables do not support their role in maintaining knee flexion in early and mid-swing.[49,50] Rather, hamstring muscles are important in decelerating the limb at the end of the swing phase,[49] and hip flexor and plantar flexor muscles are important for the acceleration and advancement of the limb through the swing phase.[50] As with any therapeutic intervention, the focus of the EMGBF treatment session should be guided by the goal of decreasing movement dysfunction. Therefore, treatment should be directed around realistic movement behaviors under relevant environmental contexts as soon as possible.

Continuing with the previous example, Colborne and colleagues have used EMGBF and joint angle feedback in patients with stroke[37] and EMGBF in patients with cerebral palsy[51] to retrain the activation of the plantar flexor muscles during walking. Colborne and colleagues, recognizing the importance of adequate push-off from the ankle for successful walking and wanting to apply EMGBF during a functionally relevant task to maximize carryover, designed a therapeutic intervention to address this issue.[32]

Biofeedback training during gait following stroke has been used for years; however, most research and subsequent clinical applications focused on targeting the dorsiflexor muscles to address the problem of footdrop.[52] This approach remains useful today. The plantar flexor muscles' role in force generation may not have been the focus of most interventions because of the prevailing treatment approaches of the time, which emphasized reduction of abnormal tone and the reluctance of the proponents of these approaches to improve the force-generating capacity of muscles presumed to be spastic.[42]

In the case of adult hemiplegic gait, Colborne, Olney, and Griffin[37] found the application of ankle angle feedback in conjunction with EMGBF from the paretic soleus muscle improved push-off impulse. Biofeedback training was superior to regular PT, and the training effect was maintained at follow-up. An auditory tone was provided when the threshold level targets from the soleus muscle and the ankle angle were met. Additionally, patients could monitor their performance on a visual display; however, an auditory cue was preferred because patients needed to focus their vision on the environment.[37] These researchers hypothesized that the patients monitored their responses for each stride and may or may not have had adequate time to use the feedback within the same stride. The subjects may have used knowledge of the results from the previous stride to modify in a feed-forward manner the ankle responses of the subsequent stride.[37] In the application of EMGBF from triceps sura muscles in children with cerebral palsy,[51] greater ankle power for push-off and total positive work at the hip and ankle were demonstrated. This improved push-off subsequently resulted in a decrease in stance time.

Another motor learning issue is the nature and frequency of feedback provided to the patient. Examples of the nature of BF include the muscle EMG activity during EMGBF, weight from a scale or force from a force platform during force (kinetic) feedback, and displacement or position during motion (kinematic) feedback. The frequency of feedback can range from a constant schedule to eventually complete removal of extrinsic feedback. Frequent feedback during recruitment is probably important early in training because the patient may still be learning how to produce the desired response. One could argue that most patients with neurologic problems may be in the verbal–cognitive or early motor stage of learning early in training.[1] If this is true, guidance and frequent feedback may be necessary. As treatment progresses, however, and the patient becomes more skilled in activating and relaxing the muscle in isolation, during movements or both, feedback should be gradually taken away. Too much feedback for too long a period of time may result in dependence on the feedback and could limit learning.[1] Specific schedules for fading feedback have not been identified when EMGBF is used; however, research has started to address this issue with other forms of extrinsic feedback, such as force feedback, to learn partial weight bearing.[53]

### Inhibition or Relaxation

The goal here is to induce and maintain a relaxed state of muscle activation by progressively shaping muscle EMG activity downward.[3] Inhibition or relaxation generally refers to decreasing excessive EMG activity secondary to a neurologic disorder, which results in abnormal increases in muscle tone (spasticity), or decreasing a state of hyperarousal of the muscle secondary to an acute or chronic pain syndrome or abnormal posture resulting from a pain syndrome.

In the presence of spastic muscle, a small interelectrode distance may be preferable early in training in order to minimize excessive EMG feedback.[3] With a small interelectrode distance, the EMG signal reflects only a small portion of the hyperactive muscle and may be easier for the patient to monitor and begin to control than if the interelectrode distance were wide. As discussed earlier, however, the adjustment of interelectrode distance must be considered in light of surrounding musculature that could contaminate the signal. The threshold level or goal should be just below the baseline level in which the muscle is producing feedback so that the patient may begin to inhibit the muscle with elevated activity and receive feedback on the success of the relaxation effort.

As stated previously, traditional neurotherapeutic approaches advocated decreasing spasticity as a necessary prerequisite for normal movement capability. However, recent studies have questioned the need to perform inhibition training first following a cortical lesion. Gowland and colleagues investigated the role impaired antagonist inhibition played in arm movements of patients with hemiplegia,[54] essentially testing Bobath's[42] contention that spasticity is a primary movement problem. Using a variety of upper extremity movements of differing complexity, a range of performance from the subjects was identified. Those subjects who could not perform a particular task exhibited significantly lower muscle EMG activity than those subjects who could.[54] These authors concluded that abnormal agonist–antagonist cocontraction was not the reason for impaired arm movements in these subjects, but rather, inadequate recruitment of the agonist muscles.[54] These findings would support focusing on recruitment training of weak agonists and deemphasizing inhibition training, which has traditionally been performed before recruitment.

More recently, Wolf and colleagues compared recruitment up-training using EMGBF to conventional training (similar exercise training only without BF) for overcoming active and passive elbow extension restrictions. Biofeedback and non-BF training were equally effective in improving active elbow extension in this group of subjects although the BF group demonstrated a significant improvement in triceps muscle EMG activity.[55] Improvements in active elbow extension occurred despite the presence of biceps–triceps muscle cocontraction in upper extremity movements where shoulder elevation was an additional component (during reaching). Within the limitations of this study, these findings support emphasizing recruitment training and further support Gowland's and colleagues conclusions.[54] Efforts have begun to address inhibition of excessive muscle activity at the level of the spinal stretch reflex.[56] Taken collectively, research in these areas may prove to further enhance cost benefit as treatment approaches more specifically focus on the patient's actual motor control problem. Such information should be considered in the design of therapeutic interventions when EMGBF is part of a comprehensive treatment plan.

EMGBF is also used in the treatment of excessive EMG activity because of pain[57] as well as during general relaxation training.[58] For general relaxation, the patient should first develop an awareness of muscle activity. There are several adjunctive approaches that can be used with BF to promote a relaxation effect. Two popular methods include progressive relaxation[59] and autogenic training.[58] Progressive relaxation, consists of a series of 7- to 10-sec isometric contractions following an instruction to "tense" a muscle or group by the clinician. This tensing activity is followed by a "relax" instruction, which is sustained for approximately 20 to 40 sec. This tensing–relaxing activity is usually performed in a comfortable position while systematically progressing throughout major muscles of the body. Autogenic training[58] emphasizes feelings of limb heaviness and warmth through a series of instructions provided by the clinician. The goal is to increase awareness of the limb and promote a state of relaxation. Training should start with a general relaxation approach using a nonthreatening area of the body such as the forearm. The frontalis muscle, a good muscle for relaxation training, may be targeted in later sessions.[58] Suggested guidelines for moving the patient through the session exist.[58] Early in the session, the patient should try to understand what makes the auditory or visual signals increase and decrease. Moving adjacent areas of the body will help reinforce this. The majority of the session should be focused on the relaxation effect itself. Using autogenic training or progressive relaxation approaches in conjunction with EMGBF may be useful in this regard.[58] At the end of a session, the clinician should try to assist the patient in identifying the feeling of low arousal. The patient should be encouraged to try to incorporate this feeling or the relaxation exercises into his or her daily activities.[58]

The clinician should be aware that relaxation methods and EMGBF may affect the relaxation response through different mechanisms.[60] In a review article, Lehrer and colleagues examined the literature on a variety of stress management EMG techniques, including progressive relaxation, autogenic training, and EMGBF. Their conclusions have implications as to the nature of the impairment or disability a patient may present. That is, EMGBF, focusing at the muscle level, may be more beneficial for impairments with a muscular origin (eg, tension headache) as compared to impairments with an anxiety or phobia component.[60] In this connection, impairments with an autonomic component may benefit from autonomic-related BF (temperature, blood pressure) versus other forms of BF.[60]

Chronic low back pain is a specific impairment that has been studied with regard to EMGBF.[7,61,62] Patients have pain and subsequently heightened levels of muscle EMG activity related to postures or movements that then can be the focus of treatment application.[3] Some patients with chronic low back and temporomandibular pain may also have difficulty discriminating levels of muscle activity during voluntary efforts.[63] In a study, these patients and healthy controls were asked to perform muscle contractions of differing levels of activity of the erector spinae and masseter muscles. All patients were less accurate as compared with subjects without pain and perceived higher muscle EMG activity as less muscle tension.[63] This difference in accuracy was true regardless of the targeted muscle. This study suggests that these patients have deficits in perceptions of muscle tension and that procedures that increase patient awareness of muscle activity such as EMGBF may be useful.

To address this issue for patients with low back pain, positioning should begin in a comfortable or recumbent position in order to establish a general relaxation response. Recording from the low back erector spinae muscles is relatively straightforward. Cram, Kasman, and Holtz recommend a 2-cm interelectrode distance with active electrodes placed 2 cm lateral to the spinal column.[25] The iliac crest can be used to identify the third lumbar level. There are advantages and disadvantages to parallel or serial placement, but the parallel approach appears to be generally accepted. More importantly, interelectrode distance and electrode movement can occur with forward or backward bending.[40] Any electrode movement should be monitored by the physical therapist throughout the treatment intervention. As training progresses, so should the posture, eventually attaining lower levels of muscle (paraspinal) EMG during static postures such as sitting or standing and during functional movements such as sit-to-stand transfers and bending. Targeting paraspinal muscles has been successful in decreasing excessive EMG activity in these patients.[62] In a case report, Jones and Wolf identified improvements in ROM of spinal joints and subjective reports of pain with BF training.[7] Although Nouwen did not find concomitant decreases in pain with decreases in paraspinal muscle EMG activity,[62] Flor, Haag, and Turk found positive long-term results using EMGBF.[61]

## OUTCOME MEASURES

The incorporation of a specific example of a documentation form into this chapter is of little use because most clinical settings have specific policies and standards related to documentation. However, the following areas are useful to include for completeness of documentation for third-party payers and to ensure reproducibility for colleagues assisting with the patient's treatment session. These areas include:

- Treatment goal(s) and how BF addresses a given impairment or disability
- Nature of treatment, that is, recruitment versus relaxation and how either is being addressed through patient position, specific activities, and shaping procedures
- Muscle(s) targeted
- Electrode type, size, placement, and interelectrode distance
- Any relevant BF unit settings such as sensitivity and time constant as well as preferred choice of feedback (auditory or visual)
- The length or number of trials the patient is performing in a given treatment session

Some computerized BF systems include software that will provide reports related to the treatment sessions. EMGBF outputs are primarily at the impairment level. Documentation on how many microvolts of EMG activity were achieved in a treatment session can show and support short-term progress, but identifying a that muscle is either overactive or underactive will not support the use of EMGBF in a comprehensive treatment plan. Ultimately, documentation must be directed toward demonstration of functional deficits and functional gains. A skilled clinician should identify and support the need for EMGBF in light of a functional deficit or disability.

## VALUE-ADDED BENEFIT AND COST BENEFIT

There is additional (capital expense) cost associated with EMGBF when using computerized technology. However, with the increase in use of technology in the clinical setting and continued decline in personal computer costs, this equipment is comparable to other electrotherapeutic modalities or computerized technology purchased and used by physical therapists. The provision of BF may require one-to-one clinician–patient interaction. However, some patients may be trained to use this independently in the clinic or while at home as part of a home exercise program. The average clinician can expect to add approximately 5 minutes in equipment and patient (unit and electrodes) preparation. In a health care environment that is increasingly stressing delegation of many tasks to physical therapist assistants and on-the-job–trained personnel, the physical therapist's time and cost have become more significant factors. This time–cost factor, however, is not unique to the application of EMGBF. Equipment preparation and patient setup may be delegated to physical therapist assistants or other support personnel when deemed appropriate by the physical therapist. This delegation could potentially decrease the time the physical therapist is involved in nonproductive activity.

## EFFICACY

Studies examining the effect of EMGBF in patients with musculoskeletal or neurologic problems have produced favorable results. Only a small sample of these studies has been identified in this chapter. AHCPR clinical practice guidelines such as those addressing the assessment and treatment of urinary incontinence[33] support the efficacy of BF to improve muscle performance in patients with this problem. AHCPR guidelines for the management of acute low back problems[64] failed to recognize BF as a recommended adjunctive treatment. However, BF for this specific population has not been adequately studied to this point.[64] Research on the efficacy of EMGBF in the chronic condition has been more favorable.

The inconclusive findings for the use of BF from the Post-Stroke Clinical Practice Guidelines[65] is largely a result of conflicting findings of meta-analyses. When examining the effect of EMGBF on neurologic improvement in patients with hemiparesis, Schleenbaker and Mainous found an overall significantly positive effect. A positive aspect of this meta-analysis is that these researchers focused on functional measures.[66] A subsequent meta-analysis by Glanz and colleagues reviewed only randomized controlled trials and used change in joint ROM in the paretic limb as the measurement of interest. Most of the studies reviewed by these researchers demonstrated favorable results for the use of EMGBF; however, when pooled together, there was a nonsignificant effect size.[67] Caution must be used when interpreting these findings on the applicability of EMGBF in this patient population because the meta-analysis examined ROM only as an outcome variable, and the researchers also warned that the possibility of a type II error may exist.[67] A type II error essentially means that there is the possibility that no significant difference was found when one may actually exist.[68]

Two additional meta-analyses on the effect of EMGBF on post-stroke rehabilitation outcomes were recently performed by Moreland and Thomson[69] and Moreland, Thomson, and Fuoco.[70] Moreland and Thomson used strict criteria for study inclusion, measured impairment and function outcomes, and compared EMGBF with conventional therapy. This meta-analysis found that EMGBF was at least as effective as conventional therapy in improving upper extremity performance. In the invited commentary to this article,[69] Wolf emphasized the importance of the inclusion of EMGBF within a treatment program rather than in isolation and that its use to monitor results and progress with therapy actually supports cost-effective treatment. A previous article by Wolf, Edwards, and Shutter demonstrated this potential benefit.[14]

Moreland, Thomson, and Fuoco examined impairment and functional outcome measures, including ankle muscle force (strength), ankle angle ROM, gait quality, ankle angle during gait, stride length, and gait speed.[70] The strongest and most positive finding from this review was that EMGBF is superior to conventional therapy alone for improving ankle dorsiflexor muscle force (strength). The meta-analysis also detected a positive effect of EMGBF on gait quality. Some but not all studies demonstrated a positive effect for gait speed and ankle range of motion. The authors concluded that further research is required to conclusively demonstrate a significant effect regarding these variables.[70]

## TRENDS

Some insurance companies may not reimburse physical therapists for BF treatments when used alone and for purely relaxation purposes. Some companies, like Medicare, may cover BF if it is part of a comprehensive neuromuscular reeducation regimen. According to the *Coding and Payment Guide for the Physical Therapist*, "Biofeedback therapy is covered by Medicare when it is reasonable and necessary for reeducation of specific muscle groups or for treating pathological muscle abnormalities of spasticity, incapacitating muscle spasm or weakness and when conventional treatments such as heat, cold, massage, exercise, and support have not been successful."[71]

Although some research has compared EMGBF alone against traditional treatments, clinically, such isolation is not appropriate.[3]

Changing the perception that EMGBF is a stand-alone therapy and identifying it as a component of a comprehensive treatment plan is the first step in identifying any potential cost benefit. Rethinking the use of EMGBF in light of recent information from the movement sciences may also prove fruitful in providing cost-effective EMGBF-assisted therapeutic exercise.

# Summary

This chapter reviewed major considerations in the application of BF generally, and EMGBF specifically. This information was highlighted in the context of the WHO's impairment, disability, and handicaps classification system[26] and the recently published *Guide to Physical Therapist Practice*.[2] In this connection, major impairments and disabilities amenable to BF were described. Muscle EMG signal processing was summarized and electrode application was reviewed. Recruitment and relaxation interventions were discussed in light of the available literature. Aspects of motor learning principles were discussed in the context of these treatment interventions. Finally, the efficacy of BF was addressed and available Clinical Practice Guidelines were incorporated to support the potential benefit the application of BF may have when included into a comprehensive physical therapy plan.

## CASE STUDY

## THERAPEUTIC USE OF BIOFEEDBACK

### ■ Examination

A middle-aged, otherwise healthy male with left hemiparesis following a cerebrovascular accident (CVA) was receiving a comprehensive inpatient rehabilitation program that included physical therapy (PT). Specific tests and measures including arousal, attention and cognition, gait, locomotion and balance, motor function, muscle performance, posture, sensory integrity, and ROM[2] were performed by the physical therapist to identify impairments and functional limitations.

### ■ Evaluation/Diagnosis/Prognosis

The examination revealed deficits in multiple areas associated with the applied tests and measures. This individual exhibited impair-

**CASE STUDY** *continued*

ments in muscle performance, motor function, posture, and sensory integrity. Of particular concern during early physical therapy sessions was a functional limitation in transferring from a seated position to standing. This required moderate assistance by the physical therapist. Through evaluation of the examination findings, the physical therapist hypothesized that an altered initial condition (initial state of the system and interaction with the environment)[23] was one stage of movement in which impairments limited the sit-to-stand transfer. An altered sitting postural alignment secondary to decreased force generation of the trunk musculature and increased resistance to passive movement, which increased effort in maintaining a vertically erect sitting position, were hypothesized as contributing influences to the altered initial conditions. The altered initial condition was confirmed during interdisciplinary patient care meetings and believed to be affecting the initiation of and participation in other functional tasks associated with basic daily care.

As part of the prognosis process, the physical therapist determined that targeting this problem might provide the initial postural alignment necessary for the ability to initiate the sit-to-stand transfer. To improve sitting posture, the physical therapy plan of care included EMGBF to the right and left paraspinal musculature concomitant with visual feedback of sitting position provided by a mirror. Goals consistent with the use of EMGBF[2] included (1) improving performance of physical tasks (in this case, sit-to-stand) and (2) improving motor function and muscle performance (force-generating capacity and unwanted trunk extensor muscle activity). This individual's initial conditions were expected to improve, through the application of this electrotherapeutic modality in conjunction with the therapeutic exercise program, to a point where a stable, symmetric, and vertical sitting position was consistently achieved.

### ■ Intervention

EMGBF was used because it could improve posture through assisting in the appropriate contraction of the paraspinal muscles and the minimization of unwanted muscle EMG activity. The goal was to achieve a relatively symmetric activation (and relaxation) of the right and left paraspinal muscles while sitting and while maintaining a symmetric, vertical sitting position. Patient instruction included the general goal of the treatment (normal postural alignment in sitting) and the EMGBF goal (symmetric activity of the right and left paraspinal muscles during sitting), the application of electrodes, and the type of feedback that would be provided. Electrodes were applied bilaterally following a brief skin preparation approximately 2 to 3 cm from the spinous processes at the thoracolumbar level. A wider interelectrode distance (greater than 4 cm) was believed to be warranted for more general monitoring of the paraspinal muscles in this example. This distance is in contrast to that which would be used for specific muscle reeducation such as monitoring paraspinal EMG activity at a specific segment or segments of the lumbar spine in patients with low back pain. A ground electrode was applied adjacent to the recording electrodes.

Because the postural goal during the application of EMGBF was for a more vertically erect, symmetric sitting position, the physical therapist used a mirror to provide visual feedback of the head and trunk position in conjunction with information from the EMGBF equipment. In this connection, instantaneous auditory feedback was used to represent the change in paraspinal muscle EMG activity so that the patient could use vision to attend to his sitting posture in the mirror. The patient was able to identify the effect that active postural adjustments (including trunk positioning and changes in pelvic orientation) had on changes in sitting posture. He was also able to use the auditory information from the BF unit in conjunction with the visual feedback from the mirror to modify muscle activity in the targeted muscles. Initially, simple trunk movements laterally and anteroposteriorly were used to help the patient identify changes in muscle EMG activity in the targeted muscles.

Training sessions, which supplemented the daily physical therapy treatment, were conducted several times a week and lasted 15 to 20 min. As training progressed, the patient gained an appreciation for recruitment of these muscles as well as an improved ability to maintain relatively symmetrical paraspinal muscle EMG activity levels as he attempted to maintain an appropriate sitting position. At this point, the physical therapist faded the auditory feedback. Despite decreasing the frequency of feedback to the patient, paraspinal muscle activity monitoring continued for several sessions in order for the physical therapist to evaluate the success with which activation and inhibition were maintained. The frequency of using the mirror to provide visual feedback of sitting posture was also decreased as part of regular physical therapy sessions.

### ■ Outcomes

The primary outcome related to the application of EMGBF in this example was the improved quasi-static sitting balance and associated normal postural alignment. The initial conditions (postural set and ability to interact with the environment) were optimized sufficiently

**CASE STUDY** *continued*

in order for the subsequent initiation and execution of a sit-to-stand transfer to be carried out with less assistance by the physical therapist. Note, however, that treating the initial conditions identified in this example was necessary but insufficient for the successful completion of a sit-to-stand transfer. Additional neurotherapeutic exercise was performed in order to address the impact inpairments in muscle performance and motor function had on the successful execution of this functional task.

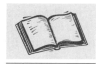

## REVIEW QUESTIONS

1. For motor control problems such as impaired reaching, abnormal sitting posture, and asymmetric weight bearing, what information (feedback) might be important to the patient? Under what conditions might EMGBF, force feedback, or motion feedback be indicated?

2. What are the major processes involved in taking a raw EMG signal and presenting it to the patient in the form of auditory or visual feedback?

3. When would an electrode placement with a small interelectrode distance be indicated? Contrast this to a wider interelectrode distance and the consequences of changing this distance.

4. What factors are important to consider when adjusting the gain or sensitivity of the BF device?

5. What are the implications of part/whole task transfer and frequency of feedback in the application of EMGBF during a therapeutic intervention?

## References

1. Schmidt RA. Motor Learning & Performance: From Principles to Practice. Champaign, IL, Human Kinetics, pp 227–259, 1991.

2. Guide to Physical Therapist Practice. Alexandria, VA, American Physical Therapy Association, 1997.

3. Wolf SL. Electromyographic biofeedback: An overview. In Nelson RM, Currier DP (eds), Clinical Electrotherapy (2nd ed). Norwalk, CT, Appleton & Lange, pp 361–383, 1991.

4. Basmajian JV. Introduction: Principles and Background. In Basmajian JV (ed), Biofeedback: Principles and Practice for Clinicians (3rd ed). Baltimore, MD, Williams & Wilkins, pp 1–4, 1989.

5. Binder-Macleod SA. Electromyographic biofeedback to improve voluntary motor control. In Robinson AJ, Snyder-Mackler LS (eds), Clinical Electrophysiology: Electrotherapy and Electrophysiologic Testing (2nd ed). Baltimore, MD, Williams & Wilkins, pp 433–450, 1995.

6. King AC, Ahles TA, Martin JE, White R. EMG biofeedback-controlled exercise in chronic arthritic knee pain. Arch Phys Med Rehabil, 65:341–343, 1984.

7. Jones AL, Wolf SL. Treating chronic low back pain: EMG biofeedback training during movement. Phys Ther, 60:58–63, 1980.

8. Krebs DE. Clinical electromyographic feedback following meniscectomy. Phys Ther, 61:1017–1021, 1981.

9. Draper V. Electromyographic biofeedback and recovery of quadriceps femoris muscle function following anterior cruciate ligament reconstruction. Phys Ther, 70:11–17, 1990.

10. Ince LP, Leon MS. Biofeedback treatment of upper extremity dysfunction in Guillain-Barré syndrome. Arch Phys Med Rehabil, 67:30–33, 1986.

11. Basmajian JV. Biofeedback in rehabilitation: A review of principles and practice. Arch Phys Med Rehabil, 62:469–475, 1981.

12. Wolf SL. Electromyographic biofeedback applications to stroke patients: A critical review. Phys Ther, 63:1448–1459, 1983.

13. Brucker BS, Bulaeva NV. Biofeedback effect on electromyography responses in patients with spinal cord injury. Arch Phys Med Rehabil, 77:133–137, 1996.

14. Wolf SL, Edwards DI, Shutter LA. Concurrent assessment of muscle activity (CAMA): A procedural approach to assess treatment goals. Phys Ther, 66:218–224, 1986.

15. Wolf SL, Hudson JE. Feedback signal based upon force and time delay: Modification of the Krusen limb load monitor. Phys Ther, 60:1289–1290, 1980.

16. Nichols DS. Balance retraining after stroke using force platform biofeedback. Phys Ther, 77:553–558 1997.

17. Lieper CI, Miller A, Lang J, Herman R. Sensory feedback for head control in cerebral palsy. Phys Ther, 61:512–518, 1981.

18. Bjork L, Wetzel A. A positional biofeedback device for sitting balance. Phys Ther, 63:1460–1461, 1983.

19. Hogue RE, McCandless S. Genu recurvatum: Auditory biofeedback treatment for adult patients with stroke or head injuries. Arch Phys Med Rehabil, 64:368–370, 1983.

20. Todorov E, Shadmehr R, Bizzi E. Augmented feedback presented in a virtual environment accelerates learning of a difficult motor task. J Motor Behav, 29(2):147–158, 1997.

21. Enoka RM. Neuromechanical Basis of Kinesiology. Champaign, IL, Human Kinetics, pp 119–149, 1988.

22. McComas AJ. Skeletal Muscle: Form and Function. Champaign, IL, Human Kinetics, pp 37–46, 1996.

23. Hedman LD, Rogers MW, Hanke TA. Neurologic entry level education: Linking the foundation science of motor control with physical therapy interventions for movement dysfunction. Neurology Report, 20(1):9–13, 1996.

24. Harvey RF, Jellinek HM. Functional performance assessment: A program approach. Arch Phys Med Rehabil, 62:456–461, 1981.

25. Cram JR, Kasman GS, Holtz J. Introduction to Surface Electromyography. Gaithersburg, MD, Aspen Publications, pp 59, 153–172, 223–235, 1998.

26. International Classification of Impairments, Disabilities, and Handicaps. Geneva, World Health Organization, pp 23–31, 1980.

27. Wolf SL, Baker MP, Kelly JL. EMG biofeedback in stroke: Effects of patient characteristics. Arch Phys Med Rehabil, 60:96–102, 1979.

28. Wolf SL, Binder-Macleod SA. Electromyographic biofeedback applications to the hemiplegic patient: Changes in upper extremity neuromuscular and functional status. Phys Ther, 63: 1393-1403, 1983.

29. Kegel AH. Progressive resistance exercise in the functional restoration of the perineal muscles. Am J Obstet Gynecol, 56:238–248, 1948.

30. McDowell BJ, Burgio KL, Dombrowski M, Locher JL, Rodriguez E. An interdisciplinary approach to the assessment and behavioral treatment of urinary incontinence in geriatric outpatients. J Am Geriatr Soc, 40:370–374, 1992.

31. Burns PA, Pranikoff K, Nochajski T, Desotelle P, Harwood MK. Treatment of stress incontinence with pelvic floor exercises and biofeedback. J Am Geriatr Soc, 38:341–344, 1990.

32. Burgio KL, Engel BT. Biofeedback-assisted behavioral training for elderly men and women. J Am Geriatr Soc, 38:338–340, 1990.

33. Fantl JA, Newman DK, Colling J et al. Urinary Incontinence in Adults: Acute and Chronic Management. Clinical Practice Guidelines No. 2, 1996 Update. Rockville, MD, U.S. Department of Health and Human Services. Public Health Service, Agency for Health Care Policy and Research. AHCPR Publication No. 96-0682, March 1996.

34. Loeb GE, Gans C. Electromyography for Experimentalists. Chicago, IL, University of Chicago Press, pp 21–22, 1986.

35. Robinson AJ, Kellogg R. Clinical Electrophysiologic Assessment. In Robinson AJ, Snyder-Mackler LS (eds), Clinical Electrophysiology: Electrotherapy and Electrophysiologic Testing (2nd ed). Baltimore, MD, Williams & Wilkins, pp 359–432, 1995.

36. Basmajian JV, DeLuca CJ. Muscles Alive: Their Functions Revealed by Electromyography (5th ed). Baltimore, MD, Williams and Wilkins, pp 95–96, 1985.

37. Colborne GR, Olney SJ, Griffin MP. Feedback of ankle joint angle and soleus EMG in rehabilitation of hemiplegic gait. Arch Phys Med Rehabil, 74:1100–1106, 1993.

38. LeCraw DE, Wolf SL. Electromyographic biofeedback (EMGBF) for neuromuscular relaxation and re-education. In Gersh MR (ed). Electrotherapy in Rehabilitation. Philadelphia, PA, F.A. Davis, pp 291–327, 1992.

39. Basmajian JV, Blumenstein R. Electrode placement in electromyographic biofeedback. In Basmajian JV (ed), Biofeedback: Principles and Practice for Clinicians (3rd ed). Baltimore, MD, Williams & Wilkins, pp 369–382, 1989.

40. Zedke M, Kumar S, Narayan Y. Comparison of surface EMG signals between electrode types, interelectrode distances and electrode orienta-

tions in isometric exercise of the erector spinae muscle. Electromyogr Clin Neurophysiol, 37:439–447, 1997.

41. LeCraw DE. Biofeedback in stroke rehabilitation. In Basmajian JV (ed), Biofeedback: Principles and Practice for Clinicians (3rd ed). Baltimore, MD, Williams & Wilkins, pp 105–117, 1989.

42. Bobath B. Adult Hemiplegia: Evaluation and Treatment (3rd ed). Oxford, Butterworth-Heinemann, 1990.

43. Sawner KA, LaVigne JM. Brunnstrom's Movement Therapy in Hemiplegia: A Neurophysiological Approach (2nd ed). New York, NY, J.B. Lippincott, 1992.

44. Knott M, Voss DE. Proprioceptive Neuromuscular Facilitation: Patterns and Techniques, 2nd ed. New York, NY, Harper & Row, 1968.

45. Gordon J. Assumptions underlying physical therapy inteventions: theoretical and historical perspecives. In Carr JH, and Shepherd RB (eds). Movement Science: Foundations for Physical Therapy in Rehabilitation. Rockville, MD, Aspen Publication, pp 1–30, 1987.

46. Horak FB. Assumptions underlying motor control for neurologic rehabilitation. In Lister MJ (ed), Contemporary Management of Motor Control Problems: Proceedings of the II Step Conference. Alexandria, VA, Foundation for Physical Therapy, pp 11–28, 1991.

47. Tries J. EMG feedback for the treatment of upper-extremity dysfunction: can it be effective? Biofeedback and Self-Regulation, 14(1):21–53, 1989.

48. Olney SJ, Richards C. Hemiparetic gait following stroke. Part 1: Characteristics. Gait & Posture, 4:136–148, 1996.

49. Cappozzo A. The mechanics of human walking. In Patla A (ed), Adaptability of Human Gait. North-Holland, Elsevier Science Publications, pp 167–186, 1991.

50. Winter DA. Biomechanical motor patterns in normal walking. J Motor Behav, 15(4):302–330, 1983.

51. Colborne GR, Wright V, Naumann S. Feedback of triceps surae EMG in gait of children with cerebral palsy: A controlled study. Arch Phys Med Rehabil, 75:40–45, 1994.

52. Basmajian JV, Kukulka CG, Narayan MG, Takebe K. Biofeedback treatment of foot-drop after stroke compared with standard rehabilitation technique: Effects on voluntary control and strength. Arch Phys Med Rehabil, 56:231–236, 1975.

53. Winstein CJ, Pohl PS, Cardinale C et al. Learning a partial-weight bearing skill: Effectiveness of two forms of feedback. Phys Ther, 76:985–993, 1996.

54. Gowland C, deBruin H, Basmajian JV et al. Agonist and antagonist activity during voluntary upper limb movement in patients with stroke. Phys Ther, 72:624–633, 1992.

55. Wolf SL, Catlin PA, Blanton S et al. Overcoming limitations in elbow movement in the presence of antagonist hyperactivity. Phys Ther, 74:826–835, 1994.

56. Segal RL. Plasticity in the central nervous system: Operant conditioning of the spinal stretch reflex. Top Stroke Rehabil, 3(4):76–87, 1997.

57. Johnson HE, Hockersmith V. Therapeutic electromyography in chronic back pain. In Basmajian JV (ed), Biofeedback: Principles and Practice

for Clinicians (3rd ed). Baltimore, MD, Williams & Wilkins, pp 311–316, 1989.

58. Soyva JM. Autogenic training and biofeedback combined: A reliable method for the induction of general relaxation. In Basmajian JV (ed), Biofeedback: Principles and Practice for Clinicians (3rd ed). Baltimore, MD, Williams & Wilkins, pp 169–186, 1989.

59. Jacobsen E. Progressive Relaxation (2nd ed). Chicago, IL, University of Chicago Press, 1938.

60. Lehrer PM, Carr R, Sargunaraj D, Woolfolk RL. Stress management techniques: Are they all equivalent, or do they have specific effects? Biofeedback and Self-Regulation, 19(4):353–401, 1994.

61. Flor H, Haag G, Turk DC. Long-term efficacy of EMG biofeedback for chronic rheumatic back pain. Pain, 27:195–202, 1986.

62. Nouwen A. EMG biofeedback used to reduce standing levels of paraspinal muscle tension in chronic low back pain. Pain, 17:353–360, 1983.

63. Flor H, Schugens MM, Birbaumer N. Discrimination of muscle tension in chronic pain patients and healthy controls. Biofeedback and Self-Regulation, 17(3):165–177, 1992.

64. Bigos S, Bowyer O, Braen G et al. Acute Low Back Problems in Adults. Clinical Practice Guidelines No. 14. AHCPR Publication No. 95-0642. Rockville, MD, Agency for Health Care Policy and Research, Public Health Service, U.S. Department of Health and Human Services, December 1994.

65. Gresham GE, Duncan PW, Strason WB et al. Post-Stroke Rehabilitation. Clinical Practice Guidelines No. 16. Rockville, MD, U.S. Department of Health and Human Services. Public Health Service, Agency for Health Care Policy and Research. AHCPR Publication No. 95-0662, May 1995.

66. Schleenbaker RE, Mainous III AG. Electromyographic biofeedback for neuromuscular reeducation in the hemiplegic stroke patient: a meta-analysis. Arch Phys Med Rehabil, 74:1301–1304, 1993.

67. Glanz M, Klawansky S, Stason W et al. Biofeedback therapy in poststroke rehabilitation: a meta-analysis of the randomized controlled trials. Arch Phys Med Rehabil, 76:508–515, 1995.

68. Portney LG, Watkins MP. Foundations of Clinical Research: Applications to Practice, Norwalk, CT, Appleton & Lange, pp 177–179, 1993.

69. Moreland J, Thomson MA. Efficacy of electromyographic biofeedback compared with conventional physical therapy for upper-extremity function in patients following stroke: A research overview and meta-analysis. Phys Ther, 74:534–547, 1994.

70. Moreland JD, Thomson MA, Fuoco AR. Electromyographic biofeedback to improve lower extremity function after stroke: A meta-analysis. Arch Phys Med Rehabil, 79:134–140, 1998.

71. Coding and Payment Guide for the Physical Therapist. Reston, VA, St. Anthony's, 1997.

# 12

# Electrophysiologic Evaluation: An Overview

David E. Nestor and Roger M. Nelson

## Introduction

The majority of the content of this book deals with the electrophysiologic aspects of treatment; for example, the use of neuromuscular electrical stimulation (NMES) on innervated and denervated muscle, the use of high-voltage stimulation in the treatment of disease and injury, and the use of NMES to increase muscle force. This chapter takes the electophysiologic process in a different direction; we now use the electrophysiologic phenomena present in muscles and nerves to evaluate the functional integrity of the neuromuscular system. **Electrophysiologic evaluation** may be defined (broadly) as encompassing the observation, recording, analysis, and interpretation of bioelectric muscle and nerve potentials, detected by means of surface or needle electrodes, for the purpose of evaluating the integrity of the neuromusculoskeletal system.

Electrophysiologic evaluation may be divided into two major components: evoked potentials and voluntary potentials. Major components of both are reviewed in this chapter. The objective of this chapter is to raise the reader's level of comprehension of the role that electrophysiologic evaluation plays in the practice of physical therapy. Electrophysiologic evaluation tests are often called diagnostic tests by some members of the health professions. Electrophysiologic evaluation results do not give a clinical diagnosis of the patient's illness. There are no waveforms that are pathognomonic of specific disease entities. Electrophysiologic evaluation aids in diagnosis insofar as the evidence of abnormality of the motor unit that it provides is or is not compatible with the clinical diagnosis under consideration. The electrophysiologic evaluation results must be integrated with results of other tests, the clinical examination, and the history in arriving at the final diagnosis.

The referring physician must combine the results of the electrophysiologic evaluation and the results of other tests in order to make a final diagnosis. Electrophysiologic test results may be likened to the mosaic tiles that make up a mosaic picture. Without all of the mosaic tiles in place, a complete picture will not be evident. Similarly, the referring physician will need to use all of the tests to arrive at the final diagnosis.

This chapter begins with a description of evoked potentials and ends with a discussion of voluntary potentials. The intent of the chapter is not to make the reader proficient in the areas presented. Rather, an overview of the specialty field of electrophysiologic evaluation is presented in order to make the reader aware of the use of this physical therapy practice area.

## EVOKED POTENTIALS

The term *evoked* implies that some outside influence has caused a change in the excitable cell. (Recall Chapter 1 and the discussion of the excitable cell.) The cell discharges with an action potential when a critical threshold level is reached. In evoked potentials, the critical level of depolarization is used to evaluate the functional integrity of the neuromuscular system by externally controlling the discharge of the cell structure. The key ingredient in evoked potentials is the factor of control. The examiner has control over the amount, timing, and electrophysical characteristics of the stimulation. The examiner allows only one physiologic response to vary. For example, neural conduction is the response variable to nerve electrostimulation. Therefore, any abnormal calculated neural conduction value is assumed to be the result of a disease process or injury.

There are four major categories of evoked responses currently used in the clinical setting: (1) motor nerve conduction; (2) sensory nerve conduction; (3) electronic reflex testing; and (4) centrally recorded evoked responses. Motor nerve conduction studies use the information of the motor component of the peripheral nerve bundle. Sensory nerve studies use information from the large sensory fibers of the peripheral nerve bundles. These studies form the bulk of the evoked potential analysis used in the electrophysiologic evaluation process. Electronic reflex testing uses information from the proximal portions of the peripheral nervous system. The distal portion of the peripheral nervous system is used as the carrier in determining conduction along the proximal portion of the nervous system. Centrally recorded evoked potentials use the distal, proximal, and central portions of the nervous system to record, transmit, and distribute the response to the brain.

## Motor Nerve Conduction Velocity Studies

The peripheral nerve bundle conducts both afferent and efferent information. Afferent information travels from the periphery to the central nervous system (CNS) for interpretation and processing; the afferent system is predominantly feedback. Efferent information begins in the central nervous system, eventually exiting the ventral root of the spinal cord and terminating on the peripheral components. The majority of efferent axons are from alpha motor neurons that innervate the peripheral components, such as voluntary striated skeletal muscle. Motor nerve conduction velocity (MNCV) studies seek to estimate the rate of movement of the induced impulse along the alpha motor neurons by an indirect method.

The method used to estimate conduction of motor nerve action potential impulses is indirect, because the alpha motor neuron impulses are not directly measured; rather, the response of alpha motor neurons to NMES is recorded from skeletal muscle. The result of alpha motor neuron response to stimulation is the evoked skeletal muscle action potential. The evoked response is recorded from a skeletal muscle innervated by that group of alpha motor neurons. It should be remembered that NMES of the peripheral nerve bundle causes depolarization and a subsequent synchronous volley of action potentials along both efferent and afferent nerve bundles. The selective recording of the motor response from the associated skeletal muscle allows an estimation of the impulse's rate of travel along the alpha motor axons, as well as an estimation of the number of motor units participating in the evoked muscle action potential.

The technique for performing motor nerve conduction studies includes the recording of the motor response from a superficially located skeletal muscle innervated by the peripheral nerve being studied. The muscle must be superficial, distal to the site of stimulation, and innervated only by that particular peripheral nerve. When the nerve is stimulated, an evoked muscle response is obtained. This response is called an evoked compound muscle action potential. When the nerve is electrically stimulated, a stimulus artifact is instantly introduced on the left-hand side of the oscilloscope (Figure 12–1). The latency is expressed in milliseconds and represents the time delay from stimulus artifact to the beginning of the evoked muscle action potential. The latency reflects the amount of time that the impulse takes to move from the site of stimulation to the muscle.

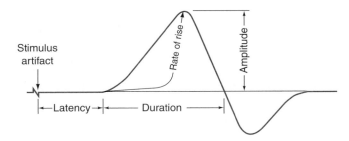

FIGURE 12–1. Schematic rendition of an evoked muscle action potential resulting from supramaximal electrical stimulation.

Latency is commonly measured from the stimulus artifact to the beginning of the evoked muscle action potential. The measurement of latency reflects the conduction of the induced impulse along the largest and fastest motor axons in the peripheral nerve. Terminal latency cannot be computed into a velocity segment for motor nerve conduction studies. Simply recording the terminal latency is not sufficient to calculate **velocity,** which is a ratio of time divided by distance. The measurement of distance from the site of stimulation to the recording electrode on the muscle is inaccurate. Many physiologic factors make such a measurement inappropriate. For example, as the action potential (impulses) reaches the terminal branch, the nerve starts to arborize, conduction slows as nerve diameter decreases, the actual distance of terminal branches is unknown, and the time for neurotransmitter activation at the neuromuscular junction is unknown.

A solution to the problem of terminal latency is to have an additional site at which to stimulate the nerve. If an additional site is available, the distal site latency may be subtracted from the more proximal latency, leaving the residual latency, which reflects conduction time along the nerve segment. Using the basic principle of two sites of stimulation along the nerve, the conduction of the motor portion of the peripheral nerve complex may be estimated (Figure 12–2) for as many anatomic segments as the examined nerve allows.

Some important technical points to remember when performing motor nerve conduction studies are to maintain (1) the same shape and negative phase amplitude of the evoked muscle action potential at all sites of stimulation; (2) close proximity of stimulating electrodes to the peripheral nerve bundle; and (3) a supramaximal evoked muscle action potential at all stimulation sites.

Most of the peripheral nerves in the human body that have a motor component have had motor nerve conduction velocities calculated and reported. An example of the technical procedures used

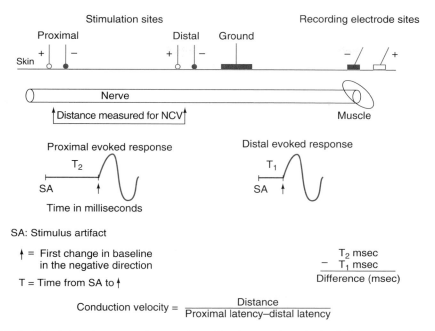

FIGURE 12–2. Calculation of motor conduction velocity. Conduction velocity (m/sec) of a nerve can be calculated by measuring the distance (mm) between two stimulation sites and dividing by the difference in latency (msec) from the more proximal stimulus and the latency (msec) of the distal stimulus.

to perform a motor nerve conduction study is shown in Table 12–1 and Figures 12–3 and 12–4. Evoked muscle action potential responses from all sites *should* be similar in waveform, amplitude, and duration of response.

Wrist site stimulation voltage, stimulus pulse duration, or both, should be increased gradually and monitored carefully as a high-voltage, long-pulse-duration stimulation at the wrist may volume conduct to the adjacent ulnar nerve at the wrist, eliciting a short-latency volume-conducted ulnar response.

The clinical response should be carefully observed to avoid mistaking an ulnar for a median nerve response. At the wrist, median nerve stimulation elicits thumb palmar **abduction** and opposition, while ulnar nerve stimulation elicits thumb **adduction** and metacarpophalangeal flexion. At the above-elbow and axilla stimulation sites, median stimulation elicits wrist flexion in radial deviation involving the flexor carpi radialis muscle, while ulnar nerve stimulation involves wrist flexion in ulnar deviation by contraction of the flexor carpi ulnaris muscle. Palpation of the tendons may help to distinguish the two contractions.

---

### TABLE 12–1. PROCEDURE FOR MEDIAN MOTOR NERVE CONDUCTION

**Electromyograph Instrument Characteristics**

Filter settings/frequency response: 10–10,000 Hz
Sweep speed: 2–5 msec/div
Sensitivity/gain: 1000–5000 µV/div

**Patient Position (Figure 12–3)**

The patient is positioned supine with arm abducted approximately 45 degrees. The forearm is fully supinated and the wrist is in a neutral position.

**Electrode Placement (Figure 12–3)**

Active (recording) electrode: The active recording electrode is positioned directly over the anatomic center of the abductor pollicis brevis muscle. The electrode is placed one-half the distance between the metacarpophalangeal joint of the thumb and the midpoint of the distal wrist crease.

Reference electrode: The reference electrode is positioned off the abductor pollicis brevis muscle on the distal phalanx of the thumb over bone or tendon.

Ground electrode: The ground electrode should be firmly positioned on the dorsum of the hand between the recording and stimulating electrodes.

**Electrostimulation (Figure 12–4)**

Transcutaneous electrostimulation is performed at the appropriate anatomic sites in the following order.

S1: Distal stimulation is performed at the wrist between the palmaris longus and flexor carpi radialis muscle tendons.

S2: Stimulation above the elbow is performed proximal and medial to the antecubital space and proximal to the elbow crease between the belly of the biceps muscle and the medial head of the triceps muscle. The stimulator should be positioned just lateral to the brachial artery to minimize the possibility of inadvertent electrostimulation of the ulnar nerve.

S3: Proximal stimulation is performed in the axilla at least 10 cm proximal to the above elbow site and immediately lateral and anterior to the brachial artery.

---

The wrist should be maintained in a standard position while measuring forearm distance. Wrist flexion decreases while wrist extension increases the distance. All distance measurements should be taken with a metal tape measure. The measurement of distance should approximate the anatomic course of the nerve being tested.

In clinical practice, the median, ulnar, common peroneal, and posterior tibial nerves are most often assessed. (Normal values are published in most textbooks, ie, Kimura, Johnson, Oh, Smorto, Echternach; see the bibliography at the end of the chapter.)

## Sensory Conduction

The estimation of conduction in the sensory segment of the peripheral nerve bundle follows the same basic paradigm as the motor component; with the sensory segment, however, the skin (dermis)

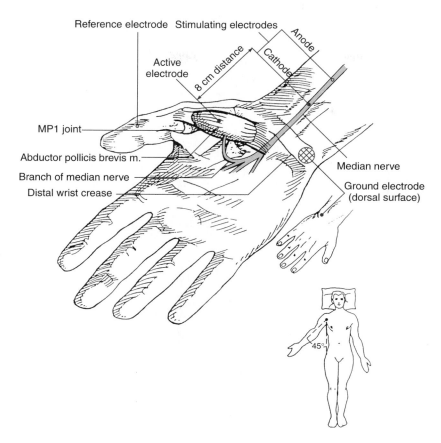

**FIGURE 12–3.** Body position of subject receiving median motor nerve conduction study showing location of recording and distal stimulating electrodes and ground.

and not the muscle becomes the effector organ. Unlike the muscle, the skin has the ability to be both effector and receptor. The two methods for sensory conduction are orthodromic and antidromic.

**Orthodromic conduction** refers to the normal way in which a physiologic response travels. For example, the dermis of the skin is stimulated, thereby initiating a response by the cutaneous receptors of light touch. These receptors have endings in the dermis of the skin and conduct impulses to the CNS by way of the dorsal root. The impulse generated by dermal stimulation is recorded by surface electrodes over the peripheral nerve bundle at a superficial point. An example of the technical procedures used to perform an orthodromic sensory conduction study is shown in Table 12–2 and Figure 12–5. A low stimulation amplitude is usually adequate to elicit an orthodromic

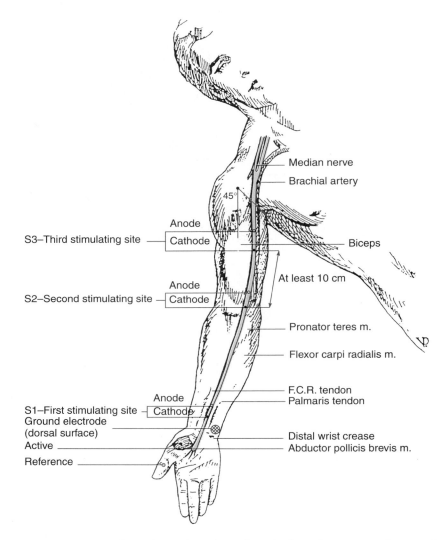

FIGURE 12–4. Location of recording and stimulating electrodes for median motor conduction study.

sensory response. The possibility of obtaining a spurious motor response is decreased using the orthodromic technique. Motor response and volume conduction effects may be lessened by decreasing NMES amplitude, decreasing pulse duration, or both, of the applied electrostimulation. *Special concern:* Care must be taken to maintain a separation between the stimulating cathode and anode on the index finger. Do not allow conducting gel to bridge the interelectrode space.

## TABLE 12–2. PROCEDURE FOR ORTHODROMIC MEDIAN SENSORY NERVE CONDUCTION

**Electromyograph Instrument Characteristics**

Filter settings/frequency response: 20–2000 Hz
Sweep speed: 1–2 msec/div
Sensitivity/gain: 5–10 μV/div

**Patient Position (Figure 12–5)**

The patient is positioned supine with arm abducted approximately 45 degrees. The forearm is fully supinated, the wrist is in a neutral position. The fingers may flex slightly when in a resting position.

**Electrode Placement (Figure 12–5)**

Active (recording) electrode: The active recording electrode will be positioned on the skin directly over the cathode (distal) stimulation site used for evoking the median nerve motor response at the wrist.
Reference electrode: The reference electrode will be positioned 2 to 3 cm proximal to the active electrode. This electrode will be positioned so that it is directly over the anode (proximal) stimulating site used for evoking the median nerve motor response at the wrist.
Ground electrode: The ground electrode should be firmly positioned on the dorsum of the hand between the active and stimulating electrodes.

**Electrostimulation (Figure 12–5)**

Transcutaneous electrostimulation is performed as follows. Stimulation is applied over the digital nerve via electrodes attached to the index finger. The cathode is positioned at the midpoint of the proximal phalanx of the index finger and the anode is positioned at or about the distal phalangeal joint line. A distance of no less than 10 cm, but not more than 14 cm, is maintained between the stimulating cathode on the index finger and the active electrode at the wrist.

**Antidromic conduction** is the stimulation of the nerve bundle and subsequent recording of the distal impulse over the dermis of the skin. An example of the technical procedures used to perform an antidromic sensory conduction study is shown in Table 12–3 and Figure 12–6. A low stimulation amplitude is usually adequate to elicit the antidromic sensory response. Motor response and volume conduction effects may be lessened by decreasing electrostimulation amplitude, decreasing pulse duration, or both, of the applied electrostimulation. (NOTE: Motor responses from hand muscles and volume conduction are more of a technical problem when utilizing antidromic techniques than when using orthodromic techniques.) *Special concern:* Care must be taken to maintain a separation between the active and reference electrodes on the index finger. Do not allow conducting gel to bridge the interelectrode space.

The following differences exist between the sensory evoked action potential and the evoked muscle action potential:

1. Sensory potential is much smaller in amplitude than is muscle evoked potential.

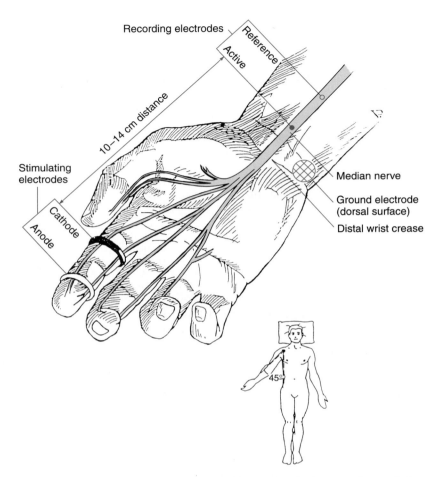

FIGURE 12–5. Body position and location of recording, stimulating, and ground electrodes for orthodromic median sensory nerve conduction study.

2. Sensory potential has a single negative phase, whereas muscle evoked potential is biphasic.

3. Sensory potential is usually a single characteristic that may be used to determine latency and, if desired, to compute a velocity. Recall that evoked muscle action potential includes components that involve terminal conduction and myoneural junctional delay. Sensory nerve endings have no junctional delay at the distal portions, because the sensory endings in the dermis are dendrites rather than terminal branches.

4. The last difference revolves about the physiologic response; the evoked potential results from the combined excitation of

---

**TABLE 12–3. PROCEDURE FOR ANTIDROMIC MEDIAN SENSORY NERVE CONDUCTION**

---

**Electromyograph Instrument Characteristics**

Filter settings/frequency response: 20–2000 Hz
Sweep speed: 1–2 msec/div
Sensitivity/gain: 5–20 μV/div

**Patient Position (Figure 12–6)**

The patient is positioned supine with arm abducted approximately 45 degrees. The forearm is fully supinated, the wrist is in a neutral postion. The fingers may flex slightly when in a resting position.

**Electrode Placement (Figure 12–6)**

Active (recording) electrode: The active recording electrode is attached to the index finger at the midpoint of the distance between the phalangeal flexion crease and the web space of the index finger so that a distance of at least 10 cm, but not more than 14 cm, is maintained between the stimulating electrode and the active electrode.
Reference electrode: The reference electrode is positioned at or about the distal interphalangeal flexion crease of the index finger so that a distance of at least 3 cm is maintained between the active and reference electrode.
Ground electrode: The ground electrode should be firmly positioned on the skin of the dorsum of the hand between the active and stimulating electrodes.

**Electrostimulation (Figure 12–6)**

Transcutaneous electrostimulation is performed as follows. Stimulation is performed at the wrist between the palmaris longus and flexor carpi radialis muscle tendons proximal to the transverse carpal ligament.

---

skeletal muscle fibers, whereas the sensory potential represents the neural excitability of the low-threshold, large-diameter, cutaneous sensory neurons.

## Clinical Use of Motor and Sensory Conduction Studies

The ability to estimate the velocity of motor conduction helps to delineate a systemic problem from a local one. Velocity in systemic problems is generally decreased for all nerves tested. In disease and injury states, the lower-extremity nerves usually exhibit earlier changes in motor nerve conduction than do those of the upper extremities. A local problem of decreased nerve conduction may be described by the example of a peripheral nerve sustaining a compressive force in an anatomic area where the nerve is bordered by uncompromising structures. When the nerve is bound between bone and connective tissue, the conduction of the induced stimulus is slower at the compressive site because of the increased internal resistance of the axis cylinder. The nerve may be compressed at any site, but certain anatomic areas have a predilection for compression.

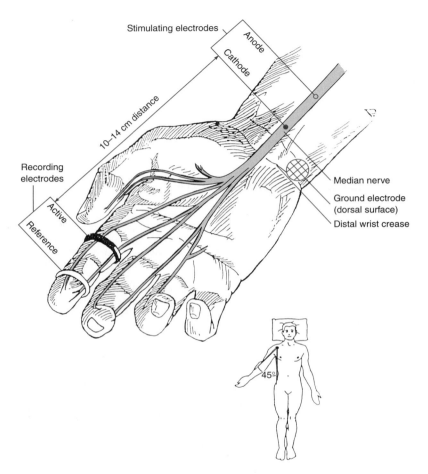

**FIGURE 12–6.** Body position and location of recording, stimulating, and ground electrodes for antidromic median sensory nerve conduction study.

For example, a common site for median nerve compression is in the area of the wrist, as the median nerve passes through the carpal tunnel. When the nerve is compressed at a distal site, both motor and sensory distal latencies are prolonged. The computed velocity segments are unaltered. Compression tends to affect conduction along the sensory nerves prior to the motor nerve. Part of the physiologic reason for earlier changes in sensory axons relates to the relative lack of myelin coating surrounding the sensory axons. Compressive alteration is more difficult to obtain in a motor axon because of the concentric rings of myelin surrounding it.

When a peripheral nerve bundle is damaged by disease, both motor and sensory nerve evoked components may illustrate physiologic alterations in both computed velocity and evoked waveform characteristics. Each reported indicator of motor nerve conduction, such as amplitude, duration of the evoked muscle action potential, and latency of response, plays a part in the overall evaluation of the patient. The determination of the anatomic area, the degree of involvement, and the possible prognosis of the process may be estimated by using all of the elements listed above as common to the motor nerve conduction velocity segment. The differentiation of local versus systemic nerve involvement may be evaluated by sensory and motor nerve conduction techniques. For example, if the ulnar nerve is compressed at the elbow without metabolic compromise of the axon, the motor nerve conduction velocity computed for the segment below the elbow would be within normal limits. The computed velocity above the elbow, however, would be slower than for the segment below the elbow. In addition to the slower velocity component, a change in the evoked muscle action potential may also be evident. The amplitude of the potential, resulting from stimulation above the elbow, would be diminished compared to the stimulation below the elbow.

The patient who has a systemic disease involving the peripheral nerves would tend to exhibit different findings in motor nerve conduction studies. For example, the individual who has diabetes may illustrate changes of slowing in motor nerve conduction velocity of approximately 20 percent, with an accompanied increase in negative phase duration for the evoked muscle action potential but with no decrease in negative phase amplitude. The patient with chronic alcoholism illustrates little or no change in computed motor nerve conduction velocity but may exhibit changes in negative phase amplitude of the evoked muscle action potential.

Similarly, sensory evoked action potentials present information to the investigator about the functional integrity of the sensory component of the peripheral nerve complex. As mentioned earlier, the sensory axons are more susceptible to focal-type compression and to systemic neuropathic changes than are motor axons. Therefore, focal compressive changes occur earlier in the sensory axons than in the motor axons. Recall that motor axons have concentric rings of myelin, whereas sensory axons have a disorganized myelin sheath. Compression or systemic disease (or both) that affects the myelin will influence the sensory axons prior to affecting the motor axons. Results of sensory conduction studies confirm the subjective description by the patient of earlier temporal involvement by illustrating the alterations in sensory conduction and sensory evoked potential characteristics prior to changes in the motor nerve conduction components.

The major problem surrounding both motor and sensory nerve conduction studies remains the fact that both techniques measure only the distal component of the peripheral nerve. For example, the median nerve may be measured in motor and sensory conduction from the anterior cervical triangle to the wrist. Conduction proximal to the anterior cervical triangle is not possible with standard techniques. The following section amplifies upon the electrophysiologic assessment technique used to evaluate the conduction of the evoked response through the proximal arc in the neural segment.

## Electronic Reflex Testing

The reflex arcs that normally occur in the intact physiologic state, the H reflex, F wave, and blink reflex, will now be reviewed. The F wave is not a reflex in the strict form of the definition, but a recurrent response to NMES, and it has the ability to assess proximal conduction.

The term *evoked* implies that some control is exerted over the physiologic situation. In electronic reflex testing, control is expressed by the NMES characteristics used. The term *reflex* implies that a synapse is included in the arc and that some direct control over the physiologic sequence is masked.

### H Reflex

The "H" in H reflex is in honor of Hoffman, who, in 1918, described a monosynaptic, electrically induced equivalent of the tendon tap response. Hoffman reasoned that a tendon, when subjected to a brief and sudden stretch, produces a small, brief muscle contraction after an intervening time period. He hypothesized that NMES of the afferent peripheral nerve carrying neurons involved in the tendon tap response would cause the same type of response. He recorded a response both to tendon tap and to NMES of the nerve proximal to the muscle. The same small-muscle response was obtained with both stimuli.

The tendon tap causes a mechanical stretch of the muscle and of the associated, parallel-arranged muscle spindles. The stretch of the muscle spindles causes a volley of neural impulses up the afferent arc along the IA afferent nerves, through the dorsal-root ganglia to the spinal cord, where the IA afferent nerves synapse directly on the homonomous anterior horn cells. The excitation causes a twitch response of the extrafusal fibers associated with that spindle complex.

The electrically induced H-reflex response bypasses the short spindle stretch and directly depolarizes the large IA fibers proximal to the muscle. For example, the soleus muscle in the lower extremity is innervated by the posterior tibial nerve. The posterior tibial nerve is stimulated in the popliteal fossa proximal to the soleus muscle. The afferent volley of impulses follows the same course as when the response is mechanically induced. The major difference between the tendon tap and NMES is the level of external control that the evaluator has over the physiologic response. The latter is controlled, with all characteristics of stimulation chosen by the examiner. The response from the extrafusal fibers is synchronous and is recorded by surface electrodes over the soleus muscle. The time interval from stimulus delivery to response recording is approximately 30 msec.

Two components make up the H-reflex arc: The afferent arc is along the IA fibers, while the efferent arc is along the alpha motor neurons. Because the H reflex indicates a response to IA nerve fibers, and because those nerve fibers are the afferent arc of muscle spindles, it follows that the H reflex is found only in those muscles that have an abundance of muscle spindles. Muscles that contain slow-twitch fibers have an abundance of spindles and commonly illustrate the appearance of an H reflex.

### CLINICAL USE OF H REFLEX

The $S_1$ nerve root innervates the soleus muscle, which is composed predominantly of slow-twitch motor units. The proximal conduction of afferent impulses occurs along the IA fibers, through the dorsal root to the alpha motor neurons, which pass out of the $S_1$ foramen to innervate the soleus. The H reflex is used to assess proximal conduction; for example, the conduction of the impulse through the dorsal root into the dorsal portion of the spinal cord and then through the ventral root at $S_1$ to the muscle. Compression at the neural foramen will cause a concomitant slowing of the reflex latency. Assessing proximal conduction through the $S_1$ nerve root is thought to be possible with the H reflex.

## F Wave

Unlike the H reflex, the F wave does not have separate afferent and efferent arcs. Rather, the F wave has both afferent and efferent arcs in the same peripheral nerve. The alpha motor neuron serves both functions. The suspected physiologic mechanism for the F wave is described as an afferent volley composed of antidromic stimuli followed by a reverberation of the impulse once it reaches the anterior horn cell. The alpha motor neuron is stimulated at a distal site, and the induced stimulus travels in an orthodromic fashion to the muscle. At the same time, an antidromic impulse travels to the anterior horn cell of that nerve. Once the antidromic impulse reaches the axon hillock, it is thought to reverberate and cause an orthodromic volley of impulses back to the muscle. The time for the F wave is approximately 30 msec in the upper extremities and 40 to 50 msec in the lower extremities. Unlike the H reflex, the F wave is apparent upon maximal NMES. The F wave is inconsistent in its appearance and must be calculated on at least ten successive responses. The F wave is not a reflex, because no reflex arc is used. The F wave is simply a reverberating response to supramaximal NMES of the alpha motor neurons.

### CLINICAL USE OF F WAVE

The F wave, like the H reflex, is a measure of proximal conduction. The F wave may be obtained from most muscles upon appropriate neural stimulation. (Recall that the H reflex is present only in muscles with a high proportion of muscle spindles.) Those muscles that have a predominance of slow-twitch motor units have high spindle indexes. Since the F-wave response is possible from a variety of muscles and from muscles that have few or no spindles, the results of the F-wave test are useful in determining proximal conduction delays along many spinal segments. A comparison of proximal conduction components is useful when entrapment of the nerve at the vertebral foramen is expected. The latency of the F wave is also an important measure when comparing proximal conduction along a peripheral nerve to distal conduction along the same nerve. A comparison of proximal and distal conduction components is useful in ruling out polyneuropathic conditions, in which distal segments of the nerve begin to die back before the proximal segments in the natural course of the disease process.

## Blink Reflex

The blink reflex is a facial muscle response to stimulation of the trigeminal nerve at the supraorbital notch. The stimulation may be a mechanical tap to the glabella or may be NMES of the trigeminal nerve. With both forms of stimulation, the observed response is the defensive reflex of eyelid closure by contraction of the orbicularis oculi muscle. The mechanical tap cannot be controlled or sufficiently modulated; therefore, the use of NMES is preferred. Electrostimulation of the trigeminal nerve causes a reflex contraction of the orbicularis oculi muscle. In bilateral recording from the orbicularis oculi muscle, the observed response to NMES is composed of two distinct waveforms. The first component, or waveform, is called the $R_1$ response. The $R_2$ component is the second evoked potential noted. It is less well organized than the $R_1$ potential. The latency of the $R_2$ potential is consistent, but the duration and amplitude tend to vary, indicating the need for an average value for amplitude on both the ipsilateral and contralateral sides of stimulation.

The blink reflex is unlike the H reflex and F wave. The difference lies in the fact that one electrostimulation causes two distinct responses of the orbicularis oculi muscle. The first response ($R_1$)

represents the conduction along the trigeminal nerve and the immediate activation of the facial nerve. The second response ($R_2$) represents the time of conduction along the trigeminal pontine relay and facial nerve. The presumed reason for the inconsistent response of $R_2$ is the excitability of the interneuron pool at the pontine level, the axonal conduction of both the trigeminal and facial nerves, and the synaptic transmission throughout the reflex arc.

### CLINICAL USE OF BLINK REFLEX

The use of the blink reflex in the clinical setting provides the clinician with information about the afferent (trigeminal) and efferent (facial) arcs of the nerves. An important portion is the efferent arc formed by the facial nerve. The proximal portion of the facial nerve may be examined with the blink reflex. Recall that the nerve-excitability test for facial nerve paralysis will only present information about the distal portion of the facial nerve. The proximal portion lies within the stylomastoid foramen. Since Bell's palsy is thought to involve the proximal portion of the facial nerve, the blink reflex may be the test of choice for evaluating the functional integrity of the nerve. The second component of the blink reflex ($R_2$) represents proximal facial nerve conduction. Therefore, increased $R_2$ delay, decreased amplitude of $R_2$, or a lack of response of $R_2$ may indicate facial nerve compromise proximal to the stylomastoid foramen.

Electronic reflex testing uses evoked responses to evaluate the proximal component of the peripheral nervous system. The principles of evoked responses, controlled by known characteristics of NMES, allow for the evaluation of conduction of both afferent and efferent neural segments. A response, whether or not it is delayed in character, must be kept in perspective. The blink response is the result of a reflex action on the part of neurons, interneurons, and synapses. Since the response is a reflex and involves many possible sources of error, a negative result in one of these studies alone is not conclusive of a pathologic implication. Reflex testing should be considered one tile in the overall mosaic that is developed for that patient.

## Centrally Recorded Evoked Potentials

Motor and sensory nerve conduction studies, and electronic reflex testing, form the majority of evoked potentials used by individuals in electrophysiologic evaluation. Assessment of an integrated, functional, and complete nervous system includes the evaluation of **distal peripheral nerve conduction,** proximal conduction through reflex function and the CNS, through scalp-recorded evoked potentials.

There are three major types of centrally evoked responses currently used by clinicians in electrophysiologic evaluation: somatosensory evoked potentials, brainstem auditory evoked potentials, and visual evoked potentials. All of the centrally recorded evoked potentials are useful in studying CNS dysfunction. The following discussion should be viewed as descriptive only and not as an in-depth or practical explication of this field.

Viewed in a historical perspective, central scalp–recorded evoked potentials are a recent form of evoked potentials, when compared (for example) to motor and sensory nerve conduction studies or electronic reflex testing. The central scalp recording of evoked potentials is possible only through the use of the computer and the averaging abilities of the digital systems. The increased level of sophistication in electrical technology has enabled the development of centrally evoked potentials.

### Somatosensory Evoked Potentials

When the distal portion of the peripheral nerve is electrostimulated at a minimal motor threshold, a volley of sensory impulses is known to be generated. The minimal motor threshold is used to standardize the excitation threshold of the sensory axons. (Recall that threshold-to-sensory stimulation is less than that of the motor threshold.)

The volley of orthodromic sensory potentials travels through the dorsal root ganglia into the spinal cord, where the sensory terminal branches form excitatory synapses with central nervous system dendrites, which (in turn) travel centrally and eventually terminate on the contralateral region of the postcentral gyrus of the sensory cortex. Using a specific configuration of surface electrodes placed on the contralateral scalp, the wave of depolarization may be recorded by averaging at least 1000 successive stimuli. A series of positive and negative waveforms is recorded, each described by its relative location from the beginning point.

#### CLINICAL USE OF SOMATOSENSORY EVOKED POTENTIALS

Many disorders of the central nervous system do not result in symptoms in the early stages. Recorded somatosensory evoked potentials (SSEPs) often illustrate slowing in velocity segments at the central portion of the evoked waveforms. Monitoring spinal trauma cases in order to ascertain the degree of cord transection is another clinical use of SSEPs. Somatosensory evoked potentials are present even during the spinal shock stage, when reflex function is depressed. The qualitative role of SSEPs is useful to the clinical neurologist when findings from other tests are inconclusive.

### Brainstem Auditory Evoked Potentials

In the early 1970s, the ability to record autitory evoked responses from scalp-recording techniques was first reported. The use of a brief click was the source of auditory-nerve depolarization. The computer-averaging technique is the same for brainstem auditory evoked potentials (BAEPs) as with SSEPs, except that the stimulus source is a click of monaural quality applied to one ear, while the other ear receives a masking noise. The surface recording electrodes are placed on the ipsilateral vertex and are amplified up to 1 million times. An average of 1000 to 2000 click stimuli are used to obtain the desired signal from the brain. Since the gain of the amplifier is very high, the artifacts that might be produced by swallowing, moving, or any muscle contraction must be minimized. Therefore, BAEPs are often conducted as part of a sleep study.

### CLINICAL USE OF BRAINSTEM AUDITORY EVOKED POTENTIALS

In clinical neurology, BAEPs are used to assess hearing loss that results from peripheral mechanisms. In patients in whom a progression of hearing loss is noted and in whom acoustic neuromas are expected, BAEPs are sensitive as an initial screening test. BAEPs are also used for patients who are suspected of suffering from a demyelinating disease. The ability to confirm a diagnosis of multiple sclerosis with just symptoms and signs is about 50 percent accurate. In those patients without symptoms and signs, the percentage drops dramatically (to 19 percent).

A valuable aspect of BAEPs is their ability to document those lesions that are unsuspected in the early stages of multiple sclerosis. Validation of the early changes of BAEPs with a diagnosis of multiple sclerosis continues by concurrent validation process. Brainstem auditory evoked potentials have other uses in clinical neurology; for example, the evaluation of both the location and the extent of damage caused by intrinsic brainstem tumors, the evaluation of brain death, and the surgical monitoring of potentials during neurosurgical procedures in the region of the posterior fossa.

### Visual Evoked Potentials

Visual evoked potentials (VEPs) are useful when the underlying process of damage and assessment of the neurologic area of a visual problem is difficult to determine. The ability to objectively evaluate the function of the visual pathway without conscious cooperation from the patient is helpful when patients present visual problems without a diagnosis. Visual evoked potentials are also useful in detecting compromise of the optic nerve in the early stages of dysfunction. The objective nature of the test, along with the ability to perform VEPs without conscious cooperation on the part of the patient, make it possible to differentiate functional loss of sight from actual (organic) loss of sight. Visual evoked potentials have been effective in determining early demyelinating disease, especially the early stage of multiple sclerosis.

The VEP technique requires all of the special hardware and software noted for other evoked potentials, and in addition requires an accurate, sharply focused visual stimulus in order to produce a synchronous volley of afferent visual stimuli. Unlike SSEPs and BAEPs, where 1000 to 2000 repetitive stimuli are needed, only 100 or 200 stimuli are required to obtain adequate VEPs. The VEP technique requires that the scalp-located surface electrodes be placed over the occipital area. The VEP response results from the type of original stimulus projected by the video display terminal. The examiner may record the response from stimulation of one eye independently or of both visual pathways at once. If separate responses for each eye are needed, careful attention must be given to maintenance of the same amplitude and latency recording characteristics.

### CLINICAL USE OF VISUAL EVOKED POTENTIALS

Visual evoked potentials are used in the clinical setting to test for demyelinating disease of the optic nerve. The predominant feature in demyelination of the optic nerve is a shift in the latency to the prolonged region of normal latency. VEPs are also used in patients with various CNS dysfunctions as an aid to early detection of the accompanying decline in visual impairment. Changes are noted in either the latencies or the characteristics of the waveforms.

Visual evoked potentials are also useful in delineating the patient suffering from hysterical blindness. If VEPs are well formed along the segment examined, and if the latencies are within the normal limits ascribed according to age and gender data limits in the presence of a visual acuity beyond 20/120, the blindness is not organic.

## VOLUNTARY POTENTIALS

Voluntary potential electrical activity comes from muscle fiber membranes during a volitional contraction of a skeletal muscle. The potentials are recorded by a sterile needle electrode inserted in the muscle. The use of a needle electrode is essential to the proper recording and subsequent display of the action potentials. The needle electrode enables the examiner to move throughout a muscle in order to sample action potentials from all aspects of the muscle. (Recall that the motor unit distribution in a muscle is in a mosaic-like pattern.) The muscle fibers of the motor unit are distributed throughout a relatively large portion of the muscle. The needle electrode allows the movement of the recording electrode to approximate the source of the action potential.

The action potential recorded from a motor unit within a muscle that is actively contracting has certain morphometric characteristics. The structural component of the voluntary motor unit action potential depends on the size of the motor unit, the histologic type of muscle fiber, and the density of the motor unit structure within the muscle (Figures 12–7 and 12–8). The size of the motor unit depends on the function of the muscle. For example, a muscle that has one joint to act on, and that performs postural, sustained contractions, will have fewer muscle fibers per motor unit than a muscle with the opposite functional need characteristics.

The decreased size of the small motor unit will yield a small amplitude recorded action potential. The type of muscle fiber will also yield an action potential with a particular size. A fast motor unit will have muscle fiber membranes that are larger and that conduct the action potential along the muscle fiber membrane faster than the membranes of a slow motor unit. The larger muscle fiber mem-

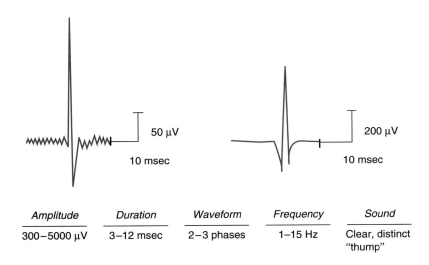

| Amplitude | Duration | Waveform | Frequency | Sound |
|---|---|---|---|---|
| 300–5000 µV | 3–12 msec | 2–3 phases | 1–15 Hz | Clear, distinct "thump" |

FIGURE 12–7. The motor unit consists of the anterior horn cell, its axon, neuromuscular junction, and all muscle fibers it innervates. A motor unit action potential is the synchronous discharge of all muscle fibers innervated by the anterior horn cell. They occur during volitional activity. Initial deflection may be either positive or negative. The amplitude of the motor unit action potential is dependent upon the number of motor unit muscle fibers in close proximity to the recording electrode. The rate of rise of the motor unit action potential is dependent upon the closeness of the recording electrode to the active muscle fibers. The motor unit action potential duration is dependent upon the relative density of the muscle fibers in the recording area. Duration of motor unit action potentials increases as intramuscular temperature decreases. Duration of motor unit action potentials also increases with age. The percentage of polyphasic motor unit action potentials increases with a decrease in temperature and with muscle fatigue.

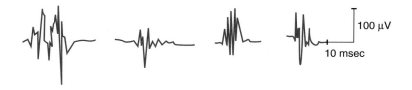

| Amplitude | Duration | Waveform | Frequency | Sound |
|-----------|----------|----------|-----------|-------|
| 20–5000 µV | 2–25 msec | 5–25 phases | 2–30 Hz | Rough/rasping |

FIGURE 12–8. Polyphasic potentials. Complex motor unit action potential with multiple phases; probably results from the asynchronous discharge of muscle fibers in the motor unit; represents the electrical expression of a motor unit undergoing reorganization. Polyphasics are observed in partial compressive neuropathies and in muscular dystrophy. Initial deflection may be either positive or negative. They occur during volitional activity. High-amplitude long-duration (HALD) polyphasic potentials are usually seen in long-standing chronic neuropathies.

branes will yield a larger amplitude, a faster rise-time response, and a shorter-duration action potential than a slow motor unit. The relative density of motor units within a muscle will also affect the recorded morphometric characteristics of the muscle action potential. Because of the high specificity of the muscle function, a muscle with motor units that are closely spaced will have recorded action potentials of short durations and of relatively low amplitudes.

Several factors must be accounted for when analyzing the shape, size, and duration of the recorded voluntary muscle action potentials. The major consideration is the relative proximity of the recording electrode to the active muscle fibers. The rise time of the action potential decreases in an exponential fashion when distance from the active muscle fiber increases by 10 percent from the recording electrode. The rise time is crucial in the estimation of the overall shape of the waveform. A slow rise time will both increase the duration and decrease the amplitude. A short rise time in the recorded muscle action potential is indicated by the crispness in sound heard from the speaker.

## ELECTROMYOGRAPHY

The term *voluntary* implies the use of some conscious effort on the part of the subject to perform a function. In that subcategory of electrophysiologic evaluation called **electromyography (EMG),** the patient is asked to move a particular muscle so that voluntary potentials in the form of motor units might be recorded, displayed, and subsequently analyzed. Strictly defined, the term *electromyography* involves both the recording of action potentials from muscle fibers under conditions of voluntary movement and the observance of spontaneous action potentials, if any, recorded from muscle fibers at rest.

A typical electromyographic evaluation of a skeletal muscle by a needle electrode includes the use of four distinct and separate processes: electrode insertion, oscilloscope observation during rest, oscilloscope observation of voluntary motor unit action potentials during minimal contraction, and oscilloscope observation during a level of muscle contractions graded from weak to strong. An example of the technical procedures used to perform clinical electromyography is shown in Table 12–4.

Initially, the evaluator must choose a series of skeletal muscles to test. The muscles are chosen on the basis of nerve root distribution and peripheral nerve innervation. Once a muscle is chosen, the area of skin overlying that muscle is cleansed by rubbing it with a sterile pad containing a 70 percent isopropyl alcohol solution. (NOTE: Universal precautions to prevent blood-borne infections will be used during all EMG testing.) The needle is inserted into the muscle, and the oscilloscope is observed while the muscle is at rest and while the needle is moved about. A muscle that is in a state of irritability will react to the movement of a needle electrode by having an increased time period of injury potentials during the needle's movement. The insertional activity or injury potentials are in the form of a burst of short-duration potentials that persist for less than a few milliseconds. If a muscle is irritable because of some injury to the neural supply system, the length of time of insertional activity increases as the needle is moved in the muscle. Insertional activity is a subjective measure, however; because it lacks an objective scale, it should not be used by itself to evaluate muscle health.

When voluntary contraction at low levels of force takes place, the action potentials that result are evaluated for shape, size, duration, and firing rate. The shape of the voluntary motor unit should be two or three phases. The investigator must know the morphometric and histochemical constituents of the muscle being examined. The size or amplitude of the muscle action potential is related to muscle size, histologic type, and expected motor unit density. At least 10 to 15 voluntary motor units should be examined for their duration, amplitude, and phase number in at least eight different anatomic areas of the skeletal muscle.

Recruitment of motor units and judgment of the interference pattern is the last area that the examiner assesses in the electromyographic assessment of the skeletal muscle. The examiner requests that the patient voluntarily contract the skeletal muscle in an isomet-

## TABLE 12–4. PROCEDURE FOR CLINICAL EMG

**Introduction**

1. Decide on distribution of:
   - Nerve root
   - Plexus
   - Peripheral nerve
2. Know location of the anatomic structures in no. 1, above.
3. Decide on representative muscles in decision of no. 1, above.
4. Know the action and function of the muscle.
5. Know the specificity of muscle function.
6. Know the cross-sectional anatomy of the muscle.
7. Know the relative mass of the muscle.
8. NOTE:
   - Use latex gloves and protective eyewear for all routine electromyographic studies.
   - Use latex gloves, protective eyewear, and gown for all electromyographic studies performed on patients with human immunodeficiency virus (HIV).

**Motor Unit Observation**

Machine settings:
   Gain = 100–200 μV/div
   Filter = 10,000 Hz high, 10 Hz low
   Sweep = 10–20 msec/div

Patient preapartion:

1. Cleanse the skin overlying the muscle with a sterile alcohol pad.
2. While cleaning the skin, feel the consistency of the target muscle.
3. Insert the sterile needle electrode through the skin to a point just under the dermal layer.
4. Switch the preamplifier to the "ON" position.
5. Move the needle into the muscle using a brisk, probing movement.
6. While moving the needle, observe the relative presence and the amount of spontaneous, insertional activity.
7. Stop electrode movement and observe (sight and sound) for other spontaneous activity.
8. Ask the patient to perform a minimal voluntary isometric muscle contraction (keep in mind the muscle testing position and muscle function).
9. While under minimal voluntary isometric contraction, observe the motor units which are in close proximity to the recording electrode:
   - A rapid rise time and resultant high-frequency "click" is heard when a motor unit is close to the recording electrode.
   - The amplitude of the voluntary motor unit potential is measured from the largest negative peak to the largest positive peak of the motor unit being observed when the recording electrode is near that motor unit.
10. Observe the voluntary motor unit action potential for its shape (phases), amplitude, and duration.
11. Observe and measure (according to no. 10, above) two or three voluntary motor units in each area of the msucle being tested.
12. Move the needle further into the muscle and repeat steps 6 through 11.
13. Sample additional sites in the muscle by using the quadrant position technique and evaluate 4 to 8 levels and sites in each muscle being tested.

**Recruitment and Interference Evaluation**

EMG machine settings:
   Gain = 500–1000 μV/div
   Filter = 10,000 Hz high, 10 Hz low
   Sweep = 20–50 msec/div

Patient preparation:

1. Move the needle electrode to the anatomic cross-sectional center of the muscle.
2. Request the patient to gradually increase the force of voluntary isometric muscle activity until maximum effort is accomplished.
3. Observe the voluntary motor unit action potentials for:
   - Motor unit recruitment pattern, small to large (poor–fair–good)
   - Interference pattern—decreased number of motor units firing rapidly: incomplete, decreased, full.

ric manner; that is, with a progressively increasing level of muscle tension without limb movement. The motor units that begin to discharge as the tension levels become progressively greater should be of higher and higher amplitude. This condition results from the recruitment of larger motor units, with progressively increasing amplitudes, as tension requirements increase. In addition to increasing the amplitude of motor unit discharge, the active units should also increase in their firing rate. Recruitment pattern is a qualitative or quantitative description or both of the sequence of appearance of motor unit action potentials with increasing force of voluntary muscle contraction. **Interference pattern** is a term used to identify the relative firing frequency of discharging motor units.

The normal sequence of events that occurs in response to the gradual increase in muscle tension involves motor units discharging and gradually increasing in their discharge rate. The rate of discharge increase is fixed; when a motor unit cannot discharge faster, a fusion frequency is reached, so another physiologic method is used to increase tension: New and larger motor units are recruited. The larger motor units will discharge at their preferred frequency, with the smaller units continuing to discharge at their fusion freqency. The result of the old, quickly discharging motor units and the new, larger motor units is a gradual disappearance of the EMG electronic display baseline. The electromyographer observes increases in amplitude and in the motor unit interference pattern. The gradual increase in amplitude (because of motor unit recruitment) and the increase in the baseline disruption (because of an increase in the discharge frequency) account for the proper physiologic sequencing of available motor units in normal muscle.

## Spontaneous Activity

Electrical silence is noted when a needle electrode is placed in a healthy muscle that is not actively contracting. At rest, healthy muscle will not yield any form of electrical membrane potentials. If a muscle loses its innervation in a rapid fashion, such as with a ligation or a significant and rapid compression of the peripheral nerve supply, the muscle is without neuronal supply and, after 14 to 21 days, begins to fibrillate continuously.

The fibrillation occurs because the muscle membrane becomes increasingly sensitive to acetylcholine. The receptor sites along the muscle membrane, normally dormant in the innervated state, become active and highly sensitive to small amounts of acetylcholine. The electrical membrane potentials spontaneously released by the muscle membranes are of short duration and low amplitude; they are called **fibrillation potentials.** (See Figure 12–9.) Denervation fib-

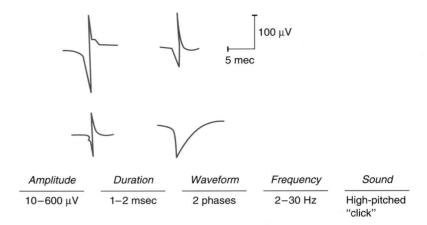

| Amplitude | Duration | Waveform | Frequency | Sound |
|-----------|----------|----------|-----------|-------|
| 10–600 μV | 1–2 msec | 2 phases | 2–30 Hz | High-pitched "click" |

FIGURE 12–9. Fibrillation potentials. Represents spontaneous, repetitive discharge of a single muscle fiber. *Initial deflection is positive.* It indicates altered muscle membrane excitability and an unstable muscle membrane that depolarizes in a variety of circumstances, and may result from denervation (separation of muscle from nerve), metabolic dysfunction (altered electrolyte state), inflammatory diseases (polymyositis), trauma (injection sites), or lack of trophic influence (stroke or spinal cord injury).

rillation potentials occur in a muscle that is at rest. Upon attempts at voluntary muscle contraction, no active motor units are observed.

There are other forms of spontaneous activity in muscle that are indicative of neural dysfunction. (See Figures 12–10 through 12–12.) All types of activity remain spontaneous, in that they occur without volitional effort. Refer to the bibliography at the end of this chapter for a complete description of each of the spontaneous forms of activity, along with their pathologic implications.)

| Amplitude | Duration | Waveform | Frequency | Sound |
|-----------|----------|----------|-----------|-------|
| 30–4000 μV | 2–10 msec | 2 phases | 2–100 Hz | Dull "thud" |

FIGURE 12–10. Positive sharp wave potentials. Positive sharp waves may represent asynchronous discharge of a number of denervated muscle fibers. They reflect an altered muscle membrane excitability. *Initial deflection is positive.* Its shape is the most constant of all EMG potentials. They appear spontaneously at rest and are not predictable. They are seen in both neuropathies and myopathies.

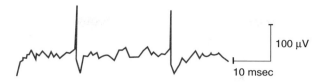

| Amplitude | Duration | Waveform | Frequency | Sound |
|-----------|----------|----------|-----------|-------|
| 25–250 µV | 1–4 msec | 2 phases | 30–150 Hz | High-pitched noise |

FIGURE 12–11. Endplate potentials. Endplate potentials are produced when the EMG needle electrode comes into contact with nerve fibrils within the muscle. Patients complain of increased pain when these potentials are present. Slight needle movement should relieve the pain, eliminate the endplate "noise," and clear the screen display of these potentials. *Initial deflection is negative.*

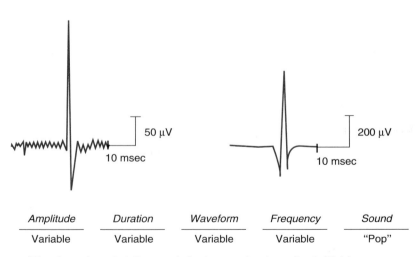

| Amplitude | Duration | Waveform | Frequency | Sound |
|-----------|----------|----------|-----------|-------|
| Variable | Variable | Variable | Variable | "Pop" |

(Waveform characteristics are similar to normal motor unit potentials)

FIGURE 12–12. Fasciculation potentials. Fasciculations are seen in patients with and without neuromuscular disease. Fasciculation potentials may be either benign or pathologic. Pathologic significance is best determined by the coexistence of fibrillation and positive sharp waves in the same muscle. Waveform configuration is the same as the normal motor unit action potential. Initial deflection may be either positive or negative.

## ELECTROPHYSIOLOGIC EVALUATION

The preceding material has provided the elements involved in electrophysiologic evaluation of the patient with a suspected neurologic disorder. The actual evaluation for specific neurologic disorders has not been discussed. Specific tests must be correctly chosen, and the proper nerves and muscles must be selected for study, in order to optimize the results and their ultimate interpretation. The evaluation process begins with a physical examination to determine the possible site or sites of neural injury. The choice of nerves and muscles examined may change as the electrophysiologic evaluation proceeds.

Usually, motor nerve conduction (latency, velocity, amplitude) studies are performed first, followed by sensory nerve studies (latency, amplitude). Which muscles are tested depends upon the peripheral nerve innervation and the root level of the muscles. The addition of reflex testing and evoked potential analysis depends upon the pathologic findings of the earlier electrophysiologic procedures. The use of centrally recorded evoked potentials depends on the pathologic results of peripheral nerve conduction studies and electric reflex testing. Clinical electromyography completes the assessment.

# Summary

A testing hierarchy is established that allows for the development of evoked potential and EMG procedures to answer the questions: Is the patient suffering from a dysfunction in the neuromusculoskeletal system? If yes, where is the lesion? Is the lesion at the nerve root, plexus, peripheral nerve, neuromusculoskeletal junction, or muscle? The electrophysiologic evaluation must answer these questions. A sample NCV-EMG study is provided in appendix A to illustrate a typical electrophysiologic evaluation.

# Appendix A

**Patient:**  **Age/DOB:** 10-05-62  **Physician:**
**Patient ID:** 05198-000  **Test By:**
**Sex:** Male  **Ref Phys**:

## Nerve Conduction Report:
### Motor Nerves

| Nerve | Site | Onset Lat (ms) | Norm Onset | Norm Peak | Amplitude | Norm Amp | Seg Name | Delta (ms) | Distance (cm) | Velocity (m/s) | Norm Vel |
|---|---|---|---|---|---|---|---|---|---|---|---|
| R Median | APB | | | | O-P (mV) | | | O | | | |
| | Wrist | 4.88 | <4.2 | | 4.89 | >5.0 | Elbow-Wrist | 5.16 | 27.00 | 52.4 | >50.0 |
| | Elbow | 10.03 | | | 5.01 | | | | | | |
| R Ulnar | ADM | | | | O-P (mV) | | | O | | | |
| | Wrist | 2.72 | <3.5 | | 9.14 | >3.0 | BElbow-wrist | 4.50 | 28.00 | 62.2 | >53.0 |
| | BElbow | 7.22 | | | 9.82 | | AElbow-BElbow | 3.42 | 22.00 | 64.3 | >53.0 |
| | AElbow | 10.64 | | | 9.47 | | | | | | |

### Sensory Nerves

| Nerve | Site | Onset Lat (ms) | Peak Lat (ms) | Norm Peak | Amplitude | Seg Name | Delta (ms) | Distance (cm) | Velocity (m/s) |
|---|---|---|---|---|---|---|---|---|---|
| R Radial | IDI | | | | P-T (μV) | | P | | |
| | Wrist | 1.50 | 2.00 | < 2.5 | 27.16 | Wrist-IDI | 2.00 | 10.00 | 50.0 |
| R Med | Wrist | | | | P-T (μV) | | P | | |
| Orth | 2 Dig | 3.47 | 4.44 | < 3.5 | 14.46 | 2 Dig-Wrist | 4.44 | 14.00 | 31.5 |
| | Palm | 1.59 | 1.94 | | 19.44 | Palm-Wrist | 1.94 | 8.00 | 41.3 |
| R Ulnar | 5thDig | | | | P-T (μV) | | P | | |
| | Wrist | 2.38 | 3.06 | <3.0 | 4.36 | Wrist-Digit5 | 3.06 | 12.00 | 39.2 |
| R DorsCut | Digit5 | | | | P-T (μV) | | P | | |
| | Wrist | 1.41 | 2.16 | <2.5 | 5.28 | Wrist-Digit5 | 2.16 | 12.00 | 55.7 |

### F/H Report:

| Nerve | Muscle | Lat1 (ms) | Lat2 (ms) | Lat2 – Lat1 (ms) |
|---|---|---|---|---|
| R Median F | APB | 33.20 | | 33.20 |
| R Ulnar F | ADM | 29.69 | | 29.69 |

### EMG Report:

| Side | Muscle | Nerve | Root | INS | FIBS | PSW | AMP | DUR | PHS | REC | IP | Comment |
|---|---|---|---|---|---|---|---|---|---|---|---|---|
| R | APB | Median | C8-T1 | Nml | Nml | Nml | Nml | Nml | 3 | Reduced | 75% | |
| R | 1stDor Int | Ulnar | C8-T1 | Nml | Nml | Nml | Nml | Nml | 2 | Nml | Nml | |
| R | PronatorTer | Median | C6-7 | Nml | Nml | Nml | Nml | Nml | 2 | Nml | Nml | |
| R | Biceps | Musc | C5–6 | Nml | Nml | Nml | Nml | Nml | 2 | Nml | Nml | |
| R | Triceps | Radial | C6–7–8 | Nml | Nml | Nml | Nml | Nml | 2 | Nml | Nml | |
| R | Brachiorad | Radial | C5–6 | Nml | Nml | Nml | Nml | Nml | 2 | Nml | Nml | |

### History
Pt. c/o right hand numbness; sometimes first three digits and sometimes last three digits. History of right wrist fracture when 10 years old. IDDM for three years.

### Summary:
The right median motor and sensory distal latencies were prolonged. The right ulnar sensory distal latency was mildly delayed. The right median F-wave latency was prolonged. Remaining motor, sensory, and F-wave values were WNL. Sterile, disposable, monopolar electrode studies of selected right upper extremity muscles reveal brief insertional activity, silence at rest with mild motor unit changes and recruitment/interference alternations in the right APB. No active, acute denervation signs were observed. No peripheral neuropathy, radiculopathy, or myopathy signs were noted.

### Impression:
NCV/EMG findings suggest neuropathic involvement of the right median nerve at the wrist. Early ulnar sensory involvement was also noted.

# REVIEW QUESTIONS

1. Electrophysiologic evaluation uses surface and needle electrodes to assess the integrity of the neuromuscular system. Discuss the use of surface and needle electrodes to record evoked potentials and voluntary potentials.

2. Discuss how the electrophysiologic evaluation is a "functional" assessment of the neuromuscular system.

3. Discuss the "functional" relationship between the findings of the physical examination and the findings of the electrophysiologic evaluation.

4. Compare electrophysiologic evaluation ("functional" assessment) to the "structural" assessment of the neuromuscular skeletal system using x-ray, magnetic resonance imaging (MRI), computed tomography (CT) scan, or myelogram, or all.

5. List the four major categories of evoked responses. Briefly discuss the region(s) of the neuromuscular system (distal, proximal, both distal and proximal) being assessed with evoked potentials.

6. Define afferent and efferent transmission of neural impulses.

7. Describe the procedures required to perform a motor nerve conduction velocity study.

8. Describe the procedures required to perform an orthodromic sensory conduction study.

9. Describe the procedures required to perform an antidromic sensory conduction study.

10. Motor conduction velocity studies require two stimulation sites, whereas sensory conduction studies require only one site of stimulation. Describe the neuromuscular and neuroanatomic basis for the need for two-site stimulation to perform the motor conduction studies.

11. Describe how motor and sensory conduction studies may be used to differentiate systemic neuromuscular dysfunction from a local one (ie, a peripheral entrapment versus demyelinating disease process).

12. Describe the procedures required to complete the H-reflex evoked potential study and discuss the clinical use of the H reflex.

13. Describe the procedures required to complete the F-wave evoked potential study and discuss the clinical significance of the F wave.

14. List the differences and similarities between the H-reflex and F-wave evoked potential procedures.

15. List two centrally recorded evoked potentials and describe their clinical use.

16. List the components of a motor unit and describe the characteristics (amplitude, duration, waveform, frequency, sound) of normal motor units as they are recorded and displayed during electromyography of voluntary (volitional) contraction of skeletal muscle.

17. Describe the four distinct and separate processes required to conduct a typical needle electrode EMG evaluation of skeletal muscle.

18. List three forms of spontaneous EMG activity and discuss the clinical significance of each waveform.

19. The electrophysiologic evaluation, evoked potentials, and voluntary potentials may be used to assist the referring physician in determining if the patient is suffering from which of the following?
    A. Peripheral neuropathy
    B. Peripheral entrapment
    C. Dysfunction of the myoneural junction
    D. Plexopathy
    E. Radiculopathy
    F. Myopathy
    G. Myelopathy
    H. All of the above

## Bibliography

Aminoff M. Electromyography in Clinical Practice (2nd ed). New York, NY, Churchill Livingstone, 1987.

Aminoff M. Electrodiagnosis in Clinical Neurology. New York, NY, Churchill Livingstone, 1980.

Ashbury A, Johnson P. Pathology of the Peripheral Nerve. Philadelphia, PA, W.B. Saunders, 1978.

Bradley W. Disorders of Periperal Nerves (2nd ed). Oxford, Blackwell, 1985.

Brooke, M. A Clinician's View of Neuromuscular Diseases (2nd ed). Baltimore, MD, Williams & Wilkins, 1985.

Brown W. The Physiological and the Technical Basis of Electromyography. New York, NY, Churchill Livingstone, 1985.

Chu-Andrews J. Electrodiagnosis, An Anatomic and Clinical Approach. Philadelphia, PA, J.B. Lippincott, 1986.

Cohen H, Brumlik J. A Manual of Electroneuromyography (2nd ed). New York, NY, Harper & Row, 1976.

Currier DF, Nelson RM (eds). Dynamics of Human Biologic Tissues. Philadelphia, PA, F.A. Davis, 1992.

Dawson D, Hallett M, Millender L. Entrapment Neuropathies. Boston, MA, Little, Brown, 1983.

Delagi EF, Perotto A, Iazetti J, Morrison D. Anatomic Guide for the Electromyographer. Springfield, MO, Charles C Thomas, 1980.

DeLisa J, Lee H, Baran E et al. Manual of Nerve Conduction Velocity & Clinical Neurophysiology (3rd ed). New York, NY, Raven Press, 1994.

DeLisa J, Mackenzie K, Baran E. Manual of Nerve Conduction Velocity and Somatosensory Evoked Potentials. New York, NY, Raven Press, 1982.

Desmedt J (ed). New Developments in Electromyography and Clinical Neurophysiology. London, Basel, Karger, 1973. Volumes 1, 2, 3.

Desmedt J (ed). Clinical Uses of Cerebral, Brainstem and Spinal Somatosensory EP's. London, Basel, Karger, 1979.

DHHS (NIOSH) Publication No. 90-113. Manual for Performing Motor & Sensory Neuronal Conduction in Adult Humans, 1990.

DHHS (NIOCH) Publication No. 91-100. Selected Topics in Surface Electromyography for Use in the Occupational Setting: An Expert Perspective. Soderberg G (ed), 1992.

Dyck PJ, Thomas JE, Lambert EH (eds). Peripheral Neuropathy. Philadelphia, PA, W.B. Saunders, 1975, Volumes 1 and 2.

Echternach J. Introduction to Electromyography and Nerve Conduction Testing: A Laboratory Manual. Thorofare, NJ, Slack Inc., 1994.

Electromyography: International Journal of Electromyography Abstracts. Louvain, Belgium, Nauwelaerts Publishing House, 1989.

Goodgold J. Anatomical Correlates of Clinical Electromyography. Baltimore, MD, Williams & Wilkins, 1974.

Goodgold J, Eberstein A. Electrodiagnosis of Neuromuscular Disease. Baltimore, MD, Williams & Wilkins, 1983.

Hammer K. Nerve Conduction Studies. Springfield, MO, Charles C Thomas, 1982.

Hoppenfeld S. Physical Examination of the Spine and Extremities. New York, NY, Appleton-Century-Crofts, 1976.

Hoppenfeld S. Orthopaedic Neurology. Philadelphia, PA, J.B. Lippincott, 1972.

Jabre J, Hackett E. EMG Manual. Springfield, MO, Charles C Thomas, 1983.

Johnson E. Practical Electromyography (2nd ed). Baltimore, MD, Williams & Wilkins, 1988.

Kimura J. Electrodiagnosis in Disease of Nerve and Muscle (2nd ed). Philadelphia, PA, F.A. Davis, 1989.

Kopell H, Thompson W. Peripheral Entrapment Neuropathies. Huntington, NY, Robert E. Krieger, 1976.

Leffert R. Brachial Plexus Injuries. New York, NY, Churchill Livingstone, 1985.

Lenman J, Richie A. Clinical Electromyography, 2nd ed. Philadelphia, PA, J.B. Lippincott, 1978.

Liveson J, Ma D. Laboratory Reference for Clinical Neurophysiology. Philadelphia, F.A. Davis, 1992.

Liveson J, Spielholtz N. Peripheral Neurology (2nd ed). Philadelphia, PA, F.A. Davis, 1991.

Loeb G, Gans C. Electromyography for Experimentalists. Chicago, IL, University of Chicago Press, 1986.

Ludin H. Electromyography. New York, NY, Thieme-Stratton, 1980.

Ma D, Liveson J. Nerve Conduction Handbook. Philadelphia, PA, F.A. Davis, 1983.

McComas A. Neuromuscular Function and Disorders. London, Butterworths, 1977.

Mayo Clinic and Mayo Clinic Foundation. Clinical Examinations in Neurology (4th ed). Philadelphia, PA, W.B. Saunders, 1971.

Oh S. Clinical Electromyography, Nerve Conduction Studies. Baltimore, MD, University Park Press, 1984.

Oh S. Electromyography: Neuromuscular Transmission Studies. Baltimore, Williams & Wilkins, 1988.

Omer GE, Spinner M. Management of Peripheral Nerve Problems. Philadelphia, PA, W.B. Saunders, 1980.

Patten J. Neurological Differential Diagnosis. New York, NY, Springer-Verlag, 1977.

Rosenfalck P. Electromyography: Sensory and Motor Conduction Findings in Normal Subjects. Copenhagen, Laboratory of Clinical Neurophysiology Rigshospitalet, 1975.

Schaumburg H, Spencer P. The Neurology and Neuropathology of the Occupational Neuropathies. J Occup Med, 18:789, 1976.

Schaumburg H, Spencer P, Thomas P. Disorders of Peripheral Nerves (2nd ed). Philadelphia, PA, F.A. Davis, 1991.

Shahani B (ed). Electromyography in CNS Disorders: Central EMG. Boston, MA, Butterworth, 1984.

Smorto M, Basmajian J. Electrodiagnosis. A Handbook for Neurologist. Hagerstown, MD, Harper & Row, 1977.

Smorto M, Basmajian J. Clinical Electromyography. An Introduction to Nerve Conduction Tests (2nd ed). Baltimore, MD, Williams & Wilkins, 1990.

Snyder-Mackler L, Robinson A. Clinical Electrophysiology: Electrotherapy and Electrophysiologic Testing (2nd ed). Baltimore, MD, Williams & Wilkins, 1995.

Spinner M. Injuries to the Major Branches of Peripheral Nerves of the Forearm. Philadelphia, PA, W.B. Saunders, 1978.

Stalberg E, Young R (eds). Neurology Clinical Neurophysiology. Boston, MA, Butterworths International Medical Reviews, 1981.

Stewart J. Focal Peripheral Neuropathies. New York, NY, Elsevier, 1987.

Sumner A. The Physiology of Peripheral Nerve Disease. Philadelphia, PA, W.B. Saunders, 1980.

Sunderland S. Nerves and Nerve Injuries (2nd ed). Edinburgh, E & S Livingston, 1978.

Vinken P, Bruyn G. Diseases of Nerves: Handbook of Clinical Neurology, Part 7. Amsterdam, North Holland Publishing Co, 1970.

Weller R, Cervos-Navarro J. Pathology of Peripheral Nerves. London, Butterworths, 1977.

Wolf S. Electrotherapy. New York, NY, Churchill Livingstone, 1981.

# Index

Page numbers followed by *f* or *t* indicate figures or tables, respectively.

# *Also From Appleton & Lange*

**Patient Care Skills**
*Fourth Edition*
Minor & Minor
1998, ISBN 0-8385-8157-9, A8157-8

**Geriatric Physical Therapy**
*A Clinical Approach*
*Second Edition*
Bottomley & Lewis
1999, ISBN 0-8385-3138-5, A3138-3

**Rehabilitation in Sports Medicine**
*A Comprehensive Guide*
*Canavan*
1998, ISBN 0-8385-8313-X, A8313-7

**Physical Examination of the Spine and Extremities**
Hoppenfeld
1976, ISBN 0-8385-7853-5, A7853-3

**Manual for Physical Agents**
*Fifth Edition*
Hayes
1999, ISBN 0-8385-6128-4, A6128-1

**Foundations of Clinical Research**
*Applications to Practice*
*Second Edition*
Portney & Watkins
1999, ISBN 0-8385-2695-0, A2695-3

**Spinal Rehabilitation**
Stude
1999, ISBN 0-8385-3685-9, A3685-3

**Prosthetics and Orthotics**
*Second Edition*
Shurr & Cook
1999, ISBN 0-8385-8133-1, A8133-9

**Pathophysiology**
*A Self-Instructional Program*
Burns
1998, ISBN 0-8385-8084-X, A8084-4

**The Terminology of Health and Medicine**
*A Self-Instructional Program*
Rice
1998, ISBN 0-8385-6260-4, A6260-2

**Medical Terminology**
*With Human Anatomy*
*Fourth Edition*
Rice
1998, ISBN 0-8385-6274-4, A6274-3

**MedWorks**
*Anatomy & Physiology*
Victory Technology
ISBN 0-8385-6377-5

**How to Examine the Nervous System**
*Third Edition*
Ross
1998, ISBN 0-8385-3852-5

**MedArt**
*Anatomy & Physiology Images*
Victory Technology
ISBN 0-8385-6366-X

To order or for more information, visit your local health science bookstore, call Appleton & Lange at 1-800-423-1359, or visit our website at www.appletonlange.com.